POCKET NOTEBOOK

Pocket
NEPHROLOGY

Edited by
WOOIN AHN
JAI RADHAKRISHNAN

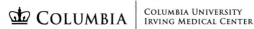

COLUMBIA | COLUMBIA UNIVERSITY
IRVING MEDICAL CENTER

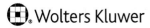 Wolters Kluwer

Philadelphia · Baltimore · New York · London
Buenos Aires · Hong Kong · Sydney · Tokyo

Acquisitions Editor: Robin Najar
Development Editor: Ariel S. Winter
Editorial Coordinator: Cody P. Adams
Senior Production Project Manager: Alicia Jackson
Team Lead, Design: Steve Druding
Senior Manufacturing Coordinator: Beth Welsh
Prepress Vendor: Aptara, Inc.

Copyright © 2020 Wolters Kluwer.

9 8 7 6 5 4 3

Printed in the United States of America

978-1-4963-5192-0
Library of Congress Cataloging-in-Publication Data
available upon request

Library of Congress Control Number: 2019910695

shop.lww.com

CONTRIBUTING AUTHORS

Wooin Ahn, MD, PhD
Assistant Professor of Medicine, Columbia University Vagelos College of Physicians and Surgeons

Gerald B. Appel, MD
Professor of Medicine, Columbia University Vagelos College of Physicians and Surgeons
Director, Glomerular Kidney Center, New York-Presbyterian Hospital/Columbia University Irving Medical Center

Rachel Arakawa, MD
Clinical Fellow, New York-Presbyterian Hospital/Columbia University Irving Medical Center

Rupali S. Avasare, MD
Assistant Professor of Medicine, Oregon Health & Science University

Yorg Azzi, MD
Assistant Professor of Medicine, Department of Medicine, Albert Einstein Medical School

Vasanthi Balaraman, MD
Assistant Professor, Department of Surgery, University of Tennessee Health Science Center
Transplant Nephrologist/Physician, Department of Surgery, Methodist University Hospital

Andrew Beenken, MD, PhD
Postdoctoral Clinical Fellow, Columbia University Vagelos College of Physicians and Surgeons

David Bennett, MD
Attending Nephrologist, Department of Medicine, Bridgeport Hospital

Andrew S. Bomback, MD, MPH
Associate Professor of Medicine, Columbia University Vagelos College of Physicians and Surgeons

Pietro Canetta, MD, MSc
Assistant Professor of Medicine, Columbia University Vagelos College of Physicians and Surgeons

Jae Hyung Chang, MD
Assistant Professor of Medicine, Columbia University Vagelos College of Physicians and Surgeons

Efren A. Chavez Morales, MD
Clinical Fellow, New York-Presbyterian Hospital/Columbia University Irving Medical Center

Jen-Tse Cheng, MD
Assistant Professor of Clinical Medicine (retired), Columbia University Vagelos College of Physicians and Surgeons
Chief (retired), Division of Nephrology and Hypertension, Harlem Hospital Center

Russell J. Crew, MD
Assistant Professor of Medicine, Columbia University Vagelos College of Physicians and Surgeons

Yelena Drexler, MD
Assistant Professor, University of Miami

Geoffrey K. Dube, MD
Assistant Professor of Medicine, Columbia University Vagelos College of Physicians and Surgeons

Hilda Elena Fernandez, MD, MSCE
Assistant Professor of Medicine, Columbia University Vagelos College of Physicians and Surgeons

Abdallah S. Geara, MD
Assistant Professor of Clinical Medicine, University of Pennsylvania

Jonathan Hogan, MD
Assistant Professor, University of Pennsylvania

S. Ali Husain, MD, MPH
Assistant Professor of Medicine, Columbia University Vagelos College of Physicians and Surgeons

Sean D. Kalloo, MD, MBA
Assistant Professor of Medicine (in Radiology), Columbia University Vagelos College of Physicians and Surgeons

Jeanne Kamal, MD
Instructor in Medicine, Columbia University Vagelos College of Physicians and Surgeons

Pascale Khairallah, MD
Clinical Fellow, New York-Presbyterian Hospital/Columbia University Irving Medical Center

Minesh Khatri, MD
Clinical Assistant Professor, State University of New York at Stony Brook

Krzysztof Kiryluk, MD, MS
Associate Professor of Medicine, Columbia University College of Physicians & Surgeons

Mark W. Kozicky, MD
Adjunct Assistant Clinical Professor, Department of Medical Education/Medicine, Lake Erie College of Osteopathic Medicine
Assistant Program Directory, Department of Internal Medicine/Nephrology, St. John's Riverside Hospital

Wai Lang Lau, MD
Assistant Professor, University of Florida

Hila Milo Rasouly, PhD
Associate Research Scientist, Columbia University Vagelos College of Physicians and Surgeons

Sumit Mohan, MD, MPH
Associate Professor of Medicine and Epidemiology, Columbia University Vagelos College of Physicians and Surgeons and Mailman School of Public Health

Heather Morris, MD
Assistant Professor of Medicine, Columbia University Vagelos College of Physicians and Surgeons

Maria Berenice Nava, MD
Nephrologist, Department of Medicine, Kaiser Permanente (San Diego, California)

Jordan Gabriela Nestor, MD
Postdoctoral Clinical Fellow, Columbia University Vagelos College of Physicians and Surgeons

Thomas Nickolas, MD, MS
Associate Professor of Medicine, Columbia University Vagelos College of Physicians and Surgeons

Akshta Pai, MD, MPH
Assistant Professor, Division of Immunology and Organ Transplantation, Division of Renal Disease and Hypertension, McGovern Medical School, The University of Texas Health Sciences Center at Houston

Yonatan Peleg, MD
Clinical Fellow, New York-Presbyterian Hospital/Columbia University Irving Medical Center

Jai Radhakrishnan, MD, MS
Professor of Medicine, Columbia University Vagelos College of Physicians and Surgeons

Maya K. Rao, MD
Assistant Professor of Medicine, Columbia University Vagelos College of Physicians and Surgeons

Renu Regunathan-Shenk, MD
Assistant Professor, George Washington University

Dominick Santoriello, MD
Assistant Professor of Pathology and Cell Biology, Columbia University Vagelos College of Physicians and Surgeons

Shayan Shirazian, MD
Assistant Professor of Medicine, Columbia University Vagelos College of Physicians and Surgeons

Eric Siddall, MD
Assistant Professor of Medicine, Columbia University Vagelos College of Physicians and Surgeons

Meghan E. Sise, MD, MS
Assistant Professor of Medicine, Department of Medicine, Harvard Medical School

Jacob Sam Stevens, MD
Instructor in Medicine, Columbia University Vagelos College of Physicians and Surgeons

Zachary H. Taxin, MD
Internal Medicine Resident, New York-Presbyterian Hospital/Columbia University Medical Center

Demetra Tsapepas, PharmD, BCPS
Assistant Professor of Clinical Surgical Sciences, Columbia University Vagelos College of Physicians and Surgeons
Director of Quality and Research in Transplantation, Department of Transplantation, New York-Presbyterian Hospital/Columbia University Irving Medical Center

Anthony M. Valeri, MD
Professor of Medicine, Columbia University Vagelos College of Physicians and Surgeons

Hector Alvarado Verduzco, MD
Clinical Fellow, New York-Presbyterian Hospital/Columbia University Irving Medical Center

Romina Wahab, MD
Assistant Professor of Medicine, Columbia University Vagelos College of Physicians and Surgeons

PREFACE

Pocket Nephrology joins the Pocket Notebook series as a complete resource for topics related to renal kidney physiology and pathophysiology designed as a first bedside reference for the busy clinicians. This book is intended for medical students, internal medicine and nephrology trainees as well as seasoned clinicians involved in the care of patients with kidney disease. The book is divided into two sections. The first part discusses the general approach to disorders of the kidney. The second part of book will address individual topics under each of the following categories: Electrolytes and Acid–Base Balance, Tubular, Interstitial and Cystic Diseases, Extrarenal Diseases, Glomerular and Vascular Diseases, Hypertension, Renal Replacement Therapy, and Transplantation. Individual topics are written to make pertinent information readily available to clinicians in order to facilitate evidence-based patient care.

WOOIN AHN AND JAI RADHAKRISHNAN

CONTENTS

CLINICAL MANIFESTATIONS

Wooin Ahn, Jai Radhakrishnan, Abdallah S. Geara, Yonatan Peleg, Romina Wahab, Eric Siddall, Jonathan Hogan, Minesh Khatri, Shayan Shirazian, Hilda Elena Fernandez

DIAGNOSIS

S. Ali Husain, Anthony M. Valeri, Wooin Ahn, Jen-Tse Cheng, David Bennett, Dominick Santoriello, Hila Milo Rasouly

TREATMENT AND TOXIN

Minesh Khatri, Hector Alvarado Verduzco, Wooin Ahn, Demetra Tsapepas, Jai Radhakrishnan, Jacob Sam Stevens, Geoffrey K. Dube, Yorg Azzi, Anthony M. Valeri

ELECTROLYTES AND ACID BASE BALANCE

Abdallah S. Geara, Zachary H. Taxin, Wooin Ahn

TUBULAR, INTERSTITIAL, AND CYSTIC DISEASES

Minesh Khatri, Jacob Sam Stevens, Jai Radhakrishnan,
Wooin Ahn, Krzysztof Kiryluk

EXTRARENAL DISEASES

Hilda Elena Fernandez

GLOMERULAR AND VASCULAR DISEASES

Renu Regunathan-Shenk, Pietro Canetta, Rupali S. Avasare, Wailang Lau,
Gerald B. Appel, Jordan Gabriela Nestor

HYPERTENSION

Yelena Drexler, Andrew S. Bomback

SPECIFIC TOPICS

Russell J. Crew, Geoffrey K. Dube, Shayan Shirazian, Maria Berenice Nava, Meghan E. Sise, Jordan Gabriela Nestor, Wooin Ahn, Andrew Beenken, Maya K. Rao, Jai Radhakrishnan, Abdallah S. Geara, S. Ali Husain, Rachel Arakawa, Thomas Nickolas, Minesh Khatri, Vasanthi Balaraman, Jae Hyung Chang, Mark W. Kozicky

RENAL REPLACEMENT THERAPY

Anthony M. Valeri, Wooin Ahn, Efren A. Chavez Morales, Sean D. Kalloo, Sumit Mohan, Pascale Khairallah

TRANSPLANTATION

Vasanthi Balaraman, Jae Hyung Chang, Jeanne Kamal, Sumit Mohan, Heather Morris, Akshta Pai, Russell J. Crew, Dominick Santoriello, Yorg Azzi, Geoffrey K. Dube, Yelena Drexler, Andrew S. Bomback, Hilda Elena Fernandez

PHOTO INSETS

Jen-Tse Cheng, Dominick Santoriello

APPENDIX

ABBREVIATIONS

INDEX

PROTEINURIA

- Proteinuria: protein in urine >150 mg/d
- ↑ ESRD risk w/ UACR 20–200 mg/g in men and 30–300 mg/g in women ×13.0; UACR >200 mg/g in men and >300 mg/g in women ×47.2 (JASN 2009;20:1069)
- Albuminuria ↑ ESRD, all-cause and cardiovascular mortality (Lancet 2010;375:2073)

Urinary Proteins		
Protein	Nl Value/Size	Remarks
Tamm–Horsfall protein (THP; uromodulin)	9–35 mg/d 85 kD	Synthesized and secreted in TAL Defense against UTI; inhibit Ca crystallization The matrix of various casts, including LC cast Gene mutation causes ADTKD
Albumin	<20 mg/d 69 kD	Predominant serum protein Very small proportion is filtered and reabsorbed
Retinol-binding protein (RBP)	<163 µg/d 21 kD	Urine level is ↑ in early stage of graft failure (AJT 2013;13:676)
α-1 microglobulin	<19 mg/d 27 kD	Heme-binding protein with antioxidant activity
β-2 microglobulin	<300 µg/L (24-hr level not established) 12 kD	Synthesized in all nuclear cells Component of class I MHC Serum level is elevated in MM, lymphoma, and has prognostic value; renal dysfunction ↑ Precursor of Aβ2M (dialysis related) amyloid
Other minor proteins (kD): myoglobin (18), hemoglobin (64), Cystatin C (13), κ (22.5) and λ (45) light chain, vitamin D–binding protein (58), polypeptides		

Low–Molecular-Weight (LMW) Proteins

- Proteins of a size smaller than albumin; RBP, α-1, β-2 microglobulin and Ig light chain
- Freely filtered in the glomerulus
- Megalin–cubilin–amnionless complex in PT reabsorbs albumin and LMW proteins
- ↑ urinary LMW protein (tubular proteinuria) suggests proximal tubule dysfunction

Workup

Evaluation of Proteinuria		
Test	Pros	Cons
Dipstick: reaction w/ tetra-bromophenol blue	Sensitive to albumin Rapid, cheap Possible home monitoring	Insensitive to LMW proteins Semiquantitative: affected by urine concentration False (+): pH >9 w/ urea splitting organisms, iodinated contrast
Random protein to creatinine ratio (UPCR)	Convenient Correlates w/ 24-hr (NEJM 1983;309:1543)	Diurnal variation
Random albumin to creatinine ratio (UACR)	Sensitive in detecting glomerular lesion	Diurnal variation More expensive than UPCR Miss nonalbumin proteinuria
24-hr urine protein	Gold standard Can ✓CrCl together Not affected by diurnal variation	Cumbersome Over- or under-collection: ✓ w/ creatinine for adequacy

- Initial proteinuria workup: ✓ both UPCR and UACR
- Spot urine albumin/protein ratio: < 0.4: tubulointerstitial (NDT 2012;27:1534); <0.25: light chain cast nephropathy in monoclonal gammopathy (CJASN 2012;7:1964)
- Sulfosalicylic acid (SSA): semiquantitatively detects all proteins including LC; add 3% SSA to urine ✓ turbidity; false (+) w/ iodinated contrast, PCN, and ceph.

Assay Sensitivity of Various Proteins and Substances					
Assay	Albumin	LMW Proteins	Light Chain	Lysozyme	Iodinated Contrast
Dipstick	+	+/−	+/−	+	+
SSA	+	+	+	+	+
Total protein	+	+	+	+	+
Albumin	+	−	−	−	−

- Transient proteinuria: caused by fever, extreme cold, seizure, and exercise
- Orthostatic proteinuria: common in child and adolescents; benign condition

GLOMERULAR PROTEINURIA

- Loss of glomerular filtration barrier; albuminuria: hallmark of glomerular damage
- Infection, exercise can cause transient glomerular proteinuria
- Moderately increased (A2, formerly micro-) albuminuria: 30–300 mg/g or 3–30 mg/mmol
- Severely increased (A3, formerly macro-) albuminuria: >300 mg/g or 30 mg/mmol
- Tool to monitor glomerular diseases: ↓ proteinuria w/ stable renal function = remission

General Management

- Low sodium diet: more effective than dual RAASi *(BMJ 2011;343:d4366)*
- ACEi or ARB; non-DHP CCB *(KI 2004;65:1991)*
- BP goal: 125/75 vs 140/90 in 24-hr UPCR >0.22 a/w ↓ CKD progression (HR 0.73) *(AASK NEJM 2010;363:918)*; in ≥1 g/d proteinuria a/w ↓ ESRD after 14 yr (HR 0.59) *(JASN 2017;28:671)*

TUBULAR PROTEINURIA

- Proximal tubular damage → inability of absorption of filtered LMW protein
- Can be missed w/ dipstick (discordance between UPCR and dipstick)

Acquired Causes

- ATN, tubulointerstitial diseases
- Light chain proximal tubulopathy: m/c cause of acquired Fanconi syndrome
- Heavy metals (lead, cadmium, mercury, copper), ifosfamide, tenofovir

Cystinosis

- AR mutations of *CTNS* gene encoding lysosomal protein **cystinosin**; cystine accumulation in proximal tubular cells; m/c cause of inherited Fanconi syndrome

Dent Disease

- Type 1: x-linked defect in *CLCN5* gene encoding Cl^-/H^+ exchanger, **CLC-5**, expressed in the PT and CD intercalated cells → ↓ cubilin and megalin expression → LMW proteinuria
- Type 2: x-linked defect in *OCRL* gene encoding 4,5-bisphophate 5-phosphatase
- PT damage (unclear mechanism): aminoaciduria, glycosuria, phosphaturia, and hypercalciuria; CaOx/CaP nephrolithiasis/nephrocalcinosis; FGGS *(CJASN 2013;8:1979)*
- Biopsy: FGGS (83%), mild segmental FPE (57%), focal interstitial fibrosis (60%), interstitial lymphocytic infiltrate (53%), tubular damage (70%) *(CJASN 2016;11:2168)*

Rare Genetic Causes of Tubular Proteinuria

- Donnai-Barrow/facio-oculo-acoustico-renal syndromes: AR mutation of LDL receptor protein 2 (**megalin**). Hypertelorism, myopia, hearing loss, and proteinuria
- Gräsbeck–Imerslund disease: AR defect in either **cubilin** or **amnionless**. Megaloblastic anemia; B_{12} absorption is mediated by cubilin amnionless complex

OVERFLOW PROTEINURIA

- The amount of filtered protein exceeding reabsorption capacity
- Causes: light chain cast nephropathy, rhabdomyolysis (myoglobulin, β on UPEP), hemolysis (hemoglobulin), lysozyme-induced nephropathy

Lysozyme-Induced Nephropathy *(AJKD 2009;54:159)*

- Lysozyme (muramidase): small (15 kD) cationic protein produced by monocytes and macrophages; filtered by glomeruli and reabsorbed in the PT, causing injury
- Chronic myelomonocytic leukemia (CMML): neoplasm producing mature monocytes; chronic monocytic leukemia, multiple myeloma, sarcoidosis *(AJKD 2012;59:xxxiii)*
- ↑ γ region in SPEP w/ (−) SIEP; (+) urine dipstick protein; ↑ serum, urine lysozyme
- AKI, hypokalemia
- LM: eosinophilic protein granules in PT; EM: large prominent lysosomes in PT
- Tx: treatment of primary disease

PROTEINURIA AFTER KIDNEY TRANSPLANTATION

- Albuminuria (>proteinuria) predicts renal outcome after txp *(AJKD 2011;57:733)*
- Proteinuria is a/w cardiovascular morbidity and mortality *(Transplantation 2002;73:1345)*
- Proteinuria from native kidney rapidly declines after txp *(AJT 2006;6:1660)*
- Causes: transplant glomerulopathy, *de novo* or recurrent glomerular disease, acute rejection
- Biopsy unexplained proteinuria ≥3 g/d *(KDIGO; AJT 2009;9 Suppl 3:S1)*

HEMATURIA

- **Hematuria:** ≥3 RBC/HPF on a properly collected specimen (avoid during menstruation)
- Dipstick ⊕, sediment ⊖ for RBC: not hematuria; consider myo- or hemoglobinuria, semen
- **Hemoglobinuria:** caused by any intravascular hemolysis (eg, MAHA, transfusion reaction, and PNH) with **hemosiderinuria** (Prussian blue ⊕ tubular cells), ↓ haptoglobin, ↑ LDH May cause Prussian blue ⊕ hemosiderin deposit in PT (AJKD 2010;56:780)
- Prevalence of hematuria: 2.5–18% in healthy individuals
- Persistent asymptomatic microscopic hematuria: ×18.5 risk of ESRD (JAMA 2011;306:729)

Causes of Hematuria	
Origin	**Selected Causes**
Glomerular	IgAN/IgAV, thin basement membrane disease, Alport syndrome Warfarin-related nephropathy, Loin pain hematuria syndrome, TMA Any other glomerular diseases including DN (41%) (Nephron Clin Pract 2008;109:c119) and MCD (29%) (CJASN 2007;2:445)
Nonglomerular renal	Interstitial nephritis, papillary necrosis, pyelonephritis, BKV infection Cystic diseases (PKD, acquired cystic kidney disease), Benign mass Malignancy (RCC, lymphoma, metastatic cancer) Hypercalciuria, hyperuricosuria
Nonrenal urinary tract	Nephro/urolithiasis, trauma (catheterization, instrumentation) Prostatitis, BPH, endometriosis, malignancy (TCC, SCC, prostate) Cystitis (infection, chemical, eg, CYC-associated), urethritis
Vascular	Renal artery thromboembolism, renal vein thrombosis, renal AVM

History

Relevant History for Hematuria Evaluation	
History	**Potential Causes**
AKI	RPGN, intratubular RBC casts (eg, IgAN)
CKD	Acquired cystic kidney disease
Blood clot	Nonglomerular origin
Recent upper respiratory infection	Postinfectious GN, IgA nephropathy
Sensorineural hearing loss, retinopathy, lenticonus	Alport syndrome
Heavy exercise	Exercise-induced hematuria/hemolysis
Recent renal procedure or injury	Renal arteriovenous malformation (AVM)
Unilateral flank pain	Stone, renal infarction, pyelonephritis
Irritative voiding symptoms (frequency, urgency, dysuria), suprapubic pain	Bladder cancer, cystitis
Increased sexual activity, perineal pain, dysuria, terminal hematuria	Prostatitis
Cyclic hematuria a/w menstruation	Endometriosis of urinary tract
Blunt trauma a/w lower rib fractures	Traumatic renal injuries
Excessive anticoagulation	Anticoagulant-related nephropathy
Travel/residence in Africa, the Middle East	Schistosoma hematobium cystitis
Sickle cell disease	Renal infarction, papillary necrosis
Sickle cell trait	Renal medullary carcinoma

- Antithrombotics ↑ hematuria-related complications, bladder ca dx (JAMA 2017;318:1260); should continue hematuria w/u for underlying causes (Arch IM 1994;154:649)

Gross Hematuria Timing Pattern and Potential Sites	
Timing	**Potential Site of Bleeding**
At the beginning	Urethra
At the end	Prostate gland or the trigonal area of the bladder
Throughout	Bladder, ureter or kidney

Workup

- Urine dipstick: detects peroxidase activity of Hb; myoglobin has pseudoperoxidase activity; ascorbic acid can induce false $\ominus$
- Urine sediment: ≥3 RBC/HPF; RBC casts, dysmorphic RBC → glomerular; supernatant is clear in hematuria; extreme pH (<5 or >8) can cause RBC lysis
- Proteinuria >0.5 g/d → glomerular; hematuria doesn't cause significant proteinuria
- If >10 RBC/HPF + 2 g/d proteinuria, 93% glomerular, 83% GN (NDT 2018;33:1397)
- Urine albumin/protein >0.59, w/ urine protein ≥5 → glomerular origin (AJKD 2008;52:235)
- Urocrit (hematocrit test of urine) >1% → urologic
- Urine culture: if $\oplus$, re-evaluate 6 wk after treatment
- Renal U/S: blood clot can cause hydronephrosis; Doppler study detects AVM
- Stone protocol (low radiation) CT w/o contrast only if stone is likely cause
- CT urography and cystoscopy if risk factor of urinary malignancy w/o obvious other causes (J Urol 2012;188:2473). Re-evaluate after resolution of other causes

Risk Factors of Urinary Tract Malignancy (J Urol 2012;188:2473; Ann IM 2016;164:488)
Male, >50 y/o, past or current smoking, analgesic abuse
Exposure to benzenes or aromatic amines, alkylating agents, aristolochic acid
Gross hematuria (even if self-limited), urologic disorder or disease
Irritative voiding symptoms (dysuria, urgency, and frequency)
Pelvic irradiation, chronic UTI, chronic indwelling foreign body

  - Cystoscopy: identify bleeding source and ureter laterality; eg, unilateral ureter bleeding excludes glomerular origin
  - CT urography: CT w/o contrast (stone, calcification, unenhanced baseline); contrast renal parenchymal phase (enhancing renal mass); excretory phase (collecting system evaluation)
- Cytology: very low sensitivity; not recommended for initial workup (Ann IM 2016;164:488)
- 24-hour urine study: detect hypercalciuria, hyperuricosuria

Possible Causes of AKI in Hematuria

- Gross and glomerular: intratubular RBC cast and ATN; common in IgAN
- Microscopic and glomerular: crescentic GN, vascular lesion (vasculitis, TMA)
- Gross and non-glomerular: blood clot causing urinary tract obstruction

Treatment

- Glomerular hematuria: consider ACEi or ARB, kidney biopsy
  Can serve as marker of activity predicting future relapse (CJASN 2018;13:251)
- Nonglomerular origin gross hematuria: generous fluid intake to prevent blood clot obstruction of the ureter or bladder; bladder irrigation if refractory
- If urologic workup is negative, ✓annual urinalysis. After 2 negative annual urinalyses, no further urinalyses are necessary (J Urol 2012;188:2473)

EXERCISE-INDUCED HEMATURIA

- Direct trauma to the kidneys +/− bladder in contact sports; renal ischemia d/t ↑ blood flow to muscles and nutcracker syndrome in noncontact sports
- Gross or microscopic hematuria after strenuous exercise; resolves w/i 1 wk w/ rest
- Tx: observation; if persists after 1 wk of rest r/o other causes
- ≠ Exercise-induced hemolysis, aka march hemoglobinuria or runner's hemolysis: presents w/ intravascular hemolysis, hemoglobinuria (dipstick $\oplus$, sediment $\ominus$)
  Hemosiderinuria (Prussian blue $\oplus$ tubular cells), urine iron loss → IDA

NUTCRACKER SYNDROME

- Left renal vein (LRV) entrapment between SMA and aorta → LRV HTN → rupture of thin vein into collecting system → hematuria; can be complicated by left RVT
- Gross or microscopic hematuria +/− left flank pain in children and Asians
- Dx: doppler U/S, MRA of LRV
- Tx: stent; transposition of the SMA or LRV, autotransplantation of left kidney

LOIN PAIN HEMATURIA SYNDROME

- Glomerular hypertension or GBM instability, causing capillary rupture into renal tubules and tubular obstruction (AJKD 2006;47:419)
- Recurrent uni- or bilateral flank pain, microscopic or gross, w/ nl renal function
- Urine sediment: dysmorphic RBCs. Kidney bx: RBCs or RBC casts in the tubules
- Tx: ACEi/ARB; analgesics, celiac plexus block, kidney autotransplantation, renal denervation (AJKD 2017;69:156). Unilateral nephrectomy not recommended d/t frequent relapses in the contralateral kidney

RENAL ARTERIOVENOUS MALFORMATION (AVM)

- A communication between the intrarenal artery and vein
- Usually congenital. Acquired forms, called AVF, caused by trauma or kidney bx (4–18%)
- Hematuria, renal colic, hypertension (↑ renin secretion from hypoperfusion distal to the AVM), ↓ renal function decline, CHF
- Dx: doppler study, CT angiography, MR angiography, and digital subtraction angiography
- Tx: observation, embolization, total or partial nephrectomy

POLYURIA

- UOP >3 L/d; commonly w/ nocturia (inability to concentrate the urine overnight)
- A patient with normal cognition and normal thirst reflex will try to compensate for polyuria and usually keep serum Na and osmolality within the normal range

Etiologies of Polyuria	
Osmotic diuresis	Glycosuria, sodium diuresis Urea diuresis: improving AKI, high prot diet, tissue catabolism, parenteral nutrition
1° polydipsia	High free water intake d/t psychiatric illness, hypothalamic lesions (thirst center)
CDI: defect in ADH secretion	Idiopathic, trauma, pituitary surgery, ischemic, familial
NDI: renal resistance to ADH	Hereditary: mutations of AVPR2 (X-linked), aquaporin-2 (AD or AR) Hypercalcemia, hypokalemia Lithium (chronic), cidofovir, foscarnet, vasopressin antagonists, ifosfamide, demeclocycline
Gestational DI	Release of vasopressinase from the placenta during pregnancy
Others	Sickle cell disease/trait, Sjögren's, bilateral obstructive uropathy, Bartter's, cystinosis

Workup

- Na >145 + low U_{osm} (<P_{osm}) → diabetes insipidus (DI)

  Water restriction test (WRT) is not necessary and desmopressin challenge can be done to differentiate between central DI (CDI) and nephrogenic DI (NDI).
- WRT differentiates between the different etiologies:

  Step 1: restrict water intake and measure UOP and U_{osm} Q1h; [Na] and P_{osm} Q2h

  Step 2: stop WRT and proceed to step 3 when U_{osm} >600; U_{osm} stable for 3 hr; Na >145 or P_{osm} >300

  Step 3: desmopressin challenge: measure U_{osm} and UOP every 30 min following desmopressin 10 mcg IN or 4 mcg SC or IV
- ✓ Plasma and urine ADH levels if the response to the WRT is nonconclusive

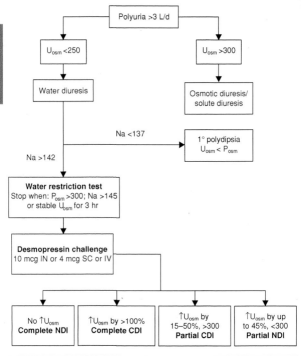

Laboratory Profiles of the Different Polyuria Etiologies			
	Baseline	WRT	Desmopressin Challenge
Osmotic diuresis	↑ Na (>142) ↑ U_{osm} (>300)	Not needed	Not needed
1° polydipsia	↓ Na (<137) ↓ U_{osm}	↑ U_{osm} (>500)	Similar to NDI
CDI, Gestational DI	↑ Na (>142) ↓ U_{osm}	↑ Na; ↑ P_{osm} $U_{osm} < P_{osm}$	↑ U_{osm} >100% in complete CDI
NDI	↑ Na (>142) ↓ U_{osm}	↑ Na; ↑ P_{osm} $U_{osm} < P_{osm}$	Submaximal or no change in U_{osm} in complete NDI (U_{osm} <300)

- Copeptin (C-terminal segment of vasopressin prohormone) level after 3% NaCl 250 mL
  may differentiate 1° polydipsia from CDI (*NEJM* 2018;379:428).
  Copeptin/P_{Na} ≥0.02 pmol/L: 1° polydipsia; <0.02 pmol/L: partial CDI
  Basal copeptin <2.6 pmol/L: complete CDI
- 1° polydipsia can induce partial NDI (decrease urea accumulation in the medullary
  interstitium → defect of the corticomedullary gradient)

CENTRAL DIABETES INSIPIDUS (CDI)

Pathogenesis
- ↓ release of antidiuretic hormone (ADH) (or AVP) from the hypothalamus
- Idiopathic or autoimmune (30–50%)
- Hypothalamic lesions: tumor, infiltrative disease (eg, Langerhans cell histiocytosis,
  sarcoidosis, GPA, and autoimmune lymphocytic hypophysitis), trauma, surgery
- Autoimmune disease: IgG4-related disease, GPA

- Familial: AR or AD mutations in ADH gene
  - Wolfram syndrome (DIDMOAD): AR mutation of *WFS1* encoding wolframin, endoplasmic reticulum protein. Manifestations: <u>DI</u>, <u>DM</u>, optic atrophy and <u>deafness</u>; hydronephrosis
- Congenital hypopituitarism, septo-optic dysplasia
- Post-SVT: transient (↑ left atrial and systemic pressure → ↓ secretion of ADH)

Clinical Manifestations
- Polyuria, polydipsia, nocturia, predilection for iced water; abrupt onset
- Na high normal (>142), no to mild increase of U_{osm} with WRT, no change to mild response to desmopressin (U_{osm} <300)
- Low free mineral density (is not corrected by desmopressin therapy)
- During pregnancy, asymptomatic patients with partial CDI start to have symptoms due to vasopressinases released from the placenta
- Surgical or traumatic damage of the hypothalamus has triphasic response: initial polyuric phase (1–5 d ↓ ADH release), antidiuretic phase (6–11 d; release of ADH by degenerating posterior pituitary) followed by permanent CDI or resolution (most cases are not permanent)

Treatment
- Desmopressin: 0.1- or 0.2-mg tablet or 5–10 mcg of the nasal spray preferably at bedtime (to decrease the nocturia), titrate up depending on the nocturia, Na should be measured within 24–48 hours to check for hyponatremia (patient should be educated to decrease free water intake)
- The response to the IN desmopressin is more predictable than the PO
- Thiazide diuretics and NSAIDs (used mainly in DI)
- Other drugs (less effective, more toxic): chlorpropamide and carbamazepine (enhances renal response to ADH) and clofibrate (↑ ADH release)
- A low-solute (mostly low-sodium, low-protein) diet: for patients with partial and mild DI

NEPHROGENIC DIABETES INSIPIDUS (NDI)

Pathogenesis
- Hereditary NDI: V2 receptor (*AVPR2*) (X-linked) and aquaporin-2 gene (AD, AR)
- Chronic lithium toxicity: dysfunction of the aquaporin-2 in the principal cells
- Hypercalcemia and hypokalemia: interference with the countercurrent mechanism; ↓ aquaporin-2 expression
- Mild NDI (elderly, AKI, CKD): interference with the countercurrent mechanism
- Postobstructive AKI, sickle cell disease or trait, PCKD, renal amyloidosis, Sjogren's
- Drugs: vasopressin antagonists, cidofovir, foscarnet, amphotericin B, demeclocycline, ifosfamide, ofloxacin, orlistat, and didanosine
- Hereditary tubular syndrome: Bartter's, cystinosis, familial hypomagnesemia with hypercalciuria and nephrocalcinosis

Clinical Manifestations
- Polyuria, polydipsia, nocturia; gradual onset
- Na >142, no or mild ↑ U_{osm} with WRT, no or mild response to desmopressin (U_{osm} <300)

Treatment
- A low-solute (mostly low-sodium <2.3 g/d, low-protein ≤1 g/kg/d) diet is sufficient in most patients with intact thirst response; medical therapy is only for patient intolerant to polyuria/polydipsia
- Thiazides diuretics: (1) volume depletion → proximal sodium reabsorption → ↓ UOP; (2) inhibition of the urine concentration in the DCT
- Amiloride: added thiazide (corrects thiazide-induced potassium wasting) or in lithium-induced NDI (blocks lithium entry through ENaC in the collecting tubule cells)
- NSAIDs: inhibition of renal PG synthesis, mainly for Bartter-like syndromes
- Desmopressin can help in some cases of partial NDI

GESTATIONAL DIABETES INSIPIDUS (*J Obstet Gynaecol Can* 2010;32:225)

- Polyuria can be due to release of vasopressinase from the placenta
- Same lab pattern as central DI
- Polyuria response to desmopressin (DDAVP) since it is not inactivated by the vasopressinase (arginine vasopressin is degraded by vasopressinase)
- Transient condition; treatment is by increasing access to free water +/– desmopressin

URINARY SYMPTOMS

Causes and Associated Conditions of Urine Change	
Red, smoky brown, cola-color	Glomerular hematuria If no RBC on sediment: myoglobinuria, hemoglobinuria
Bright red, pink	Nonglomerular hematuria Beets, blackberries, rhubarb, food coloring, fava beans Phenazopyridine (pyridium), phenytoin, phenolphthalein, rifampin, doxorubicin, deferoxamine, chloroquine, ibuprofen, methyldopa
Brown	Levodopa, metronidazole, nitrofurantoin, iron sorbitol, chloroquine, methyldopa Alkaptonuria: turns dark brown if left standing/alkalinization
Orange	Bilirubin from hepatocellular or obstructive jaundice
Green or blue	Methylene blue, amitriptyline, indomethacin, triamterene Propofol (Lancet 2009;373:1462); UTI of pseudomonas
Pink or reddish orange	Uric acid crystal (Intensive Care Med 2013;39:389; KI 2012;81:1281)
Bright yellow	Riboflavin (vit B_2)
Purple	Porphyria (↑ porphobilinogen, porphyrins), UTI with E. coli, Klebsiella pneumoniae, Providencia rettgeri, Proteus mirabilis (Clin Interv Aging 2008;3:729)
Black	Disseminated melanoma (NEJM 2019;380:1166), alkaptonuria (homogentisic acid)
Turbid, milky	WBCs, bacteria, fungi; chyluria (KI 2006;70:1518) Crystals: uric acid, Ca pyrophosphates and indinavir
Foamy	Heavy albuminuria in NS; yellow foam from bilirubin

REDUCED URINE OUTPUT

Determinants of Urine Output (UOP)
- **Renal function** (glomerular filtration): UOP can be preserved in advanced kidney injury as in nonoliguric AKI or stage V CKD
- **Tubular reabsorption:** directed by ADH-mediated water reabsorption
  - U_{osm}: 60–1,200 mOsmol/kg; correlate with ADH activity
- **Urine solute** (mOsmol/d): affected by diet and protein catabolism. 600–900 with usual diet
  - If U_{osm} is fixed at 150 (eg, nephrogenic DI), solute intake should be decreased
  Solute load 600: UOP 600/150 = 4 L
  Solute load 900: UOP 900/150 = 6 L: may lose more water, increasing [Na]
  - If U_{osm} is fixed at 300 (eg, SIADH), solute intake should be increased
  Solute load 600: UOP 600/300 = 2 L: may retain water, decreasing [Na]
  Solute load 900: UOP 900/300 = 3 L

Oliguria
- Used to define and stage AKI along with creatinine elevation

Definitions of Oliguria and UOP Criteria in AKI	
Conventional	<400 or 500 cc/d If solute load is 600 mOsmol/d and kidney can maximally concentrate urine (1,200 mOsmol/kg), UOP will be 500 mL
RIFLE (Critical Care 2004;8:R204)	Risk: <0.5 mL/kg/hr for 6 hr Injury: <0.5 mL/kg/hr for ≥12 hr Failure: <0.3 mL/kg/hr for ≥24 hr or anuria for ≥12 hr
AKIN (Crit Care 2007;11:R31, KDIGO AKI 2012)	Stage 1: <0.5 mL/kg/hr for 6–12 hr Stage 2: <0.5 mL/kg/hr for ≥12 hr Stage 3: <0.3 mL/kg/hr for ≥24 hr or anuria for ≥12 hr

- Consecutive oliguria for a shorter (3–5 hr) period may predict AKI risk (CJASN 2014;9:1168)
- Oliguria is a/w ↑ mortality (KI 2011;80:760), ↑ dialysis requirement, >90 d dialysis and hospital mortality c/t nonoliguric AKI (Nephron Clin Prac 2010;115:c59)
- Diuretic use for conversion from oliguria to nonoliguric AKI is a/w worse outcome (JAMA 2002;288:2547); consider only in volume overload not requiring RRT otherwise
- In RRT requiring AKI, urine output at initial cessation of CRRT without diuretics is the best predictor of renal recovery (Crit Care Med 2009;37:2576)
  Can ✓ CrCl when UOP >30 mL/hr (720 mL/d) (NEJM 2008;359:7)

Anuria

- UOP <100 mL/d; severe AKI, eg, shock, RPGN, renal infarct, bilateral urinary obstruction

URINARY RETENTION

- Definition: inability to voluntarily pass urine
- Normal postvoid residual volume is <50 mL in <65 yo, <100 mL in ≥65 yo
- 24% of hospitalized ≥70 yo patients have urinary retention >150 mL (Am J Med 2015;128:77)
- Acute: predominantly in elderly men a/w prostatic enlargement
- Chronic: postvoid residual > 300 mL that persisted for >6 mo and documented on 2 or more separate occasions (AUA J Urol 2017;198:153)

Causes

- Bladder outlet obstruction: BPH (m/c in ♂), constipation, malignancy (prostate, bladder), urethral stricture, urolithiasis, phimosis, paraphimosis, blood clots (nonglomerular hematuria, eg, kidney biopsy), urethral diverticulum
  ♀: organ prolapse (eg, cystocele or rectocele), fibroids obstructing the urethra
- Underactive bladder: autonomic dysfunction (DM, Parkinson disease), spinal cord injury, stroke, medications with antimuscarinic property

Medications a/w Urinary Retention (J Am Geriatr Soc 2012;60;616; Emerg Med Pract 2014;16:1)	
Antimuscarinic	Darifenacin, fesoterodine, flavoxate, oxybutynin, solifenacin, tolterodine, trospium Inhaled ipratropium, tiotropium (♂ only) (Arch IM 2011;171:914)
Antihistamines	Brompheniramine, carbinoxamine, chlorpheniramine, clemastine, cyproheptadine, dimenhydrinate, diphenhydramine, doxepin, doxylamine, hydroxyzine, loratadine, meclizine
Antipsychotics	Chlorpromazine, clozapine, fluphenazine, loxapine, methotrimeprazine (levomepromazine), perphenazine, pimozide, prochlorperazine, promethazine, thioridazine, thiothixene, trifluoperazine Atypical antipsychotics (quetiapine, risperidone, olanzapine) a/w AKI (×1.73), urinary retention (×1.98) (Ann IM 2014;161:242)
Antidepressant	Amitriptyline, amoxapine, clomipramine, desipramine, doxepin, imipramine, nortriptyline, paroxetine, protriptyline, trimipramine
Antiparkinson	Benztropine, trihexyphenidyl
Muscle relaxants	Carisoprodol, cyclobenzaprine, orphenadrine, tizanidine
Antispasmodics	Atropine, belladonna alkaloids, dicyclomine, homatropine, hyoscyamine products, propantheline, scopolamine
Antiemetics	Hydroxyzine, meclizine, promethazine, scopolamine
Sympathomimetics (α-agonist)	Ephedrine sulfate, phenylephrine, phenylpropanolamine, pseudoephedrine

Diagnosis and Workup

- Bladder scan: postvoid >300 cc diagnostic; 150–300 cc possible retention
- Bladder and renal U/S to r/o hydronephrosis; BMP, urinalysis, urine culture
- CKD and hydronephrosis regarded as high risk → further work, eg, urodynamic study (AUA J Urol 2017;198:153)

Treatment and Monitoring

- Urinary catheterization: sometimes also diagnostic; indwelling or intermittent
- Bladder decompression may cause transient hypotension
- Monitor postobstructive diuresis and hypernatremia
- Treat UTI: common complication

NOCTURIA

- Nocturia: the need to wake at night ≥1 for voiding; ≥×2/night a/w impaired quality of life (Eur Urol 2010;57:488)
- Nocturnal polyuria: nocturnal UOP >33% of daily UOP in >65 yo (>20% in younger adults) of daily UOP w/o global polyuria (>3 L/d)

Causes and Pathogenesis

- Global polyuria (>3 L/d): osmotic (DM, salt) or water (DI) diuresis, primary polydipsia
- Nocturnal polyuria:
  Volume overload (CKD, NS, liver cirrhosis, CHF): supine position → mobilization of fluid from the LE to trunk → fluid shift into vascular space → ↑ natriuretic peptide
  Aging: blunted diurnal variation of vasopressin: high at night in normal

Pelvic floor dysfunction: position change may ↓ pelvic floor musculature support
Autonomic dysfunction (eg, Parkinson disease): ↓ sympathetic activity
Evening dose diuretics; excessive drinking in the evening
- Low bladder capacity: postvoid residual (BPH), bladder irritation (cystitis), bladder wall fibrosis/surgery/cancer/stone/detrusor overactivity
- Sleep apnea (Intern Med 2016;55:901): wake up d/t sleep disorder ± ↑ natriuretic peptide

Clinical Manifestations
- Low QoL, fall, fracture, death (J Urol 2010;184:1413; J Urol 2011;185:571), depression (Urology 2007;69:691)

Workup
- Frequency volume chart: r/o polyuria
- STOP-BANG for sleep apnea (Sleep Med Rev 2017;36:57)

Treatment
- Avoid fluid intake (esp. caffeine and alcohol), diuretics in the evening
- Furosemide 6 hr before bedtime (Br J Urol 1998;81:215)
- Desmopressin: ↓ nocturia (Cochrane Database Syst Rev 2017;10:CD012059)
- CPAP in sleep apnea: ↓ nocturia, nocturnal UOP (Urology 2015;85:333)

LOWER URINARY TRACT SYMPTOMS (LUTS) (J Urol 2013;189:S93)

Types of LUTS (NEJM 2012;367:248)		
	Obstructive Symptoms	**Storage Symptoms**
Symptoms	Incomplete emptying, weak stream, hesitancy, delay in initiation, intermittency, involuntary interruption, straining, terminal dribbling	Frequency, nocturia, bladder pain Overactive bladder: urgency ± urge incontinence
Causes	All causes of bladder outlet obstruction including: BPH, prostate cancer (♂) Urethral stricture	BPH, prostatitis, epididymitis (♂) Bladder: cystitis, cancer Low bladder capacity, ureterovesical reflux, urethral and meatal stricture Spinal cord injury
Symptomatic treatments	**α-1 antagonist** (-osin): doxaz-, teraz-, alfuz-*, tamsul-*, silod-* s/e: (orthostatic) hypotension; **α-1a** selective drugs (*) may have less ↓ BP	**Antimuscarinic:** oxybutynin, tolterodine, darifenacin, solifenacin, fesoterodine, trospium s/e: urinary/gastric retention, ↑ HR, dry mouth, blurred vision, dementia and brain atrophy (JAMA Neurol 2016;73:721)

- Evaluate for polyuria (>3 L/d), nocturnal polyuria, urethritis, and UTI (cystitis)

Dysuria
- ♀ >> ♂; common causes include cystitis, urethritis, vaginitis, and prostatitis
- Common organisms causing urethritis (♀): N. gonorrhoeae, Chlamydia, Mycoplasma genitalium, Trichomonas vaginalis, HSV
- Irritative symptoms (urgency, urge incontinence, frequency, dysuria, nocturia) + hematuria: risk factors of bladder cancer; ✓cystoscopy (ACP Ann IM 2016;164:4488)
- Interstitial cystitis/bladder pain syndrome: bladder pain, pressure, discomfort a/w LUTS of >6 wk, w/o infection or other identifiable causes (Neurourol Urodyn 2009;28:274)

URINARY INCONTINENCE

Urinary Incontinence (ACP Guideline Ann IM 2014;161:429)		
	Stress Incontinence	**Urge Incontinence**
Symptom	Small amount urine loss w/ exertion, sneezing, coughing or laughing Daytime/standing position only	Large amount urine loss w/o prediction Day and night urgency and frequency
Causes	Weakened support structures of the urethra Age, obesity, pregnancy, repetitive pelvic floor stress Vaginal delivery (JAMA 2018;320:2438) Radical prostatectomy > TURP	Bladder irritation: infection, inflammation, stone, cancer Stroke, spinal cord injury

Workup		Urine culture Cystoscopy, urodynamic study
Treatment	Pelvic floor muscle training Weight loss/bariatric surgery if overweight (JAMA IM 2015;175:1378) Midurethral sling (NEJM 2013;369:1124)	Bladder training Antimuscarinic Mirabegron: β-3 agonist s/e: HTN

- **Overflow incontinence**: incomplete emptying d/t underactive bladder ± outlet obstruction

FLUID IMBALANCE

Fluid Intake
- Water and food intake ~25–35 mL/kg/d → ± climate, habits, level of physical activity
- CHO oxidation 200–300 mL/d

Body Fluid Compartments

Estimation by Percentage of Ideal Body Weight (IBW)			
Body Fluid Compartment	Young Male	Elderly Male, Young Female	Elderly Female
Total body water (TBW)	60	50	45
Intracellular fluid (ICF): 2/3 of TBW	40	33	30
Extracellular fluid (ECF): 1/3 of TBW	20	16.7	15
Interstitial fluid: 3/4 of ECF	15	12.5	11.3
Intravascular fluid: 1/4 of ECF	5	4.2	3.8

- Transcellular (1–2 L): synovial, peritoneal, pericardial, intraocular, and CSF

Measurement of Body Fluid Volumes	
Volume	Indicators
TBW	Deuterium, tritium, antipyrine
Extracellular	^{22}Na, ^{125}I-iothalamate, thiosulfate, inulin
Intracellular	Calculate = TBW − extracellular volume
Plasma	^{125}I-albumin, Evans blue dye
Blood volume	^{51}Cr-labeled RBCs; calculate = plasma volume/(1-Hct)
Interstitial fluid	Calculate = extracellular − plasma volume

Fluid Loss
- Insensible: respiratory tract, skin 500–700 mL/d → ↑ extensive burns, cold weather, fever, tachypnea, open wounds, ↑ metabolism (>10-fold)
- Sweat: hypotonic, highly variable ~100 mL/d → ↑ exercise, hot climate (1–2 L/hr)
- Feces/GI: ~150 mL/d; ↑ diarrhea, NGT drainage fistula
- Urine: main regulator, multiple mechanisms (0.5–20 L/d); also regulates Na, Cl, K 0.5 L to excrete 600 mOsm with maximal ADH activity (1,200 mOsm/L)

Sodium and Water Imbalance

Manifestation of Salt and Water Imbalance		
	Salt	Water
Deficit	Volume depletion	Dehydration/Hypernatremia
Excess	Volume overload	Hyponatremia

DEHYDRATION

- Effective osmoles: cannot cross cell membranes w/o transporter activity eg, Na, K, glcuose, and mannitol
- Ineffective osmoles: freely cross cell membranes, do not affect transmembrane water flow, eg, urea and alcohol
- **Osmolality:** the milliosmoles of solutes per 1 kg of water. It is the same through ICF and ECF since water (via aquaporins) can freely traverse plasma membrane Calculated $P_{osm} = 2 \times [Na] + [glucose\ (mg/dL)]/18 + [BUN\ (mg/dL)]/2.8$

- **Tonicity:** the ratio of plasma effective osmoles (solutes that do not cross membrane barriers) to plasma water. It dictates the movement of water across a membrane. Approximately $2 \times [Na] + [glucose (mg/dL)]/18$
- **Dehydration:** a loss of TBW, resulting in hypertonicity; $\neq$ volume depletion
- **Hypernatremia:** [Na] >145, mainly from water deficit, rarely from total body Na or K increase with relative TBW deficit.
- High urea is hyperosmolar, but not hypertonic; hypernatremia is hyperosmolar and hypertonic

Pathophysiology

- Changes in plasma tonicity >280–289 mOsm/kg are sensed in hypothalamus
  → thirst sensation/water intake and **ADH** go up in a linear manner
  → ADH acts on the V2 receptor on the outer and inner medullary collecting duct resulting in luminal AQP channel placement in a cAMP-dependent manner
  → ↑ water absorption → ↓ tonicity → hypothalamic stimulus is turned off
- Water deficit results from decreased thirst/water intake +/– decreased renal concentrating capacity (**DI**), although the former is the more common mechanism
- Increased plasma osmolality → water shift from the intracellular to the extracellular space → cellular shrinkage
- In hypernatremia/hypertonicity, brain cells generate osmolytes to increase intracellular osmolality and counter the increase in extracellular osmolality. **If hypernatremia correction is rapid, iatrogenic cerebral edema can occur** due to the delayed decrease in intracellular osmolality in brain cells.

Clinical Manifestations

- Thirst, oliguria, anorexia, N/V, generalized weakness, fatigue, lethargy, irritability, confusion
- Severity of neurologic symptoms related to rate of rise of [Na] than absolute value
- Signs: dry mucous membranes, longitudinal tongue furrows, seizures, coma, ICH (in infants)
- Hypernatremia, ↑ U_{osm}, ↑ Urine specific gravity, relative polycythemia

Workup

- Determine the patient's overall sodium balance (volume status)

Salt and Water Balance and Mechanisms in Hypernatremia			
Volume Status	**Salt**	**Water**	**Mechanism**
Hypovolemic	↓	↓↓	Loss of hypotonic fluids
Euvolemic	–	↓	Loss of electrolyte free water
Hypervolemic	↑	–	Excessive salt intake

- Hypovolemic hypernatremia (negative sodium balance): loss of hypotonic fluids
  U_{Na} >20: renal loss; diuretics, post-ATN, post-obstructive, osmotic
  U_{Na} <20: extra-renal loss; vomiting, diarrhea, enterocutaneous fistula, sweating, burns
- Euvolemic hypernatremia (normal sodium balance): loss of electrolyte free water
  U_{osm} <300: renal loss, complete DI
  U_{osm} 300–600: renal loss, partial DI, compensated diuresis
  U_{osm} >700–800: extra-renal (cutaneous, respiratory) losses, primary hypodipsia, limited H_2O access, post seizures, severe exercise

Causes of Diabetes Insipidus (DI)	
ADH-dependent DI	**ADH-independent DI**
Exogenous vasopressin ↑ U_{osm}	Exogenous vasopressin does not ↑ U_{osm}
CDI: congenital, trauma, neurosurgery, CNS tumor, infiltrative, hypoxia encephalopathy, hemorrhage, CNS infection, aneurysm Gestational DI: vasopressinase mediated	Hereditary NDI: X-linked recessive, complete or partial Acquired NDI: ↑ Ca, ↓ K, lithium, demeclocycline, amphotericin B, foscarnet, methoxyflurane, vaptans, chronic interstitial kidney disease d/t medullary cystic disease, sickle cell disease, amyloid, Sjögren's, malnutrition

Hypernatremia Not Caused by Total Body Water Deficit

- Hypervolemic (positive sodium balance): least common; often iatrogenic after receiving hypertonic fluids, salt poisoning, rarely due to mineralocorticoid excess
- Intracellular water shift: electroshock-induced seizures and severe exercise, transient

Treatment

- Identify and treat underlying cause and replete water deficit
- CDI: desmopressin

- NDI:
  Thiazide: (1) mild volume depletion → ↑ reabsorption → ↓ tubular fluid and urine volume; (2) NCC-independent aquaporin 2 expression *(AJP Renal 2014;306:F525)*
  Low Na and protein diets: decreased urine output and water loss
  NSAID: PGE$_2$ ↓ AQP2 expression; desmopressin if partial
- Positive sodium balance: diuretics/dialysis; loop diuretics ↑ electrolyte free water loss as well as natriuresis and thus requires ongoing free water replacement

VOLUME DEPLETION

Definitions
- **Volume depletion: a deficit in ECF volume,** caused by loss or sequestration of sodium containing fluids
- Effective arterial blood volume: required to maintain effective tissue perfusion
  In nonedematous states, it is proportion to ECF volume
  In edematous states, ECF and effective arterial blood volume are not proportionate

Pathophysiology

Control Mechanisms of Extracellular Fluid		
Component	**Regulation**	**Effect**
Response to ECF volume Deficit		
Renin-Angiotensin-Aldosterone System (RAAS)	↑ renin release at JG apparatus granular cells by: 1. ↓ perfusion pressure at afferent arteriole by baroreceptor 2. ↓ NaCl delivery to macula densa in the TALH 3. β-adrenergic receptor activation	Sodium reabsorption Vasoconstriction
SNS	Activated by ↓ perfusion pressure/stretch at carotid sinus and aorta	↑ HR, BP RAAS activation
ADH	Nonosmotic release of ADH All ↑ release of ADH	Water retention Vasopressor effect
Response to ECF volume Excess		
Natriuretic Peptides	Released by stretch at atria and LV	Sodium excretion ↓ renin release

Etiologies
- GI: vomiting, diarrhea, bleeding, external drainage (while on avg only 150 cc/d, 3–6 L/d are generated by GI tract, normally all resorbed, if GI pathology lose ability to resorb and become volume depleted)
- Renal: diuretics, osmotic diuresis, salt wasting nephropathies, hypoaldosteronism
  In healthy kidney, 120–180 L/day filtered across glomerulus with >98% resorbed, if there is even a mild tubulopathy with even a slight ↓ in resorptive capacity, this will result in volume depletion (seen in chronic interstitial diseases)
- Skin: 1–2 L/hr can occur in hot/dry climate; burn
- Hemorrhage; sequestration into a third space: GI catastrophes (pancreatitis, obstruction, peritonitis), crush injuries

Clinical Manifestations
- Weight loss, orthostatic dizziness, oliguria, muscle cramps, agitation, thirst, confusion
- Orthostatic hypotension, ↑ HR: progress to supine hypotension ↑ HR
- Diminished skin turgor (less reliable in the elderly), delayed capillary refill
- Organ ischemia: nonocclusive mesenteric ischemia
- Hypovolemic shock: cold, clammy extremities, cyanosis, pulsus paradoxus (↓ SBP ≥10 during inspiration; DDx: cardiac tamponade, constrictive pericarditis)

Laboratory Findings of Volume Depletion	
↑ Cr	False (−): low muscle mass and liver cirrhosis
↑↑ BUN, BUN/Cr >20	↑ urea reabsorption in proximal tubule False (+): steroid, GIB, tetracycline
↓ Na	↑ ADH activity; masked by accompanied dehydration False (+): SIADH, HF, cirrhosis, NS, CKD, 1° polydipsia
↑ Hb, albumin	Hemoconcentration; masked by accompanied anemia, hypoalbuminemia

↓ U_{Na} <20	↑ Na reabsorption in renal tubules
	False (–):
	• Salt wasting from diuretics or underlying renal disease
	• High rate of water reabsorption
	• Metabolic alkalosis from vomiting: HCO_3^- is excreted and pulls Na with it, ✓urinary chloride
	False (+): HF, cirrhosis, NS
↑ U_{osm}	↑ ADH; False (+): dehydration

Diagnosis
- Fluid responsiveness: improvement of stroke volume and cardiac index by fluid is diagnostic of volume depletion; prediction prior to fluid administration is challenging
- History taking including weight change
- Physical examination: insensitive (JAMA 1999;281:1022; J Crit Care 2013;28:537.e1)

Static Assessments
- CVP: did not predict fluid responsiveness (Chest 2008;134:172; Crit Care Med 2013;41:1774)
- PAC/PCWP-guided therapy in CHF (ESCAPE JAMA 2005;294:1625), ARDS (JAMA 2003;290:2713), and acute lung injury (NEJM 2006;354:2213) didn't improve outcome

Dynamic Assessments: may be more indicative of volume responsiveness and potentially improve clinical outcome (Crit Care Med 2017;45:1538)
- Pulse pressure variation (PPV) (AJRCCM 2000;162:134; Crit Care Med 2009;37:2642)
- Stroke volume variation (SVV) (Br J Anaesth 2008;101:761; Anesth Analg. 2009;108:513)
- Passive leg raising: semi-recumbent position with 45° elevation of upper part of body → lower upper body and elevate leg at 45° x 1 min: brings 300–500 cc to the heart; ↑ CO and ↓ SVV and PPV predicts fluid responsiveness (Ann Intensive Care 2011;1:1; Crit Care Res Pract 2012; 2012:513480)
- IVC respiratory variation (Intensive Care Med 2004;30:1834; Intensive Care Med 2004;30:1740)

Management
- Rapid 1–2 L of isotonic fluid to restore tissue perfusion if there is evidence of shock
- Not possible to precisely predict the total fluid deficit for a given patient, clinical signs such as BP, MAP, UOP, MS, peripheral perfusion can guide adequacy of resuscitation

VOLUME OVERLOAD

Background and Clinical Implication
- Volume overload: sodium excess and expanded ECF volume
- a/w longer ICU stay and mortality (Crit Care 2013;17:R288)
- In septic shock, a/w ↑ mortality (VASST Crit Care Med 2011;39:259)
- In decompensated HF, hemoconcentration (absence of volume overload, measured by ↑ protein, albumin, Hct by diuresis) is a/w ↓ eGFR, ↑ survival (Circulation 2010;122:265)
- In acute lung injury, conservative management targeting CVP <4, PCWP <8 was a/w improved oxygenation index increasing ventilator-free and ICU free days c/t liberal management targeting CVP 10–14 or PCWP 14–18 (FACTT NEJM 2006;354:2564).
- In AKI a/w ↑ mortality x2.07 (KI 2009;76:422), ↓ renal recovery (KI 2009;76:422; NDT 2012;27:956)
- In CKD a/w rapid progression (AJKD 2014;63:68)
- Volume overload at the RRT initiation is a/w mortality (Crit Care 2012;16:R197)
- Hemodilution may lead to underestimation of the severity of AKI (Crit Care 2010;14:R82)

Pathophysiology
- Appropriate response: ↑ stretch at cardiac receptors (atria and ventricle) → atria release ANP, ventricles release BNP → natriuresis.
- **Heart failure:** ↓ cardiac output → ↓ perfusion pressure → low effective arterial blood volume → ↑ SNS and RAAS activation
- **Cirrhosis:** vasodilatation → ↓ perfusion pressure → low effective arterial blood volume → ↑ SNS and RAAS activation
- **Nephrotic syndrome:** ↓ oncotic pressure → ↓ tissue perfusion → low effective arterial blood volume → ↑ SNS and RAAS activation (underfill); 1° Na retention (overfill)
- Chronic kidney disease: blunted response to rapid sodium intake

Clinical Manifestations
- ↑ weight, ↑ BP, JVD, orthopnea, paroxysmal nocturnal dyspnea, nocturia
- Peripheral edema: pretibial and ankle in ambulatory; sacral in bedridden patients; periorbital edema in nephrotic syndrome

Manifestations of Fluid Overload in Organs	
Lungs	Pulmonary edema (rales), pleural effusion
CVS	↑ filling pressure, ↓ cardiac output, conduction disturbances, vasodilation
GI	Ascites, gut edema, malabsorption
Liver	Congestive hepatopathy
Skin, soft tissue	Wound infection, poor wound healing, pressure ulcer
CNS	Cerebral edema, delirium
Kidney	Interstitial edema, ↑ renal venous congestion → ↓ renal function

- Hyponatremia: ↓ tissue perfusion in HF, cirrhosis → ↑ ADH
- Hypoalbuminemia: ↑ urinary loss in the NS, ↓ synthesis in cirrhosis, dilutional; dilutional anemia
- ↑ BNP, NT-proBNP: cleared by kidney; less reliable in CKD
- ↑ PCWP >22 mmHg
- Thoracic ultrasound: B lines (aka comet-tail images) *(Chest 2005;127:1690)*

Management

- Monitor volume status; ✓daily fluid balance and weight
- Address underlying cause and treat appropriately
  HF: neurohormonal blockade
  Cirrhosis: anti-virals/immunosuppression depending of etiology
  NS: immunosuppression/RAAS inhibition
- Low salt diet: restrict dietary Na intake to <2 g (87 mEq) per day
- Avoid drugs that foster sodium retention as able such as NSAIDs, nonspecific vasodilators, high-dose β-blockers or central α-agonists
- Diuretics based on underlying conditions
- Adjust dose to achieve threshold dose: if weight loss is not achieved, can ✓24-hr urine urinary Na excretion OR 1–2 hr post loop diuretic FE_{Na}
  - If U_{Na} >100 mEq/d or FE_{Na} >2%: effective diuretics; if not losing weight, restrict salt intake
  - If U_{Na} <100 mEq/d or FE_{Na} <2%: ineffective diuretics; ↑ diuretic dose
- In severe hypoalbuminemia (eg, cirrhosis with ascites or nephrotic syndrome), albumin-assisted diuresis may be used *(JASN 2001;12:1010; Saudi J Kidney Dis Transpl 2012: 23;371)*
- In decompensated HF, it is essential to have enough BP to ensure tubular delivery of furosemide *(NEJM 2011;364:797)*. Inotrope-assisted diuresis can be considered in low output and congestive status in severe LV systolic dysfunction
- Dialysis initiation

FLUID IMBALANCE IN ESRD

Background

- Volume depletion: a/w loss of vascular access and residual renal function *(CJASN 2010;5:1255)*; hypotension, death *(JASN 2015;26:724)*
- Volume overload: a/w LVH and death *(Circulation 2009;119:671; JASN 2017;28:2491)*
- Postdialysis weight >2 kg above and below are a/w mortality *(CJASN 2015;10:808)*

Dry Weight (DW)

- Weight that the patient needs to achieve at the end of dialysis with minimal symptoms or signs of hypovolemia or hypervolemia
- Normal blood pressure s/p iHD can be used to assess euvolemia, but this requires the patient to not be on any other antihypertensive which is rare in HD patients
- Needs to be re-evaluated periodically to follow flesh weight change
- Over-estimated DW: may cause pulmonary edema and HTN
- Under-estimated DW: weakness, cramps, and hypotension

DW Assessment

- Clinical evaluation: edema (peripheral, pulmonary); absence does not r/o overload
- Bioimpedance: applying electrodes to the skin and estimating volume status by measuring resistance encountered by an electrical current passed through the body's tissues; not FDA approved in the U.S. *(NDT 2008;23:808, KI 2014;86:489)*

Relative Blood (or Plasma) Volume Monitoring
- Blood volume estimation with continuous hematocrit (Hct) measurement
  Volume overload: continuous transfer of fluid from interstitial to intravascular compartment during UF → stable Hct, flat curve
  Volume depletion: refill rate from the interstitium to intervascular space lags behind the UF rate → ↑ Hct, "blood volume" drop
- More hospitalization and mortality than conventional care (JASN 2005;16:2162)
- No ↓ intradialytic hypotension (CJASN 2017;12:1831)

Management (AJKD 2014;64:685)
- The normalization of the ECF volume is a primary goal of dialysis ("volume first")
- In HD, fluid removal should be gradual: ↓ interdialytic weight gain, treatment duration ≥4 hr, UF rate <10–13 mL/kg/hr; excessive UF during routine HD associated with morbidity and mortality (DOPPS KI 2006;69:1222; HEMO KI 2011;79:250; AJKD 2016;68:911)
- Avoiding intradialytic sodium loading: sodium profiling ↑ mortality (CJASN 2019;14:385)
- Dietary counseling: low sodium diet; fluid restriction
- High-dose loop diuretics: if urine output >~200 cc/d; ↓ interdialytic weight gain, UF amount, and intradialytic hypotension (CJASN 2019;14:95)

HYPOTENSION

- Absolute (SBP <90, MAP <65) or relative (drop in SBP >40 from baseline)
- Not synonymous with shock

HYPOTENSION-INDUCED AKI

- Autoregulation: hypotension, ↓ perfusion pressure → PG-mediated afferent arteriole dilation, and angiotensin II (AII)–mediated efferent arteriole constriction → maintain GFR
- NSAIDs and RASi impair autoregulatory mechanisms
- If perfusion pressure drops below the autoregulatory range, endogenous vasoconstrictors and endothelial cell injury ↑ afferent arteriolar resistance → ↓ glomerular capillary pressure → ↓ GFR
- If autoregulation is impaired, renal perfusion is dependent on MAP (KI 1994;46:318)
- Systemic arterial vasodilation from distributive shock (eg, sepsis) and liver cirrhosis ↓ renal perfusion and GFR +/− systemic hypotension
- Persistent renal hypoperfusion leads to tubular cell injury/ATN

SHOCK

- State of tissue hypoxia due to inadequate oxygen delivery or impaired oxygen utilization
- Most commonly occurs when there is reduced tissue perfusion in setting of hypotension
- Multiple types of shock often coexist

Types of Shock and Physiologic Characteristics (Parameter)

Types: Causes	Preload (PCWP)	Pump Function (CO)	Afterload (SVR)	Tissue Perfusion (S_vO_2)
Hypovolemic: fluid loss, hemorrhage	↓	NL or ↓	↑	NL or ↓
Distributive/Vasodilatory: septic, anaphylactic, neurogenic, adrenal insufficiency, thyroid dysfunction, burns, trauma, pancreatitis, postoperative vasoplegia	NL or ↓	NL or ↑	↓	↑
Cardiogenic: MI, CHF, arrhythmia, valve rupture, VSD, critical valvular stenosis, dissection, myocarditis	↑	↓	↑	↓
Obstructive: tension pneumothorax, pulmonary embolism, pulmonary hypertension crisis, cardiac tamponade	NL or ↓	NL or ↓	↑	variable

Clinical Manifestations
- Hypotension, tachycardia, altered mental status, tachypnea, oliguria, cool clammy, or warm/vasodilated depending on etiology of shock
- Exam: mucous membrane, rashes, JVD, murmurs/rubs, lungs crackles/breath sounds/ hyperinflation, tense or soft abdomen, LE edema, cap refill

Workup
- Lactate, cardiac enzymes, renal/liver function, CBC and differential, coagulation parameters, ABG, natriuretic peptides
- ECG, CXR, TTE, infectious cultures, bedside ultrasound, additional imaging as needed
- No benefit to the routine use of pulmonary artery catheter monitoring for shock or ARDS (JAMA 2003;290:2713; NEJM 2006;254:2213), high-risk surgical patients requiring ICU stay (NEJM 2003;348:5); no large studies examining use in cardiogenic shock

General Treatment
- Treat <u>underlying etiology of shock</u> while providing resuscitation: fluid, vasopressors, inotropes based on hemodynamic assessment

Fluid Resuscitation in Septic Shock
- 30 mL/kg IV crystalloid in the first 3 hr (Intensive Care Med 2017;43:304; JAMA 2017;317:847)
- Balanced crystalloid is particularly beneficial in sepsis (NEJM 2018;378:829)
- Early goal-directed therapy (EGDT): fluids, vasopressors, blood transfusions, and inotropes with target MAP ≥65, CVP 8–12, central venous O_2 sat ≥70% within the first 6 hr
  - ↓ hospital mortality from 46.5–30.5% c/t usual care (Rivers protocol NEJM 2001;345:1368)
- However, 3 large multicenter RCTs (ProCESS NEJM 2014;370:1683; ARISE NEJM 2014;371:1496; ProMISe NEJM 2015;372:1301) and the prospective patient-level meta-analysis of these RCTs (PRISM NEJM 2017;376:2223) failed to show lower mortality with EGDT (Likely reflects early recognition of sepsis and early antibiotics/fluids in most patients since EGDT trial)
- Can trend lactate clearance (≥10%/2 hr) instead of central venous O_2 (JAMA 2010;303:739)
- No mortality difference in targeting MAP 65–70 vs 70–85 in septic shock; in pre-specified subgroup of patients with chronic HTN, higher MAP group had less renal dysfunction and less need for RRT than lower MAP group (SEPSISPAM NEJM 2014;370:1583)
- Transfuse PRBC only when Hgb <7 in adults, unless active MI or acute hemorrhage (TRICC NEJM 1999;340:409; TRISS NEJM 2014;371:1381)
- Albumin: consider if substantial amounts of crystalloids required (Intensive Care Med 2017;43:304)
- Avoid fluid overload: a/w ↑ mortality (VASST Crit Care Med 2011;39:259)

Steroids in Septic Shock
- Initially showed benefit (JAMA 2002;288:862) but not replicated in subsequent trials (CORTICUS NEJM 2008;358:111; ADRENAL NEJM 2018;378:809)
- Hydrocortisone + fludrocortisone ↓ 90 day mortality (APROCCHSS NEJM 2018;378:797)
- Small benefits in mortality, length of ICU and hospital stay (Crit Care Med 2018;46:1411)
- Avoid routine use; hydrocortisone 200 mg IV per day if hemodynamic stability not achieved with fluid resuscitation and vasopressors alone (Intensive Care Med 2017;43:304)
- Steroids are indicated in patients on chronic steroid therapy or adrenal dysfunction
- s/e: neuromuscular weakness, hypernatremia

Properties of Vasopressors and Inotropes					
Drug	Receptors	Dilation	Constriction	Inotropy	Chronotropy
Vasopressors					
Dopamine					
1–3 mcg/kg/min	DA >> β1	+	+	+	+
3–10 mcg/kg/min	β1 > β2, DA > α1	–	++	++	++
>10 mcg/kg/min	α1 > β1 >>> β2	–	+++	+++	++
Epinephrine					
1–20 mcg/min	α1, α2, β1 > β2	+	++++	++++	++++
Norepinephrine					
1–40 mcg/min	α1, α2 >> β1	–	++++	++	+
Phenylephrine					
10–400 mcg/min	α1 >>> α2	–	++++	–	–
Vasopressin					
0.04 U/min	V1/ V2	–	+++	–	–
Inotropes					
Dobutamine					
2–20 mcg/kg/min	β1 > β2	++	–	+++	++
Milrinone					
0.125–0.5 mcg/ kg/min	cAMP PDE-3 inhibitor	+++	–	++	+

DA: dopamine, α1: α-1 adrenergic, α2: α-2 adrenergic, β1: β-1 adrenergic, β2: β-2 adrenergic, V: vasopressin, PDE-3: Phosphodiesterase-3

- Vasopressors generally improve GFR (J Physiol 1981;321:21; CJASN 2008;3:546)
- Norepinephrine: preferred over dopamine as first-line: no overall mortality difference but more arrhythmias with dopamine (SOAP II NEJM 2010;362:779)
- Vasopressin or epinephrine: can be added to norepinephrine to meet MAP target
- Epinephrine ≈ norepinephrine for achieving MAP goal (Intensive Care Med 2008;34:2226)
- Phenylephrine vs other vasopressors on clinical outcomes in shock not well studied
- Angiotensin II (Giapreza®): in vasodilatory shock, ↑ MAP, ↓ SOFA score (NEJM 2017;377:419); in AKI requiring RRT, ↓ 28-d mortality and ↑ RRT liberation (Crit Care Med 2018;46:949)
- Low-dose dopamine: does not prevent AKI; may worsen renal perfusion (KI 2006;69:1669)

Vasopressors in Septic Shock

- Mortality was lowest when begun 1–6 hr after onset with IV fluid (Crit Care Med 2014;42:2158)
- Every hour of delayed norepinephrine was a/w ↑ 5.3% mortality (Crit Care 2014;18:532)
- Norepinephrine: 1st choice (Intensive Care Med 2017;43:304; JAMA 2017;317:847)
- Vasopressin at 0.03 U/min added to low-dose norepinephrine: no difference in mortality c/t high-dose norepinephrine; mortality benefit seen in a pre-specified subgroup of less severe septic shock on 5–14 mcg/min norepinephrine (VASST NEJM 2008;358:877)
- Vasopressin (up to 0.06 U/min) vs Norepinephrine: no difference in kidney failure-free days or death, but vasopressin group had less use of RRT (VANISH JAMA 2016;316:509)
- Norepinephrine + dobutamine vs epinephrine: no difference in mortality (Lancet 2007;370:676)

Inotropes

- May be added to vasopressors for shock when the etiology is primarily cardiogenic or significant cardiac contribution in mixed shock states (eg, septic/cardiogenic shock, obstructive/cardiogenic shock in a large acute pulmonary embolus)
- Use often prompted by low central venous O$_2$ sat despite vasopressor support
- Milrinone dose should be adjusted for reduced kidney function

RENAL REPLACEMENT THERAPY IN SHOCK

- CRRT: more likely to ↓ fluid accumulation than HD (KI 2009;76:422)

Timing of RRT

- In multicenter trial on AKI (KDIGO 3) requiring mechanical ventilation early vs delayed RRT showed no mortality benefit at 60 d (AKIKI NEJM 2016;375:122). Post-hoc analysis in ARDS or septic shock, no benefit of early RRT (AJRCCM 2018;198:58)
- In single-center trial on AKI (KDIGO 2–3) and NGAL >150 ng/mL, early RRT was a/w ↓ 90 day mortality (ELAIN JAMA 2016;315:2190), ↓ 1-yr mortality and ↑ renal recovery (JASN 2018;29:1011)
- In multicenter trial on AKI (RIFLE failure stage) with septic shock, early RRT not a/w mortality reduction. 62% of delayed group did not require RRT (NEJM 2018;379:1431)

ORTHOSTATIC HYPOTENSION (OH)

- Physiologic response to standing: the pooling of 500–1,000 mL of blood in the lower extremities and splanchnic circulation → ↓ venous return to the heart and ↓ cardiac output and BP → ↑ sympathetic outflow (baroreceptor reflex) → ↑ peripheral vascular resistance, venous return, cardiac output, and BP
- OH: postural reduction in SBP ≥20 or DBP ≥10 w/i 3 min of standing
- BP fall w/i 1 min was a/w dizziness, fracture, syncope, and death (JAMA IM 2017;177:1316)
- Delayed OH: OH after 3 min of standing; a/w Parkinson disease (Neurology 2015;85:1362)
- Postural tachycardia syndrome (POTS): ↑ HR ≥30 beats/min w/i 10 min of standing or head-up tilt in the absence of OH
- Postprandial hypotension: BP reduction within 1–2 hr after a meal

Causes

- Volume depletion: fluid loss, overdiuresis, overdialysis; adrenal insufficiency, anemia
- Autonomic dysfunction: amyloidosis, DM, Parkinson disease, multiple system atrophy
- Drugs: all antihypertensives, α1-blockers (for BPH or HTN), trazodone, SSRI, MAOi, TCA, vasodilators (including PDE5 inhibitors)

Clinical Manifestations

- Dizziness, weakness, palpitations, blurred vision, fall, syncope, fall
- Sometimes asymptomatic due to autoregulation of the cerebral blood flow

Treatment

- Volume repletion, d/c of causing drugs; avoid rapid postural change
- Compression stockings, abdominal binder
- Fludrocortisone: mineralocorticoid; s/e: supine HTN, hypokalemia, sodium retention
- Midodrine: α1-agonist
  s/e: supine HTN, urinary retention, piloerection, scalp pruritus and paresthesia, bradycardia, bowel ischemia (Crit Care Med 2018;46:e628)
- Droxidopa: norepinephrine precursor; less supine HTN than midodrine (Ann Pharmacother 2018;52:1182)

Familial Dysautonomia

- Ashkenazi Jewish, AR, mutation of IKBKAP, orthostatic hypotension, supine HTN, ↑ CKD
- 19% of alive pts at age 25 required dialysis (AJKD 2006;48:780); KT is an option (CJASN 2010;5:1676)

EDEMA

- Edema occurs when there is sodium retention by the kidney with resultant expansion of the interstitial space
- The sodium retention by the kidney can be 1° (renin and aldosterone are suppressed) or 2° (renin and aldosterone are increased d/t a hemodynamic stimulus)
- In 2° renal sodium retention, the stimulus can be an absolute decrease in the intra-vascular volume (as with disorders of capillary leakage) or due to arterial underfilling. Disorders of arterial underfilling are characterized by an increase in total blood volume, but an inadequate arterial perfusing volume
- Mechanical causes of edema tend to cause edema that is localized (ie, to an extremity) in contradistinction to other conditions in which it is more generalized

Causes (*causes that do not respond to diuretics)
- **Primary renal sodium retention**
  - CKD/ESRD, nephrotic syndrome (NS, majority) (KI 2012;82:635), thiazolidinediones
- **Secondary renal sodium retention**
  - **Arterial underfilling** (JASN 2007;18:2028)
    HF of various etiologies (including constrictive pericarditis), cirrhosis, pregnancy
    Severe hypoalbuminemia, usually <2.0, of diverse causes (generally a/w relative or absolute hypotension)
    NS (minority) (KI 2012;82:635)
    Protein losing enteropathy, kwashiorkor, severe chronic illness (particularly infection)
  - **Decreased arteriolar tone** causing increased capillary pressure
    *Vasodilator antihypertensive medications: minoxidil, hydralazine, dihydropyridine Calcium channel blockers (Curr Cardiol Rep 2002;4:479)
  - **Increased capillary permeability**
    *Sepsis, *pre-eclampsia, *pancreatitis
    *Capillary leak syndromes (KI 2017;92:37)
    Idiopathic systemic capillary leak syndrome (SCLS) aka Clarkson disease
    Drug-induced (IL-2, IL-11, IL-12, gemcitabine, OKT-3, alemtuzumab and rituximab in hematologic malignancies)
    Engraftment syndrome, graft-vs-host disease following allogeneic BMT
    Differentiation syndrome, ovarian hyperstimulation syndrome
    Hemophagocytic lymphohistiocytosis, viral hemorrhagic fever
- Unknown: hypothyroid/myxedema-exact mechanism is unclear, but it is characterized by
  - ↑ plasma volume, ↓ cardiac output, and ↓ GFR
- Mechanical causes: *lymphedema, *venous obstruction, or insufficiency

Clinical Manifestations
- Edema will be unilateral/localized in mechanical causes and symmetric in other causes
- In nonmechanical causes, extremity edema may coexist with serous cavity effusions (pleural, pericardial, peritoneal) or pulmonary edema

Workup
- History and physical: relevant new medications; evidence of heart failure, cirrhosis, NS
- NS and CKD: serum creatinine, urine protein: creatinine ratio, serum albumin
- Liver disease: coagulation studies and albumin, abdominal ultrasound
- Heart failure: B-type natriuretic peptide, cardiac ultrasound
- Myxedema: TSH, free T4
- Venous insufficiency: venous LE U/S to evaluate competence of venous valves
- Further evaluation for uncommon causes as dictated by the clinical presentation

Treatment of Edema	
Cause	Treatment
1° renal Na retention, arterial underfilling	Loop diuretics +/− thiazide diuretics
Severe hypoalbuminemia (<2) with poor response to diuretics/volume depletion	IV albumin (to achieve serum albumin >2.0) + loop diuretics +/− thiazides
Mechanical causes	Address mechanical cause
Others	Treat underlying disease

Definition and Pathogenesis

- Proteinuria: >3.5 g/d or >3 g/g by urine protein to Cr ratio (UPCR) due to podocyte injury
- Hypoalbuminemia (<3.5 g/dL): urinary losses + tubular metabolism > hepatic synthesis
- Edema: 1° Na retention (overfilling) ± ↓ oncotic pressre (underfilling)/RAAS activation
- Hyperlipidemia (cholesterol and/or TG): not required to fulfill the criteria for NS; low plasma oncotic pressure leads to ↑ LDL, ↑ angiopoietin-like 4 → ↑ TG (Nat Med 2014;20:37)
- NS is a phenotype (not a disease); microscopic hematuria, AKI possible (overlapping features with nephritic syndrome)

Etiologies

- Primary podocyte/GBM injury: MCD, FSGS, MN. Some cases of IgAN, MPGN
- Glomerular injury d/t systemic diseases: DM (nephrotic range proteinuria > NS), amyloidosis, lupus nephritis (esp. class V)

Epidemiology

- ≤18 yo: MCD > MPGN > FSGS (KI 1978:13:159)
- 18–60 yo: FSGS = MN > MCD > LN > DN > IgAN
- ≥60 yo: MN > amyloid > MCD > FSGS > DM > IgAN (ACKD 2012:19:61)
- ≥80 yo: MCD > MN > amyloid > FSGS > IgAN > DM (ACKD 2012:19:61)

Extra-Renal Clinical Manifestations

- Hypercoagulability: unclear mechanism; adults > children; venous > arterial thromboses; MN > other diseases; risk factors: Alb <2.8, heavy proteinuria (CJASN 2012;7:513)
- Pleural effusion: transdates pattern as in cirrhosis, CHF, constrictive pericarditis
- Ascites: serum ascites albumin gradient <1.1 as in peritonitis, peritoneal carcinomatosis
- Gut edema: N/V, abdominal discomfort; pericardial effusion
- ↑ TSH: thyroxine-binding globulins loss from proteinuria
- Vitamin D deficiency: vitamin D–binding protein loss in urine
- Infection, hypogammaglobulinemia: antibody loss in urine

Nephrotic Syndrome–Associated Conditions	
NSAIDs, penicillamine	MCD, MN
Lithium, IFN, pamidronate, HIV	MCD, Collapsing FSGS
Rifampin, ampicillin, EBV, syphilis, ehrlichiosis, mycoplasma Hodgkin lymphoma, thymoma, atopy/eczema	MCD
Strongyloides stercoralis (KI Rep 2018;3:14)	MCD, Tip FSGS
Heroin, anabolic steroids, sirolimus, HCV DAA (Hepatology 2017;66:658) CMV, SV40, parvovirus B19, leishmaniasis, filariasis HLH/Macrophage activation syndrome, cerebral arteritis, adult-onset Still disease, MCTD, multiple myeloma, SCD, acute monoblastic leukemia, polycythemia vera, essential thrombocythemia, primary myelofibrosis	FSGS
Gold, mercury, captopril; HBV, syphilis, Malaria, SLE, RA Malignancy (lung, colon, breast, prostate, uterus, gastric)	MN
Chronic osteomyelitis, tuberculosis, RCC, RA, IBD Familial Mediterranean fever, hidradenitis suppurativa	AA amyloidosis

Workup and Diagnosis

- Kidney bx required in most cases
- Lab: hepatitis B and C serologies, HIV, ANA, C3, C4, SPEP with IFE, kappa/lambda free light chain assay, UPEP with IFE, Hb A1c, anti-PLA2R Ab
- In diabetics, consider kidney biopsy if rapidly progressive kidney disease, extra-renal symptoms c/w systemic disease, (+) serologies, and in patients with short duration of DM

Management of Complications

- Volume overload: loop, thiazdes, MRBs diuretics PO (absorption may be reduced from gut edema) or IV; IV diuretics + IV albumin if severe/refractory
- Hypertension: goal <130/80, use RAAS blockade if persistent proteinuria
- Hypercoagulability: prophylactic anticoagulation if bleeding risk is low and serum alb <2.8 for MN (KI 2013;85:1412). Role of prophylactic anticoagulation for other NS etiologies uncertain, but could be considered if serum alb <2.0
- Hyperlipidemia: statins if persistent due to ↑ HMG-CoA reductase activity and risk of coronary heart disease in NS (KI 1993;44:638)
- Hypothyroidism: treat unless resolves with management of NS

GLOMERULONEPHRITIS (GN)

Definition and Renal Manifestations

- Microscopic or gross hematuria: dysmorphic RBCs/acanthocytes, RBC casts on sediment
- Azotemia, HTN common; proteinuria, usually subnephrotic (<3.5 g/d), can also have nephrotic range proteinuria (overlapping presentation with NS)
- GN is a *phenotype* of inflammatory glomerular disease, not a specific disease

Diagnosis

- Based on kidney bx and clinical history/labs
- Proliferation (mesangial, endocapillary, extracapillary/crescents) common on bx
- Glomerular injury secondary to systemic diseases: eg, infections such as endocarditis, SLE, ANCA-associated vasculitis, Henoch–Schönlein purpura, Goodpasture syndrome
- Lab workup depending on clinical presentation: C3, C4, ANA, hepatitis B and C serologies, ANCA (including anti-MPO and anti–PR-3 Ab titers), anti-GBM Ab, HIV, SPEP/IFE, serum kappa/lambda free light chain assay, cryoglobulins, RF, and blood culture

Common Serum Complement Changes in GN	
Low Complement	Normal Complement
Immune complex–mediated MPGN, lupus nephritis	Pauci-immune GN
Infection-related GN, cryoglobulinemic GN, C3G	Anti-GBM dz
PGNMID, MIDD (esp, heavy chain), immunotactoid GN	IgA nephritis, fibrillary GN

Epidemiology (Differs by Sex and Race) (*CJASN 2017;12:614*)

- ≤18 yo: LN > IgAN > ANCA > anti-GBM dz, Alport's
- 18–60 yo: LN > IgAN > ANCA > anti-GBM dz, Alport's
- 60–80 yo: ANCA > IgAN > LN > fibrillary GN > anti-GBM dz, Alport's
- ≥80 yo: ANCA > IgAN > LN ≈ fibrillary GN ≈ anti-GBM dz ≈ Alport's
- Male: IgAN > ANCA > LN > FGN > TBM lesion > GBM > Alport's > ITGN
- Female: LN >> ANCA ≈ IgAN > TBM lesion > FGN > GBM > Alport's > ITGN

Extra-Renal Manifestations

Extra-Renal Manifestations of Systemic Diseases That Cause GN	
Disease	Extra-Renal Presentation
IgA Vasculitis (IgAV, aka HSP)	Skin: urticaria, ecchymoses, maculae, palpable purpura GI: Abd pain, GIB, nausea, vomiting MSK: arthralgias, arthritis
Systemic lupus erythematosus (SLE)	Constitutional: fever, malaise, weight loss Skin: malar rash, discoid lupus Lung: pleuritis; cardiac: pericarditis GI: abdominal pain, GIB MSK: arthralgias, arthritis; neuro: confusion, seizure, stroke
ANCA-associated vasculitis	Constitutional: fever, malaise, weight loss Skin: palpable purpura Lung: cavities, nodules, pulmonary hemoorrhage, cough GI: abdominal pain, GIB MSK: arthralgias, arthritis; neuro: mononeuritis multiplex ENT: rhinosinusitis, hearing loss, cartilage destruction
Anti-GBM dz	Pulmonary hemorrhage
Alport syndrome	ENT: sensorineural hearing loss Eyes: lens, retinal and corneal defects
Cryoglobulinemic GN	Skin: palpable purpura, ulcers Neuro: neuropathy MSK: arthralgias, arthritis, myalgias

RAPIDLY PROGRESSIVE GLOMERULONEPHRITIS (RPGN)

- Clinical presentation of inflammatory glomerular disease with rapidly worsening kidney function over days, weeks, or months → associated with poor prognosis if untreated
- Causes: ANCA-associated vasculitis, anti-GBM dz, lupus nephritis, IgAN/IgAV, infection-related GN (especially endocarditis)
- Crescents (extracapillary proliferation) often seen on kidney bx in RPGN cases

- Requires rapid diagnosis (kidney bx) and treatment
- If awaiting biopsy, empiric treatment with pulse IV glucocorticoids (methylprednisolone 500–1,000 mg/d × 3 days): will not change biopsy results
- PLEX: consider in DAH and severe AKI

THROMBOTIC MICROANGIOPATHY

- Endothelial damage → microangiopathic hemolytic anemia (MAHA), platelet aggregation and consumption in small vessel → organ damage

Causes (NEJM 2014;371:654)
- Infection: enterohemorrhagic E. coli (Shiga toxin), Shigella dysenteriae, S. pneumonia, Influenza A/H1N1, HIV, EBV, CMV, M. pneumoniae, Bordetella pertussis, Parvovirus B19
- TTP: hereditary or autoimmune ADAMTS13 deficiency
- Atypical HUS: hereditary or autoimmune disorders of complement regulation
- Pregnancy or postpartum: (pre)eclampsia, HELLP syndrome
- Transplantation: solid organ, bone marrow or stem-cell transplantation
- Metabolic: cobalamin C (vitamin B_{12}) def (Lancet 2015;386:1011; Pediatr Nephrol 2015;30:1203)
- Autoimmune: SLE, APS, scleroderma renal crisis (SRC, in systemic sclerosis type)
- Malignancies: metastatic adenocarcinoma, monoclonal gammopathy (KI 2017;91:691)
- Malignant hypertension
- Drugs: CNI, gemcitabine, quinine, ticlopidine, anti-VEGF therapy (NEJM 2008;358:1129)
- Genetic: DGKE (Nat Genet 2013;45:531; CJASN 2015;10:1011), INF2 (JASN 2016;4:1084)

Clinical Manifestation and Diagnosis
- Hematologic TMA: MAHA (↑ retic count, ↑ LDH, ↓ haptoglobin, ↑ indirect bilirubin, schistocytes on peripheral blood smear) + thrombocytopenia (<150 or >25% ↓ from baseline) + organ dysfunction
- Renal TMA: AKI, proteinuria, glomerular hematuria, hematologic TMA, hypertension
- Not all renal TMA has all features of hematologic TMA
- Biopsy: fibrin thrombi (when acute), endotheliosis, mesangiolysis, intimal edema, "onion skinning" (myocyte proliferation) of vessel walls; glomeruloid body (organized thrombus, specific for APLA), capillary loop duplication, subendothelial electrolucent material on EM (in chronic)
  SRC and malignant hypertension: vascular damage predominantly

Extra-Renal Manifestations (Front Pediatr 2014;2:97; KI 2017;91:539)
- Neurologic: irritability, mental status change, stroke, focal deficits, seizure, coma
- GI: N/V, bloody diarrhea, pancreatitis, liver injury
- Skin: purpura, small vessel vasculopathy, gangrene
- Cardiac: cardiomyopathy, MI, myocarditis, CHF, occlusive CAD
- Others: pulmonary hemorrhage, rhabdomyolysis

TMA Workup	
Cause, Clues	Workup
All TMA	Culture studies, HIV, homocysteine, methylmalonic acid: cobalamin C deficiency Paraprotein studies: SPEP, sIFE, serum FLC
HUS: diarrhea (D)+	Stool studies for STEC EHEC
aHUS: no other history or family h/o TMA	Complement studies: C3, C4, CH50, gene mutations/autoantibodies; ✓ if KT being considered
TTP	ADAMTS13: activity, inhibitor and antigen
SLE	ANA, aCL Ab, β2GP-1 Ab, lupus anticoagulant
Scleroderma	RNA polymerase III ab, skin exam
Malignant HTN	Retinal exam, TTE, and ECG (for LVH)
Preeclampsia / HELLP	LFTs, fetal monitoring, placental ultrasound

Treatment
- Empiric: PLEX if no obvious etiology identified, CS if low suspicion of scleroderma or infection; stop potential offending agents

TMA Treatment When Etiology Known	
Cause	Treatment
HUS: D+	Supportive care: fluid/electrolyte management, dialysis if needed
aHUS	PLEX, eculizumab (NEJM 2013;23:2169); CS, rituximab if autoAb+
TTP	CS, plasma infusion/PLEX, cyclosporine, or rituximab if refractory. Splenectomy rarely needed
Autoimmune	Immunosuppression for SLE, ACEi for SRC, anticoagulation for APS
Malignant HTN	Aggressive blood pressure control
(Pre)eclampsia	Deliver baby → consider alternative dx if TMA does not improve

ACUTE KIDNEY INJURY (AKI)

Background and Epidemiology
- Overall global incidence 22% in hospitalized patients (CJASN 2013;8:1482)
- Up to 67% of ICU patients (Crit Care 2006;10:R73)
- Up to 50% in septic shock; associated mortality ~70% (KDIGO AKI 2012)
- **Risk factors:** volume depletion, age, hypoalbuminemia, female, CKD, DM, ↓ EF, cardiac surgery, chronic liver disease, malignancy (KDIGO AKI 2012)

Definition
- Sudden loss of kidney function, clinically manifested as ↑ creatinine +/− ↓ UOP

AKI Staging (KDIGO AKI 2012)		
Stage	Creatinine	Urine Output (UOP)
1	↑ 0.3 in 48 hr or ↑ to 1.5–1.99x baseline w/i 7 d	<0.5 cc/kg/hr for >6–12 hr
2	↑ to 2.0–2.99x baseline w/i 7 d	<0.5 cc/kg/hr for ≥12 hr
3	↑ to ≥3x baseline w/i 7 d; OR increase in Cr to ≥4.0; OR need for RRT	<0.3 cc/kg/hr for ≥24 hr or anuria for ≥12 hr

- More advanced stages associated with worse outcomes an mortality

---

CAUSES OF AKI

- **Causes of anuric renal failure:** usually due to severe shock, RPGN, bilateral (or single if one kidney) renal artery or urinary obstruction

Prenal: ↓ effective arterial volume
- Hypovolemia, cirrhosis, early shock of any etiology before progressing to ATN, cardiorenal (CHF, AS, RV dysfunction), abdominal compartment syndrome, hepatorenal syndrome, hypercalcemia, capillary leak syndrome

Intrarenal
- Glomeruli: GN, look out for RPGN
  Anti-GBM disease
  Immune complex: infection-related GN, SLE, cryo, IgAN, IgAV/HSP, endocarditis
  Pauci-immune: ANCA-associated (GPA, MPA)
  Thrombotic: TMA (TTP/HUS, DIC, complement/drug-mediated TMA, antiphospholipid antibody syndrome, preeclampsia/HELLP, malignancy)
- Vasculature: TMA (malignant HTN, scleroderma renal crisis), emboli (eg, cholesterol), renal artery occlusion, renal vein thrombosis, polyarteritis nodosa
- Tubules: ATN (sepsis, ischemia, toxins), light chain cast nephropathy,
  Crystal induced: urate from tumor lysis, PO_4 from oral and possibly enema (KJ 2016;90:13)
- Interstitium (AIN):
  Drugs (70%) especially antibiotics, NSAIDs, PPIs
  Infections (many bacterial incl staph, strep, syphilis, Legionella; viruses; mycobacteria)
  Autoimmune diseases (SLE, Sjögren's, IgG4 vasculitis, sarcoidosis)
  Miscellaneous (TINU syndrome, lymphoma)

Postrenal
- Stones, BPH/prostate cancer, retroperitoneal fibrosis, bladder/pelvic malignancies, transitional cell carcinoma, fungus balls, blood clots, papillary necrosis with sloughed tissue causing obstruction

WORKUP OF AKI

History and Physical Examination
- Hypotension: absolute or relative vs baseline
- Drugs: NSAIDs, diuretics, ACEi/ARB, PPI, antibiotics, herbal remedies/ illicit drug
- Volume depletion: diarrhea, poor PO intake
- Infection/sepsis, IV contrast
- Recent surgery/arterial catheterization: cholesterol emboli
- Markers of volume status: BP, skin turgor, mucous membranes, JVD, edema, rales
- Changes in urine output (oliguria), hematuria
- Rashes/joint pain: vasculitis, endocarditis, AIN
- Respiratory symptoms: pulmonary renal syndrome, eg, ANCA, anti-GBM, SLE, cryo

Initial Laboratory Workup
- ✓ on most patients: BMP, LFTs, Ca, PO₄, albumin, CPK, UA with microscopy and sediment, spot urine protein/sodium/urea/creatinine, CBC with differential
- **BUN/Creatinine ratio**: normal roughly 10:1
  - >20:1 suggests prerenal because hypovolemia causes ↑ reabsorption of sodium and water in proximal tubule, and urea follows passively
  - <20:1 suggests intrinsic renal disease
  - False ↑ BUN: steroids, GI bleeding from increased urea production; creatinine ↓ with low muscle mass (eg, elderly, cirrhotics)
  - False ↓ BUN: low protein intake;
  - ↑ creatinine release from rhabdomyolysis or impaired tubular creatinine secretion (eg, trimethoprim, cimetidine)
- **FE_Na:** used to distinguish prerenal from other causes
  - <1% (prerenal); 1–2% (prerenal or intrarenal); >2% (intrarenal or obstruction)
  - <1% cutoff for prerenal only applies for marked ↓ GFR, prerenal physiology with normal kidney function can have FE_Na <0.1%
  - Caveats: nonprerenal <1% can occur with contrast nephropathy, rhabdomyolysis, GN, ATN in background of severe prerenal state (eg, cirrhosis, CHF); prerenal with >1% can occur with background CKD or diuretic therapy
  - FE_Na accounts for water handling, better than urine sodium alone
- **FE_Urea:** likely better than FE_Na on diuretics *(Nephron Clin Pract 2010;114:c145)*

Laboratory Findings of Prerenal AKI and ATN		
Measurement	**Prerenal**	**ATN**
BUN/Cr ratio	>20:1	<20:1
Urine sediment	Bland or hyaline casts	Renal tubular epithelial cells, "muddy brown casts," granular casts
Urine specific gravity	>1.020	~1.010
Urine osmolality	>500	<350
Urine sodium	<10–20	>20–40
FE_Na	<1%	>2%
FE_Urea	<35%	>35%

- **Urine sediment:** utility controversial; considerable inter-operator variability; polarized light to see crystals, lipid droplets in NS (maltese crosses)

Urine Sediment Findings and Significance	
Finding	**Significance**
RBC	**Nonglomerular:** stones, tumor, exercise, menses, infection, interstitial cystitis, transient, AVM, papillary necrosis, PKD, medullary sponge, hypercalciuria **Glomerular:** GN, thin basement membrane nephropathy, Alport's
Dysmorphic RBC	GN, loin-pain hematuria syndrome; acanthocytes are subtype with 98% specificity for GN *(KI 1991; 40:115)*
RBC casts	GN usually, less commonly AIN *(AJKD 2012; 60:330)*
WBC	AIN, TB, schistosomiasis, fungal, stone, tumor, infection, interstitial cystitis *(NEJM 2015;372:1048)*
WBC casts	AIN, GN, pyelonephritis Only 3% of AIN with WBC casts *(AJKD 2014; 64:558)*

Crystals (AJKD 2016;67:954)	Medications: acyclovir, indinavir, sulfamethoxazole, sulfadiazine, methotrexate, amoxicillin, ciprofloxacin
	CaOx: ethylene glycol, hypercalciuria, enteric or primary hyperoxaluria, orlistat, vitamin C
	CaP: phosphate nephropathy; alkaline pH
	Uric acid: hyperuricemia, urate nephropathy, tumor lysis; acidic pH
	Cystinuria; Struvite: Mg-ammonium-phosphate, "triple phosphate"; with urease splitting bacteria, alkaline pH
Renal tubular epithelial cell casts	ATN Any RTEC or granular casts may predict ATN with sensitivity 83% and specificity 77% (CJASN 2008; 3:1615)
Granular casts	Derived from degenerated epithelial cell casts; "muddy brown casts" are pigmented version (ATN, hyperbilirubinemia)
Hyaline casts	Nonspecific; seen in healthy and disease states
Waxy casts	Degenerated granular casts; nonspecific, seen in both chronic and acute disease

- **Urinalysis**
  Specific gravity can approx urine osmolality; ~ 1.010 ~ 300 mOsms/kg (intrinsic disease, >1.020 with prerenal disease); discordance with large, heavy molecules (contrast, glucose) which ↑ sp gravity more than osmolality
  (+) blood w/o RBC: myoglobin (rhabdomyolysis, ✓CK), Hb (✓blood smear, hemolysis)
  (+) proteinuria only detects albumin (and usually only >300 mg/g creat, previously known as "macroalbuminuria"); if discordance between dipstick proteinuria and quantified proteinuria, then likely LMW proteins or paraproteins present; sulfosalicylic acid can be added to detect nonalbumin proteinuria
  (+) glucose with serum glucose <180 suggests proximal tubular defect (aminoglycosides, paraprotein disease, heavy metals, cisplatin, tenofovir) or SGLT2 inhibitor
- **Quantified proteinuria**
  Spot UPCR or UACR; approximates 24-hour urine protein or albumin excretion if daily creatinine excretion is ~1 g/d (can significantly underestimate or overestimate daily proteinuria in large/muscular or low muscle mass/elderly, respectively)
  Spot ratio can also be inaccurate when serum creatinine is fluctuating
  Nevertheless 24-hour urine collection not usually needed in AKI
  Quantify proteinuria even if dipstick protein negative to evaluate for nonalbumin proteinuria (eg, paraproteins in multiple myeloma)
  % urine albumin excretion <25% may predict cast nephropathy in dysproteinemic kidney disease (CJASN 2012;7:1964)
  AKI on CKD—proteinuria may be due to the chronic process, and not acute (eg, ATN in patient with pre-existing diabetic nephropathy)
- **CBC with differential**
  Eosinophilia may suggest AIN, atheroembolic disease
  Significant anemia can suggest CKD, TMA (especially if thrombocytopenia), multiple myeloma, hemolysis (and pigment-related injury)
  Thrombocytopenia can suggest TMA (eg, TTP, HUS, DIC), SLE, antiphospholipid antibody syndrome, cirrhosis; ✓ smear for schistocytes if anemic, coags
  Leukocytosis can suggest sepsis, myeloproliferative disorder
- **Calcium**
  ↑: can cause AKI (prerenal, ATN); or clue for multiple myeloma, sarcoidosis, malignancy
  ↓: CKD, hyperphosphatemia; pancreatitis, tumor lysis, rhabdomyolysis
- **Serum albumin**
  If low, in nephrotic range proteinuria, suggests primary NS
  Very low levels (<2.8) in NS can increase risk of thrombosis, including renal vein thrombosis (especially with primary membranous nephropathy)
  Large gap between total protein and albumin level suggests paraprotein disease

Radiographic Testing

- Renal ultrasound (preferred) or noncontrast CT in most patients to r/o obstruction
  Small kidneys (<9 cm) suggests chronicity (except with diabetes)
  Large kidneys (>11–12 cm) suggests AIN, diabetes, amyloid, PKD, lymphoma, HIVAN, renal vein thrombosis
- Echogenicity not a reliable indicator of CKD (CJASN 2014;9:373)
- Asymmetric kidneys suggest unilateral renovascular or congenital disease

- **Paraprotein workup –** ✓ SPEP/IFE, serum free light chains, UPEP
  Get if > age 50 w/ unexplained AKI; or manifestations of MM, amyloidosis, etc
- **Serum uric acid:** ↑ in any renal disease due to decreased renal clearance; especially ↑ in tumor lysis, rhabdomyolysis, myeloproliferative disorders, acute urate nephropathy
  If ↑ out of proportion to renal failure (ie, >15) then could be cause rather than effect of kidney disease; urine uric acid:creatinine ratio >1 suggestive of this
  If acute urate nephropathy suspected, treatment is IV saline, rasburicase, XOI
- **If suspecting glomerular disease:** serologic workup can include hepatitis B/C, ANCA, ANA, dsDNA, C3, C4, cryo, anti-GBM, SPEP/IFE, serum free light chains, UPEP, HIV, blood cultures; ultimately need kidney biopsy to confirm
- **Novel biomarkers for ATN** (not yet clinically available)
  Urine neutrophil gelatinase-associated lipocalin (NGAL) (Ann IM 2008;148:810)
  Urine kidney injury molecule-1 (KIM-1) (KI 2008;73:1008)

Indications for Kidney Biopsy in AKI

- Unresolving AKI; suspected GN; AIN for which steroid treatment is being considered

Common Patterns Associated with Acute or Subacute Kidney Diseases	
Findings	**Possible Diagnosis**
Acellular urine, minimal proteinuria (<1 g)	Prerenal and ATN most likely, AIN also possible (even without pyuria or proteinuria), obstruction, crystal disease (oxalate, urate, phosphate nephropathy), cast nephropathy
Nephrotic range proteinuria, +/– microhematuria	NS w/ ATN (usually minimal change), FSGS (especially collapsing), amyloid and other paraprotein-related glomerulopathy, renal vein thrombosis (especially MN)
Pyuria with minimal proteinuria (<1 g)	Infection, AIN, atheroemboli
Subnephrotic proteinuria and cellular urine	Inflammatory glomerulonephritis (immune-complex such as SLE/infection related/IgA, anti-GBM, ANCA), TMA, malignant HTN, PAN
Pulmonary–renal syndromes	ATN from sepsis (pneumonia), ANCA, anti-GBM, SLE, cryo, AIN from pulmonary infection (Legionella, TB, Streptococcus) or the antibiotics used for treatment, infection-related GN, AKI with volume overload and pulmonary edema, scleroderma, sarcoidosis, drugs (PTU, cocaine), IgAV (rare pulmonary hemorrhage), IgAN (hematuria following URI), C3G following URI
Dermatology–renal syndromes	Vasculitis (ANCA, SLE, cryo, PAN, HSP), AIN, endocarditis, infection-related (cellulitis), scleroderma, atheroemboli, hep C (porphyria), amyloidosis (purpura), HIV (Kaposi sarcoma, eosinophilic folliculitis)
Low complements	SLE, infection-related, cryo, C3G, other MPGN, IgG4-related disease, endocarditis, atheroembolism

PREVENTION OF AKI

- **General preventive measures:** minimize nephrotoxins (eg, contrast, NSAIDs), volume depletion, hypotension; renally dose medications
- No single medication consistently shown to prevent septic or ischemic ATN
  Low-dose dopamine ineffective and potentially even harmful (KI 2006;69:1669)
  Fenoldopam ↓ AKI but not RRT/mortality; needs more data (Crit Care 2015;19:449)
  Atrial natriuretic peptide (ANP) with mixed results (CJASN 2009;4:261)
- Remote ischemic preconditioning safe but uncertain efficacy; meta-analysis negative, do not recommend currently for ischemic ATN (Cochrane Database Syst Rev 2017;CD010777)
- Off pump cardiac surgery did not ↓ rates of AKI requiring dialysis (NEJM 2013;368:1179)
- Withholding ACEi/ARB prior to surgery of uncertain benefit, may prevent peri-op hypotension, but need RCT to determine effect on hard outcomes
- Aminoglycosides: once-daily dosing reduces AKI without affecting efficacy (Am J Health Syst Pharm 1996; 53:1141); gentamicin > tobramycin > amikacin, in decreasing toxicity

Fluid Resuscitation
- Use crystalloids over colloids; balanced crystalloids reduced kidney events vs NS in ICU (NEJM 2018;378:829) and non-ICU settings (NEJM 2018; 378:819)

Contrast Nephropathy
- Use low/iso-osmolar agents, minimal contrast dose, peri-procedure normal saline if pulmonary status ok
- Conflicting data on NAC, likely not beneficial (NEJM 2018; 378:603–14); isotonic sodium bicarbonate not beneficial over NS (NEJM 2018; 378:603)

MANAGEMENT OF AKI

- Mainly supportive; control of underlying process (eg, sepsis, volume depletion, RPGN)
- No single medication shown to improve outcomes after septic/ischemic ATN
- Loop diuretics can be used to manage volume while awaiting recovery, but does not hasten renal recovery and should not be used to delay dialysis if indicated

Renal Replacement Therapy
- **Indications:** acidosis/hyperkalemia/volume overload refractory to medications, uremia (pericardial effusion, ΔMS), certain ingestions
- **Modalities:**
  - Continuous renal replacement therapy (CRRT), intermittent HD (iHD), slow low efficiency dialysis (SLED); no modality proven to be superior (JAMA 2008;299:793)
  - Hemofiltration may improve clearance of middle molecules but no improvement in outcomes over hemodialysis (Crit Care 2012;16:R146)
  - CRRT or SLED preferred over iHD if patient is hemodynamically unstable, or with increased intracranial pressure (less dramatic osmotic shifts than iHD)
- **Dose:** 3x/wk noninferior to 6x/wk for iHD, effluent rate of 20 cc/kg/hr noninferior to 35 cc/kg/hr for CRRT (NEJM 2008;359:7); aim for modestly higher effluent rate for CRRT as interruptions will limit actual delivered dose compared to prescribed dose; weekly Kt/V ≥3.9 for intermittent or extended daily dialysis (KDIGO AKI 2012)
- **Timing of RRT:** most evidence does not suggest mortality benefit for early vs delayed initiation of RRT (AKIKI NEJM 2016;375:122; NEJM 2018;379:1431); no specific BUN or Cr threshold when to start

PROGNOSIS OF AKI

- Depends on severity and duration of injury, baseline function, comorbidities
- Furosemide stress test: 1–1.5 mg/kg of furosemide; increased urine output predicts more favorable outcome, but does not alter outcome (JASN 2015;26:2023)
- Nonoliguric ATN generally w/ better prognosis, possibly d/t less severe injury and better volume status; positive fluid balance w/ AKI a/w worse outcomes (Crit Care Med 2012;40:1753)
- Full extent of recovery with ATN occurs usually by 6–12 wk
- Up to 1/3 of all AKI is "transient" (recovery w/i 3 days), but still a/w ↑ hospital mortality vs no AKI (NDT 2010;25:1833)
- ↑ mortality in survivors of AKI (rate ratio 2.59) (AJKD 2009; 53:961)
- Cardiac surgery: AKI ↑ long-term mortality, even w/ complete AKI recovery (Circulation 2009;119:2444)
- Long-term mortality in survivors of AKI worse if renal function doesn't normalize (46% vs 83%) (Crit Care 2012;16:R13)
- AKI increases risk for CKD (HR 8.8), ESRD (HR 3.1), mortality (HR 2.0) (KI 2012;81:442)
- ICU: hospital mortality ↑ with ↑ severity of AKI; 8.8–26.3% range (Crit Care 2006;10:R73)
- 35% hospital mortality, 49% 6-month mortality in AKI requiring RRT in Finland ICUs (Crit Care 2012;16: R13); 47% hospital mortality, 65% 1 yr mortality in another study in AKI requiring RRT in ICU

CHRONIC KIDNEY DISEASE (CKD)

Definition
- CKD: presence of kidney damage or ↓ kidney function (eGFR <60) for ≥3 mo (AJKD 2002;39:S1)
- Kidney damage: UACR >30 mg/g, active urine sediment, kidney transplant, or abnormalities on biopsy or imaging (Lancet 2012;379:165)
- Staging risk stratifies pts and aids in management (AJKD 2002;39:S1)

CKD Staging (G: GFR category; A: albuminuria category)					
G	**GFR (mL/min/1.73 m²)**			**A**	**AER (mg/d)**
G1	≥90 + kidney damage			**A1**	<30
G2	60–89 + kidney damage			**A2**	30–300
G3a	45–59	**G4**	15–29	**A3**	>300
G3b	30–44	**G5**	<15		

- Stages are classified into risk categories (based on mortality, CV mortality, and ESRD risk)
- All G3b, G4, G5, and A3 pts are consider at high or very high risk (KDIGO CKD 2012)

Epidemiology (2018 USRDS annual data report)
- Prevalence of pre-dialysis CKD (1–5) was ~14.8% of the U.S. population in 2013–2016
- Stage 3 (6.4%) the most prevalent
- Females > males (16.7% vs 12.9%); CKD ↑ w/ age (32.2% of adults >60).
- <10% of CKD pts aware of disease (AJN 2012;35:191), 57% awareness in stage 4 CKD

Causes
- Prerenal, intrinsic (vascular, glomerular, and tubulointerstitial) or postrenal.
- Urinalysis and renal ultrasound (U/S) can differentiate

Etiologies of CKD			
Category	**Possible Causes**	**Urinalysis**	**Renal U/S**
Prerenal	Chronic CHF Chronic cirrhosis	Minimal protein, bland sediment	
Vascular	HTN (APOL1) Renal vascular disease TMA	Minimal protein, bland sediment	Small kidneys excluding DM
Glomerular	Chronic glomerular disease DM (m/c cause of CKD)	(+) protein, +/– RBCs	HIV, DM: large kidneys
Tubulointerstitial	Inherited disease: cystic kidney disease eg, PKD, CAKUT Infiltrative disease Chronic TIN	(+) protein <2 g/d, +/– WBCs	PKD: large cystic kidneys DM, infiltrative disease: large kidneys
Postrenal	Obstructive uropathy RP fibrosis	Minimal protein	(+) hydronephrosis RP fibrosis: +/– hydro

- 36% w/ CKD have DM, 31% HTN, and 40% CV disease (2018 USRDS annual data report)

CV and All-Cause Mortality of CKD
- CKD a/w traditional CAD risk factors such as HTN, DM, smoking, HLD, older age, and the metabolic syndrome (JASN 2005;16:529)
- ↓ eGFR, ↑ UACR = **independent** risk factors for CV and all-cause mortality (Arch IM 2007;167:2490; JASN 2002;13:745)
- CKD is CAD risk equivalent → risk factor reduction is needed (Circulation 2003;108:2154)
- Nontraditional CAD risk factors: anemia (Am J Cardiol 2008;102:266), inflammation (JASN 2004;15:538), +calcium balance (NDT 2006;21:2464), CKD-MBD (NDT 2006;21:2464)
- Proportion of CV deaths, infections, DM complications ↑ w/ eGFR (JASN 2015;26:2504)

Progression to ESRD
- Injury → Adaptive hyperfiltration initially ↓ Cr → eventually CKD progression
- Rate of transition 3 + 4 CKD → ESRD: 1.5%/yr (Ann IM 2004;141: 95)
- Pts with uncontrolled HTN, DM, and CKD lose ~12 mL/min GFR/yr. When treated ~4 mL/min GFR/yr (KI 2001;59:702)
- 2- and 5-yr kidney failure risk can be predicted with 4 or 8 variables (JAMA 2011;305:1553; JAMA 2016;315:164, available at QxMD®)

GENERAL CKD TREATMENT

Evaluate Etiology and Treat Reversible Causes
- d/c potential nephrotoxins; prerenal: hold diuretics, NSAIDs, RASi
- Renal U/S to ✓ for obstruction

If Not Reversible Goals Should Be
- Slow progression; adjust medications by eGFR; management of complications
- Refer to nephrology when GFR <30, UACR ≥300 mg/g, glomerular hematuria, or CKD of unknown etiology; prepare for RRT

CKD TREATMENT TO SLOW PROGRESSION

Blood Pressure and Proteinuria Control in Nondiabetic CKD
- In nonproteinuric CKD pts, SBP >130 a/w ↑ CKD progression (Ann IM 2015;162:258)
- ↓ BP in nonproteinuric CKD pts has not slowed CKD progression but ↓ mortality (JASN 2017;28:2812)
- In proteinuric CKD pts, ↓ BP (SBP 110–129) ↓ CKD progression (Ann IM 2003;139:244)
- In nondiabetic CKD pts w/ proteinuria ≥500 mg/day, ACEi ↓ CKD progression vs other antihypertensives (JASN 2007;18:1959).
- RASi ↓ CKD progression in proteinuric pts independent of BP (Lancet 1998;352:1252).
- RASi ↓ CKD progression in advanced, proteinuric CKD (NEJM 2006;354:131)
- Combo ACEi + ARB did not ↓ CKD progression or ↓ mortality; ↑ serious adverse events (ONTARGET Lancet 2008;372:547)

Blood Pressure and Proteinuria Control in Diabetic CKD
- 10 mmHg ↓ SBP ↓ 12% renal failure, and ↓ 5 mmHg ↓ CV events (BMJ 2000;321:412)
- RASi > other anti-HTNsve meds ↓ CKD progression (JASN 2001;345:851)
- RASi ↓ CKD progression independent of BP effect (NEJM 1993;329:1456; NEJM 2001;345:861)
- Combo ACEi and ARB did not ↓ CKD progression or ↓ mortality; ↑ serious adverse events (VA-NEPHRON-D NEJM 2013;369:1892)

Glycemic Control in Diabetic CKD
- In T1DM, intensive glucose treatment to near-normal levels may ↓ CKD progression (DCCT/EDIC NEJM 2011;365:2366)
- In T2DM, HbA1c of 7.0% vs 7.9% ↓ CKD progression (UKPDS Lancet 1998;352:837)
- SGLT-2 inhibitors ↓ CKD progression in T2DM (EMPA-REG OUTCOME NEJM 2016;375:323) ↓ kidney failure and CV events (CREDENCE NEJM 2019;380:2295)
- Treat to goal HbA1c ~ 7.0% to ↓ CKD progression (AJKD 2012;60:850)

Other Treatments
- Low protein intake ~0.8 g/kg/d may ↓ related deaths (Cochrane Database Syst Rev 2009;CD001892)
- Smoking cessation: ↓ CKD progression 16 (JASN 2004;15:S58)
- NaHCO₃ PO 600 mg TID (if [HCO₃] 16–20) ↑ to target [HCO₃] ≥23 ↓ CKD progression and improves nutritional status (JASN 2009;20:2075)
- Multifactorial therapy (diet, exercise, smoking cessation, ACEi, and statins) ↓ CKD progression (NEJM 2003;348:383)

TREATMENT OF CKD COMPLICATIONS

Treatment of CKD Complications (KDIGO CKD 2013; KDIGO 2012 Anemia; KDIGO 2017 MBD)	
Volume overload	Diuretics: thiazides less effective when eGFR <20, use loop diuretics in advanced CKD; Low (<2 g) sodium diet (KDIGO CKD 2012)
HTN/ Proteinuria	>85% of CKD pts have HTN (AJKD 2010;55:441–51)
	If proteinuria treat with RASi, then MRAs (JAMA 2015;314:884), then nondihydropyridine CCBs (KI 1996;50:1641)
	Low sodium diet potentiates antihypertensives and antiproteinuric effects of RASi (Diabetes Care 2002;25:663)
	Treat to UPCR goal <500–1,000 mg/g (AJKD 2004;43:S1)
HLD	Statins ↓ CV risks in nondialysis CKD (Lancet 2011;377:2181)

Hyperkalemia	Emergency if K^+ >6.5, symptoms or ECG changes: stabilize cardiac myocytes (IV Ca^+) then shift K (insulin + glucose, IV bicarbonate, β2-adrenergic agonists) then eliminate from the body (diuretics +/– saline, sodium polystyrene sulfonate) Lower K^+ if nonoliguric or planning surgery: low K diet, stop offending agents (eg, ACEI/ARB, NSAIDs), $NaHCO_3$, diuretics, cation exchangers GI cation exchangers • Patiromer, s/e: ↓ Mg^+, binds other meds (NEJM 2015;372:211) • Sodium zirconium cyclosilicate: exchanges Na^+ and H^+ for K^+ s/e: edema (HARMONIZE JAMA 2014;312:2223) • Avoid Kayexalate +/– sorbitol unless life-threatening hyperkalemia given risk of colonic necrosis
Platelet dysfunction	↑ BT d/t uremic toxins, anemia, ↑ platelet NO synthesis Correct if active bleeding or invasive procedure (eg, kidney biopsy) Tx: DDAVP 0.3 mcg/kg IV 1 hr prior to invasive procedure, heparin-free HD or PD, tx anemia to Hb > 10 with resistant bleeding add cryoprecipitate
Malnutrition	Caused by uremia-related anorexia, decreased intestinal absorption and digestion, and metabolic acidosis Maintain diet w/ 30–35 kcal/kg/d and 0.8–1.0 g/kg/d protein Check dry weights and serum albumin if decreasing → start dialysis
Anemia Background	↓ EPO production by the kidney; normocytic normochromic [Hb] <13.0 in males and <12.0 in females. ↑ prevalence w/ CKD progression: 1% eGFR 60, 9% eGFR 30, 33–67% eGFR 15 (Arch IM 2002;162:1401) ✓RBC indices, retic count, iron, TIBC, ferritin, WBC w/ diff, platelets, and B_{12} and folate if MCV >100 If anemia + off ESA, monitor every 3 mo
Anemia – Iron	Iron deficiency + if TSat ≤20% or ferritin ≤100 ng/mL Iron may ↑ Hb if TSat ≤30% and ferritin ≤500 ng/mL Oral iron: 65-mg elemental iron QD or QOD (1–3 mo trial) IV iron (iron dextran, ferric carboxymaltose, sodium ferric gluconate complex, ferumoxytol, iron sucrose, ferric pyrophosphate citrate) if severe deficiency or no ↑ Hb w/ oral iron
Anemia – ESA	Address correctable causes of anemia prior to ESA Treating anemia to near-normal Hb in pre-dialysis CKD with darbe ↑ stroke (TREAT NEJM 2009;361:2019) Consider ESAs if Hb <10 to prevent blood transfusion Goal Hb 10–11.5 Don't use if malignancy, severe HTN, recent stroke
CKD-MBD Background	PO_4 retention, ↓ Ca, ↓ calcitriol, ↑ FGF-23 and ↓ klotho 1st step: PO_4 retention → ↑ PTH (AJKD 1997;30:809) ↑ PTH, ↓ calcitriol when eGFR <60 (CJASN 2009;4:186, KI 2007;71:31) ↑ PO_4 when eGFR <30 (PO_4 controlled at higher eGFR due to ↑ FGF-23 and PTH (JASN 2005;16:2205)
CKD-MBD Treatment	✓serial PO_4, Ca, and PTH levels. Imaging, bx not yet used for tx Tx Phos to normal w/ diet and phos binders Non–Ca-based phos binders > Ca-based (Lancet 2013;382:1268) If PTH ↑ing → correct ↑ PO_4, ↓ Ca, ↓ vitamin D Calcitriol or vitamin D analogs if severe and worsening ↑ PTH No vitamin D (nutritional or active) if Ca ≥9.5 or ↑ PO_4

END-STAGE RENAL DISEASE (ESRD)

Definition (2018 USRDS Annual Data Report)
- Defined by CMS as a condition in which regular long-term dialysis or KT is necessary to maintain life. ESRD includes chronic HD, PD, or s/p kidney transplant
- Results from the progression of CKD or if AKI persists for ≥3 mo

Epidemiology (2015–2018 USRDS Annual Data Report)
- The USRDS database contains UTD info on epidemiology
- 726,331 prevalent ESRD cases; 124,675 incident cases in 2016
- ESRD prevalence is 9.5× in American Indians/Alaska Natives, 3.7× in Blacks, 1.5× Native Hawaiians/Pacific Islanders, and 1.3× Asians than Whites
- Prevalent ESRD with DM ~40%; ↑ cognitive impairment in HD (Neurology 2006;67:216)

- Prevalence of depression in ESRD pts is 30–40% (KI 2013;84:179)
- 35.4% with little or no pre-ESRD nephrology care; mean eGFR at dialysis initiation 9.

Renal Replacement Therapy (2018 USRDS Annual Data Report)

- 87.3% incident ESRD pts receive HD, 9.7% PD, and 2.8% a preemptive kidney transplant
- 63.1% prevalent ESRD pts receive HD, 7.0% PD, and 29.6% have a kidney transplant
- In 2015, home dialysis (HHD or PD) accounted for 8.6% of prevalent dialysis pts
- 80% use a catheter at HD initiation
- 62.8% HD pts use an AVF, 80% were using an AVF or AVG at 1 yr after initiation
- 39% of AVFs fail to mature; median time to first use of AVF is 108 days

Prognosis of ESRD (2017–2018 USRDS Annual Data Report)

3-Yr Survival in ESRD (2018 USRDS Annual Data Report)				
	LDKT (%)	DDKT (%)	PD (%)	HD (%)
ESRD	91	86	70	57
Age-, sex-matched general population	98	98	95	92

- Survival: transplantation w/o dialysis > transplantation after dialysis
- Mortality ≥65 yr ↑ 7× than general population
- ESRD pts are hospitalized ~ 2x/yr
- 48% of deaths in dialysis 2/2 CV causes (arrhythmias, cardiac arrest, CHF, AMI, ASHD)
- ↑ mortality on Monday or Tuesday after a long weekend (NEJM 2011;365:1099)
- Statins do not ↓ CV risk (SHARP Lancet 2011;377:2181)
- ↓ K+ HD bath a/w arrhythmias (KI 1980;17:811)
- Medicare spending on ESRD in 2016 was $35.4 billion (7.2% of overall budget).
  $28 billion on HD and $90,971/pt/yr. PD costs < HD per pt

Treatment of ESRD	
Diet, exercise (AJKD 2000;35:S17)	Sodium, potassium, phosphorus, and liquid restriction Protein intake for HD and PD = 1.2–1.3 g/kg/d Energy intake for HD and PD = 35 kcal/kg if <60 yo and 30–35 kcal/kg if ≥ 60 (AJKD 2000;35:S1) Exercise is a/w improved health outcomes (AJKD 2014;64:383)
Adequate dialysis (KDOQI AJKD 2015;66:884; AJKD 2006;48:S98)	Target a delivered Kt/V of 1.2 per HD session. No ↑ benefits from ↑ Kt/V$_{urea}$ (HEMO NEJM 2002;347:2010) Minimum of 3 hr HD with a biocompatible membrane For PD, target a minimum Kt/V$_{urea}$ of 1.7/wk (residual kidney function + PD clearance) No ↑ from ↑ Kt/V$_{urea}$ (ADMEX JASN 2002;13:1307)
Volume Overload	Optimize dry weight Chronic fluid overload ↑ mortality (CJASN 2015;10:808) ↑ ultrafiltration rates (>10 mL/hr/kg) ↑ CV mortality (KI 2011;79:250)
HTN	SBP <120 and SBP ≥150 ↑ mortality (JASN 2006;17:513) ↓ BP with antihypertensives ↓ CV events (Hypertension 2009;53:860) No RCTs of BP targets in ESRD Tx: 1st step is ↓ dry weight to achieve euvolemia. Target 0.5 kg ↓ per session. Then consider medication: βB, RASi, DHP CCB β-blocker ↓ CV event, hospitalizations in HD pts w/ LVH (NDT 2014;29:672) In PD, RASi preserves residual renal function (AJKD 2004;43:1056)
Hyperkalemia	Emergency if K+ >6.5, symptoms or ECG changes: stabilize cardiac mycoytes, shift K+, then emergency dialysis Urgency if K 5.5–6.5: stabilize, shift, then urgent dialysis w/in 6–12 hr For dialysis pts with chronic ↑ K+, use GI cation exchangers Avoid low K+ HD bath: ↑ arrhythmias (KI 1980;17:811)
Anemia (KDIGO Anemia 2012)	Evaluate monthly; IV iron if TSAT <30% and ferritin <500 ng/mL and no active systemic infections ESAs when Hb 9.0–10.0; stop ESAs when Hb >11.5
CKD-MBD (KDIGO MBD 2017)	Evaluate PO$_4$, Ca, and PTH levels serially Treat ↑ PO$_4$ w/ diet and binders; restrict dose of Ca-based binders Non–Ca-containing PO$_4$ binders: sevelamer, lanthanum, ferric citrate, sucroferric oxyhydroxide Dialysate [calcium] 2.5–3.0 mEq/L Maintain PTH at 2–9 × ULN of assay w/ calcimimetics or vitamin D analogs; severe ↑ PTH: parathyroidectomy

TRANSITION OF CARE FOR YOUNG ADULTS

- 90% of adolescents and young adults (AYA) w/ special health care needs survive into adulthood. Adult services have increasing numbers of AYA who have either transitioned from pediatric care or presented directly to adult services.
- Medication adherence worsens posttransfer *(Pediatr Nephrol 2009;24:1055)*
- 17–24 yo txp recipients have higher graft failure rate than older *(Transplantation 2011;92:1237)*
- Some childhood onset renal diseases have new clinical manifestations in adulthood, eg, cystinosis: DM, myopathy, pulmonary, and CNS dysfunction *(Front Pediatr 2017;31:191)*
- Childhood kidney disease even w/ nl renal function is a/w adult ESRD *(NEJM 2018;378:428)*
- AYA w/ CKD has impaired sense of self-worth, perceive a precarious future, and feel limited in their physical and psychosocial capacities *(AJKD 2013 61:375)*

Health Care Transition (HCT)

- Purposeful, planned efforts to address the biopsychological needs of early adolescents (11–15 yo), late adolescents (16–18 yo), and emerging adults (18–25 yo)
- Goal is to ensure AYA obtain self-management knowledge and skills necessary to manage their daily treatment needs as independently as possible and become a literate health consumer *(J Pediatr Nurs 2017;35:160)*

Transfer of Care

- Dual process of locating & arranging 1°, specialty, & interdisciplinary providers who provide care to AYA as their eligibility provided by pediatric providers ends
- Actual shift from pediatric to adult care

Consensus Statement From ISN and IPNA *(KI 2011;80:704)*

- Only transfer AYA following assessment of transition process and AYA preparedness
- Health Care Transition Process should:
  - Include key support: parents, family, or significant others
  - Offer opportunity of informal visit to adult service prior to transfer
  - Tools to aid in acquisition of disease self-management skills
- Transfer from Pediatric to Adult Nephrology
  - Individualized transition plan, agreed upon jointly by AYA and medical team
  - Should take place during a period *without* crisis
  - Take into account treatment plans by other subspecialties
  - Take place with due consideration of financial factors, with adequate preparation

TRANSITION STEPS

Extended HCT Preparation (12–18 yo)

- Plan of care with measureable outcome, with detailed timeline
- HCT coordinator to "champion"/lead transition, coordinate referrals, health care coverage
- Age of majority (18 yo or on graduation from high school in AK, NV, OH, TN, UT, VA, WI) needs to be considered, discussion of guardianship, HIPAA
- Discuss changing role of parent from 1° caregiver to that of coach/consultant, AYA as CEO of own health

Transfer of Care Period (18–21 yo)

- Pediatric providers can provide resources for adult providers
- Direct handoff between pediatric and adult providers, with a Transfer Summary
- Transfer Summary: comprehensive written and verbal summary of all multidisciplinary aspects of young person's care: medical, Nursing, Dietary, Social and Educational

Post HCT/Transfer of Care Period (>18 yo)

- Documentation that transfer has taken place and AYA connected with adult providers
- Assessment of AYA knowledge & skills; identify and adult 1° care provider and dentist
- Review an emergency plan, whom to contact if ill or needs refills
- Assess ongoing insurance coverage—referral to Financial Coordinators
- Discuss future goals with AYA alone and with support system
- Introduction of AYA to key clinic staff; consultation letter to referring pediatric provider

Knowledge and Skills Assessment Tools	
Got Transition/Center for Health Care Transition Improvement	http://www.gottransition.org/
U. North Carolina STARx Program	https://pediatrics.med.unc.edu/transition
Transition Readiness Assessment Questionnaire	https://www.etsu.edu/com/pediatrics/traq

PURPOSES OF RENAL FUNCTION ASSESSMENT

- CKD staging: allows adherence to stage-specific management guidelines
  - Reduced renal function is one marker of kidney damage along with: albuminuria, abnormal urine sediment (eg, glomerular hematuria), renal tubular disorders, abnormal pathology, abnormal imaging (eg, polycystic or dysplastic kidneys or cortical scarring), and kidney transplantation (KDIGO CKD 2012)
- Medication dosing adjustments based on renal function
- Prognosis: eGFR associated with renal outcomes (development of ESRD), cardiovascular outcomes, and all-cause death (NEJM 2013;369:932)
- Transplantation donor evaluation

MEASURED GLOMERULAR FILTRATION RATE (mGFR)

- Administration of exogenous filtration markers (inulin, iohexol, iothalamate, EDTA) followed by serial measurements of blood/urine concentrations over time
- Most accurate assessment of renal function; impractical for routine use d/t cost, complexity
- Does not provide a quantification of tubular function

CREATININE

- Organic cation, metabolic byproduct of creatine from muscle and dietary meat
- Not reabsorbed or metabolized by kidney
- Secreted by organic cation transporters in PCT
- Increased secretion in late stages of CKD

Conditions That Change Serum Creatinine	
↓ Creatinine	↑ Creatinine
↑ GFR ↓ Generation: ↓ muscle mass (limb loss, cachexia, cirrhosis, lower extremes of height) ↑ Secretion: hypoalbuminemia in NS (NDT 2005;20:707)	↓ GFR ↑ Generation: ↑ muscle mass/bodybuilder, upper extremes of height ↑ Intake: creatine, high meat diet ↓ Secretion: cimetidine, trimethoprim, pyrimethamine, dolutegravir, rilpivirine, cobicistat, ritonavir, amiodarone, dronedarone, ranolazine Peritoneal reabsorption: uroperitoneum from bladder rupture (NDT 2006;21:1119), ureter leak Cross reactivity in alkaline picrate method: acetoacetate in DKA, cefoxitin, flucytosine

RENAL FUNCTION IN CKD

Creatinine-based Estimated GFR (eGFR)
- In steady state, creatinine level can estimate GFR by MDRD or CKD-EPI equations
- Use Cr, sex, age, and race to calculate eGFR
- Decreased precision at higher levels of GFR (CKD-EPI better than MDRD), and possibly in advanced age and race other than white/black

Blood Urea Nitrogen (BUN)
- Filtered but passively reabsorbed in the proximal tubule
- Rises more than creatinine in volume depletion or renal hyperperfusion
- Not affected by above conditions affecting creatinine level, but overall a less reliable indicator of kidney function
- GFR-independent ↑ BUN: GI bleed, corticosteroids, high protein intake, catabolic state (fever, burns)
- GFR-independent ↓ BUN: low protein intake/malnutrition, liver disease

Cystatin C–based eGFR
- Endogenous protease inhibitor produced by most nucleated cells at stable rate
- Cystatin C generation displays less interperson variability than Cr
- Affected by smoking, thyroid disease, corticosteroid use
- Alternative CKD-EPI equation using both cystatin C and creatinine performs best (NEJM 2012;367:20)
- Other Cr-based eGFR formulas (CAPA, BIS) not shown to outperform CKD-EPI (JASN 2015;1982)
- Limitation: cystatin C assays not as well standardized as for Cr

Timed Cr Clearance (C_{cr}) and Urea Clearance (C_{urea})
- Measurement of serum Cr and urea and timed urine Cr, urea and volume
- Practical alternative to measure GFR in patients for whom eGFR is inadequate (eg, kidney donors, prior to chemotherapy)
- C_{urea}: underestimates GFR due to passive reabsorption of urea in the PCT
- C_{cr}: overestimates GFR due to secretion of creatinine in the PCT
- Mean of C_{urea} and C_{cr}: partially adjusts for these limitations
- Limited by accuracy of urinary collection: over- or undercollection can lead to extremely inaccurate estimates

Estimated CrCl (Cockcroft–Gault Equation)
- CrCl (mL/min) = [(140 − age) × weight in kg × 0.85 (if female)]/(72 × SCr)
- Less accurate estimation of GFR than eGFR, should not be used in routine clinical practice for CKD identification and staging
- Many drug dosing recommendations are based on CrCl instead of eGFR

Nuclear Renogram
- Can be used to estimate the relative contribution of each kidney to overall renal function (eg, prior to nephrectomy)

RENAL FUNCTION ON RENAL REPLACEMENT THERAPY

- Residual kidney function for patients on HD/PD assessed using timed urine collection of creatinine and urea
- May be able to use serum β-trace protein, β2-microglobulin, cystatin C rather than using collection, but not common practice (KI 2016;89:1099)

RENAL FUNCTION IN AKI

- Cannot use eGFR in AKI b/c Cr not at steady state (ΔCr lags behind ΔGFR)
- Changes in UOP may be informative, but cannot be relied upon since UOP can be preserved even after large decrease in GFR
- Kinetic GFR estimate (KeGFR) uses rate of Cr change to estimate GFR when Cr is not at steady state (JASN 2013;24:877; available at QxMD®)

URINE STUDY

URINE DIPSTICK

- Should wait for 30 s–1 min before reading
- Urine dipstick is semiquantitative assay

Specific Gravity (SG): relative weight (mass) to water
- Osmolality is concentration of dissociated solute particle number
- Each 0.001 rise from 1 ≈ ↑ 30–35 mOsm/kg when urine solutes are Na, K, NH_4, urea only
- SG overestimates osmolality when urine contains heavy solutes: glucose, protein, contrast
- SG underestimates osmolality after saline diuresis (Am J Med Sci 2002;323:39)

Interpretation of SG		
1.008–1.012	Isosthenuria	Similar SG of plasma Possible concentration defect in ATN, CKD
<1.008	Low SG (hyposthenuria)	↓ ADH: DI, 1° polydipsia; intact diluting capacity, impending Na rise w/ water restriction
>1.012	High SG	↑ ADH: dehydration, volume depletion

pH (normal: 5.5–6.5)
- <5.5 in metabolic alkalosis: nonbicarbonate nonreabsorbable anions, eg, ticarcillin, carbenicillin, piperacillin (CJASN 2019;14:306)
- ↓: metabolic acidosis, ↑ protein diet, volume depletion (↑ aldo-induced ↑ H$^+$ excretion)
- ↑: vegetarian diet, urease (urea → CO_2 + NH_3)-forming bacteria, ATN
  >8: urea splitting organism
  >6.5: bicarbonate in urine; high pH suggests N/V in hypokalemia (Am J Med 2017;130:846)
  >5.5 in NAGMA: dRTA, hypokalemia (↑ ammoniagenesis), toluene
Protein (normal: negative)
- Trace, 5–20 mg/dL; 1+, 30 mg/dL; 2+, 100 mg/dL; 3+, 300 mg/dL; 4+, >2,000 mg/dL
- <1+ rules out urine albumin creatinine ratio (UACR) ≥300 mg/g (AJKD 2011;58:19)
- Highly sensitive to albumin, but cannot detect microalbuminuria (<3 mg/dL)

- Less sensitive to globulin or light chains. Suspect BJP when a dipstick test shows trace to 1+ protein yet a turbidity test for urine protein shows 3+ proteinuria
- (+) in renal impairment, suggestive of glomerular injury
- (−) in renal impairment, suggestive of tubulointerstitial injury
- False (+): buffered alkaline urine

Blood (normal: negative)
- Detects pseudoperoxidase activity of hemoglobin and myoglobin
- Punctate staining: 1–4 RBC/HPF hematuria
- Homogeneous staining: free hemoglobin or myoglobin; False (−): ascorbic acid

Leukocyte Esterase (normal: negative)
- 5–15 WBC/HPF will give a positive granulocyte esterase reaction
- Lymphocytes in chyluria will not produce a positive test
- False (+): contamination with vaginal fluid

Nitrite (normal: negative)
- Urine nitrate is converted by nitrate reductase of *Enterobacteriaceae*
- (−) with non-*Enterobacteriaceae* bacteria; False (+): dipsticks exposed to humidity

Glucose (normal: negative)
- Glucose oxidase reaction, allowing semiquantitation for glycosuria
- (+): hyperglycemia >180, proximal tubular dysfunction (Fanconi syndrome), SGLT-2 inhibitor or mutation, familial renal glucosuria (*CJASN* 2010;5:133)
- False (−): ascorbic acid

Ketones (normal: negative)
- Detects acetoacetate and acetone. Does not react with β-hydroxybutyrate (dominant ketoacid in alcoholic ketoacidosis).

Bilirubin (normal: negative)
- Detects conjugated bilirubin; small fraction that is not reabsorbed in the PT
- Unconjugated bilirubin binds to albumin and does not pass glomerulus
- (+): obstructive or hepatocellular jaundice
- False (+): chlorpromazine, phenazopyridine; delta bilirubin (albumin bound bilirubin) in prolonged cholestasis
- False (−): ascorbic acid

Urobilinogen (normal: 0.2–1 mg/dL)
- Conjugated bilirubin is metabolized to urobilinogen by bacteria in the colon
- Not reliable for detection of porphobilinogen in porphyria
- ↑: hepatocellular jaundice, hemolysis; (−): obstructive jaundice

---

URINE SEDIMENT EXAMINATION BY MICROSCOPE

Procedure
- Spin 12 mL of clean catch urine in a centrifuge tube at 3,000 rpm for 5 min
- Completely invert the centrifuge tube. Resuspend the sediment in the urine that drains back down from the side of the tube. Flick the bottom of the tube to mix the sediment. Aspirate the sediment with a clean disposable pipette, place a drop of sediment onto a microscope slide, and cover with a cover slip.
- Examine the sediment (wet mount) with subdued light by partially closing the iris diaphragm and lowering the condenser of the microscope until optimum contrast is achieved. The fine adjustment of the microscope should be continuously adjusted up and down to see the depth of the object as well as other structures that maybe on a different plane.
- Scan the entire cover slip under lower magnification (×100) and then turn to the high-power magnification (×400) to identify specific cells and casts. Pay special attention to the edge of the coverslip where many casts tend to accumulate.
- Quantify and report casts as number/low-power field (LPF)
- Quantify and report cells as number per high-power field (HPF)
- Stains are useful in specific instances:
  - Sedi-Stain: cellular elements; Gram stain: bacteria or fungi
  - Hansel stain (a modified Wright stain): eosinophils and other cellular elements
  - Sudan III stain: oval fat bodies (OFB), fat globules, and fatty casts

Urine Sediment Findings	
Findings	**Comments and Possible Causes or Associated Conditions**
Cells	
RBCs	Dysmorphic: glomerular, eg, glomerulonephritis, vasculitis Isomorphic: extraglomerular, eg, interstitial nephritis, UTI, trauma, stone, or tumor
WBCs	UTI, interstitial nephritis, glomerulonephritis
Epithelial cells	Desquamated cells from renal tubules, urinary bladder, vaginal epithelium, urethra, or foreskin
Oval fat bodies	Sloughed renal tubular cells containing lipid droplets, typically seen in nephrotic syndrome but may be seen in polycystic kidney disease and Fabry disease
Bubble cells	Vacuolated renal tubular cells seen in acute tubular injury or tubular necrosis (*JASN* 1991;1:999)
Casts: cylindrical structures in the tubule lumen; Tamm–Horsfall protein is matrix	
RBC or Hb casts	GN, vasculitis
WBC casts	Interstitial nephritis, pyelonephritis or GN
Fatty casts	Nephrotic syndrome
Tubular cell casts	Renal tubular injury/ATN
Granular casts	Dark muddy brown granular cast is a/w ATN
Waxy casts	Advanced renal disease
Hyaline casts	Benign
Crystals: solid particle with a geometric shape (*NEJM* 2016;3745:2465)	
Calcium oxalate dihydrate or monohydrate	Envelope or needle shaped Ethylene glycol poisoning (*NEJM* 2017;377:1467; *Am J Med* 1988;84:145), hyperoxaluria, hypercalciuria
Calcium phosphate dihydrate (brushite)	Asymmetrical rod-shaped aggregates; in hypercalciuria, renal stone disease
Uric acid	Rhombic plates or rosettes. In many forms in acid urine, seen in healthy individuals; in patients with gout, hyperuricosuria, after recurrent seizure, after propofol anesthesia, renal stone disease, and heat stress-related Mesoamerican nephropathy
Cystine	Hexagonal; Cystinuria: ↓ PT reabsorption ≠ cystinosis
Triple phosphate (struvite)	Coffin lid shaped in infected urine or alkaline urine; infected renal stone disease
Sulfa drug	Sheaves of needles on sulfadiazine in volume depletion
Indinavir	Starburst form in HIV patients (*Ann IM* 1997;127:119)
Acyclovir	Needle-shaped crystals in sediment or inside WBCs; Valacyclovir or acyclovir toxicity
Bacteria	UTI, contamination, or overgrowth after prolonged standing
Yeasts or Fungi	UTI, contaminations; prolonged indwelling Foley catheter

URINE LABORATORY TESTS (*CJASN* 2019;14:306)

Random Spot Urine Collection
- Convenient; affected by diurnal variation; both random and timed always need Cr level

Timed Urine Collection
- 24-hr: gold standard for many tests, but susceptible to over- or undercollection
- Creatinine should be checked together to monitor collection adequacy
- If nonrenal excretion is negligible and not produced or metabolized in body, reflects intake in steady state
- Can be used for concentration; eg, UPEP

Urine Creatinine, Spot (Random)
- Should be checked with other quantitative spot urine assays to correct the effect of urine volume or to consider the amount of glomerular filtration, eg, Fractional excretion (FE) and random protein/creatinine ratio
- Higher than in the serum. Used when suspected urine leak, eg, urinoma d/t post-transplant fluid collection or kidney trauma, urinothorax (pleural effusion from urine)

Urine Creatinine, 24-hr
- Significant variation in 24-hr values suggests over- or undercollection

Estimated 24-hr Urine Creatinine Level (mg/kg) (Nephron 1976;16:31)						
= 28 − (0.2 × age)						
Age	**20**	**30**	**40**	**50**	**60**	**70**
Male	24	22	20	18	16	14
Female (×0.85)	20.4	18.7	17	15.3	13.6	11.9

- Can be used to calculate CrCl (≠ eGFR due to tubular creatinine secretion)

Urine Osmolality (U$_{osm}$, mOsm/kg): ADH Activity

- Number of solute particles per unit volume; mainly Na and K salts and urea
- Correlates with aquaporin-2 activity controlled by ADH
- Ranges 60–1,200 to maintain plasma osmolality within 275–290 and extracellular volume
- Aging is a/w decreased concentration and diluting capacity; range decreased to 100–800

Urine Osmoles, 24-hr

- 600–900 mOsmol/d with normal diet and renal function
- Low urine osmoles: low protein, low sodium diet (beer, tea and toast), malnutrition; CHO and alcohol ↓ endogenous protein catabolism; ↓ water excretion (JASN 2008;19:1076)
- High urine osmoles: osmotic diuresis (hypernatremia), salt wasting (hyponatremia)

Urine Protein and Albumin

- Random: protein or albumin (mg/dL)/Cr (mg/dL) ≈ 24-hr protein or albumin (g) excretion
- 24-hr: gold standard for proteinuria evaluation

Fractional Excretion (FE)

- The percent of filtered solute that is excreted in the urine
- Used to evaluate renal handling of the solute excluding the effect of water reabsorption
- FE of solute X = Quantity of X excreted in the urine/Quantity of X filtered
$$= (U_x \times V)/(S_x \times CrCl) = (U_x/S_x)/(U_{cr}/S_{cr})$$
  U_x: urine concentration of X; S_x: serum concentration of X; V: urine volume
- Depending on solute, filtered fraction should be considered, eg, 0.7 × serum Mg is filtered d/t protein binding

Urine Sodium (U$_{Na}$)

- Sodium avidity (low level): reflects RAAS activation and sodium reabsorption
- 24-hr: approximate measurement of dietary sodium intake; nonrenal excretion is variable >10 mEq/d; 87 mmol = 2 g; 100 mmol = 2.3 g
- U$_{Na}$/U$_K$ <1 in mineralocorticoid excess (hypovolemia, hyperkalemia)

Fractional Excretion of Sodium (FE$_{Na}$)

- In AKI <1%: volume depletion, CHF, liver cirrhosis/HRS, nephrotic syndrome, severe burn Vasoconstriction: iodine CIN, rhabdomyolysis/hemolysis, sepsis (Crit Care 2013;17:R234), acute urinary obstruction, acute GN, acute allograft rejection
- ↑ by diuretics: furosemide can achieve ~8% of FE$_{Na}$ (Int Urol Nephrol 2010;42:273) If <8%, other site inhibition would be necessary, eg, thiazide

Urine Urea Nitrogen (U$_{UN}$)

- FE$_{urea}$: ↓ in volume depletion (d/t ↑ reabsorption) and adrenal insufficiency; not affected by diuretic
- Urea clearance: used to estimate residual kidney function in dialysis patients
- Protein catabolic rate (PCR, protein equivalent of nitrogen appearance) can estimate protein intake if nitrogen balance is even and protein catabolism is not significant (steady BUN with steady renal function)

Daily Nitrogen Balance	
Input	**Output**
Protein intake	Urine urea nitrogen
Endogenous protein catabolism	Nonurea nitrogen excretion (g, nonurea urinary nitrogen + fecal urea excretion) ≈ 0.031 × weight (kg) (KI 1985;27:58)
Protein (nitrogen) intake ≈ urine urea nitrogen + nonurea nitrogen excretion × 6.25 to convert nitrogen (g) to protein (g)	
eg, 60 kg, U$_{UN}$ 7 g/d: weight normalized PCR = [(7 + 0.031 × 60) × 6.25]/60 = 0.92 g/kg/d	

Fractional Excretion of Uric Acid (FE$_{UA}$)

- ↓ in volume depletion d/t ↑ reabsorption; not affected by diuretic use
- >12% in SIADH (JCEM 2008;93:2991), thiazide-induced hyponatremia (JCI 2017;127:3367)

Urine Chloride (U_Cl)

- Low U_{Cl} in metabolic alkalosis: Cl responsive requiring NaCl
  U_{Na} may ↑ due to other anions: bicarbonate, ticarcillin, carbenicillin, piperacillin
- High U_{Cl} in metabolic acidosis due to NH_4^+
- In hypokalemia U_{Na}/U_{Cl} >1.6 suggests N/V, <0.7 suggests laxative (Am J Med 2017;130:846)

Urine Anion Gap (UAG) and Urine Osmolal Gap (UOG)

- Used to estimate NH_4^+ renal excretion in NAGMA: NH_4^+ <40 mmol/d is c/w dRTA

Urine Anion Gap (mEq/L or mmol/L) = U_{Na} + U_K − U_{Cl}	
Negative	**Positive**
Appropriate distal tubule NH_4^+ excretion: • GI HCO_3 loss (diarrhea) • Ingestion of NH_4Cl • pRTA due to ↑ unmeasured cation (NH_4^+) w/o significant change of unmeasured anion → unmeasured cation (NH_4^+, Ca^{2+}, Mg^{2+}) >unmeasured anion (HCO_3^-, SO_4^-, PO_4^-, other organic anions) (NEJM 1988;318:594)	Inappropriate NH_4^+ excretion in NAGMA: dRTA and type 4 RTA Appropriate NH_4^+ excretion with ↑ unmeasured anions in NAGMA: • Bicarbonate (alkali therapy for pRTA) • β-hydroxybutyrate and acetoacetate • Hippurate (toluene) • D-lactate (D-lactic acidosis) • 5-oxoproline (acetaminophen) Typical Western diet (10–90 mEq/L) w/o NAGMA (Am J Med Sci 1986;292:198) Respiratory alkalosis: can be used to differentiate from NAGMA when ABG is unavailable (AJKD 2017;70:440)

Urine Osmolal Gap (mOsmol/kg) = Measured U_{osm} − Calculated U_{osm}	
Calculated U_{osm} = (2 × [U_{Na} + U_K]) + [U_{urea} (mg/dL)]/2.8 + [$U_{glucose}$ (mg/dL)]/18	
>200–400	**<150**
Appropriate NH_4^+ excretion in: GI HCO_3 loss (diarrhea), pRTA Urease–producing bacteria: formation of NH_4^+ in the bladder or container Osmotically active solutes: mannitol, methanol, ethylene glycol	Inappropriate NH_4^+ excretion w/ NAGMA: dRTA and type 4 RTA Healthy individual w/o metabolic acidosis: 10–100

- In advanced CKD, UAG is a poor surrogate for NH_4^+ excretion (CJASN 2018;13:205)

Solute-free Water Clearance (C_{H_2O})

- Urine flow (V) = Osmolal clearance (C_{osm}) + Free water clearance (C_{H_2O})
- C_{osm}: the volume needed to excrete all solutes at the concentration of plasma osmolality
  $$C_{osm} = V × U_{osm}/P_{osm}$$
- C_{H_2O}: a theoretical volume of solute-free water that is added to or reabsorbed from the iso-osmolal urine to create either a dilute (hypo-osmolal) or concentrated (hyperosmolal) urine
  $$C_{H_2O} = V − C_{osm} = V − (V × U_{osm}/P_{osm}) = V × (1 − U_{osm}/P_{osm})$$
- U_{osm}/P_{osm} determines the direction of solute-free water flow: excretion vs reabsorption
- U_{osm}/P_{osm} <1.0, dilute, (+) C_{H_2O}, the addition of a solute-free water to the iso-osmolal urine
- U_{osm}/P_{osm} >1.0, concentrated, (−) C_{H_2O}, reabsorption of solute-free water from the iso-osmolal urine

Electrolyte-free Water Clearance ($C^e_{H_2O}$)

- Since the calculation of C_{H_2O} has included ineffective osmoles such as urea, which plays no role in transmembrane water movement and body fluid tonicity, C_{H_2O} may not be accurate in reflecting renal excretion or reabsorption of electrolyte-free water
- Instead, evaluation and calculation of $C^e_{H_2O}$ will provide a more accurate assessment of renal response to change in water metabolism (Am J Med 1986;81:1033)
- $C^e_{H_2O} = V × [1 − (U_{Na} + U_K)/P_{Na}]$
- In a patient on high protein feeding who develops polyuria and hypernatremia from urea osmotic diuresis, the C_{H_2O} value may remain (−), as a result of high urea content causing U_{osm} > P_{osm}, thus suggesting continued reabsorption of free water. However, the calculation of $C^e_{H_2O}$ will give a (+) value and accurately indicates continued renal loss of electrolyte-free water with resultant development of hypernatremia, requiring free water replacement
- $(U_{Na} + U_K)/P_{Na}$ for bed side evaluation of patients with hyponatremia or hypernatremia
  - $(U_{Na} + U_K)/P_{Na}$ ≥1.0: zero or (−) $C^e_{H_2O}$, no loss of electrolyte-free water
  - $(U_{Na} + U_K)/P_{Na}$ <0.5: (+) $C^e_{H_2O}$, renal excretion of significant amount of electrolyte-free water (Am J Med Sci 2000;319:240)

Urine Laboratory Tests in Appropriate and Inappropriate Renal Handling

Urine Lab	Appropriate	Inappropriate	Causes of Inappropriate Renal Handling
Volume Depletion			
U_{Na}	<20	>40	Tubular injury, salt wasting, diuretics, adrenal insufficiency, metabolic alkalosis: Na coupled w/ HCO_3^- excretion; AGMA: Na coupled w/ organic anions
$U_{Na}/(U_{cr}/S_{cr})$	<1	>1	
FE_{Na} (%)	<1	>2	
U_{Cl} (mEq/L)	<15–25	>40	Tubular injury, salt wasting, diuretics, NAGMA: Cl coupled w/ NH_4^+ excretion
FE_{urea} (%)	<35	>50–65	PT injury, acetazolamide, osmotic diuresis (mannitol, glucose), sepsis, elderly
U_{urea}/BUN	>20	<10	High protein diet and catabolism
FE_{UA} (%)	<12	>20	PT injury
U_{osm}	>500	<350	Tubular injury, loop diuretic
U_{cr}/S_{cr}	>40	<20	Inefficient water reabsorption from tubular injury
U_{osm}/S_{osm}	>1.4–2	<1–1.2	
Specific gravity	>1.020	<1.012	
Hyponatremia			
U_{osm}	<100	>100	SIADH, severe renal failure, thiazides, volume depletion, salt wasting
Hypernatremia			
U_{osm}	>700–800	<700–800	DI, diuresis (osmotic, loop)
Hypokalemia			
U_K (mEq/L)	<15–25	>30–40	Hyperaldosteronism, Vomiting, NGT, Mg deficiency, dRTA, pRTA, DKA
24-hr U_K (mEq/d)	<20–25	>30	
U_K/U_{cr} (mEq/g)	<13–20	>13	
TTKG	<2–3	>4–7	
Hyperkalemia			
U_K (mEq/L)	>20–30	<20	Hypoaldosteronism
24-hr U_K (mEq/d)	>40	<30	↓ Na delivery to CD
U_K/U_{cr} (mEq/g)	>30–200	<30	Type4 RTA
TTKG	>7–11	<3–6	PHA1, PHA2
Hypercalcemia			
24-hr FE_{Ca} (%)	>2	<1	Familial hypocalciuric hypercalcemia, (Thiazide, milk-alkali syndrome)
24-hr Ca (mg/d)	>200	<100	
U_{Ca}/U_{Cr} (g/g)	>0.01	<0.01	
Hypophosphatemia			
FE_{PO4}	<5%	>5%	Hyperparathyroidism, Vit D def, Oncogenic osteomalacia: ↑ FGF23 pRTA, Hereditary hypophosphatemic rickets
24-hr PO_4 (mg/d)	<100	>100	
Hyperphosphatemia			
FE_{PO4}	>15%	<15%	Hypoparathyroidism
Hypomagnesemia			
FE_{Mg} (use 0.7 × serum Mg)	<2%	>2%	Renal wasting
24-hr Mg (mg/d)	<10	>10–30	

IMAGING

RENAL ULTRASOUND (U/S) (CJASN 2014;9:382)

Indications

- Used to evaluate AKI, CKD, and as a guide for percutaneous renal biopsy
- Can detect renal cysts, nephrolithiasis, nephrocalcinosis, hydronephrosis, ADPKD, postkidney transplantation perinephric fluid collection (urinoma, hematoma, lymphocele)
- Can detect nonrenal abnormalities: fluid collection, BPH, bladder retention

Kidney Size

Normal Kidney Length (mm, 10th–90th percentile) (AJR 1993;160:83)						
	All	30s	40s	50s	60s	70s
Left	101–123	104–128	103–123	102–125	100–122	94–120
Right	98–122	101–124	100–123	100–122	95–120	91–118

- Small (bilateral): CKD, renal scarring
- Large (bilateral): hyperfiltration (obesity, diabetic nephropathy), interstitial nephritis (AIN, IgG4-related disease), interstitial infiltration (lymphoma, amyloidosis, sarcoidosis), HIVAN, ADPKD w/ multiple cysts
- Asymmetric (>1 cm discrepancy): hypertrophy from contralateral kidney dysfunction, pyelonephritis, RAS, renal infarction, renal vein thrombosis, congenital abnormality of the kidney and urologic tract

Echogenicity: normally equal to or less than spleen and liver; sinus is echogenic

- Echogenic kidney with combined length <20 cm a/w severe disease (KI 2005;67:1515)
- Increased cortical echogenicity (>spleen, liver without fatty liver changes) Alteration/intrinsic histologic damage: interstitial inflammation and tubular atrophy
- Increased medullary echogenicity with normal cortex: medullary nephrocalcinosis, Tamm–Horsfall protein in tubules, sickle cell disease, medullary sponge kidney
- Decreased cortical echogenicity: acute cortical necrosis, edema

Other Possible Markers of CKD

- Kidney volume (NDT 2009;24:1690); Cortical thickness (AJR 2010;195:W146)

Hydronephrosis

- Dilation of renal pelvis; high sensitivity for urinary tract obstruction
- False (+): diuresis with nephrogenic DI, pregnancy, renal cysts, congenital megacalyces, calyceal diverticula, parapelvic cyst, transplanted graft (when it is mild)
- False (–): volume depletion, early acute obstruction, RP fibrosis, staghorn calculi, infiltrative metastasis; can re ✓ after fluid; consider retrograde pyelography
- If finding is different from clinical suspicion, can ✓ radionuclide scan or CT

Cystic and Solid Mass

- Simple cysts: sharply demarcated with thin smooth walls, anechoic content, and strong posterior wall echo; no further imaging is necessary
- Complex cysts: calcifications, septations, mural nodules, internal echoes; majority are not malignancy; still need contrast CT or MRI to try to exclude malignancy
- Solid mass: need contrast CT or MRI

Duplex Doppler Ultrasound

- Check flow of renal artery and veins: assessment for RAS and RVT
- RAS: main renal artery to aortic peak systolic velocity ratio >3.5
- RVT: reversed diastolic flow, absent venous flow, thrombus in venous lumen, ↑ RI
- Ureteral jets, urine flow into the bladder rules out complete ureteral obstruction

$$\text{Resistive index (RI)} = \frac{(\text{peak systolic velocity} - \text{end diastolic velocity})}{\text{peak systolic velocity}}$$

0.56–0.66: normal

>0.85: nonspecific sign of microvascular compromise, eg, graft rejection, ATN, ureteral obstruction, pyelonephritis

CT SCAN

Indications
- Noncontrast CT: for urinary stone (more sensitive than contrast CT in detecting small stones), hydronephrosis (attenuation: renal parenchyma > urine > sinus fat), localization of obstruction, chronicity of renal disease (cortical thinning)
- Contrast CT: for complex cyst (for Bosniak criteria), mass, cancer staging, renal/perinephric abscess, retroperitoneal fibrosis, RAS, RVT, papillary or cortical necrosis, infarction, adrenal masses
- CT urography (w/o and w/ contrast): for hematuria with high-risk urothelial cancer

CT Findings
- Calcification: stones, nephrocalcinosis; cortex (cortical necrosis, chronic GN), medulla (tubular pathology, medullary sponge kidney, papillary necrosis)
- Perinephric/periureteral stranding: nonspecific sign of urinary obstruction, inflammation
- **Pseudotumor:** various conditions can mimic malignancy *(AJR 2007;188:1380)*
  Developmental: prominent columns of Bertin, Dromedary hump, persistent fetal lobulation
  Infectious: focal pyelonephritis (√DMSA scan), abscess, scarring
  Inflammatory: xanthogranulomatous pyelonephritis, sarcoidosis, malakoplakia, IgG4-RD
  Vascular: AVM, hematoma, extramedullary hematopoiesis

MRI AND MRA

- For complex cyst, mass (esp, small lesion), RAS, pregnancy with any indication of CT scan
- s/e: gadolinium-induced nephrogenic systemic fibrosis (NSF)
- In pts with stage 4–5 CKD, macrocyclic or newer linear (gadobenate dimeglumine and gadoxetate disodium) gadolinium-based contrast agents (GBCA) can be administered when GBCA-enhanced MRI is considered necessary and no alternative test is available *(Can Assoc Radiol J 2018;69:136)*
- MRA without contrast, such as phase contrast MRA is available

---

RADIONUCLIDE RENAL SCAN

Radiotracers Used for Renal Scan		
Radiotracer	Function	Clinical Use
^{99m}Tc-DTPA	Glomerular filtration	GFR measurement Urinary tract obstruction
^{99m}Tc-MAG3	Tubular secretion: by the PCT	Split renal function; Urinary tract obstruction Evaluate effective renal plasma flow Used when renal function is reduced
^{99m}Tc-DMSA	Tubular retention: binds to the -SH groups of PCT	Split renal function Cortical scarring or infarction; VUR Focal pyelonephritis vs cancer

^{99m}Tc-DMSA, technetium 99m-labeled dimercaptosuccinate
^{99m}Tc-DTPA, technetium 99m-labeled diethylenetriaminepentaacetic acid

- Split radionuclide renal scan: predict postnephrectomy dialysis requirement
- Furosemide renal scan: ^{99m}Tc-DTPA; ^{99m}Tc-MAG3 if reduced renal function; delayed renal pelvis clearance in urinary tract obstruction
- Captopril renal scan: ^{99m}Tc-DTPA; use ^{99m}Tc-MAG3 if reduced renal function; can show peak activity delay or ↓ GFR in the kidney with RAS

OTHER IMAGING TESTS

Angiography
- Definitive test for and, for some diseases, treatment of vascular abnormalities: RAS, FMD, large and medium (eg, polyarteritis nodosa) vessel vasculitis
- Risk of CIN (in CKD) and cholesterol atheroemboli

Pyelography
- For suspicious ureteral obstruction in the absence of hydronephrosis on U/S or CT and proper renal contrast excretion is not expected due to AKI
- Retrograde: contrast into distal ureter or bladder orifice performed by urologist along with cystoscopy

- Anterograde: contrast injection into collecting system; performed by interventional radiologist along with therapeutic nephrostomy
- Complications: upper urinary tract infection

Voiding Cystourethrography
- To diagnose and evaluate vesicoureteral reflux
- Radionuclide cystogram can be used for follow-up evaluation for less radiation exposure

Positron Emission Tomography (PET)
- cyst infection in ADPKD (NDT 2008;23:404) and renal graft PTLD (Haematologica 2013;98:771)

Plain Abdominal Radiography
- Can detect radiopaque stone, nephrocalcinosis, and other calcification

Intravenous Pyelogram
- evaluation of upper urinary tract in hematuria, flank pain, and stone disease
- Replaced by noncontrast CT scan

RENAL BIOPSY

Indications of Renal Biopsy (bx)
- RPGN; proteinuria >1 g/d (with proteinuria >0.5); unexplained renal impairment

Impact of Biopsy on Diagnosis and Management				
Diagnosis (BMC Nephrol 2009;10:11)		**Bx Affected Management** (NDT 1994;9:1255)	
Predicted diagnosis confirmed	29%	Nephrotic range proteinuria	86%
One of differential diagnosis	14%	Acute kidney injury	71%
Unexpected diagnosis	15%	Chronic kidney disease	45%
Bx done to assess ase severity	29%	Hematuria and proteinuria	32%
Nondiagnostic	11%	Subnephrotic proteinuria	12%
Technical failure	2%	Hematuria alone	3%
		Overall	42%

Absolute Contraindications to Percutaneous Renal Biopsy
- Uncooperative patient or inability to follow instructions during bx, uncontrolled severe HTN (>180/120), uncorrectable bleeding diathesis

Relative Contraindications to Renal Biopsy
- Inability to provide informed consent, recent antiplatelet or anticoagulant therapy, Hb <8.0, platelet <100, INR >1.5, ↑ aPTT, liver cirrhosis
- Echogenic small kidneys (<10 cm) (KI 2005;67:1515), solitary kidney, multiple bilateral cysts, hydronephrosis, horseshoe kidney, ESRD, UTI, pyelonephritis, or perirenal abscess/infection, pregnancy after 32 wk gestation
- Inability to stop anticoagulation (eg, w/i 3 mo after prosthetic heart valve)

Preparation: Admit High-Risk Patients
- Emergent bx is a/w major complications (3.7 vs 0.5% w/ elective) (NDT 2008;23:356)
- Hold ASA, dipyridamole, clopidogrel, NSAIDs, UFH, LMWH, GP IIb/IIIa inhibitors, omega 3 fatty acids (NDT Plus 2011;4:270) if clinically indicated
- Prebiopsy Labs: CBC, PT, aPTT, type and screen, factor X if AL amyloid is suspected
- If Hb <8.0, blood transfusion or hospitalization; BP <140/90; anxiolytic prn
- If factor X def, FFP, Prothrombin complex concentrate 3-factor (II, IX, X, eg, Bebulin, Profilnine) (AJH 2014;89:1153) or 4-factor (II, VII, IX, X, eg, Beriplex, Octaplex, Kcentra)

Antiplatelets and NSAIDs
- Antiplatelets and NSAIDs (vs d/c 5 d before) ↑ ≥1.0 Hb drop, no difference in the need for blood transfusion, surgical or radiological intervention (NDT 2008;23:3566)
- ASA within 10 d of bx did not increase risk of major bleeding (AJR 2010;194:784)
- NSAIDs (esp, one w/ long half-life) ↑ bleeding; Renal impairment ↓ clearance

Half-Life of NSAIDs (Arch IM 1991;151:1963)			
0–3 hr	fenoprofen, ibuprofen, meclofenamate sodium, tolmetin	4–5 hr	indomethacin, ketoprofen
6–15 hr	diflunisal, naproxen, sulindac	>15 hr	piroxicam
NSAIDs should be stopped ~5 half-lives for complete elimination			

- Hold antiplatelets for 7–10 d before in low CV event risk (ACCP Chest 2012;141:e326S)
- In high-risk pts undergoing noncardiac surgery, perioperative ASA 7 d pre- to 3 d postprocedure ↓ major adverse cardiac events w/o ↑ bleeding (Br J Anaesth 2010;104:305)

Anticoagulation

Conditions with High-Risk Perioperative Thromboembolism (ACCP Chest 2012;141:e326S): stop vitamin K antagonists 5 d before the biopsy; bridge with IV UFH (stop 4–6 hr before) or LMWH (stop 24 hr before)		
Mechanical Heart Valve	**AFib**	**VTE**
Any MV prosthesis	CHADS₂ ≥5	VTE w/i 3 mo
Any caged-ball or tilting disc	Stroke or TIA w/i 3 mo	Def of protein C, protein S,
AV prosthesis	Rheumatic valvular heart	or antithrombin; APLA;
Stroke or TIA w/i 6 mo	disease	multiple abnormalities

Note: $CHADS_2 \geq 5$

Uremic Platelets

- Renal failure can cause bleeding d/t disturbances in platelet adhesion and aggregation
- Unclear if correction of the BT (bleeding time) ↓ clinical bleeding. A low Hct is a/w a ↑ BT: may be corrected by ESA or transfusion (Arch Surg 1998;133:134)
- ESA with Hct ↑ ≥30% improved platelet function in uremic patients (KI 1992;42:668)
- DDAVP 0.3 μg/kg 1 hr prior to bx ↓ hematoma (13.8% vs 30.5%) (AJKD 2011;57:850)
- BT can be shortened by HD ×2 (Clin Appl Thromb Hemost 2012;18:185), estrogen (NEJM 1986;315:731), cryoprecipitate 10 bags over 30 min, 1–12 hr (NEJM 1980;303:1318)

Ultrasound-guided Percutaneous Renal Biopsy

- No difference in complications between U/S-marked blind vs real-time U/S guided procedure and performed by nephrologists vs radiologists (BMC Nephrol 2014;15:96)
- Real-time U/S guided bx may have better tissue yield (CKJ 2015;8:151; BMC Nephrol 2014;15:96)
- Spring loaded devices w/ 14G, 16G, or 18G needles. The larger needle provide more tissue and glomeruli (KI 2000;58:390), Complication ↑ w/ 14G needle (AJKD 2012;60:62), >5 passes

CT-guided Percutaneous Renal Biopsy

- When kidney position does not support U/S-guided bx
- It does not allow direct real-time visualization (AJKD 2000;36:419).

Transjugular Biopsy

- Performed when bleeding disorders prevent conventional biopsy, for patients on mechanical ventilation, and if there is a need for both the liver and kidney
- The access is via the right internal jugular and an introducer sheather. The right renal vein is more amenable to bx because of orientation and the shorter length to access.
- Contrast (required)-induced nephropathy can happen (J Vasc Interv Radiol 2008;19:546)
- Similar yield (95.8 vs 95.5%) and major complications (1 vs 0.75%) c/w percutaneous bx (Radiology 2000;215:689); other series also showed its safety (Lancet 1990;335:1512)

Laparoscopic or Open Biopsy

- When percutaneous bx fails, for pts on chronic anticoagulation which cannot be stopped or w/ coagulopathy, religious faith (eg, Jehovah's witness), solitary kidney, multiple bilateral renal cysts, or body habitus (eg, morbid obesity, cerebral palsy) (KI 1998;54:525)

Postbiopsy Complications

Automated Biopsy Device and Real-time U/S Guidance (AJKD 2012;60:62)			
Postbiopsy Complications		**Factors on Erythrocyte Transfusion Rate**	
Macroscopic hematuria	3.5%	Age ≥40 vs <40	1.0 vs 0.2%
Need for PRBC transfusion	0.9%	Cr ≥2 vs <2	2.1 vs 0.4%
Angiographic intervention	0.6%	SBP ≥130 vs <130	1.4 vs 0.1%
Nephrectomy	0.01%	Hb <12 vs ≥12	2.6 vs 0.5%
Bladder obstruction	0.3%		
Death	0.02%		

- AVF (4–18%): rarely cause hypotension, high-output HF, and hematuria. Diagnosed w/ Doppler U/S or angio. Most spontaneously regress, but some require embolization or surgical ligation depending on size/symptoms (JASN 1994;5:1300)

- Hematoma (~4%) (*JASN* 2004;15:142), pseudoaneurysm
- Page kidney: subcapsular hematoma can cause RAS activation, HTN
- Pain: d/t subcapsular hematoma, ureteral obstruction of blood clot
- Vasovagal pseudohemorrhage: ↓ BP & HR during procedure (*JAMA* 1977;237:1259)
- AKI ↑ complications: transfusion 8%, intervention 2%, hematoma 7% (*CJASN* 2018;13:1633)

Monitoring and Postbiopsy Care
- 67% of complications occur w/i 8 hr, 11% can be seen >24 hr after biopsy (*JASN* 2004;15:142)
- Can ✓ U/S 1 hr after percutaneous bx: the absence of hematoma has a high NPV for minor (95%) or major (98%) complications (*NDT* 2009;24:2433)
- Bed rest for 4 hr; avoid heavy object lifting, jog, exercise for 1 wk
- Vital signs: BP q15min × 1 hr, q30min × 2 hr, q60min × 2 hr
- ✓ for gross hematuria; ✓CBC 4 hr postprocedure; for inpatients, CBC in following AM
- Resume antiplatelet and/or anticoagulation in 2–7 d. The exact timing for resumption of therapy should be tailored to each patient

Management of Bleeding Complications
- Bed rest, PRBC, FFP transfusion as needed
- Most patients with perinephric hematoma or hematuria will resolve spontaneously
- If unremitting gross hematuria especially with clots, a 3-way bladder irrigation catheter should be inserted and irrigation commenced
- If hemodynamic compromise, transfusion requirements or persistent gross hematuria >72 hr, CT angiogram may show the bleeding vessel or AVF, followed by selective angioembolization of the bleeding artery
- Transarterial embolization is safe; Rare complications: dissection
- Postembolization syndrome: flank pain, fever, N/V, ileus, rare w/ partial embolization

RENAL PATHOLOGY

PROCESSING OF TISSUE

Light Microscopy (LM)
- Formalin-fixed, paraffin-embedded tissue; sections cut at 2–3 μm
- Stain with hematoxylin & eosin (H&E), Periodic acid–Schiff (PAS), Jones methenamine silver (JMS), and Trichrome

Typical Color after Staining			
	PAS	**JMS**	**Trichrome**
Matrix material*	Magenta	Black	Blue
Immune material	Glassy pink	Red	Fuchsinophilic
Fibrin	Pale	Red	Bright red

*Basement membrane (BM) and mesangial matrix

- Special stain: congo red (amyloid), von Kossa (calcium phosphate deposit)

Immunofluorescence (IF)
- Zeus or Michel's transport medium; frozen and cut on cryostat
- Stain with antisera to IgG, IgM, IgA, C3, C1, albumin, fibrinogen, kappa, lambda, and C4d (transplant only)
- Special techniques: pronase IF from paraffin block (salvage, masked deposits, LCPT), IgG subtypes (IgG1–IgG4; 1 subtype favors monoclonal), COL4A (α2 and α5 chains)

Electron Microscopy (EM)
- 2.5% glutaraldehyde; 1 μm toluidine blue-stained survey section, Pb/Ur-stained section

COMMON PATTERNS OF GLOMERULAR INJURY

Definitions for Commonly Used Terms for Glomerular Injury	
Focal	Involving minority (<50%) of glomeruli
Diffuse	Involving majority (>50%) of glomeruli
Segmental	Part of glomerulus (<50%) involved
Global	Whole of glomerulus (>50%) involved

Mesangial Proliferative Glomerulonephritis
- LM: diffuse increase mesangial cells (≥3 per mesangial area)
- IF and EM: granular mesangial immune deposits
- Ddx: IgAN, LN class II, resolving IRGN, C3G

Endocapillary Proliferative Glomerulonephritis
- LM: occlusion of capillary lumina by infiltrating leukocytes and/or swollen endothelial cells
- IF and EM: subendothelial ± mesangial immune deposits
- Ddx:
  - IRGN: endocapillary neutrophils, C3-dominant IF w/ "starry-sky" pattern, subepi humps
  - Autoimmune (eg, LN): full-house IF, strong C1q staining, extraglomerular immune deposits, endothelial TRIs
  - Cryoglobulinemic: monocytes, immune thrombi
  - Others: PGNMID (monoclonal IF), IgAN, C3G

Membranoproliferative Glomerulonephritis (MPGN)
- LM: hyperlobulated glomeruli owing to increased mesangial cells and matrix, GBM double contours with cellular interposition, variable endocapillary hypercellularity

Current MPGN Classification Based on IF		
Type	IF	Etiologies
Immune complex-type: **classical** pathway mediated	Ig ≥ C3	Autoimmune: LN, Sjögren syndrome Infectious: HCV, endovascular bacterial Cryoglobulinemic: HCV, Sjögren's, LPD Dysproteinemic or idiopathic
C3 glomerulopathy: **alternative** pathway mediated	C3 ≥ 2× Ig	C3G (C3GN, DDD)
"Mimickers"	Negative (±nonspecific IgM and C3)	TMA, type III collagen glomerulopathy

Historical MPGN Classification Based on EM	
Type	EM Features
1	Mesangial and subendo
2	Mesangial ring forms and highly electron dense intramembranous
3	Mesangial and complex subendo, intramembranous, and subepi

Crescentic (Extracapillary Proliferative) Glomerulonephritis
- Focal vs diffuse; acute (cellular) vs subacute (fibrocellular) vs chronic (fibrous) crescents
- Fibrinoid necrosis (karyorrhexis, fibrin extravasation, GBM rupture) and concurrent necrotizing arteritis: usually with +ANCA
- **3 types based on IF** (overlaps can occur):
  - Pauci-immune (little or no IF staining: 85–90% +MPO- or PR3-ANCA)
  - Anti-GBM nephritis (linear IgG)
  - Immune complex-type: IRGN, LN, IgAN

Focal Segmental Glomerulosclerosis (FSGS)

Columbia Classification of FSGS			
Variant	Defining Features	Clinical Features	Associations
Collapsing	Implosive retraction of capillaries with overlying VEC hyperplasia, severe tubular injury, tubular microcysts, diffuse FPE	Primary or secondary; severe nephrotic syndrome and AKI; black racial predominance; worst prognosis	Viral infections (esp HIV), Drugs (pamidronate, INF), APOL1, acute vasoocclusion

Tip	Adhesion of tuft at tubular pole w/ foam cells, diffuse FPE	Usually primary, abrupt onset nephrotic syndrome	Usually steroid responsive, favorable prognosis
Cellular	Expansile lesion with endocapillary hypercellularity (foam cells, leukocytes)	Usually primary	
Perihilar	Hyalinosis and sclerosis centered at vascular pole, glomerulomegaly, focal FPE	Usually secondary; adaptation to glomerular hyperfiltration	Obesity, HTN, low nephron number, sickle cell
NOS	Does not meet features of above variants	m/c variant, primary or secondary	

Nodular Mesangial Sclerosing Glomerulopathy

- Most commonly diabetic glomerulosclerosis (DGS): acellular PAS+ nodules ± micro-aneurysms, capsular drop lesions (BC hyalinosis), PAS+ GBM and TBM thickening, IF/TA, arteriolar hyalinosis, arteriolosclerosis
- Idiopathic nodular glomerulosclerosis (ING, aka smoking-related glomerulopathy): seen in nondiabetic cigarette smokers → endothelial lined channels in expanded mesangium and at hilus, chronic TMA features common (mesangiolysis w/ microaneurysms, narrow GBM duplications)

Differential Diagnosis for Nodular Mesangial Expansion				
	DGS & ING	**MIDD**	**Amyloidosis**	**FGN**
PAS/JMS	+/+	+/–	–/–	–/–
Congo red	–	–	+ (Amylodiosis)	–
IF	Linear IgG and alb (GBM, TBM)	Linear κ, λ, or Ig (GBM, TBM, ves)	Smudgy Ig, κ, or λ; negative (AA, other)	Smudgy IgG, C3, κ, λ
EM	GBM thickening and ↑ mes matrix	Finely granular punctate deposits (GBM, TBM, vessels)	Randomly oriented fibrils (8–10 nm)	Randomly oriented fibrils (16–24 nm)

Membranous Nephropathy (MN)

- LM: normal GBM (stage 1) → thickened GBM with spikes (stage 2) → chain-like GBM thickening with intramembranous lucencies (stages 3–4)
- IF: granular glomerular capillary wall (subepi) staining for IgG, C3, κ, λ
- EM: small subepi immune deposits (stage 1) → intervening GBM spikes (stage 2) → incorporated into GBM by neomembrane (stage 3) → undergo resorption and become more electron lucent (stage 4)
- 1° (~80%; anti-PLA2R, 3–5% anti-THSD7A) vs 2° (autoimmune, infection [HBV, parasites, syphilis], malignancy, drugs)
- Indirect IF staining for **PLA2R**: positive in ~80% of patients with 1° MN

Thrombotic Microangiopathy (TMA)

- Early changes
  - Glomeruli: fibrin thrombi, entrapped schistocytes, endotheliosis, mesangiolysis, subendothelial "fluff," ischemic tuft retraction
  - Vessels: endothelial swelling, intraluminal and subendothelial fibrin, entrapped schistocytes, mucoid intimal edema, myointimal cellular proliferation
- Late changes
  - Glomeruli: GBM duplication, mesangial sclerosis, glomerulosclerosis
  - Vessels: concentric ("onion-skin") intimal fibrosis, organization and recanalization of intraluminal thrombi
- Etiologic considerations: dHUS, aHUS, scleroderma, APLS, malignant HTN, pre-eclampsia, drug-induced (anti-VEGF, gemcitabine, proteasome inhibitors), HIV → vascular changes of TMA predominate in malignant HTN and scleroderma

Glomerular Diseases with Organized Deposits		
Disease	Pathology	Correlation
Cryoglobulinemic GN	LM: MPGN or DPGN, abundant infiltrating monocytes, intracapillary immune thrombi IF: monoclonal Ig (type I), IgM + κ > IgG + λ (type II), polyclonal IgG + IgM (type III) EM: annular-tubular substructure (30–50 nm), may be focal Immune deposits may be spare by IF and EM b/c of aggressive phagocytosis by monocytes (pronase IF useful)	Type I: LPD Type II: HCV, Sjögren's, LPD (esp. WM), endovascular bacterial infections Type III: autoimmune conditions
Immunotactoid GN	LM: MPGN or DPGN IF: usually monoclonal IgG EM: parallel stacks of microtubules (30–50 nm)	+M-spike, B-cell lymphoproliferative disorders, ↓ C'
Fibrillary GN	LM: MPGN > MesGN > DPGN > MGN; PAS-pale silver (–) deposits; Congo red (–) IF: polyclonal IgG ("smudgy") ± C3 & C1; IgG1 & IgG4 subtypes EM: randomly oriented nonbranching fibrils that infiltrate mes and GBM (16–24 nm) IHC: DNAJB9	Idiopathic; association with HCV

Dysproteinemia-Related Renal Diseases

- Can involve all 3 renal parenchymal compartments
- Useful special techniques: congo red stain, proteomics (Alg); IgG subtypes (PGNMID); pronase IF (LCPT, masked monoclonal deposits)

Dysproteinemia-related Renal Diseases		
Disease	Pathology	Associations
LCCN	LM: hard/fractured casts, PAS-pale/negative, cellular reaction IF: κ/λ restricted staining	MM
LCPT	LM: intracellular crystals in PTC (PAS-pale, Trichrome-red) IF: >90% κ, often requires pronase IF EM: geometrically shaped or ropey crystals in PTC	Fanconi syndrome; MM, smoldering MM, MGRS
MIDD	LM: nodular mesangial sclerosis IF: linear staining involving all renal BMs; 90% κ (LCDD); can have monoclonal Ig component (HCDD, HLCDD) EM: finely granular punctate deposits in BMs	MM, smoldering MM or MGRS; ~1/3 occur w/ LCCN
AL amyloidosis	LM: amorphous eosinophilic, PAS-pale, silver negative, Congo red+ material IF: "smudgy" staining; λ > κ EM: randomly oriented nonbranching fibrils (8–10 nm)	MM, smoldering MM or MGRS
PGNMID	LM: MPGN, endocapillary proliferative GN IF: 1 IgG subclass + 1 light chain; IgG3κ m/c EM: granular electron dense deposits	Paraprotein identified in 20–30%; Ddx: type 1 cryo, ITGN

Endothelial Tubuloreticular Inclusion (TRI): "IFN footprint"

- Causes: SLE, HIV, CMV (CKJ 2014;7:174), exogenous IFN-α, β, and γ (CJASN 2010;5:607), AMR

COMMON PATTERNS OF TUBULOINTERSTITIAL INJURY

Acute Tubular Necrosis (ATN)

- Epithelial simplification, loss of PAS+ brush border, coarse clear intracytoplasmic vacuolization and enlarged nuclei with prominent nucleoli ± degenerating cellular casts
- Ddx = ischemic vs toxic tubular insults
- Histology generally non-specific except in rare instances (ie, dysmorphic mitochondria = tenofovir toxicity)

Interstitial Nephritis (Pathologic Clues)

- Interstitial inflammation and edema + tubulitis ± tubulointerstitial scarring
- ~70% allergic/drug-induced (interstitial eosinophils)
- ~20% autoimmune/systemic/infectious: Sjögren syndrome (plasma cell-rich), sarcoidosis (noncaseating granulomas; perivascular), IgG4-related (IgG4+ plasma cells, storiform fibrosis, TBM immune deposits by IF & EM), pyelonephritis (neutrophilic tubulitis, neutrophil casts)
- ~10% idiopathic

RENAL TRANSPLANT PATHOLOGY (Banff Criteria AJT 2018;18:293)

Acute T-cell Mediated Rejection	
Grade	Histologic Criteria
Borderline	Foci of tubulitis (t > 0) + minor interstitial inflammation (i0–1), or moderate–severe interstitial inflammation (i2–3) + mild tubulitis (t1)
IA	Interstitial inflammation involving >25% of nonscarred cortex (≥i2) + moderate tubulitis (t2)
IB	Interstitial inflammation involving >25% of nonscarred cortex (≥i2) + severe tubulitis (t3)
IIA	Mild to moderate intimal arteritis (v1) ± any i/t
IIB	Severe intimal arteritis (v2) ± any i/t
III	Transmural arteritis and/or fibrinoid necrosis (v3) ± any i/t

Chronic Active T-cell Mediated Rejection	
Grade	Histologic Criteria
IA	Interstitial inflammation involving >25% of total cortex, mainly in scarred areas (ti2–3, i-IFTA2–3) + moderate tubulitis (t2)
IB	Interstitial inflammation involving >25% of total cortex, mainly in scarred areas (ti2–3, i-IFTA2–3) + severe tubulitis (t3)
II	Chronic allograft arteriopathy (cv0–3)

Active Antibody Mediated Rejection*

1. Histologic evidence of acute tissue injury (≥1)
  • Microvascular inflammation: glomerulitis (g > 0) and/or peritubular capillaritis (ptc > 0)
  • Arteritis (v > 0)
  • Acute thrombotic microangiopathy without other apparent cause
  • Acute tubular injury without other apparent cause
2. Evidence of antibody interaction with endothelium (≥1)
  • Linear C4d staining in peritubular capillaries (C4d ≥ 2 by IF, C4d ≥ 0 by IHC)
  • At least moderate microvascular inflammation (g + ptc ≥2; g must be ≥1 if TCMR)
3. Serologic evidence of donor-specific antibodies

*All 3 criteria must be met for diagnosis.

Chronic Active Antibody Mediated Rejection*

1. Histologic evidence of chronic tissue injury (≥1)
  • Transplant glomerulopathy (cg > 0)
  • Severe peritubular capillary BM multilayering (EM)
  • Arterial intimal fibrosis w/o other apparent cause
2. Evidence of antibody interaction with endothelium (≥1)
  • Linear C4d staining in peritubular capillaries (C4d ≥ 2 by IF, C4d ≥ 0 by IHC)
  • At least moderate microvascular inflammation (g + ptc ≥2; g must be ≥1 if TCMR)
3. Serologic evidence of donor-specific antibodies

*All 3 criteria must be met for diagnosis.

GENETICS

Background (Nat Rev Nephrol 2018;14;83; NEJM 2019;380:142)
- Genetic testing has a high diagnostic yield: almost 10% for all cause CKD, >17% for patients with nephropathy of unknown origin, and >70% for pediatric cases
- Genetic diagnosis can:
  - Confirm a suspected hereditary cause
  - Discern specific subcategory of condition within broader clinical diagnosis
  - Reclassify the diagnosis and
  - Identify a molecular cause for patients with nephropathy of unknown origin
- Genetic diagnosis can affect patient management, prognosis, and have familial implications

Features of Genetic Diseases
- Early-onset: eg, congenital kidney anomaly or malformation
- Extrarenal manifestations: eg, sensory deficits, developmental problems, birth defects, facial dysmorphism; Positive family history
- Absence of clear environmental causes for kidney disease (ie, DM, CVD)
- Cautionary Note: many patients with a genetic condition do not have affected family members and do have other medical problems that can be thought to cause CKD, like diabetes, heart conditions, or hypertension

Terms Used in Genetics and Genetic Testing
- **Genetic Counseling:** a clinical consultation for individuals and their families who have genetic disease or are at risk for a disease, facilitating informed decision-making. Under current guidelines, the ordering clinician is expected to ensure informed consent.
- **Informed Consent:** required for all Genetic testing. Discussion of benefits, limitations (ie, sensitivity and specificity of the test), and risks, so the patient can decide if, when, and how he/she wants to go genetic testing
- Allele: one copy of a gene; each of us has two alleles for all genes on autosomes (and X chromosome in females), which can be identical or different
- Variant: a different allele than the reference allele, aka the allele found in the majority of the population
- Zygosity: how many variant alleles a patient has
  - Heterozygote: the patient has one variant allele and one reference allele
  - Hemizygote: variant allele of a gene on the X chromosome in male; since males have only one X, they have a single copy of the allele
  - Biallelic: 2 variant alleles for the gene
    - Homozygote = same variant;
    - Compound Heterozygote = two different variants

TYPES OF GENETIC TESTING

- Any test that can identify changes in chromosomes, genes (DNA sequencing), or proteins (biochemical tests)
- Biochemical tests are helpful for diagnosing metabolic renal diseases

Genetic Testing Modalities (Nat Rev Nephrol 2018;14;83)

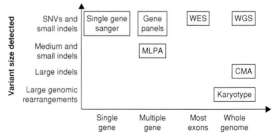

**Proportion of DNA tested in one single test
~ Odds for incidental findings**

- SNVs: single-nucleotide variants
- Indels: insertions or deletions
- Genomic rearrangements: duplications, deletions, translocations, and inversions
- Karyotype: picture of the chromosomes; count them and identify large genomic rearrangements
- Chromosomal microarray (CMA): identify genomic rearrangements such as duplications and deletions of at least 200 kb
- Multiplex ligation-dependent probe amplification (MLPA): identify relatively small deletion and duplications
- Sanger sequencing: identify variants (single-nucleotide variants [SNVs] and very small insertions or deletions) in small, targeted fragments of DNA
- Gene panels using targeted next-generation sequencing (NGS): identify variants in a predefined list of genes
- Whole-exome sequencing (WES): identify variants in the exons (protein-coding) of most genes; does not cover certain parts of the genome (eg, noncoding regions)
- Whole-genome sequencing (WGS): includes noncoding variants and better detects genomic rearrangements versus WES

BENEFITS AND RISKS OF GENETIC TESTING

Diagnosis of Renal Genetic Disease

Potential Benefits and Risks of Diagnosis	
Potential Benefits	**Potential Risks**
Diagnosis: ↓ need for further testing	↑ Medical workup: additional tests can be required to validate the genetic diagnosis
Change care: eg, initiate needed subspecialty referral, targeted workup, and/or surveillance; guide choice of therapy	Negative psychological impact: genetic findings can be uncertain, which can lead to ↑ anxiety (Nat Rev Neurosci 2013;14:488)
Identification of extrarenal anomalies	Incidental finding: relevant for nontargeted genetic testing
Family counseling: for relatives identified to be at risk of having or transmitting the disorder	
Participation in targeted clinical trials	
Incidental finding: relevant for nontargeted genetic testing	

Diagnosis of Incidental Findings

- Incidental finding: any genetic finding unrelated to the primary test indication (synonym: secondary finding). Some genes associated with diseases for which interventions preventing or lessening the disease complications exist, such that they are medically "actionable" and have been recommended for broad return (Genet Med 2017;19:249)
- Only in the case of nontargeted genetic testing

Potential Benefits and Risks of Incidental Findings	
Potential Benefits	**Potential Risks**
Change care: eg, initiate needed sub-specialty referral, targeted workup, and/or surveillance; guide choice of therapy	↑ Medical workup: the term "genetic predisposition" by definition indicates that there might be no disease YET, but it might develop in the future
Family counseling: for relatives identified to be at risk of having or transmitting the disorder	Incidental findings can require life-long medical surveillance
Participation in targeted clinical trials	Discrimination: the Genetic Information Non-Discrimination Act (GINA) protects against discrimination from employers and health insurers, but gives exemptions to certain employers, and does not include other types of insurance, including life and disability coverage
	Predictive genetic information could be used to discriminate individuals in contexts such as housing (J Law Med Ethics 2016;44:216) and child custody disputes (Curr Genet Med Rep 2016;4:98)
	Self-fulfilling prophecy: genetic diagnosis can worsen the clinical symptoms; as in ApoE and Alzheimer (Am J Psychiatry 2014;171:201) and obesity (Health Educ Behav 2016;43:337)
	Negative psychological impact: in the presence of an incidental genetic finding, the patient becomes a "patient in waiting" (J Health Soc Behav 2010;51:408)

GENETICS RESULTS INTERPRETATION (Genet Med 2015:17:405)

Criteria for Pathogenic Variants
- De novo variant: variant that is absent in the parents of the index. ↑ odds for pathogenicity
- Reported pathogenic variant: variant previously reported in patients as causing a disease
  - ↑ Odds for pathogenicity
  - The main two databases cataloguing those variants are ClinVar and HGMD
  - Caution: both have a lot of false positive variants.
- Minor allele frequency (MAF): frequency at which the allele occurs in a given population. Current population database: gnomad.broadinstitute.org includes 123,136 exome sequences and 15,496 whole-genome sequences used to calculate each allele's MAF. The rarer the variant the ↑ odds for pathogenicity.
  - Novel variant: variant not previously reported: ↑↑ odds for pathogenicity
- Deleteriousness prediction: there are many in-silico scores trying to predict the impact of a variant on the protein function (loss-of-function, gain-of-function, dominant negative effect)

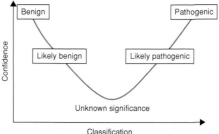

Variant Classification
- Variant classification is based on current knowledge
- Thus, all classifications can change with as new knowledge emerges
- The patient and his/her family medical histories weigh in the decision whether the variant should be considered pathogenic or not

Probabilistic Definitions
- Pathogenic (P): the variant is thought to cause a genetic disease. AKA disease-causing variants (formerly called "mutations")
- Likely Pathogenic (LP): the variant probably causes a genetic disease, but current knowledge is not sufficient to categorize it as a pathogenic variant
- Variant of unknown significance (VUS): current knowledge is NOT sufficient to categorize the variant as either benign or pathogenic
- Likely Benign (LB): the variant probably does not cause a genetic disease, but current knowledge is NOT sufficient to categorize it as a benign variant
- Benign (B): the variant is thought to not cause a genetic disease

CLINICAL GENETIC TESTING AND OTHER TYPES OF GENETIC TESTING

Genetic Research (Nat Rev Nephrol 2018:14:83)
- Aim: generate generalizable knowledge useful for future patients
- Time-line: while results from clinical testing can be returned relatively fast (test and lab dependent), research is usually unpredictable
- Results type: most research-setting are not returning VUS, and P and LP variants usually need to be validated in a clinically certified laboratory by the Clinical Laboratory Improvement Amendments (CLIA)

Direct-to-Consumer (DTC) Genetic Testing
- Aim: different DTC companies have different aims, including ancestry, as well as clinically actionable diagnosis. They usually do not offer comprehensive genetic diagnosis.
- Scope: similarly, different DTC companies are using different genetic testing modalities

USEFUL WEBSITES

- Diagnosis and management of genetic disorders:
  - GeneReviews: www.ncbi.nlm.nih.gov/books/NBK1116/
  - Orphanet: http://www.orpha.net/
  - OMIM: www.omim.org
- Identification of labs for targeted genetic tests:
  - GTR (www.ncbi.nlm.nih.gov/gtr/) and www.concertgenetics.com
- Clinical Trials: https://clinicaltrials.gov

RENAL GENETIC DISEASES

Inheritance Modes and Associated Family Patterns				
Inheritance	Variant Zygosity	Examples	Family Pattern	Family Counseling
Dominant (AD and XLD) disorders	Heterozygote or Hemizygote variant	ADPKD, BOR, MODY5, Renal coloboma syndrome	One of the parent has the disorder or the patient is the first to have the disorder in the family (de novo)	50% risk for each of the patient's kid to have the disorder
Autosomal recessive (AR) disorders	Biallelic variants	Bardet–Biedl Syndrome (BBS), Joubert syndrome, Bartter syndrome	Parents are not affected carriers Siblings may be affected (25% risk for each)	Unaffected siblings have a 66% risk to be carriers Risk for the next generation depends on the spouse's carrier status (higher risk in case of consanguinity)
X-linked recessive disorders (XLR)	Hemizygote variants	X-linked Alport syndrome, Fabry disease, Dent disease	Females are not affected. Male siblings may be affected (50% risk for each). Additional male family members may be affected on the mother's side of the family	Sisters have a 50% chance of being carriers
Mitochondrial disorders (Mito) (nuclear genes encoding mitochondrial proteins will be in the above inheritance modes)	Variants in the mitochondrial genome or depletion of the mitochondrial genome	MELAS, MERRF, Pearson syndrome, Kearns–Sayre syndrome, Leigh syndrome	Variable expressivity, depending on the proportion of affected mitochondria. Siblings may be affected, as well as additional family members on the mother's side of the family	Maternal inheritance: if proband is a female, at risk of transmitting the disorder. Sisters of affected individual at risk of transmitting the disorder.

Extrarenal Anomalies Associated with Genetic Renal Diseases (Lancet 2010;375:1287)			
Disease Group	Extrarenal Anomalies	Causal Genes	Inher.
Polycystic kidney disease (PKD)	Liver cysts, brain aneurysms	*PKD 1, PKD2; PKHD 1*	AD; AR
Tubulointerstitial kidney disease (ADTKD)	MODY5 diabetes (*HNF 1B*), anemia (*REN*), Gout	*UMOD, REN, MUC 1, HNF 1B*	AD
Ciliopathies (nephronophthisis, BBS)	Retinitis pigmentosa, polydactyly, MR, hypogenitalism, obesity	*NPHP 1-NPHP9, BBS 1-BBS 12*	AR
Congenital anomalies (CAKUT)	MODY5 diabetes (*HNF 1B*), deafness (*EYA 1*), eye anomalies (*PAX2*)	*PAX2, HNF 1B, EYA 1, SALL 1; FRAS 1, FREM2*	AD; AR
Nephrotic syndrome	Bone abnormalities, immunodeficiency, neurologic impairment, cardiomyopathy (*COQ2*)	*WT 1, TRPC6; NPHS 1-2, COQ2; MTTL 1*	AD; AR; Mito.
Alport syndrome	Hearing loss, anterior lenticonus	*COL4A3-6*	AD; AR; XLR
Tubulopathies	Short stature, eye anomalies, skeletal anomalies	*CLCN5, OCRL; SLC 12A 1, SLC 12A3*	XLR; AR
Nephrolithiasis, nephrocalcinosis	Retinopathy, peripheral neuropathy, vascular anomalies	*SLC9A3R 1; SLC3A 1, AGXT*	AD; AR

NUTRITION

- Nutrition consultation for CKD 3–5; rigorous RCT data lacking
- Cohort studies associate poor diet with incident or worsening CKD (AJKD 2013;62:267)
- Western diet more acidifying than a fruit/vegetable diet; acidosis may contribute to CKD progression, which may improve with high fruit/vegetable diet (CJASN 2013;8:371)
- Higher dietary acid load a/w ↑ prevalence of CKD (J Ren Nutr 2018;4:251)
- Western diet, high animal protein diet, and fructose consumption ↑ uric acid levels, linked to incident CKD (JASN 2008;19:1204); DASH diet a/w ↓ incident CKD (AJKD 2016;68:853)

Sodium (Na)
- High Na diets antagonize antiproteinuric effect of ACEI/ARB
- ↓ Na intake from 150→100 mEq/d ↓ BP by 2.1/1.3 in pre-HTN/stage 1 HTN; ↓ to 50 mEq/d further ↓ BP by 4.6/1.7 (DASH NEJM 2001;344:3)
- No RCT has been done in CKD looking at hard endpoints
- Low Na diets lower proteinuria and BP when added to ARB and thiazide (JASN 2008;19:999)
- Low Na diets had larger proteinuria and SBP ↓ than dual RASi (BMJ 2011;343:d4366)

Protein
- Low protein diets (0.8 g/kg/d) in CKD ND may ↓ hyperfiltration and eGFR decline
- Animal protein may lead to more hyperfiltration than vegetable protein, also contains more phosphorus than equivalent amount of vegetable protein
- Largest protein restriction RCT underpowered, inconclusive (MDRD NEJM 1994;330:877)
- Higher protein diets (1.2 g/kg/d) needed in dialysis to prevent protein-energy wasting
- Limited data suggest protein restriction safe in nephrotics (JCI 1997;99:2479)

Potassium (K)
- High K diets may ↓ BP (3.5/2.0) and stroke (24%) (BMJ 2013;346:f1378)
- High K decreases activity of NaCl cotransporter (NCC) in DCT (JASN 2016;27:981)
- Low K diet associated with salt-sensitive HTN and worsened eGFR (CJASN 2015;10:2152)

Recommended Intake in CKD/ESRD (KDIGO CKD 2012; KDOQI AJKD 2000;35:s1)	
Na	<2 g/d for CKD; insufficient evidence for <1.5 g/d (Inst Of Med Report 2013)
K	Tailor based on eGFR, K levels, and concomitant medications (eg, ACEI/ARB); usually no need for restriction for CKD 1–3 <2 g/d for HD; 3–4 g/d for PD (more efficient K removal)
Protein	Nondialysis CKD 3–5: <0.8 g/kg/d; HD/PD: 1.2 g/kg/d (NDT 2005;20:ix3)
Ca	<1,500 mg/d of elemental calcium (combined diet and medications)
PO₄	800–1,000 mg/d; ↑ bioavailability with animal and processed food sources vs vegetables; boiling foods ↓ phosphorus w/o lowering protein content
Fluids	Nondialysis: no restriction unless hyponatremic; HD/PD: 1–1.5 L/d
Fiber	No CKD guidelines; 20–35 g/d for general (US Dietary Guidelines 2015–2020)
Calories	30–35 kcal/kg; 20–30 kcal/kg in AKI (Journal of Renal Nutrition 2005;15:63)
Fats	<30% total calories from fats, <10% from saturated fats

Protein-Energy Wasting (KI 2008;73:391)
- Syndrome of muscle wasting, malnutrition, and inflammation in advanced CKD
- Associated with increased mortality and hospitalizations
- No validated criteria but some characteristics include
  BMI <23; unintentional wt loss (5% in 3 mo); body fat <10%
  Albumin <3.8; prealbumin <30 mg/dL; tot chol <100; muscle: reduced 5% in 3 mo
  Protein intake <0.8 g/kg/d (assessed by interview or calculated nPNA)
- Treatment: oral supplements, optimize dialysis prescription, treat comorbidities
  Intradialytic parenteral nutrition costly with limited data, consider if not responding to oral supplements after 2 mo; Amino acid solutions in PD (unavailable in US)
  hGH improved nutrition, QOL; limited data, experimental (JASN 2007;18:2161)

Protein Catabolic Rate (PCR, protein equivalent of nitrogen appearance rate)
- Estimates protein intake in HD patients using interdialytic BUN change; less often used in PD; significant caveats limit utility
- Formula uses interdialytic BUN change, also urinary urea losses if residual renal function; normalized to weight (nPCR), goal >1.2 g/kg/d
- Requires steady-state nitrogen balance, often not the case
  Overestimates protein intake in catabolic states, underestimates if anabolic
- Usually increases with improved dialysis (Kt/V) due to increased protein intake
- No association with mortality in US (AJKD 2004;44:39)

FLUID THERAPY

INTRAVENOUS FLUID (IVF) FOR VOLUME DEPLETION

Four Phases of Resuscitation (BJA 2014;113:740)	
Rescue	Life-threatening shock; fluid bolus >**500 mL/15 min** for a MAP 60–65
Optimization	Compensated shock; fluid challenge **100–200 mL/5–10 min** with assessment of tissue perfusion (MAP >65, CI >2.2 L/min/m², UOP >0.5 mL/kg/hr, lactate (<2 mmol/L)
Stabilization	Steady state, **maintenance** of fluid losses
De-escalation	Promote **negative balance**

- **Crystalloids:** solutions capable of passing semipermeable membrane; may be isotonic, hypertonic, hypotonic; ideal in pt with ↓ volume not from bleeding, ↓ expensive but ↑ interstitial edema; can be used for rescue and stabilization phase
- **Colloids:** high-molecular weight; draw fluid into intravascular compartment via ↑ oncotic pressure with low volume of fluid
- **Blood products:** for active bleeding, coagulopathy; improve tissue oxygenation

Composition of Crystalloids				
Fluid	Electrolyte-free H₂O/ECF Distribution (%)ᵃ	Osmolarity (mOsm/L)ᵇ	Na/Cl/K/Ca/Mg (mEq/L)	pH
D₅W	100/33	252	0/0/0/0/0	3.5–6.5
D₅¼ saline	78/50	321	34/34/0/0/0	3.5–6.5
D₅½ saline	50/66.6	406	77/77/0/0/0	3.5–6.5
0.9% NS	0/100	308	154/154/0/0/0	4.5–7
2% saline	0/100	684	342/342/0/0/0	4.5–7
3% saline	0/100	1,025	513/513/0/0/0	4.5–7
Balanced crystalloids: buffered solution containing organic anions, lactate, or acetate				
Hartmann	12/–100	278	131/111/5/4	5–7
Lactated Ringer's	13/–100	273	130/109/4/3	6–7.5
Acetate Ringer's	12/–100	276	130/112/5/5/2	6–8
Plasma-Lyteᵇ	0/100	294	140/98/5/0/3	c

ᵃ%Intravascular distribution: ¼ of ECF distribution
ᵇosmolality in intravascular space: 0.93 × osmolarity
ᶜPlasma-Lyte A pH 7.4; Plasma-Lyte 148 pH 5.5

Composition of Colloids				
Fluid	Oncotic Pressure (mmHg)	Volume Expansion (% of Administered Volume)	Na	Cl
5% albumin	20–30	70–100	145	145
25% albumin	70–100	300–500	145	145
Hydroxyethyl starch (Hetastarch) 6%	30	100–130	154	154
Dextran-40 (10%)	168–191	200	154	154
Dextran-70 (6%)	56–68	120	154	154
Gelatins (gelofusine, haemaccel): can cause anaphylaxis, not available in the US				

- **Monitoring:** individual assessment, clinical (eg, oral dryness, delayed capillary refill, neurologic symptoms, UOP); **technical findings** (passive leg raising, lactate clearance, dynamic [SVV, BPV, PPV], volumetric [ITBV, GEDV], echo [IVC, CO])

Fluid Therapy Consideration for Various Scenarios	
ICU, severe sepsis or septic shock	Balanced crystalloids; additional albumin ↓ mortality in septic shock subgroup (NEJM 2014;370:1412) Hyperchloremic (eg 0.9% NS) fluid ↑ **NAGMA, AKI/RRT, death** (Ann IM 2014;161:347; JAMA 2012;308:1566; NEJM 2018;378:829) *Early goal-directed therapy* ↓ **mortality** targeting CVP 8–12 with crystalloid or colloid, MAP ≥65 with vasoactive agents, UOP ≥0.5 mL/kg/hr, ScvO 2 70% with transfusion (NEJM 2001;345:1368) **but, not reproducible in subsequent trials** (ProCESS NEJM 2014;370:1683; ARISE NEJM 2014;371:1496; ProMISe NEJM 2015;372:1301; PRISM NEJM 2017;376:2223)
Non-ICU	Balanced crystalloids: ↓ major adverse kidney events (NEJM 2018;378:819)
Metabolic acidosis	Balanced crystalloids In AKI w/ ↑ Cr or ×2 or oliguria NaHCO₃ 4.2% (0.5 mEq/mL) to keep pH >7.3 ↓ death, RRT (Lancet 2018;392:31)
Lactic acidosis	No clear evidence for adding NaHCO₃ to correct acidemia and volume deficit, but might help to ↓ arrhythmias, ↑ response to catecholamines, ↑ CO in ↑ LV contractility
Urine alkalinization	For removal of weak acids: aspirin, phenobarbital, high dose MTX (eg, ½NS + 50–100 mEq NaHCO₃)
TCA overdose	NaHCO₃ 1–2 mEq/kg ×1–2; infusion once QRS normalized
Metabolic alkalosis with hypovolemia	0.9% NS
Hypercalcemia	0.9% NS: metabolic acidosis ↓ renal Ca reabsorption (JASN 2006;17:617)
HRS vs volume depletion	Albumin 1 g/kg/d up to 100 g × 2–3 d Avoid lactate containing fluid in severe liver dysfunction
Therapeutic paracentesis	Albumin 6–8 g/L of ascitic fluid removal
Postobstructive, post-ATN	Hypotonic fluid (eg, ½NS) to replace ½ the UOP to avoid hypernatremia
Traumatic brain injury	NS preferred to albumin (↑ mortality) (NEJM 2007;357:874) Avoid hypotonic balanced crystalloids to avoid cerebral edema Hypertonic not beneficial (JAMA 2010;304:1455) Mannitol ↑ AKI (Medicine 2015;94:e2032)
Trauma, hemorrhagic shock	Packed RBC + platelet + FFP or whole blood Permissive hypotension w/ SBP goal 80–90; avoid routine use of crystalloids (NEJM 2019;380:763)
Surgery	Balanced crystalloids (Br J Surg 2015;102:24) Major abdominal surgery: no difference in disability-free survival in restrictive (net zero fluid goal) vs liberal (10 mL/kg during induction followed by 8 mL/kg/hr) fluid resuscitation in the first 24 hr but ↑ AKI in restrictive (8.6 vs 5%) (NEJM 2018;378:2263)

FLUID THERAPY 3-3

IVF for Sodium and Water Imbalance

IVF Considerations for Sodium and Water Imbalance	
Hypovolemic hyponatremia	Hypertonic if acute or symptomatic NS otherwise with frequent labs ✓
Eu- or hypervolemic Hyponatremia	Hypertonic if acute or symptomatic; d/c cause of hyponatremia No IVF fluid initially; otherwise ✓ lab frequently
Hypovolemic hypernatremia	½ saline or D₅W + NS; after volume deficit corrected can return to oral repletion
Euvolemic hypernatremia	Enteral water (preferred) or D₅W; dextrose can lead to osmotic diuresis worsening water loss

- *Rate of Na correction goal:* <0.5 mEq/L/hr; can correct *1–2 mEq/L/hr* initially until symptoms improve if pt with severe neurologic symptoms (confusion, seizures, AMS) but do not exceed *10–12 mEq in 24 hr*
- Correction can be estimated by following equations but they are dynamic processes and does not consider loss; **needs frequent plasma Na monitoring**

Estimated Na Correction by 1 L of IVF (*NEJM* 2000;342:1581)	
$\Delta P_{Na} = (\text{Infusate}_{Na} + \text{Infusate}_K - P_{Na})/(\text{TBW} + 1)$	
Hyponatremia	**Hypernatremia**
If acute or symptomatic, use hypertonic solution 3% NaCl 100 mL (51 mEq) or 8.4% NaHCO$_3$ 50 mL (50 mEq) over 10 min ×3 as needed eg, in 70 kg young male with P_{Na} 110, 3% NaCl 100 mL will change P_{Na} by: $0.1 \times (513 - 110)/[(70 \times 0.6) + 1] \approx 0.9$ mEq/L	Free water deficit (L) = TBW × ($P_{Na}/140$) − 1] eg, in 70 kg young male with P_{Na} 150, free water deficit is 3 L Initial D$_5$W 1 L will change P_{Na} by: $1 \times (0 - 150)/[(70 \times 0.6) + 1]$ ≈ -3.5 mEq/L

- Estimated ongoing renal water losses: significant in DI (↓ U$_{osm}$), osmotic diuresis (↑ U$_{osm}$)
  - Urine output = Electrolyte clearance + Electrolyte free water clearance (C$^e_{H_2O}$)
  - Electrolyte clearance = Urine volume × [(U$_{Na}$ + U$_K$)/P$_{Na}$]
  - C$^e_{H_2O}$ = Urine volume × [1 − (U$_{Na}$ + U$_K$)/P$_{Na}$]

Interpretation of Electrolyte-free Water Clearance (C$^e_{H_2O}$)		
C$^e_{H_2O}$	Condition	Interpretation
(+): free water excretion	Hyponatremia	Will be corrected if free water intake <C$^e_{H_2O}$
	Hypernatremia	May worsen w/o water input; C$^e_{H_2O}$ should be added to estimated free water deficit
(−): free water retention	Hyponatremia	Fluid restriction only will not correct hyponatremia Consider furosemide to enhance water excretion
	Hypernatremia	May improve if there is no significant nonrenal loss C$^e_{H_2O}$ should be subtracted from free water deficit

- Nonrenal insensible losses: GI, skin, respiratory tract; *10–15 cc/kg/d* (♀), *15–20 cc/kg/d* (♂); ↑ during fever, tachypnea, burns, open wounds, diarrhea, etc.

Maintenance IVF Therapy
- When pt is NPO, to correct electrolyte imbalances, perioperatively, ventilator, cannot provide basal requirements solely with PO intake
- Goal to preserve H$_2$O/electrolyte balance and nutrition; need monitoring for volume excess (eg, edema) or depletion (eg, ↓ skin turgor, ↓ BP)
- The amount of water needed to maintain homeostasis = C$^e_{H_2O}$ + nonrenal insensible free water losses (cannot be accurately estimated) = 1,400–1,600 cc/d or 60–65 cc/hr
- Water requirement is increased in fever, GI loss
- Water requirement is decreased in oliguria, humidified air, water excess (SIADH, liver cirrhosis, CHF, and hypothyroidism)
- Electrolytes replacement: deficit + loss (renal + nonrenal)
- ✓ electrolytes: sodium level reflects water balance; others reflect their balance

Electrolyte Deficit Repletion	
Potassium	20 mEq IV or PO (equivalent w/o vomiting/diarrhea) ↑ ~0.1–0.2 mEq/L
Magnesium	2 g IV MgSO$_4$ over 30–60 min ↑ 0.4 mg/dL Administer 50% calculated dose in impaired renal function
Calcium	1 g IV Ca gluconate over 30–60 min ↑ 0.15 mg/dL Ca chloride if severe hypocalcemia: monitor for tissue extravasation
Phosphate	15 mmol sodium phosphate at rate 4–5 mmol/hr ↑ 0.4 mg/dL Administer 50% calculated dose in impaired renal function

- Dextrose 100 g (2L of 5%) ≈ 340 kcal suppress catabolism

COMPLICATIONS OF IVF THERAPY

AKI
- AKI from high Cl fluid: renal vasoconstriction and ↓ renal blood flow (*JCI* 1983;71:726)
- AKI from hydroxyethyl starch: osmotic PT injury; ↑ RRT requirement, ↑ mortality (*NEJM* 2008;358:125; 2012;367:124; *JAMA* 2013;309:678)

Rapid Sodium Correction
- Osmotic demyelination syndrome: from rapid correction of hyponatremia
- Cerebral edema: from rapid correction of hypernatremia/hypertonicity

Other Complications
- Volume overload: need careful monitoring in HF, CKD, cirrhosis, and NS
- Hyperchloremic NAGMA: from large volume high Cl fluid (eg, 0.9% NS)

- Metabolic alkalosis: large volume balanced crystalloids by metabolism of lactate or acetate to bicarbonate
- Hyperglycemia and hypokalemia: from dextrose containing fluid
- Osmotic diuresis: from large volume saline (sodium diuresis) or dextrose fluid
- Coagulopathy: dilution of clotting factors and platelets; use blood products in hemorrhage
- Anaphylaxis or anaphylactoid reaction: hydroxyethyl starch, gelatin colloids

BLOOD PRODUCTS

Blood Products	
Packed RBC	225–350 mL; should be used with platelet and FFP (1:1:1) in trauma
Whole blood	300–400 mL; can be used in trauma
FFP	200–250 mL; used in coagulopathy with active bleeding, HUS, TTP, and PLEX; needs to be ABO-identical or compatible as in blood
4-factor prothrombin complex concentrate (PCC) (*Circulation* 2013;128:1234), 3-factor PCC are alternatives if bleeding diathesis, reduced risk of volume overload and transfusion reactions

- Hb <9 is a/w death in AKI requiring dialysis (*Intensive Care Med* 2005;31:1529), still threshold for blood transfusion in AKI and CKD is unclear
- RBC transfusion is not a/w mortality in severe AKI (*Crit Care Med* 2016;44:892)

Studies on Hb Threshold for Blood Transfusion in Nontrauma Conditions	
ICU	7 vs 10: ↓ multiorgan dysfunction, MI, and pulmonary edema; ↓ mortality in less ill and <55 y/o (TRICC *NEJM* 1999;340:409)
Symptomatic CAD	10 vs 8: trend for fewer major cardiac events and deaths (*Am Heart J* 2013;165:964)
UGIB	7 vs 9: ↑ survival rate at 6 wk (*NEJM* 2013;368:11)
Septic shock	7 vs 9: no difference mortality and ischemic event (*NEJM* 2014;371:1381)
Cardiac surgery	7.5 vs 9: more deaths; no difference in serious infection or an ischemic event (*NEJM* 2015;372:997)
7.5 vs 9.5 in ICU and 8.5 in non-ICU ward: not inferior at 28 d (*NEJM* 2017;377:2133) and 6 mo (*NEJM* 2018;379:1224)

- Restrictive Hb target <7 in ICU or GIB is a/w ↓ mortality (in-hospital ×0.74, total ×0.80), rebleeding (×0.64), ACS (×0.44), pulmonary edema (×0.48), bacterial infections (×0.86) (*Am J Med* 2014;127:124)

Complications of Blood Transfusion
- Infections: bacterial or viral
- Acute allergic +/− anaphylactic reactions; delayed hemolytic transfusion reaction
- Acute hemolysis: heme pigment nephropathy
- Iron overload from chronic transfusion
- HLA alloimmunization in KT candidate (↓ by leukoreduced blood)
- Transfusion-related acute lung injury (TRALI): acute (during transfusion ~6 hr) hypoxemic respiratory distress with bilateral lung infiltrates on CXR w/o volume overload/HF/pre-existing ARDS
- Transfusion-associated circulatory overload: ↑ risk in CKD (×27), CHF (×6.6), and + fluid balance (×9.4) with ↑ mortality (×3.2) (*Am J Med* 2013;126:357.e29); prevention with slow infusion (1 mL/kg/hr) +/− diuretic use
- Hyperkalemia: released from RBC from ↑ storage time, ↑ pRBCs, irradiated; especially in massive trauma, impaired renal function and infants/newborns
- Dialyzer circuit clotting with heparin-free HD

Complications of Massive Blood Transfusion (>10 units/24 hr)
- Metabolic alkalosis: 1 mmol citrate, $C_3H_5O(COO)_3^{3-} \rightarrow$ 3 mmol HCO_3^- in liver
- Hypokalemia: d/t metabolic alkalosis; transcellular exchange of H^+ and K^+
- Hypocalcemia: citrate toxicity in liver failure; ↓ iCa

ORAL FLUID

- Requirement: vary by age, sex, pregnancy, and breast feeding status
- Water absorption in GI: Na^+/H^+ exchanger (NHE), electrochemical gradient, Na-coupled co-transport with carrier solutes (eg, glucose via SGLT-1)
- Low Na in oral fluid ↑ urine output (*Eur J Appl Physiol* 2008;103:585)

Oral Rehydration Solution (ORS)
- Indications: watery diarrhea w/o severe volume depletion/shock
- *ORS recommended by WHO*: osmolality 245 mOsm/L, glucose 13.5 g/L (75 mmol/L), Na 75 mEq/L, K 20 mEq/L, Cl 65 mEq/L, citrate 10 mmol/L, equimolar Na/glucose
- 2 phases: *rehydration* (correct in 3–4 hr by frequent, small amounts) & *maintenance*
- Advantages: lower cost, easier to administer, less invasive, ambulatory
- *Contraindications*: ∆MS, ↑ aspiration, ileus, conditions that limit GI absorption (eg, short bowel), resuscitation, severe volume depletion or vomiting

Water
- Benefits: ↓ recurrence of stones (*J Urol* 1996;155:839); ↓ cAMP, potential to slow cyst growth in ADPKD (*CJASN* 2010;5:693), ↓ recurrent UTI in premenopausal women (*JAMA IM* 2018;178:1509)
- No general benefit to support 8 glasses (2 L) of water (*JASN* 2008;19:1041)
- Complications: hyponatremia esp. in competitive runners, psychotic polydipsia, ecstasy use

PHARMACOLOGY

- Knowledge of changes in drug disposition from pharmacokinetic and pharmacodynamic alterations in the presence of reduced kidney function among patients with CKD is important to individualize pharmacotherapy and ensure optimal outcomes

PHARMACOKINETICS (ABSORPTION, DISTRIBUTION, METABOLISM, EXCRETION)

Absorption
- Absorption of a medication and subsequently bioavailability (% of medication that reaches the systemic circulation), may be altered in patients with renal disease
- CKD complications that may impact drug absorption, include: changes in GI transit time from gastroparesis, vomiting and diarrhea, alterations in gastric pH from use of acid suppressing agents (eg, proton pump inhibitors, histamine 2 antagonists)
- Phosphate binders form insoluble complexes with some medications: quinolone antibiotics

Distribution
- Distribution of medications into body compartments: plasma, water, fat, red blood cells, intracellular/extracellular binding sites, and tissue
- Volume of distribution (Vd) is a proportionality constant for the amount of drug in the body to serum concentration and can be used in clinical practice to calculate medication doses (drug concentration, mg/L*Vd, L/kg) to achieve a desired drug level
- Patients with CKD display significant alterations in Vd due to qualitative changes in tissue binding sites, competitive binding inhibition by accumulation of endogenous or exogenous substances such as uremic waste, decreased concentrations and conformational changes of albumin, and high concentrations of metabolites that accumulate and may interfere with binding of the parent compound

Vd (L/kg) of Select Medications			
Drug	Normal	ESRD	Comments
Increased			
Furosemide	0.11	0.18	Decreased plasma protein binding increases free
Phenytoin	0.64	1.4	plasma fraction
Decreased			
Digoxin	7.3	4	Uremic toxins are thought to displace drug from cellular
Ethambutol	3.7	1.6	binding sites; Reduced tissue levels of Na/K-ATPase

Metabolism
- The breakdown of medications through enzymatic pathways within the liver, gut, lungs, and plasma: oxidation, reduction, acetylation, glucuronidation, or hydrolysis
- CKD may affect hepatic drug metabolism due to accumulation of uremic toxins, increased oxidative stress from a chronic inflammatory state, and downregulation of CYP3A4 and CYP2C9 enzyme expression in the liver and intestine
- Pharmacologically active metabolites or metabolites with toxic effects may be formed
- Many drugs can stimulate or inhibit the activity of metabolizing enzymes; common pathways, inhibitors, and inducers are summarized

Major Drug Metabolizing Mechanisms			
Metabolism	Substrates	Inducers (↓ Level)	Inhibitors (↑ Level)
CYP450 3A4, 3A5	Sirolimus CsA, Tac CCB Sorafenib Sunitinib Bevacizumab Statins (except fluvastatin) Tolvaptan	Corticosteroids, Phenytoin, Phenobarbital, Rifampin/ Rifabutin/ Rifapentine Carbamazepine St. John's wort Enzalutamide Lumacaftor Mitotane Primidone Bexarotene Bosentan Dabrafenib Efavirenz Eslicarbazepine Etravirine Modafinil	CsA, Non-DHP CCB Azole antifungals: keto/flu/itra/isavu/ posa/vori Conivaptan Cobicistat Clari/teli/ erythromycin (not azithromycin) PI for HIV (-navir) Telaprevir Ima/ceri/nilo/ crizotinib Idelalisib, Ribociclib Mifepristone Nefazodone Apre/netupitant Grapefruit juice
p-glycoprotein	Tacrolimus Sirolimus Digoxin Tolvaptan	Corticosteroids	-azole antifungals: keto/flu/itra/isavu/ posa /vori, Clotrimazole, Non-DHP CCB, Erythromycin, Tolvaptan
Xanthine oxidase	AZA, 6-MP		Allopurinol, Febuxostat

Excretion

- **Excretion** is the process of removal of a drug from the body
- Primary processes: hepatobiliary excretion and renal clearance
- Hepatobiliary excretion: liver actively secretes drug and/or metabolite(s) into the bile which then gets excreted in the feces. Some agents may be reabsorbed through diffusion by the small intestine and undergo enterohepatic recirculation.
- Renal excretion: drug is filtered in the nephron → collecting ducts → urine. Compounds excreted in the urine are water soluble; agents that are lipid soluble must first be metabolized to increase water solubility.
- Renal clearance (CL_R) is a composite of glomerular filtration rate (GFR), tubular secretion ($CL_{secretion}$), and tubular reabsorption ($CL_{reabsorption}$) and is dependent on the fraction of drug that is unbound (f_u); [CL_R = (GFR*fu) + $CL_{secretion}$ − $CL_{reabsorption}$]

Proximal Tubule Drug Transporters		
Transporters	Substrates	Inhibitors
Luminal Membrane		
MATE	Creatinine Antibiotics Antivirals Cytostatics (cisplatin, topotecan) Metformin	Ritonavir Cobicistat Cimetidine Pyrimethamine Dolutegravir
OCTN	Gabapentin Carnitine	
MRP	Antivirals Cytostatics (MTX, irinotecan) Melphalan Statins (pravastatin)	
PEPT	Polymyxins β-lactam (ceph., penicillins) ACE-I (captopril, enalapril, fosinopril)	

Basolateral Membrane			

OAT	Antibiotics
	Antihypertensives
	Antivirals
	Diuretics
	MTX, paclitaxel
	NSAIDs
	Statins
	Uricosurics
	cimetidine, ranitidine
		ACE-I (captopril)
		ARB (candesartan, losartan,
		  telmisartan, valsartan)
		Statins (fluvastatin,
		  pravastatin, simvastatin)
		Cephalosporins
		Mycophenolate
		Probenecid

OCT	Creatinine Metformin Cisplatin Quinine	Dolutegravir Rilpivirine Cimetidine Quinidine Rifampicin Prazosin

MATE, multidrug and toxic compound extrusion; OCTN, organic cation/carnitine transporter; MRP, multidrug resistant protein transporter; PEPT, peptide transporter; OAT, organic anion transporter; OCT, organic cation transporter

- CKD may change drug disposition through alterations in filtration, secretion, or reabsorption
- *Secondary processes excretion through lungs, milk, sweat, tears, skin, hair, or saliva*

DRUG DOSING ADJUSTMENTS

- Estimation of creatinine clearance from clinical data (age, gender, height, weight, serum creatinine) remains the guiding factor for drug-dosage regimen design

Stepwise Approach to Dosimetry in Patients with Renal Insufficiency	
Step 1	Obtain history and relevant demographic and clinical information
Step 2	Quantitative estimate of renal function; Creatinine clearance by Cockroft-Gault Method: estimated glomerular filtration rate (eGFR), or calculated from timed urine collection
Step 3	Review medications and identify if there is a need for individualized treatment
Step 4	Determine treatment goals, calculate loading and maintenance dose by varying dose or varying interval or combination method
Step 5	Monitor parameters of drug response as well as drug levels (total drug vs free drug and peak/trough levels)
Step 6	Assess clinical response and adjust regimen based on patient's outcome

HEMODIALYSIS AND DRUG THERAPY

- Factors that affect dialyzability of medications include drug characteristics, dialysis conditions, and patients' clinical condition
- Hemodialysis units generally administer drugs after the patient has undergone dialysis to minimize the loss of drug
- **Drug-related factors** which preclude dialyzability include the molecular weight or size (>1,000 daltons), degree of protein binding (high), and distribution volume (large)
- **Dialysis prescription:** composition and surface area of the dialysis filter and blood and dialysate flow rates. High-flux membranes have a large pore size (allow passage of drugs with molecular weights of up to 20,000 daltons) and mimic the filtration characteristics of the human kidney vs conventional hemodialysis.
- Drugs extensively cleared by HD: vancomycin, atenolol, and metoprolol, angiotensin converting enzyme inhibitors (except fosinopril)

CONTINUOUS RENAL REPLACEMENT THERAPY AND DRUG THERAPY

- CRRT will remove medications by convection (unbound) and diffusion
- Little is known about drug-dosing requirements for patients receiving CRRT; however, dosing strategies can be between those used for outpatient intermittent hemodialysis using a GFR <10 up to those used in mild impairment classified as GFR 50–80

Antibiotic Dosing in Adult Patients Receiving CRRT		*(Clin Infect Dis 2005;41:1159)*	
Ampicillin–Sulbactam	3 g q12–24h*	Daptomycin	4 or 6 mg/kg q48h
Aztreonam	1–2 g q12h*	Levofloxacin	250 mg q12–24h
Cefazolin	1–2 g q12h*	Linezolid	600 mg q12h
Cefepime	1–2 g q12h*	Meropenem	1 g q12h
Ceftazidime	1–2 g q12h*	Oxacillin	2 g q4–6h
Ceftriaxone	2 g q12–24h	Piperacillin–Tazobactam	4.5 g q12h, 2.25 g q6h*
Clindamycin	600–900 mg q8h	Vancomycin	1 g q48h*
Colistin	2.5 mg/kg q48h		

*Higher doses may be necessary for CVVHD.

References

- Adjustment of drug doses in CKD and Hemodialysis (Global RPH): http://www.globalrph.com/renaldosing2.htm
- Clearance of drugs on hemodialysis (Nephrology Pharmacy Associates): http://www.just.edu.jo/DIC/Manuals/Dialysis%20of%20Drugs.pdf

RAAS INHIBITORS

Renin Angiotensin Aldosterone System (RAAS)				
Component	Release Activators	Release Inhibitors	Action Inhibitors	Comments and Actions
Renin	↓ Afferent arteriole stretch ↓ DCT Na ↑ SNS (β1)	Natriuretic peptides NSAIDs β1 blockers CNI, DN	DRI	PGE2 mediates release Converts angiotensinogen to angiotensin I
Angiotensin II (AII)	ACE Not ↑ K	ACEi	ARB	Vasoconstriction (efferent > afferent arteriole): ↑ Glom capillary pressure ↑ BP *(NEJM 2017;377:419)* ↑ Aldosterone, ADH ↑ NHE3, NCC, ENaC activity → ↑ Na reabsorption ↓ ROMK; ↑ K excretion in colon *(AJP Renal 1998;274:F275)*
Aldosterone (Aldo)	AII, ↑ K	Adrenal insufficiency, ketoconazole ACEi, ARB, heparin	MRA, ENaC inhibitors CNI DN	↑ ENaC, ↑ ROMK: ↑ Na reabsorption in CD & ↑ K⁺ and H⁺ secretion ↑ Na reabsorption by colon ↑ ROS, ↑ inflammation/fibrosis *(Nat Rev Nephrol 2013;9:459)*

- Angiotensin-converting enzyme (ACE): present at pulmonary and renal endothelium; Converts angiotensin I to angiotensin II; Kininase: degrades bradykinin
- Natriuretic peptides (ANP, BNP, CNP): released from atria (ANP) or LV (BNP); ↑ cGMP, inhibition of NHE3, NKCC2, ENaC, vasodilation, ↓ renin release, ↑ GFR
- Neprilysin (CD10): neutral endopeptidase, abundant in kidney; degrades natriuretic peptides, adrenomedullin, bradykinin, VIP, and angiotensin II

Potential Changes of RAAS Components by Medicines					
Type	Renin Level	Renin Activity	AII Level	Aldo Level	Aldo Level/Renin Activity
β1 blocker	↓	↓↓	↓	↓	↑
DRI	↑↑	↓↓	↓	↓	↑
ACEi	↑	↑↑	↓	↓	↓
ARB	↑	↑↑	↑	↓	↓
MRA	↑	↑↑	↑	↑	↓
Neprilysin inhibitor	↓	↓	↑	↑	↑

Clinical Use of ACEi and ARB

- Mild ↑ Cr: could be sign of ↓ glomerular hyperfiltration
- In CKD, ACEi use is a/w 28% ↓ mort., 39% ↓ kidney failure; 18% ↓ major CV events; ARB 30% ↓ kidney failure; 24% ↓ major CV events (AJKD 2016;67:728)
- In T2DM/DN, ARB 16–20% ↓ doubling Cr, ESRD and death (RENAAL NEJM 2001;345:861; IDNT NEJM 2001;345:851)
- ACEi or ARB is recommended for all diabetic patients with UACR >30 mg/d and nondiabetic patients with UACR >300 mg/d (KDIGO CKD 2012). Proteinuria that would quickly remit as in MCD can be monitored w/o ACEi or ARB (KDIGO GN 2012).
- In renovascular disease, ↓ death, MI, or stroke and dialysis (AHJ 2008;156:549)
- Even in predialysis CKD5, ACEi and ARB a/w ↓ dialysis, death (JAMA IM 2014;174:347)
- Supramaximal ARB ↓ proteinuria w/o lowering BP (KI 2005;68:1190; JASN 2009;20:893)
- Losartan has less maximal efficacy in BP lowering than other ARBs: losartan 100 mg <irbesartan 300 mg, valsartan 320 mg, telmisartan 80 mg, candesartan 32 mg
- Losartan ↑ uric acid excretion by inhibition of the proximal urate transporter 1 (URAT1), uric acid reabsorption mechanism (AJH 2008;21:1157)
- Use at night; improve BP (AJH 2011;24:383), ↓ DM incidence (Diabetologia 2016;59:255)
- ARBs and fosinopril are not removed by HD; other ACEi are removed by HD

Angioedema from ACEi

- Incidence is 0.68% (AJH 2004;17:103); rare with ARB (Arch IM 2012;172:1582; Am J Cardiol 2012;110:383); Usually happens w/i 1st wk of ACEi, but can happen anytime
- ↑ bradykinin mediated by ↓ ACE-mediated degradation
- Swelling of lips, tongue, face, and throat (laryngeal edema); abd pain; diarrhea
- Absence of urticaria or pruritus (Allergy Asthma Clin Immunol 2011;7 Suppl 1:S9)
- Recurrence: 46% after d/c of ACEi, 1st recurrence w/i 3 mo except 1 case (J Hypertens 2011;29:2273): should not be attributed to alternative drug, such as ARB
- Tx: d/c ACEi, airway protection; icatibant (NEJM 2015;372:418), ecallantide, C1 inhibitor concentrate, FFP

Approximate Equivalent ACEi and ARB Dose (mg, Daily Unless Specified)			
Drugs	Low	Moderate	High
Lisinopril, Fosinopril	2.5–5	10–20	30–40
Enalapril (qd–bid)	2.5–10	20	40
Enalaprilat (q6h)	0.625–1.25 q6h	2.5 q6h	5 q6h
Captopril (tid)	6.25–12.5 tid	25–50 tid	100–150 tid
Ramipril	1.25–2.5	5–10	20
Benazepril, Quinapril	5–10	20–40	80
Moexipril	7.5	15	30
Perindopril	2	4–8	16
Trandolapril	1	2–4	8
Losartan	25–50	100	—
Valsartan	40	80–160	320
Candesartan	4–8	16	32
Olmesartan	5	10–20	40
Irbesartan	75	150	300
Eprosartan	400	600–800	—
Telmisartan	20	40	80

Side Effects of ACEi and ARB

- ↑ Cr: in bilateral renal artery stenosis, HF and CKD; ✓BMP w/i 1 wk after start
- Even ↑ Cr <30% a/w ESRD, MI, HF, and death (BMJ 2017;356:j791)
- Hyperkalemia: possible in anuric HD patients (Am J Med 2002;112:110); Patiromer may be used in hyperkalemic pts on RAAS blockade (NEJM 2015;372:211)
- ACEi + ARB ↑ AKI and ↑ K in DN (NEJM 2013;369:1892)
- Teratogenicity: CNS and CVS malformation in 1st trimester (NEJM 2006;354:2443); uro-genital and renal malformation in 2nd trimester; avoid MRA and DRI
- Anemia: both ACEi and ARB (QJM 2015;108:879). Angiotensin II type 1 receptor enhance EPO-stimulated erythroid proliferation (AJM 1999;106:158); ACEi ↑ IGF-1, erythropoiesis promotor (Transplantation 1997;64:913). Used for post-txp erythrocytosis (AJT 2007;7:2350).
- Dry cough in ACEi
- PLEX reaction in ACEi; Kinin mediated; d/c 24 hr prior to PLEX (Transfusion 1994;34:891)
- No ↑ cancer (J Hypertens 2011;29:623; BMJ 2018;362:k3851)

Mineralocorticoid Receptor Antagonists (MRA)
- Addition to ACEi or ARB ↓ BP, proteinuria (*CJASN* 2009;4:542; *BMC Nephrol* 2016;17:127)
- Effective add-on drug for resistant hypertension (*Lancet* 2015;386:2059)
- ↓ mortality in NYHA II HF w/ EF <35% (*NEJM* 2011;364:11) & post-MI low EF (*NEJM* 2003;348:1309)
- In HD patients, spironolactone 50 mg bid ↓ BP (*AJKD* 2005;46:94); 50 mg qd ↑ hyperkalemia w/o changing LV mass (*KI* 2019;95:973; 2019;95:983)
- s/e: hyperkalemia esp in CKD (*JASH* 2010;4:295), ↑ Cr

Direct Renin Inhibitor (DRI)
- Aliskiren + losartan ↓ proteinuria c/w losartan only (AVOID *NEJM* 2008;358:2433)
- Addition of aliskiren to ACEi or ARB did not improve CV or renal outcome (ALTITUDE *NEJM* 2012;367:2204; 2016;374:1521)
- In HF aliskiren + ACEi ↑ Cr, ↑ K, ↓ BP w/o benefit (*NEJM* 2016;374:1521)
- s/e: hyperkalemia, ↑ Cr, angioedema

Angiotensin Receptor Neprilysin Inhibitor (ARNi): Sacubitril
- Neprilysin inhibitor ↑ natriuretic peptides, bradykinin, and angiotensin (reason ARB combination is always required); NT-proBNP is not ↑ by neprilysin inhibitor
- Indicated for symptomatic HF, NYHA II–IV w/ LVEF ≤40% despite ACEi or ARB
- HF w/ NYHA II–III on ACEi or ARB should transition to ARNi (ACC/AHA *JACC* 2017;70:776)
- Do not combine w/ ACEi for risk of angioedema (*Circulation* 2002;106:920); 36 hr washout for conversion; conversion from ARB does not require washout
- 20% ↓ CV mortality and HF hospitalization (*NEJM* 2014;371:993) and greater ↓ NT-proBNP in hospitalized pts c/w ACEi (*NEJM* 2019;389:539)
- s/e: more hypotension, less Cr ≥2.5, K >6 than ACEi (*NEJM* 2014;371:993), angioedema
- Avoid use prior to PLEX to prevent possible bradykinin-mediated reaction

NONSTEROIDAL ANTI-INFLAMMATORY DRUGS

Actions of Progstaglandins (PG) and Effects of NSAIDs	
Actions of PG	Effects of NSAIDs
Hypotension, ↓ perfusion pressure → PGI$_2$- and PGE$_2$-mediated vasodilation: mainly afferent arteriole; maintain renal perfusion when RAAS is activated	↓ Renal blood flow and GFR
High salt intake → medullary PGE$_2$ inhibits NKCC2 → natriuresis	Sodium retention/edema Hypertension ↑ Concentration ability
Volume depletion → cortical PGE$_2$ ↑ renin release from JG cells → ↑ RAAS → ↑ K excretion and BP	Hyperkalemia
PGE$_2$ ↓ AQP2 expression	↑ Concentration ability SIADH; used in NDI
Maintenance of medullary interstitial cell blood perfusion	Papillary necrosis
TxA$_2$: platelet aggregation	↑ Bleeding

- Kidney express both cyclooxygenase (COX)-1 and 2

Pharmacology of NSAIDs
- Short ½ life (<6 hr): ibuprofen, indomethacin, ketorolac, diclofenac
- Long ½ life (>6 hr): naproxen, piroxicam; phenylbutazone (a veterinary NSAID)
- Mainly metabolized by liver; Tightly bound to protein
- Topical NSAIDs can induce systemic renal effects (*NDT* 1999;14:187)

Effects on Renal Function, AKI and CKD
- Current NSAID exposure is a/w AKI w/ OR 1.73 (*BMC Nephrol* 2017;18:256); ↑ 20% of AKI and CKD (*JAMA Netw Open* 2019;2:e187896); ↑ AKI & hyperkalemia (*NDT* 2019;34:1145)
- AKI: from renal vasoconstriction, especially when combined use with diuretics and/or RAASi ↑ AKI (*KI* 2015;88:396)
- Rapid progression of CKD (*Am J Med* 2007;120:280.e1)

Other Renal Manifestations of NSAIDs

- Interstitial nephritis: acute or chronic
- ↑ K: NSAIDs used in Bartter (↑ PG pathogenic) *(NEJM 2000;343:661; JASN 2017;28:2540)* and Gitelman *(JASN 2015;26:468)*
- dRTA and ↓ K by carbonic anhydrase II inhibition *(Case Rep Crit Care 2013;875857)*
- Potentiate ADH action: can cause SIADH; used in nephrogenic DI (NDI)
- MCD, FSGS; MN *(AJKD 2013;62:1012)*
- Papillary necrosis: especially with vascular diseases, eg, sickle cell, DM
  Sloughed papillae may cause renal colic, urinary obstruction
  Contrast CT: irregular papillary tip, loss of papillae; IV urography: ring shadow
- Increased risk of pyelonephritis when used in lower UTI *(BMJ 2017;359:j4784)*
- Long-term use may be a/w RCC *(Arch IM 2011;171:1487)*

Extrarenal Clinical Manifestations

- Analgesic; anti-inflammatory effect
- ↑ BP *(Lancet 2008;371:270)*; ↓ antihypertensive effectiveness
- ↑ CV events *(NEJM 2005;352:1092; BMJ 2006;332:1302)*; even in the 1 wk of use *(Circulation 2011;123:2226; BMJ 2017;357:j1909)*
- ↑ MI: diclofenac, but not w/ naproxen; indication might matter: spondyloarthritis >OA *(Ann Rheum Dis 2018;77:1137)*; ↑ HF admission *(BMJ 2016;354:i4857)*
- Dyspepsia, peptic ulcer, and bleeding

NSAIDs Intoxication and Overdose

- Common cause of drug intoxication
- Nausea, vomiting, drowsiness, anion gap acidosis (lactic acidosis ± acidic metabolite), seizure, aplastic anemia, and granulocytosis (in phenylbutazone intoxication)
- AKI: usually reversible
- Tx: conservative; HD is ineffective d/t protein binding; may consider PLEX in severe intoxication (eg, anaphylaxis)

NSAIDs Should be Avoided in the Following Conditions

- Any use in GFR <30, prolonged use in GFR <60
- w/ lithium and RAASi *(KDIGO CKD 2012)*; HTN (especially poorly controlled) and HF
- Portal hypertension and cirrhosis *(AGA Clin Gastroenterol Hepatol 2019;17:595)*

DIURETICS

DIURETICS ACTING ON THE PROXIMAL CONVOLUTED TUBULE (PCT)

- Site of ~60–70% of Na reabsorption
- **Drugs:** carbonic anhydrase inhibitors (CAI), acetazolamide
- ↓ Na/H exchanger (NHE3) and ↑ HCO_3 excretion by 25–30% and Na is brought further downstream as the counterion *(NEJM 1954;250:759)*
- **Clinical Use:** metabolic alkalemia induced by high-dose loop diuretics in CHF, glaucoma, pseudotumor cerebri, high-altitude mountain sickness, posthypercapnea alkalemia *(Ren Physiol 1987;10:136)*
- Weak natriuretic when used alone d/t ↑ distal Na reabsorption *(NEJM 1954;250:800)*
- Effective as a natriuretic when used in combination with more distal inhibitors *(J Cardiovasc Pharmacol 1997;29:367; CMAJ 1990;123:883)*
- **PK:** usual dose is 250–500 mg daily; Secreted by OAT in PCT *(Semin Nephrol 2011;31:483)*
- **Electrolyte Effects:** metabolic acidosis, profound hypokalemia from distal nephron Na/K exchange; ensure K replete if considering use *(NEJM 1954;250:759)*

DIURETICS ACTING ON THE LOOP OF HENLE

- Site of ~25% Na reabsorption
- **Drugs:** furosemide, torsemide, bumetanide; ethacrynic acid (not sulfa-based)
- Inhibit apical Na-K-2Cl cotransporter (NKCC2) in the TAL of LOH
- **Clinical Use:** greatest natriuretic effect among the diuretics ("high ceiling" diuretic). Starting diuretic for volume management in advanced CKD, cirrhosis, CHF, and nephrosis.
- **PK:** variable PO absorption with furosemide (see table). Highly protein bound, very little filtered. Secreted by OATs in PCT *(Clin Pharm Ther 1980;27:784)*.

Pharmacokinetics of Loop Diuretics (NEJM 1998;339:387; Am J Ther 2009;16:86)				
		Equivalent Dose		
Diuretic	Oral Bioavailability (%)	PO (mg)	IV (mg)	T$_{1/2}$ (hr)
Furosemide	10–100	40	20	1.5–2
Torsemide	80–100	20	—	3–4
Bumetanide	80–100	1	1	1
Ethacrynic acid	~100%	50	50	2–4

T$_{1/2}$ significantly increases in CKD, CHF, and cirrhosis (NEJM 1998;339:387).

DIURETICS 3-13

Ceiling Doses of Furosemide (Am J Med Sci 2000;319:38): anions retained in renal failure compete with OAT		
Condition	IV (mg)	PO (mg)
eGFR 20–50	80	160
eGFR <20	200	400
CHF	40–80	80–160

- **Electrolyte Effects:** ↓ K (Δ–0.3 mEq/L) and ↓ Mg common; ↓ Na less common than in thiazides as NKCC2 inhibition ↓ medullary interstitial osm (Semin Nephrol 2011;31:542)
- **Other s/e:** hypersensitivity (sulfa-based, except ethacrynic acid), AIN (uncommon), ototoxicity (NKCC1 antagonism in inner ear; avoid concomitant aminoglycoside administration, more common with ethacrynic acid). Vascular smooth muscle relaxation with improvement in pulmonary congestion in some patients (NEJM 1973;288:1087). Can worsen LC cast nephropathy.

DIURETICS ACTING ON THE DISTAL CONVOLUTED TUBULE (DCT)

- Site of ~5% Na reabsorption
- **Drugs:** hydrochlorothiazide (HCTZ), chlorothiazide, chlorthalidone, metolazone
- Inhibit apical Na-Cl cotransporter (NCC) in the DCT
- **Clinical Use:** antihypertensive in pts with GFR >30; Edema: used in combination w/ loop diuretic for acute decompensated HF (ADHF) (JACC 2010;56:1527); Ca nephrolithiasis, nephrogenic DI (along with low solute intake)
- **PK:** blunted effect when GFR <30

Pharmacokinetics of Thiazides (JACC 2010;56:1527)			
Diuretic	Equivalent Dose (mg)	Duration of Action (hr)	Duration in CKD
HCTZ	25 (PO)	6–12	↑
Chlorthalidone	12.5 (PO)	24–72	↑
Metolazone	2.5 (PO)	12–24	↑
Chlorothiazide	250 (IV)	6–12	↑

- **Electrolyte Effects:** ↓ K (Δ–0.5–0.9 mEq/L) and ↓ Mg common
- **Other s/e:** hypersensitivity (sulfa-based), AIN (uncommon), hyperlipidemia, pancreatitis, ↓ insulin sensitivity. ↑ Li. ↑ Uric acid, gout. Some thiazide class diuretics have carbonic anhydrase inhibition (chlorothiazide, chlorthalidone, and indapamide are strongest).

Thiazide-Induced Hyponatremia (TIH)

- **Risk Factors:** old, female, low BW, low BMI, high-dose thiazide, previous h/o TIH
- common in 1st 3 mo of thiazide, risk remained high ~10 yr (Am J Med 2011;124:1064)

Mechanisms of Thiazide-Induced Hyponatremia
Lack of effects on medullary interstitial osmolality as in loop diuretic
NCC independent upregulate aquaporin-2 (AJP Renal 2014;306:F525)
Increased water intake (Ann IM 1989;110:24; J Hypertens 2015;33:627)
↓ Water clearance d/t low solute intake: Urine urea <330 mmol/d (J Hypertens 2015;33:627)
Polymorphisms of gene encoding PG transporter, EP4 ↑ aquaporin-2 (JCI 2017;127:3367)

- Low uric acid, FE$_{uric\ acid}$ >12%
- **Tx:** permanently d/c thiazide, ↑ solute intake ± fluid restriction

DIURETICS ACTING ON THE COLLECTING DUCT (CD)

- Site of ~1–2% Na reabsorption
- Mineralocorticoid-receptor blockers (MRB) and ENaC antagonists: K-sparing
- **Drugs:** spironolactone (MRB), eplerenone (MRB), amiloride (ENaC antagonist), triamterene (ENaC antagonist); Trimethoprim component of TMP/SMX inhibits ENaC
- MRBs antagonize effects of aldosterone (basolateral Na-K ATPase, apical ENaC, apical ROMK), while ENaC antagonists directly antagonize apical ENaC in principal cells in the terminal DCT, CCT, CCD (Semin Nephrol 2011;31:483)
- **Clinical Use:** as mainstay in cirrhosis and nephrosis, and as adjunctive in CHF. Can attenuate the need for K supplementation in combination diuretic regimens
- **PK:** MRBs enter cytosol via basolateral membrane. ENaC antagonists are secreted by OCT in PCT.
- **Electrolyte Effects:** ↑ K, ↓ HCO_3 (Semin Nephrol 2011;31:542)
- **Other s/e:** gynecomastia (MRBs); Triamterene can result to crystalluria and stone formation in up to 50% of patients (Clin Nephrol 1986;26:169)

Diuretic Class	Serum						Urine	
Electrolytes and Uric Acid Changes by Diuretics (Semin Nephrol 2011;31:542; AJP 2017;312:F998)	Na	K	HCO_3	Ca	Mg	Uric Acid	Ca	Mg
CAI	–	↓	↓	–	↓	–	↑	–
Loop	↑ or ↓	↓	↑	↓	↓	↑	↑	↑
Thiazide	↓	↓	↑	↑	↓	↑	↓	↑
MRB	–	↑	↓	–	–	–	–	↓
Amiloride	–	↑	↓	–	–	–	↓	↓

OTHER AGENTS WITH DIURETIC EFFECT

Vasopressin Antagonists
- **Drugs:** tolvaptan (PO), conivaptan (IV)
- Vasopressin-2 receptor antagonism blocks effect of ADH, leading to aquaresis
- **Clinical Use:** FDA approved for the treatment for hypervolemic ↓ Na and SIADH
- **PK:** dose reductions required with ketoconazole, clarithromycin, ritonavir, saquinavir, erythromycin, fluconazole, verapamil
- **Electrolyte Effects:** ↑ K, ↓ HCO_3 (Semin Nephrol 2011;31:542)
- **Other s/e:** can cause significant ↑ ALT > AST > bilirubin; Conivaptan also has V1a-receptor antagonism, can lead to variceal bleeding

Sodium Glucose Cotransporter-2 (SGLT-2) Inhibitors
- Used in T2DM; ↓ mortality, CV events, ↑ wt loss, ↓ BP, and improved renal outcomes; (NEJM 2019;380:2295; JAMA 2018;319:1580; Circulation 2016;80:2277; CJASN 2017;12:751; KI 2018;93:231)

Osmotic Agents (Arch IM 1981;141:493)
- Mannitol is filtered by glomerulus, exerts osmotic action throughout nephron
- Generally no benefit; should only be used for nondiuresis indications

BNP/ANP Potentiation (Ren Physiol Biochem 1991;14:208)
- Sacubitril: neprilysin inhibitor; ↑ natriuretic peptides; sacubitril/valsartan (Entresto®) ↓ CV mortality and HF hospitalization (NEJM 2014;371:993); in HF with NYHA II-III on ACEi or ARB should transition to ARNi (ACC/AHA JACC 2017;70:776)
- Nesiritide: recombinant human BNP; no effect on mortality and rehospitalization in ADHF (NEJM 2011;365:32); not currently recommended therapy

DIURETIC RESISTANCE (AJKD 2017;69:136)

- First assess for dietary adherence (24 hr U_{Na} <100 mmol ≈ 2.3 g) and medication adherence. Then consider alternative mechanisms for resistance (below).
- Diuretic not reaching target: too low dose, poor absorption, organic acids of uremia competing with OATs in PCT in CKD

- Blunted diuretic response (concomitant use of NSAIDs, activation of RAAS and Na retention after diuretics (*KI* 1983;24:233)), distal nephron adaptation with Na avidity
- If 24 hr U_{Na} <100 mmol, then increase PO total daily dose (dose or frequency). If no response, add distal diuretic (DCT or CD). If no response, then transition to IV.

DISEASE-SPECIFIC MANAGEMENT

Hypertension (*Semin Nephrol* 2011;31:495; *Am J Hypertens* 2016;29:1130)
- Thiazides included in 1st-line therapy recommendations by JNC-8 (*JAMA* 2014;311:507)
- Furosemide BID vs torsemide QD → similar ↓ BP in CKD-2 and -3 (*KI* 2003;64:632)

Acute Kidney Injury
- Diuretic use in critically ill patients with AKI is a/w adverse events in this group (correlation, not clearly causal); may delay initiation of RRT (PICARD *JAMA* 2002;288:2547)
- Diuretic use to achieve a negative fluid balance in patients w/ ARDS and AKI conferred a 60-d mortality benefit (FACTT *CJASN* 2011;6:966)
- "Diuretic challenges" in AKI may be trialed to manage volume overload, but requires frequent reassessment for refractoriness so as not to delay RRT
- No clear role in AKI other than volume management (Grade 2C) (KDIGO AKI 2012)

Chronic Kidney Disease (*Nature Rev Neph* 2012;8:100)
- Organic acids compete with tubular secretion by OAT, rightward shift of dose-response curve resulting in higher required doses (*JASN* 2002;13:798)
- Addition of thiazide to loop diuretic in CKD 3b and 4 results in ↓ weight, plasma volume, and BP (*Am J Med* 1982;72:929)
- In ESRD-HD, if still urinates continuing loop diuretic a/w lower IDWG, less ↑ K, and preservation of residual renal function at 1 yr (DOPPS *AJKD* 2007;49:426) and ↓ hospitalization & intradialytic hypotension (*CJASN* 2019;14:95)

Congestive Heart Failure (*Semin Nephrol* 2011;31:503)
- Diuretic resistance from several mechanisms, but afferent vasoconstriction primarily responsible for ↓ diuretic secretion (both → and ↓ shift of dose–response curve)
- Torsemide results in fewer ADHF admissions than furosemide (*Am J Med* 2001;111:513)
- For hospitalized patients, similar results in bolus vs continuous IV dosing of loop diuretics (DOSE *NEJM* 2011;364:797); however, prior study in resistant patients noted increased urine output and less ototoxicity with gtt vs bolus dosing (*JACC* 1996;28:376)
- Combination loop diuretics and thiazide can double FE_{Na} and wt loss, but ↑ risk of ↓ K, ↓ Mg, ↓ Na, ↓ BP, and worsening renal function (WRF) (*JACC* 2010;56:1527)
- Addition of metolazone vs chlorothiazide resulted in similar UOP and adverse events in diuretic resistance in ADHF (*Cardio Therap* 2015;33:42)
- In severe, refractory cases, some evidence to support the use of hypertonic therapy + high-dose loop diuretics (*Eur J Heart Fail* 2000;2:305)

Cirrhosis (*Semin Nephrol* 2011;31:503)
- Combination therapy with loop diuretic and spironolactone, usually in a 2:5 mg dose ratio (*J Clin Gastro* 1981;3 suppl 1:73; *Hepatology* 2003;38:258)
- 90% will have effective management with Na-restriction and this combination
- If CKD or OLT, need less MRB and more loop (100:80 or 100:120) given risk of ↑ K
- Loop diuretic monotherapy is not recommended, except in cases of ↑ K
- Spironolactone monotherapy if K <3.4
- Avoid ↓ K given risk of worsening hyperammonemia (intracellular acid in PCT)
- Hold diuretics for worsening encephalopathy or severe ↓ Na <120
- No role for IV therapy, even in resistant cases (more WRF with IV)
- Amiloride and triamterene less effective than spironolactone (OCTs in PCT)
- Ascites: goals of therapy depend on state of peripheral edema
  w/ peripheral edema → <2 kg/d
  w/o peripheral edema → <0.3–0.5 kg/d (consider paracentesis if symptomatic)

Nephrotic Syndrome (NS)
- Hypoalbuminemia may reduce diuretic delivery and intraluminal albuminuria may bind secreted diuretics (not confirmed in humans) (*JASN* 2000;11:1100)
- Unclear role for coadministration of albumin and furosemide (*KI* 1999;55:629) routinely. Consider albumin if signs of intravascular volume depletion (*CJASN* 2009;4:907)
- Combination with loop diuretics including thiazides, amiloride (filtered plasminogen → plasmin activates ENaC) (*JASN* 2009;20:299)

IMMUNOSUPPRESSIVE THERAPY

PRINCIPLES OF IMMUNOSUPPRESSIVE THERAPY

Glomerular Diseases

- Many glomerular diseases are mediated by immune mechanisms (KI 2014;86:905) and immunomodulating therapy is a mainstay of treatment
- Immunosuppression (IS) therapy is divided into 2 phases in some glomerular disease that relapse frequently (eg, lupus nephritis and ANCA-associated vasculitis)
  Induction therapy: intensive IS to induce remission in proliferative glomerulonephritis (eg, pulse methylprednisolone followed by cyclophosphamide)
  Maintenance therapy: after remission is induced, reduced IS is given to prevent relapse avoiding severe toxicity of IS (eg, AZA, moderate dose MMF)
- Renal dysfunction, hypogammaglobulinemia, and complement loss from proteinuria all ↑susceptibility to infection (AJKD 1994;24:427)
- Gut mucosal edema d/t NS can ↓ PO absorption of medications
- Hypoalbuminemia and proteinuria affect drug metabolism and clearance
- Regimens are tailored to the clinical syndrome being treated, patient compliance (IV or qd instead of multiple dosing if nonadherent), and comorbidities

Comorbidities and Selection of Immunomodulators in Glomerular Diseases		
Comorbidity	Avoid if Possible	May Consider
Advanced CKD	CNI	CS, MMF
DM	CS, Tac	CsA, MMF
Gout	AZA if on xanthine oxidase inhibitor	MMF
Pregnancy	MMF, CYC (contraindicated)	CS, AZA, or CNI

Kidney Transplantation

- IS can be achieved by depleting lymphocytes or blocking lymphocyte response
- T-cell activation post-Tx dependent on 3 responses:
  Signal 1: antigen–T-cell receptor interaction (via CD3 signal)
  Signal 2: costimulation with dendritic cells (via CD80/86:CD28 interaction)
  Signal 3: activation of TOR pathway → cellular proliferation (NEJM 2004;351:2715)
- **Induction therapy:** intense IS in 1st wk post-Tx; can be either lymphocyte depleting (thymoglobulin, alemtuzumab) or nondepleting (basiliximab); CS typically also given
  Risk factors for acute rejection: number of HLA mismatches; younger recipient age; older donor age; African-American race; PRA >0%; presence of DSA; blood group incompatibility; DGF; cold ischemia time >24 hr (AJT 2009;9 suppl3:S8)

Choice of Induction Based on Immunologic Risk Factors for Acute Rejection	
High-risk	Low-risk
Use lymphocyte-depleting agent (ATG more common than alemtuzumab)	Use either lymphocyte-depleting agent or IL2RA
ATG more effective than IL2RA at 1 and 5 yr at preventing acute rejection, though no difference in patient/graft survival (NEJM 2006;355:1967; 2008;359:1736)	Data are mixed whether ATG more effective at preventing rejection c/w basiliximab, though ↑adverse events with ATG (Transplantation 2009;87:1372; Lancet 2016;388:3006)
Early rejection equal between ATG and alemtuzumab, ↑late rejection with alemtuzumab (NEJM 2011;364:1909)	

- **Maintenance therapy:** ongoing IS to prevent acute rejection. Typically 2 or more. Most regimens consist of a CNI (in US ~90% Tac and ~10% CsA) and antimetabolite (in US >90% MMF), +/– CS (in US, ~67%) (AJT 2018;18 suppl1:18).
  If unable to tolerate CNI d/t severe s/e, can convert to mTORi or belatacept
- Nonadherence occurs in ~20% of KTR and is a/w ↑late acute rejection and ↓ graft survival; more common in adolescents (CJASN 2010;5:1305; Transpl Int 2005;18:1121)
- In pts at ↑risk of nonadherence, consider simplified dosing regimen of daily medications (Tac-ER, prednisone, sirolimus, and/or AZA) and/or use of monthly IV belatacept

Infection Screening Prior to IS (CJASN 2018;13:1264)

- ✓ HBsAg, anti-HBc Ab, HCV Ab, HIV Ab, strongyloides Ab
- ✓ PPD and/or IFN-gamma release assay (IGRA)
- IS can cause false (–) in many Ab-detecting and cytokine-based methods. Nucleic acid testing and both of PPD and IGRA should be considered to ↑sensitivity.

CORTICOSTEROIDS (CS)

Mechanisms of Action

- CS refers to a class of steroid hormone and the synthetic analogues that bind to glucocorticoid and mineralocorticoid receptors
- Glucocorticoids bind to the intracellular glucocorticoid receptor → binds to glucocorticoid-responsive element → gene expression regulation → ↑ anti-inflammatory protein, ↓ proinflammatory protein
- ↓ Neutrophil migration to inflammation site; ↑ neutrophil secretion of bone marrow
- Inhibition of the function of APC; Inhibition of the vasodilation; ↓ vascular permeability
- Inhibition of the synthesis of arachidonic acid → ↓ PG and LT

Formulations

Relative Activity and Action Duration of CSs (Allergy Asthma Clin Immunol 2013;9:30)			
Drugs	Glucocorticoid	Mineralocorticoid	Action Duration
Hydrocortisone	1	1	Short (8–12 hr)
Cortisone	0.8	0.8	
Prednisone	4	0.8	Intermediate (12–36 hr)
Prednisolone	4	0.8	
Methylprednisolone	5	0	
Dexamethasone	30	0	Long (36–72 hr)
Betamethasone	30	0	

- Prednisone/prednisolone 5 mg ≈ methylprednisolone 4 mg ≈ hydrocortisone 20 mg
- Physiologic cortisol: peak at 6 AM; equivalent to prednisone 5–7.5 mg/d

Clinical Use and Dose

- Dose early in AM; multiple dose may ↑ s/e (Lancet Diabetes Endocrinol 2018;6:173)
- Tapering: unnecessary if CS used <3 wk. Rapid tapering may ↑ relapse and withdrawal. No consensus on tapering method (J Rheumatol 2013;40:1646).
- RPGN: methylprednisolone 500–1,000 mg or 7–15 mg/kg IV qd ×3 d followed by high-dose PO CS, eg, prednisone 1 mg/kg qd
- Proliferative GN (eg, lupus nephritis, pauci-immune GN): high-dose CS
- Glucocorticoid responsive MCD and FSGS, IgAN: prednisone 2 mg/kg qod or 1 mg/kg qd Adult MCD may require high dose for 4 mo (CJASN 2007;2:445); Avoid use >6 mo
- Acute interstitial nephritis
- Induction and maintenance IS after KT: CS withdrawal is center dependent; 71.8% on CS 1 yr after KT in 2016 (OPTN/SRTR AJT 2018;18 suppl 1:18)
  No consensus on the optimal maintenance dose after KT (KDIGO AJT 2009;9 suppl 3:S1)
  Early steroid withdrawal after transplant performed to avoid long-term s/e of CS
  Early d/c a/w ↑ risk of recurrent GN but no ↑ in graft failure (Transplantation 2011;91:1386)
  In low-risk, early d/c a/w similar patient/graft survival & rejection rates (CJASN 2012;7:494)
  In high-risk, similar findings with early steroid withdrawal (Transplantation 2004;78:1397)
  Late steroid withdrawal after transplant a/w ↑ risk of acute rejection and graft failure
  In pts who have 1st acute rejection after steroid withdrawal, maintenance CS may ↓ risk of 2nd acute rejection and graft failure (AJT 2007;7:1948)
- Acute cellular- and antibody-mediated rejection

Pharmacology

- Metabolized by cytochrome P450 (CYP) 3A4

Infection

- Pneumonia ×5.42, candidiasis ×4.93, sepsis ×3.96, zoster ×2.37 (PLoS Med 2016;13:e1002024)
- Risk is a/w dose (Rheum Dis Clin N Am 2016;42:157)

Adrenal Insufficiency

- 3° adrenal insufficiency from withdrawal of chronic CS use; rare with <3-wk use
- Weakness, fatigue, anorexia, N/V, hyponatremia, hypotension
- Tx: ↑ dose to physiologic dose (prednisone 5–7.5 mg/d) and retry tapering; stress dose CS for surgery and shock

Osteoporosis and Fracture (NEJM 2018;379:2547)

- ↓ eGFR and ↑ albuminuria are a/w fracture (Arch IM 2007;167:133; AJKD 2016;67:218)
- Vitamin D deficiency is common in proteinuria from vitamin D binding protein loss
- CS ↓ bone formation of osteoblasts, ↑ bone resorption of osteoclasts, ↑ RANKL
- Prevention for all taking prednisone ≥2.5 mg/d for ≥3 mo (ACR Arthritis Rheumatol 2017;69:1521)

Glucocorticoid-induced Fracture Risks (ACR Arthritis Rheumatol 2017;69:1521)			
Risk	**Adults ≥40 y/o**	**Adults <40 y/o**	**Management**
Low	FRAX <10%/≤1%	None below	Ca, Vit D, lifestyle
Moderate–High	Prior osteoporotic fracture FRAX >10%/>1% Hip or spine BMD T score ≤–2.5 in ♂ ≥50 y/o and postmenopausal ♀	Prior osteoporotic fracture On prednisone ≥7.5 mg for ≥6 mo **AND** hip or spine BMD Z score <–3 or rapid bone loss ≥10%/yr	Ca, Vit D, lifestyle **PO bisphosphonate**

- If ≥40 y/o ✓FRAX (https://www.sheffield.ac.uk/FRAX/) for 10-yr risk of major osteoporotic and hip fracture
  If prednisone 5–7.5 mg/d, ✓ glucocorticoids use and use reported risks
  If prednisone >7.5 mg/d, ✓ glucocorticoids use and ×1.15 for major osteoporotic, ×1.2 for hip fracture risks
- If <40 y/o and has h/o osteoporotic fracture or has risk factors (malnutrition, significant weight loss or low body weight, hypogonadism, 2° HPT, thyroid disease, FHx of hip fracture, h/o of alcohol use [≥3 units/d] or smoking), ✓BMD w/i 6 mo of the start of CS

- All require optimal Ca (1,000–1,200 mg/d) and vitamin D (600–800 IU/d) intake
- All require lifestyle modifications: balanced diet, maintaining weight in the recommended range, smoking cessation, regular weight-bearing or resistance training exercise, limiting alcohol intake to 1–2 alcoholic beverages/d
- PO bisphosphonates (alen-, iban-, risedronate) are preferred and safer than IV

Other Side Effects
- HBV reactivation: prophylaxis (eg, entecavir 0.5 mg qd) if anti-HBcAb (+) and prednisone dose ≥10 mg/d for ≥4 wk or anti-HBcAb (+), HBsAg (+), and any dose prednisone for ≥4 wk (AGA Guideline Gastroenterology 2015;148:215)
- Hypertension, fluid retention, weight gain, DM, hyperlipidemia, avascular necrosis
- Psychosis, mood change, insomnia
- Atrophic striae, acne vulgaris, myopathy, dermal thinning, cataracts, glaucoma
- GI ulceration/bleeding: unclear association when used w/o NSAIDs (Ann IM 1991;114:735)

ADRENOCORTICOTROPIC HORMONE (ACTH)

Mechanisms of Action
- CS release; melanocortin 1 receptor activation ↓ proteinuria (JASN 2010;21:1290)

Formulations and Dose
- ACTHar® gel: porcine pituitary preparation; 80 IU/mL SC or IM ×2–3/wk
- Synacthen®: synthetic tetracosactide; 1 mg IM ×2/wk; available in Europe

Clinical Use and Side Effects
- MN (AJKD 2006;47:233), other resistant NS (Am J Nephrol 2012;36:58; CJASN 2013;8:2072)
- Cortisol level may remain low due to cortisol-binding globulin loss through proteinuria
- Similar side effects to CS

CALCINEURIN INHIBITORS (CNI)

Mechanisms of Action
- Calcineurin dephosphorylates NFAT → nuclear translocation of NFAT → Transcription of IL-2 and other cytokines and T cell signaling
- Calcineurin dephosphorylates synaptopodin → synaptopodin degradation → motile cytoskeleton of podocytes (Nat Med 2008;14:931)
- Cyclosporine A (CsA) binds to cyclophilin; tacrolimus (Tac) binds to FKBP-12: these complexes inhibit phosphatase activity of calcineurin

Clinical Use
- Maintenance immunosuppression after transplantation; Tac is superior to CsA: less acute rejection, better allograft survival (NEJM 2007;357:2562)
- MCD, FSGS, MN, class V LN (JASN 2009;20:901)
- In native kidney disease, consider avoiding use in advanced CKD, esp severe interstitial fibrosis and tubular atrophy

Formulations and Dose

- CsA modified: neoral®; capsule, solution; initial dose 9–12 mg/kg/d in 2 divided doses
- CsA nonmodified: sandimmune®; capsule, solution, IV
  Conversion from PO to IV: 1/3 of the PO dose
- Tac immediate release (IR): prograf®; start w/ 0.2 mg/kg/d in 2 divided doses
  Conversion from PO IR to SL: 1/2 of the PO dose in divided doses q12h (Transplant Proc 2010;42:4331; Pharmacotherapy 2013;33:31)
  Conversion from PO IR to IV: 1/3 – 1/5 of the PO dose as a continuous infusion over 24 hr. Its correlation with AUC is less known; SL form is preferred.
- Tac extended release (ER): Astagraf XL®, Envarsus XR®; no generic formulation
  Not interchangeable with IR and each other; time peak level and daily AUC differ among formulations. Starting conversion dose from PO IR to PO ER: total daily dose of IR = daily dose of Astagraf; dose of Envarsus XR = 70–80% total daily dose of IR (AJT 2017;17:432)
  Tac ER has similar efficacy to Tac-IR and may have fewer side effects; Envarsus XR may be a/w fewer neurologic s/e than other formulations (Clin Transplant 2015;29:796)
  No difference in allograft survival, acute rejection rates, or renal function among Tac formulations (AJT 2010;10:2632; AJKD 2016;67:648)
  Unclear whether ER formations improve adherence (AJT 2014;14:2796; 2010;10:2632)

Pharmacology and Drug Interaction

- Narrow therapeutic window; needs therapeutic drug monitoring: trough level is preferred

Target Trough Levels (ng/mL) in KT: should be individualized according to rejection risk, renal function, other immunosuppressive agents, and infection risks			
	0–3 mo	**3–6 mo**	**>6 mo**
CsA	250–350	150–250	50–150
Tac	8–12	6–10	5–8

- Unclear above level should be achieved in glomerular diseases
- Mainly metabolized by CYP 3A4 and 5; CsA inhibits CYP; avoid or use with low dose of simvastatin, lovastatin > atorvastatin; rosuvastatin, pitavastatin, and pravastatin are safer
- Due to CYP/P-glycoprotein inhibition, CsA markedly increases colchicine exposure. Use reduced dose of colchicine for prophylaxis and treatment of acute gout attacks in patients on CsA (Arthritis Rheum 2011;63:2226)
- CsA binds to lipoproteins; tac binds to albumin, α1 acid glycoprotein, and RBC; RBC exchange transfuse used for toxicity (Pediatr Nephrol 2011;26:2245)

Factors Affecting Drug Levels of CNI	
Increasing	**Decreasing**
CYP inhibitors: grapefruit juice, pomegranate juice, diltiazem, verapamil, azoles, clarithromycin, erythromycin, protease inhibitors	CYP inducers: rifampin, rifabutin, St. John wort, antiepileptics (phenytoin, barbiturates), nafcillin, cipro, imipenem, ticlopidine, octreotide
Diarrhea: intestinal CYP and p-glycoprotein inhibition (Pediatr Transplant 2005;9:315)	Cinacalcet (NDT 2008;23:1048)
Hepatic impairment	

- Rifampin, phenobarbital, & phenytoin (Case Rep Transplant 2013;2013:375263): used for toxicity

Side Effects

Side Effects of CNIs
Common Side Effects
Nephropathy: afferent vasoconstriction, tubular isometric vacuolization, arteriolar vacuolization, arteriolar hyalinosis, FSGS, TMA, striped interstitial fibrosis
Hypertension: ↑ NCC activity (Nat Med 2011;17:1304), hyperkalemia
Infections: CMV, PML, JC, BK, parvo B19, fungal
Malignancy: skin, lymphoproliferative
Neurotoxicity: tremor, headache, PRES (headache, seizure, posterior MRI lesion), CNI pain syndrome: LEx pain (Clin J Pain 2012;28:556)

More Common in CsA	More Common in Tac
Hirsutism, hyperuricemia, hyperlipidemia, hypertriglyceridemia	N/V/D, anorexia, tremor, headache, alopecia; NODAT (AJT 2007;7:1506)
Gingival hyperplasia: metronidazole (Lancet 1994;343:986) or azithromycin (Transplantation 1998;65:1611) may help	Hypomagnesemia: ↓ TRPM6 (JASN 2004;15:549); ↑ claudin-14 → ↓ paracellular Mg transport (JASN 2014;25:745)
	PTLD (AJT 2004;4:87)

mTOR Inhibitors (Sirolimus and Everolimus)

Mechanism of Action
- Binds to FKBP-12, an intracellular protein → inhibition of mammalian (or mechanistic) target of rapamycin (mTOR), serine/threonine kinase → inhibition of T cell response to cytokines → G1 cell cycle arrest → Inhibition of lymphocyte proliferation
- mTOR signaling is important in pathogenesis of tuberous sclerosis, various cancers, and antiphospholipid Ab-mediated endothelial cell injury (NEJM 2014;371:303)

Clinical Use
- Maintenance IS following KT in combination with CNI ± CS; less commonly CNI avoidance protocols. Used in <5% of recipients in the US (AJT 2018;18 Suppl1:18)
- Often avoided in early postoperative period due to delayed wound healing
- Conversion from CNI to mTORi used as CNI-sparing strategy to preserve renal function after KT and nonrenal solid organ transplantation (NRSOT)
  May be slight improvement in GFR over time but no difference on allograft survival (Transplantation 2017;10:157). KT pts with ↓ GFR or proteinuria at time of conversion less likely to benefit (Transplantation 2009;87:233).
  Baseline proteinuria also reduces chance of renal benefit with mTOR conversion after heart (J Heart Lung Transplant 2012;31:565) and lung Txp (Clin Transplant 2014;28:662). Renal function improves with conversion after liver Txp but there is an increased rate of acute rejection (Transplantation 2016;10:621).
- Switching from CNI to sirolimus ↓ Kaposi's sarcoma (NEJM 2005;352:1317) ↓ new squamous cell carcinoma (NEJM 2012;367:329) ↓ 56% risk NMSC vs CNI (BMJ 2014;349:g6679) after KT. Sirolimus but a/w higher mortality (CJASN 2016;11:1845).
- ↓ angiomyolipoma size in tuberous sclerosis or sporadic lymphangioleiomyomatosis (Lancet 2013;381:817); adjunctive therapy for breast cancer, RCC; ↓ seizure in tuberous sclerosis (Lancet 2016;388:2153)
- Sirolimus ↓ endothelial hyperplasia graft failure in APS (NEJM 2014;371:303)
- Contraindicated in pregnancy

Formulation and Dose
- Sirolimus (rapamycin): Rapamune®; start 1–5 mg qd; Loading dose can be given; trough level goal: 5–15 ng/mL
- Everolimus: Zortress®; 0.75 mg q12h; trough level goal: 3–8 ng/mL

Pharmacology
- Metabolized by CYP3A4 and P-glycoprotein
- ↑ CsA intratubular level; potentiate nephrotoxicity (KI 2006;70:1019)

Side Effects
- Proteinuria, edema, hypertension, AKI: FSGS and TMA (KI Rep 2018 2017;3:281)
- Bone marrow suppression: thrombocytopenia, anemia, leukopenia, neutropenia
- Delayed wound healing/wound dehiscence
- Angioedema when used with ACEi (CJASN 2010;5:703)
- DM, hyperlipidemia, hypertriglyceridemia, lymphoproliferative disorder
- Mucositis/stomatitis, ILD (Transplant Proc 2018;50:933)

Mycophenolate Mofetil (MMF), Mycophenolate Sodium (MPA)

Mechanisms of Action
- MMF metabolized to MPA: inhibits rate-limiting enzyme, inosine monophosphate dehydrogenase in the de novo pathway of purine synthesis; ↓ lymphocyte proliferation

Clinical Use
- Maintenance IS following KT: superior to AZA for graft survival and prevention of acute rejection (Cochrane Database Syst Rev 2015;12:CD007746)
- Lupus nephritis (LN) III and IV induction & maintenance; ANCA vasculitis induction (Ann Rheum Dis 2019;78:399) & maintenance; Interstitial nephritis (CJASN 2006;1:718)
- Contraindicated in pregnancy

Formulations and Dose

- MMF: CellCept®; PO, IV, 1,000 mg q12h for KT
  African American requires higher dose, 1,500 mg q12h (*Transplantation 1997;64:1277*)
  Oral and IV are equivalent
- Enteric-coated (EC) MPA: Myfortic®; 720 mg ≈ MMF 1,000 mg

Pharmacology and Drug Interaction

- Highly (97%) protein bound. Unbound form is active. Primarily liver clearance.

Factors Affecting Drug Levels of MMF/MPA	
Increasing	**Decreasing**
Tacrolimus Hypoalbuminemia/NS Uremia	↓ Absorption: sevelamer, Ca, Mg, iron, H₂ antagonist, PPI (*Rheumatology 2010;49:2061; AJT 2009;9:1650*) CsA: by inhibition of enterohepatic circulation CS (*KI 2002;62:1060*)

- Therapeutic drug monitoring is not routinely performed

Side Effects

- Nausea, abdominal pain, diarrhea: splitting (low frequent dose) and delayed lower GI absorption of EC MPA may lower GI intolerance; can cause colitis with similar appearance to IBD (*Histopathology 2013;63:649*), not related to dose
- Neutropenia, anemia, pure red cell aplasia, teratogenicity, pregnancy loss
- Lymphoma, hypertension, hyperglycemia, hypercholesterolemia
- Infection: esp., herpes virus; no *P. jirovecii* infection from ? protective effect (*Clin Infect Dis 2002;35:53*). Lower risk of serious infection than CYC or CS in LN (*BMC Med 2016;14:137*).

AZATHIOPRINE (AZA)

Mechanism of Action

- Metabolized to 6-mercaptopurine (6-MP) → inhibit *de novo* and salvage pathways for purine synthesis → inhibit DNA replication → inhibit lymphocyte proliferation

Clinical Use

- Maintenance for ANCA vasculitis: superior to MMF w/ more relapse (×1.69) (*JAMA 2010;304:2381*); maintenance therapy for lupus nephritis
- Maintenance immunosuppression following KT
- Relatively safer for pregnancy than MMF and cyclophosphamide

Formulations and Dose

- Imuran® (50 mg), Azasan® (75, 100 mg): 1–3 mg/kg (usually 50–150 mg/d) qd; adjust for WBC

Pharmacology and Drug Interactions

- Metabolized by xanthine oxidase or thiopurine methyltransferase (TPMT)
- TPMT deficiency: ↑ toxicity; enzyme activity, and genotype are ✓ed when initiating AZA in IBD (*AGA Gastroenterology 2017;153:827*). Not routinely ✓ed for KT or glomerular disease.
- Xanthine oxidase inhibitors (allopurinol, febuxostat) ↑ toxicity: avoid co-administration or ↓ AZA dose by 75% and monitor CBC closely

Side Effects

- Myelosuppression, hepatitis, cholestasis, pancreatitis
- Infection: bacterial, fungal, protozoal; lymphoma, PTLD

LEFLUNOMIDE

Mechanism of Action

- Metabolized to teriflunomide → noncompetitive inhibition of dihydroorotate dehydrogenase → inhibit pyrimidine synthesis in lymphocytes

Clinical Use

- Refractory BK nephropathy after KT (*Transplantation 2006;81:704; CJASN 2012;7:1003*)
- BK hemorrhagic cystitis after HSCT (*Acta Haematol 2013;130:52*); resistant CMV infection (*Case Rep Nephrol Dial 2015;5:96*)
- RA; contraindicated in pregnancy

Formulations and Dose

- Arava® (10 mg, 20 mg); Dose 20–40 mg daily; Can give loading dose 100 mg qd × 3 d
- Monitoring of drug levels not routinely performed
- Monitor CBC and LFTs; do not use if ALT >2× ULN

Pharmacology and Drug Interactions

- Active metabolite (teriflunomide) has long terminal half-life as undergoes enterohepatic recirculation; detectable levels may persist in plasma for 2 yr after discontinuation. To eliminate drug rapidly if toxicity develops, give cholestyramine 8 g tid × 11 d or activated charcoal 50 g bid × 11 d.
- May ↑ or ↓ warfarin level through interaction with CYP metabolism; monitor INR
- Due to effect on CYP2C9 may alter levels of glipizide, Celecoxib, and fluvastatin

Side Effects

- Nausea and diarrhea (may be more severe if loading dose given), rash, alopecia
- Leukopenia, anemia, thrombocytopenia: cytopenias more common if concurrent use of other marrow toxic medications. May ↑ INR in pts on warfarin.
- Hepatotoxicity (3× ↑ in AST/ALT) in up to 13%, reversible with d/c, severe liver injury and fatal liver failure are rare. More common in concurrent use of NSAIDs, MTX, or EtOH. If ALT ↑ to >2× ULN, d/c and start cholestyramine wash out (FDA Drug Safety Communication https://www.fda.gov/Drugs/DrugSafety/ucm218679).
- Hypertension: more common with concurrent NSAID use (Arch IM 1999;159:2542)
- ↑ ILD, avoid use if h/o ILD or MTX lung toxicity (Arthritis Rheum 2006;54:1435)
- Peripheral neuropathy: develops after mean 6 mo on Rx, may be reversible if discontinued early after symptoms develop (Clin Pharmacol Ther 2004;75:580)

CYCLOPHOSPHAMIDE (CYC)

Mechanism of Action

- Alkylate DNA → ↓ DNA replication, transcription → cell death of proliferating cells

Clinical Use and Dose

- Indications: induction therapy of lupus nephritis (LN) III, IV, and ANCA GN
- LN NIH IV dose is used for other aggressive forms of proliferative GN, eg, ANCA GN (JASN 1996;7:33), crescentic IgAN (NDT 2003;18:1321)
- Contraindication: pregnancy, untreated infection/malignancy, urinary retention

Cyclophosphamide Doses		
Regimen	**Initial Dose**	**Dose Adjustment**
LN NIH (Lancet 1992;340:741)	IV 0.5–1 g/m² monthly ×6	Start at 0.5 g/m²; adjust for WBC
LN Euro-Lupus (Arthritis Rheum 2002;46:2121)	IV 500 mg q2wk ×6	Not required
LN (CJASN 2009;4:1754)	PO 1–1.5 mg/kg/d (max 150 mg/d) for 2–4 mo	Required
ANCA GN (Ann IM 2009;150:670)	IV 15 mg/kg (max 1.2 g) q2–3 wk until 3 mo after remission	Cr >3.4: ↓ by 2.5 mg/kg 60–70 y/o: ↓ by 2.5 mg/kg >70 y/o: ↓ by 5 mg/kg WBC <3K: ↓ 20%; <2K: ↓ 40%
ANCA GN (Ann IM 2009;150:670)	PO 2 mg/kg/d (max 200 mg/d) until remission, 1.5 mg/kg/d ×3 mo	60–70 y/o: ↓ by 25% >70 y/o: ↓ by 50% WBC <4K: hold and restart when >4K w/ ↓ 25 mg/d
Anti-GBM disease (Ann IM 2001;134:1033)	PO 2–3 mg/kg/d	>55 y/o
MN "Modified Ponticelli regimen" (JASN 1998;9:444)	PO 2.5 mg/kg/d in mo 2,4,6 with CS in mo 1,3,5	Required
MN (NDT 2004;19:1142; BMC Nephrol 2017;18:44)	PO 1.5–2.5 mg/kg/d for 2–12 mo + prednisone ± RTX	Required

- Dose adjustment for renal function: eg, 30% for CrCl <40, 50% for CrCl <20
- Dose adjustment of age: eg, 50% for > 60 y/o; HD removes CYC: dose after HD
- High-dose regimens require dose adjustment to keep WBC >3–4K
- Mesna (2-mercaptoethane sulfonate) 60–100% of CYC dose with IV CYC to prevent hemorrhagic cystitis; no evidence of bladder cancer prevention (Arthritis Rheum 2010;62:9)

Pharmacology

- Prodrug: CYP metabolized to phosphoramide mustard (active metabolite) and acrolein
- All metabolites are excreted by urine; adjust dose for low renal function

Malignancy

Cancer Risk and Different Cumulative Dose of CYC		
Conditions	Dose	Cancer Risk
GPA (n = 293), 9.7 yr f/u (*Rheumatology* 2015;54:1345)	All	×1.9 (all cancer), ×4.0 (NMSC)
	1–36 g	×3.2 (NMSC), no ↑ in other cancer
	>36 g	×2.3 (all cancer), ×4.3 (NMSC), ×12.5 (bladder), ×31.2 (myeloid leukemia)
AAV (n = 119) 5.6 yr f/u (*Ann Rheum Dis* 2017;76:1064)	All	×3.1: Driven by NMSC
	0.1–20 g	×1.91
	>20 g	×5.06
MN (n = 127) 6 yr f/u (*CJASN* 2014;9:1066)	All (37 g)	↑ ×3.2 or ↑ annual risk 0.3–1.0%
	1–20 g	×4.5; no dose incidence correlation

NMSC, nonmelanoma skin cancer

- No established safe cut-off dose
- Prevention: lowest possible dose, lifestyle modification (eg, smoking cessation)
- Screening: at least USPSTF recommended level, urinalysis, CBC, skin exam

Other Side Effects

- Lymphopenia, agranulocytosis; Tx with G-CSF or GM-CSF
- Hemorrhagic cystitis: d/t acrolein; correlate w/ cumulative dose and duration; PO > IV p/w hematuria (microscopic or gross), bladder irritation, blood clot prevention: AM PO dosing; Mesna
- Female infertility: ovarian failure ↑ w/ age and cumulative dose (0% in <30 y/o <10 g; 100% in >40 y/o >30g) (*Arthritis Rheum* 1998;41:831)
  Prevention: GnRH agonists (leuprolide depot 3.75 mg IM, goserelin) 14 d prior to monthly CYC; ↓ amenorrhea (×0.12) in SLE (*Breast Cancer Res Treat* 2010;122:803)
  Ovarian tissue cryopreservation is an option
- Male infertility: azoospermic or severely oligospermic; 72% recover after cumulative dose <7.5 g/m^2 and 11% recover after >7.5 g/m^2 (*Cancer* 1992;70:2703)
  Sperm cryopreservation, testosterone can be used (*Ann IM* 1997;126:292; *AJKD* 2008;52:887)
- SIADH: common with high dose of hypotonic fluid (*NDT* 2010;25:1520)

ANTIBODY AGENTS

- Polyclonal Ab: IVIG, thymoglobulin

Monoclonal Ab Agents		
Chimera (75% human, -ximab)	Humanized (95% human, -zumab)	Human (100% human, -umab)
Basiliximab	Alemtuzumab, Daclizumab,	Belimumab
Rituximab	Eculizumab	Ofatumumab

- All Ab agents can be removed by PLEX; If PLEX is required, infuse Ab regimen after PLEX

Infusion (Related) Reactions

- Common with rituximab, alemtuzumab, antithymocyte globulin (ATG), IVIG
- Mechanisms: Ag–Ab interaction → cytokine release
- Fever, rigors, pruritus, flushing, dyspnea, chest discomfort, N/V/D
- Prevention: acetaminophen, diphenhydramine, and methylprednisolone pretreatment and slow infusion lower incidence
- Tx: hydrocortisone, diphenhydramine, acetaminophen; slow infusion rate

Anaphylaxis

- Rare, but fatal; reported with rituximab, ATG (*Allergy Asthma Clin Immunol* 2017;13:13)
- IgE-mediated type I hypersensitivity reaction
- Urticaria, cough, wheeze, angioedema, throat tightness (laryngeal edema), shock in addition to other symptoms of infusion related reactions
- Lab: ↑ tryptase, DIC
- Tx: d/c infusion, epinephrine 0.2–0.5 mg (1:1,000, 0.2–0.5 mL) IM, O2 ± intubation, IV fluid
- Do not rechallenge w/o proper desensitization (*J Allergy Clin Immunol* 2008;122:57)

INTRAVENOUS IMMUNE GLOBULIN (IVIG)

Mechanism of Action (*CJASN* 2016;11:332)
- Prepared from plasma pooled from healthy donors
- Binding to natural Ab, cytokines; inhibition of complement fixation; inhibition of FcR-mediated recycling of native IgG → anti-inflammatory effects, immunomodulation

Clinical Use
- Desensitization for (+) crossmatch living donor donation, ABO and HLA incompatible living donor KT with rituximab (*NEJM* 2008;359:242)
- AMR: 100 mg/kg after PLEX, followed by rituximab (*AJT* 2009;9:1099)
- Less common: refractory KT rejection: 2 g/kg (*Transplantation* 2001;72:419); BK nephritis (*Transplantation* 2006;8:117)
- Parvovirus B19 prevention and tx (*AJT* 2011;11:196) refractory CMV infection (*AJT* 2013;13:93)
- Premedications: diphenhydramine, acetaminophen

Side Effects
- AKI from osmotic proximal tubular damage with sucrose containing IVIG (*CJASN* 2006;1:844; *AJKD* 2008;51:491), hemolytic anemia: pigment nephropathy (*AJKD* 2010;55:148)
- Hyponatremia d/t water retention (*Clin Exp Nephrol* 2006;10:124), pseudohyponatremia d/t protein load (*NEJM* 1998;339:632); ✓ osm to differentiate
- Thrombosis, MI, aseptic meningitis

ANTITHYMOCYTE GLOBULIN (ATG)

Mechanism of Action
- Polyclonal Ab against human T cells: targets multiple T cell markers; lymphocyte depletion

Clinical Use, Formulation, and Dose
- 1st choice induction immunosuppression in KT in high risk for acute rejection or DGF
- ↓ Acute rejection, similar DGF c/t basiliximab (*NEJM* 2006;355:1967)
- Thymoglobulin® (rabbit origin): preferred in KT; 1.5 mg/kg for 4–10 d for induction (center-dependent); ×7 d for acute cellular rejection (IB, 2A, 2B, 3). Giving total dose as continuous infusion for induction a/w similar outcomes c/w divided daily dosing. Starting infusion intraoperatively a/w ↓ DGF compared with starting postoperatively (*Transplantation* 2008;85:1391; 2003;76:798)
- Atgam® (equine origin): 10–20 mg/kg × 8–14 d for aplastic anemia. Inferior to thymoglobulin when used for induction or treatment of acute rejection after KT (*Transplantation* 1999;67:1011; 1998;66:29)
- Premedications: methylprednisolone, diphenhydramine, acetaminophen
- Dose adjustments to keep lymphocytes <5%, absolute count ≤100; Can follow CD3, CD4
- Keep WBC ≥3, plt >75K; ↓ 50% for WBC 2–3, plt 50–75K; hold for WBC <2, plt <50K

Serum Sickness (*AJKD* 2010;55:141)
- 7–27% in KTR; ↑ with prior rabbit exposure
- Immune complex–mediated type III hypersensitivity reaction
- Clinical manifestation: arthralgia (jaw, temporomandibular joint), fever, rash, malaise
- 7–14 d after ATG initiation; clinical diagnosis
- Tx: Corticosteroids (CS) +/– PLEX

Other Side Effects
- Leukopenia, thrombocytopenia, anemia
- Infusion reactions/cytokine release: fever/chills, ↓ BP, pulmonary edema; anaphylaxis
- PTLD: more than with other induction agents (*AJT* 2007;7:2619)

ALEMTUZUMAB

Mechanism of Action
- Recombinant DNA-derived humanized monoclonal Ab against CD52
- CD52 is expressed on T cells, B cells, monocytes, macrophages, NK cells
- Lymphocyte depleting agent

Clinical Use
- Induction IS in KT (off-label): ↓ early acute rejection in low risk for rejection c/t basiliximab or thymoglobulin. Similar efficacy in high risk KT (*NEJM* 2011;364:1909) ↓ acute rejection (×0.42) c/t basiliximab induction (*Lancet* 2014;384:1684)
- ACR (off-label): may be a/w ↑ risk of infection-related death (*Transplantation* 2009;87:1092)
- Multiple sclerosis, CLL, Sezary syndrome

Formulation and Dose

- Campath®: 30 mg IV × 1–2 d for induction and acute cellular rejection
- Premedications: methylprednisolone, diphenhydramine, acetaminophen

Side Effects

- Leukopenia, pancytopenia, thrombocytopenia, anemia, infusion reactions
- HBV reactivation (high risk)
- Autoimmune thyroid disease and thrombocytopenia; not ↑ recurrent glomerular disease (*Transplantation* 2007;83:1429)
- Anti-GBM disease: a/w higher dose than standard KT dose 30 mg (*NEJM* 2008;359:768)

BASILIXIMAB/DACLIZUMAB

Mechanism of Action

- Interleukin-2 receptor antagonists (IL2RAs); Humanized monoclonal Ab against IL-2 receptor α chain (CD25) on T cells → inhibits IL-2 mediated actions
- Nonlymphocyte depleting agent

Clinical Use, Formulation, and Dose

- Basiliximab (Simulect®): 20 mg IV on d 0 and on d 3 or 4; daclizumab: withdrawn
- Induction IS in KT with low immunologic risk (eg, 2 haplotype match living donor): ↓ acute rejection rate and graft loss c/t placebo. No difference in graft loss or clinical acute rejection, ↑ biopsy-proven acute rejection at 1 yr, ↓ s/e and malignancy c/t antithymocyte globulin (*Cochrane Database Syst Rev* 2010;CD003897)
- History or expected thymoglobulin intolerance (eg, cardiopulmonary disease)

Side Effects

- Infections, lymphoproliferative disorders

BELATACEPT

Mechanism of Action

- Humanized fusion protein monoclonal Ab, CTLA-4Ig: Fc fragment of human IgG1 + extracellular domain of CTLA-4 (CD152): competitively inhibit CD28 on T cell
- CD28 on T cells binding to B7-1 (CD80) or B7-2 (CD86) on APCs → ↑ T cell activity
- CTLA-4 on T cells binding to B7-1 or B7-2 → ↓ T cell activity
- CTLA-4 is constitutively expressed on regulatory T cells

Clinical Use, Formulation, and Dose

- Nulojix®
- *De novo* IS after KT: used in combination with MMF and prednisone as CNI-sparing regimen. Higher 1-yr acute rejection rate than CsA, but higher eGFR and patient/ graft survival than CsA (*NEJM* 2016;374:333)
  10 mg/kg on d 1, 5, at the end of wk 2, 4, 8, & 12, then 5 mg/kg q4wk beginning at wk 16
- Conversion from CNI-based regimen following KT: ↑ acute rejection in 1st yr, slight ↑ eGFR at 3 yr, no difference in patient/allograft survival (*CJASN* 2011;6:430; *AJKD* 2017;69:587)
  5 mg/kg on d 1, 15, 29, 43, 57, then 5 mg/kg every 4 wk. Reduce CNI dose by 50% on d 15, discontinue d 29. Slower taper of CNI may be a/w ↓ risk of rejection. CNI should be reduced slowly every 2 wk (no reduction on d 1, 50% reduction on d 15, 80% reduction on d 23, discontinue d 29)
- ✓ EBV IgG: must be (+) due to ↑ risk of PTLD in IgG (–) pts

Side Effects

- PTLD (predominantly involving the CNS), anemia, and leukopenia
- Diarrhea, increased risk of infection: CMV, HSV, fungal, protozoal

BELIMUMAB

Mechanism of Action

- Human monoclonal Ab against the soluble form of a B cell survival factor, B cell-activating factor (BAFF, aka B lymphocyte stimulator, BLyS)

Clinical Use and Side Effects

- Approved for active autoantibody-positive SLE (*Lancet* 2011;377:721)
- ↓ Serum BLyS level but did not reduce naïve B cell number in KTR (*Lancet* 2018;391:2619)
- May lower proteinuria in lupus nephritis (*Autoimmun Rev* 2017;16:287)
- Side Effects: infusion reactions

RITUXIMAB (RTX)

Mechanism of Action

- Chimeric murine monoclonal Ab against CD20 on B lymphocytes
- Prevent SMPDL-3b downregulation in podocytopathy (Sci Transl Med 2011;3:85ra46)
- Inhibit of B cell derived IL-4 mediated proteinuria (JCI Insight 2017;81836)

Clinical Use

- ANCA vasculitis: induction (RAVE NEJM 2010;363:221; RITUXIVAS NEJM 2010;363:211) and maintenance (NEJM 2014;371:1771); refractory LN; cryoglobulinemia (Arthritis Rheum 2012;64:843), MCD, FSGS (NEMO JASN 2014;25:850), MN (MENTOR NEJM 2019;381:36; JASN 2017;28:348)
- Induction IS for (+) crossmatch living donor donation, ABO and HLA incompatible living donor KT with lymphocyte depleting agents, IVIG (NEJM 2008;359:242) and PLEX
- Antibody-mediated rejection (ABMR): with CS, IVIG, and PLEX

Formulation and Dose

- Rituxan: 1,000 mg ×2, 2 wk apart; 375 mg/m^2 ×4, weekly; 375 mg/m^2 ×1 eg, for ABMR
- Can redose if CD19(+) cell is not depleted (>5–10 cells/mm^3) or lymphocytes >1%
- ✓ HBsAg, HBsAb, HBcAb prior to administration

HBV Serology Interpretation and Rituximab Administration (Hepatology 2018;67:1560)			
HBsAg	HBsAb	HBcAb	Management
–	–	–	Administer rituximab Vaccination prior to rituximab or 6–12 mo after
–	+	–	Administer rituximab; HBV immunized
–	+	+	Administer rituximab with prophylaxis
–	–	+	✓r/o window period (HBc IgM +) Administer rituximab with prophylaxis Vaccination if not from area of intermediate or high endemicity
+	–	+	Hold rituximab; ✓ALT, HBeAg, HBV DNA Refer to hepatology

- Premedications: acetaminophen, diphenhydramine, methylprednisolone 100 mg (Arthritis Rheum 2006;54:1390)
- Slow infusion (first dose, ≥3 mo since previous dose or poorly tolerated previous infusion): Start at 50 mg/hr; ↑ by 50 mg/hr q30min; max 400 mg/hr
- Standard infusion (previously well tolerated infusion <3 mo): Start at 100 mg/hr; ↑ by 100 mg/hr q30min; max 400 mg/hr

HBV Reactivation (Hepatology 2018;67:1560; Gastroenterology 2017;152:1297)

- Reappearance or ↑ of HBV DNA or reverse seroconversion of HBsAg
- p/w impaired synthetic function (TBil >3, INR >1.5), ascites, encephalopathy, and death
- Risk factors: HBsAg (12.3% vs 1.7% w/o HBsAg), high baseline HBV DNA level, HBeAg, chronic hepB; HBsAb (–) (14% vs 5% w/ HBsAg) (Hepatology 2017;66:379)
- Rituximab ↑ risk of reactivation: 24% w/o HBsAb, 5.6% w/ HBsAb (Hepatology 2017;66:379)
- Prophylaxis: see prophylaxis chapter; Tx: HBV treatment

Progressive Multifocal Leukoencephalopathy (PML)

- Subacute demyelinating CNS infection caused by JC virus reactivation
- Multiple cases reported in HIV, hematologic malignancy, SLE and RA; Incidence 4/100,000 in rituximab-treated RA vs 0.4/100,000 in untreated RA (Joint Bone Spine 2012;79:351)
- Many cases in SLE were found w/ minimal IS w/o RTX or alkylating agent (Autoimmun Rev 2008;8:144); Rarely in GPA treated with CYC and CS (JAMA 1992;268:600)
- No report in MCD, FSGS, and MN
- Cognitive impairment, motor weakness (hemiparesis, ataxia), vision or speech problems
- Median survival in PML w/o HIV is 3 mo (Ann Neurol 2006;60:162)
- MRI: unifocal or multifocal white matter lesion; JC virus DNA in brain biopsy or CSF
- Tx: reduction of IS; allogenic BK virus specific T cells (NEJM 2018;379:1443)

Other Side Effects

- Infusion reactions: fever, chills, rash, itching, mild wheezing; 28% in MN (JASN 2012;23:1416); common with 1st dose; prevented by slow infusion and premedications Tx: slow rate or hold infusion and resume if symptoms resolve
- Anaphylaxis: urticaria, hypotension, angioedema, hypoxia, bronchospasm, stridor Tx: d/c RTX, epinephrine 0.2–0.5 mg (1:1,000, 0.2–0.5 mL) IM, O2 ± intubation, IV fluid Ofatumumab: human monoclonal CD20 Ab; successfully used after anaphylaxis associated with rituximab (NEJM 2018;378:92)
- Rarely pulmonary infiltrates, ARDS, MI, VF, cardiogenic shock, or death

- Serum sickness (Semin Arthritis Rheum 2015;45:334): fever, rash, arthralgia; type III hypersensitivity reaction 7–21 d after infusion; low complement; Tx: CS
- Blunted immune response to vaccination (JACI 2011;128:1295)
- Hypogammaglobulinemia: esp low IgM; ↑ with repeated cycle (J Rheumatol 2010;37:558)
- Leukopenia (even 3–6 mo after administration), anemia
- Not a/w ↑ malignancy (Ann Rheum Dis 2017;76:1064)

ECULIZUMAB

Mechanism of Action
- Monoclonal Ab against C5; inhibition of C5 cleavage to C5a (neutrophil chemoattractant) and C5b (component of membrane attack complex)

Clinical Use and Dose
- Monitoring (goal): CH50 (<10% of nl), alternative pathway hemolytic activity/AH50 (M 10% of nl), eculizumab trough level (50–100 mcg/mL); sC5b-9 may remain detectable, not recommended for monitoring (KI 2017;91:539)
- aHUS: IV eculizumab 900 mg weekly ×4, 1,200 mg 1 wk later, then every 2 wk; supplemental 600 mg w/i 60 min after each TPE
- PNH: IV eculizumab 600 mg weekly ×4, 900 mg 1 wk later, then every 2 wk
- Off-label use: C3G (CJASN 2012;7:748), refractory APS (Arthritis Rheum 2012;64:2719; Case Rep Hematol 2014;704371); recurrence prevention of APS after KT (NEJM 2010;362:1744)
- Off-label use: prevention and treatment of acute AMR (Transplantation 2019;PMID: 30801549), chronic AMR (AJT 2017;17:682) and desensitization (AJT 2011;11:2405)

Prophylaxis (Curr Opin Infect Dis 2016;29:319)
- Meningococcal vaccination: **both** polysaccharide quadrivalent and serogroup B vaccines (can be given simultaneously at different sites) >2 wk prior to the 1st dose; if <2 wk, give penicillin VK 250–500 mg bid or ciprofloxacin 500 mg qd until 4 wk after last vaccine
  - Meningococcal polysaccharide quadrivalent conjugate vaccine (MenACWY): MCV4-D (Menactra®) or MCV4-CRM (Menveo®), 2 doses, 8 wk apart; boost every 5 yr
  - Meningococcal serogroup B vaccine (MenB): MenB-4C (Bexsero®, 2 doses 1 mo apart) or MenB-FHbp (Trumenba®, 0, 2, and 6 mo) (MMWR 2015;64:608)
- Pneumococcal vaccine: PCV13 and PPSV23; Haemophilus influenzae vaccine

Side Effects
- Infection: encapsulated bacteria esp, meningococcus (MMWR 2016;65:696)
- IgG2 and IgG4 κ staining of eculizumab: not pathogenic (JASN 2012;23:1229)

PROPHYLAXIS

VACCINATIONS

- CKD (AJKD 2012;59:356), NS (AJKD 1994;24:427), and immunosuppression (IS) ↑ risk of infection
- IS decreases efficacy of the vaccine: eg, it takes ~1 yr to regain immune response after rituximab (J Allergy Clin Immunol 2011;1288:1295); it may take longer depending on disease: eg, ANCA (Arthritis Res Ther 2017;19:101)
- More vaccines are recommended than non-CKD population; vaccination should be started prior to IS and progression to advanced CKD

Recommendation Based on Vaccine Type (IDSA CID 2014;58:309; AJT 2013;13 Suppl 4:311)		
	Inactivated Vaccines	Live Vaccines
Vaccine	PCV13, PPSV23, Tdap/Td Inactivated influenza, RZV, HPV	MMR, Varicella, ZVL
Prior to IS/KT	Ideally ≥2 wk prior to the initiation	Ideally ≥4 wk prior to the initiation
During IS	Recommended if indicated	Contraindicated
After KT	Recommended if indicated Usually 2–6 mo after KT If influenza outbreak, 1 mo after KT (AJT 2011;11:2020)	Contraindicated
Household and close contacts	Recommended if indicated	Recommended if indicated If rash develops after ZVL or varicella, avoid contact and consider antiviral prophylaxis

Vaccination Indication (R: Recommended; X: Contraindicated)		
http://www.cdc.gov/vaccines, (KDIGO CKD 2012; IDSA CID 2014;58:309; AJT 2013;13 Suppl 4:311)		
Vaccine	CKD	On IS/KTR
Influenza, inactive	R: annually	
Tdap/Td	R: Tdap ×1, Td q10y	
MMR	R if born in 1957 or later	X
Varicella	R if born in 1980 or late	X
RZV	R if ≥50 y/o	Insufficient data
HPV	R if ♀ ≤26 y/o ♂ ≤21 y/o	
Pneumococcal	R	
HBV	R for eGFR <30	

Zoster Vaccine
- Recombinant zoster vaccine (RZV, Shingrix®) is recommended for nonimmunosuppressed ≥50 y/o regardless of past zoster infection or zoster vaccine live (ZVL) vaccination history
- RZV: contains adjuvant suspension that boosts T-cell function. Theoretical graft rejection and glomerular disease flare up were not well studied.
- ZVL: is contraindicated in pts on IS and KTR. Disseminated zoster on low level IS (MMWR 2017;66:763) and a fatal case (BMJ Case Rep 2016;PMID 27147629) reported.

Pneumococcal Vaccine
- Recommended for all adult CKD including <65 y/o, pts on IS and KTR

Pneumococcal Vaccine in CKD (eGFR <30) and Immunocompromised States	
Prior Vaccine	Indicated Vaccine
None	PCV13 → PPSV23 ≥8 wk later then 2nd PPSV23 ≥5 yr later
1 dose of PPSV23	PCV13 ≥1 yr after the PPSV23 then PPSV23 ≥8 wk after PCV13 and ≥5 yr after the 1st PPSV23
2 doses of PPSV23	PCV13 ≥1 yr after the most recent dose of PPSV23
PCV13	PPSV23 ≥8 wk after PCV13 then 2nd PPSV23 ≥5 yr after the 1st PPSV23
PCV13 and 1 dose of PPSV23	2nd PPSV23 ≥8 wk after PCV13 and ≥5 yr after the 1st PPSV23

- If the most recent dose of PPSV23 was at age <65 yr, at age ≥65 yr, administer a dose of PPSV23 ≥8 wk after PCV13 and ≥5 yr after the last dose of PPSV23
- PCV13 to PPSV23 interval should be ≥1 yr for those indicated only by age ≥65

Hepatitis B Vaccine
- CKD patients have reduced immune response to vaccination: 50–60% vs 90% in non-CKD (AJKD 1998;32:1041); require higher dose
- ✓ Anti-HBsAb 1–2 mo after series in (pre)dialysis and immunocompromised patients
  If anti-HBsAb <10 mIU/mL, repeat another series
  If annual anti-HBs Ab falls to <10 mIU/mL, Recombivax HB® or Engerix-B® 40 mcg ×1
- Surveillance in HD: monthly HbsAg if anti-HBs Ab <10 mIU/mL
  HBsAg could be (+) after vaccination; do not ✓ w/i 3–4 wk (JASN 1996;7:1228)
  (+) HBsAg: use dedicated machine at isolated room
  Unknown HBsAg: bleach disinfection of dialysis machine

Recommended HBV Vaccination Dose (mcg) and Schedule (mo)			
Conditions	Recombivax HB®	Engerix-B®	Heplisav-B®
Non-CKD	10; 0, 1, 6	20; 0, 1, 6	20; 0, 1
Immunocompromised	40; 0, 1, 6	40; 0, 1, 6	Insufficient data
(Pre)dialysis	40; 0, 1, 6	40; 0, 1, 2, 6	Insufficient data

Antimicrobial Prophylaxis for Patients on Immunomodulators	
CMV (AJT 2013;13 Suppl 4:93)	After KT, Valganciclovir (adjusted for CrCl) for at least 6 mo in high risk (D+/R−) and 3 mo in intermediate risk (R+); consider 3 mo in low risk (D−/R−) Also prevent HSV1, HSV2, EBV, VZV, HHV6,7,8
Pneumocystis jirovecii	After KT, TMP/SMZ SS (80/400 mg) qd × 1 yr (prevents also UTI, listeria, and nocardia infection) If sulfa allergy, dapsone 100 mg qd (✓G6PD before; s/e: methemoglobinemia) (Cancer 2011;117:3484) or atovaquone 1,500 mg qd (AJT 2013;13 Suppl 4:272) No consensus in IS use for nontransplantation setting. One recommendation is TMP/SMZ DS (160/800 mg) ×3/wk in pts receiving an equivalent of prednisone >16 mg qd × ≥8 wk (NEJM 2004;350:2487; Rheum Dis Clin N Am 2016;42:157)
Candida (AJT 2009;9 suppl 3:62)	After KT, fluconazole or clotrimazole (may ↑ CNI and mTORi level; monitor level), or nystatin 4–6 mL bid. Total prophylaxis for 1–3 mo.
Latent TB (AJT 2013;13 Suppl 4:68)	If positive PPD or IGRA (QuantiFERON gold®) Isoniazid 300 mg qd × 9 mo with pyridoxine 25–50 mg qd or Rifampin 10 mg/kg (max 600) × 4 mo (NEJM 2018;379:440); may ↓ CNI level: monitor level of CNI

PROPHYLAXIS 3-29

HBV PROPHYLAXIS (Gastroenterology 2015;148:215; AJT 2015;15:1162)

HBV Reactivation Risk and Management in anti-HBcAb (+) Patients (AGA Guideline Gastroenterology 2015;148:215; Gastroenterology 2017;152:1297)			
Category	HBsAg[a]	Immunomodulator	Management
High (>10%)	+ or −	Rituximab, ofatumumab, alemtuzumab	Prophylaxis
	+	Prednisone >20 mg/d	
	+	Prednisone 10–20 mg/d Prednisone <10 mg/d for ≥4 wk	
Moderate (1–10%)	+	CNI	Prophylaxis or Monitor[b]
	−	CNI	
	−	Prednisone >20 mg/d	
Low (<1%)	+ or −	Azathioprine	Monitor[b]
	+	Prednisone <10 mg/d for <4 wk	
	−	Prednisone <20 mg/d	

[a]If HBsAg (+), consider obtaining hepatology consult; HBV DNA ≥2,000 U/mL and ALT elevation: Chronic hepatitis B requiring treatment

[b]Monitor: ✓HBsAg, ALT, HBV DNA q3mo

- Regimen:
  Entecavir 0.5 mg qd (if CrCl 30–50 q48h; if CrCl 10–30 q72h; if CrCl <10 qwk)
  Tenofovir alafenamide (TAF): 25 mg qd (avoid if CrCl <15); better renal function than TDF (Lancet Gastroenterol Hepatol 2016;1:185; J Hepatol 2018;68:672)
  Tenofovir disoproxil fumarate (TDF): avoid for proximal tubulopathy
  Lamivudine: avoid for resistance
- Start: 2–4 wk before initiation of IS
- End: ≥12 mo of last dose of B cell-depleting agent (eg, rituximab) or ≥6 mo others; reactivation beyond 12 mo has been reported in malignancy (Leuk Res 2018;50:46)
- Prophylaxis is a/w 87% and 83% reduction of reactivation and hepatitis flares, respectively (Gastroenterology 2015;148:221); reactivation rarer with HBsAg (−) pts (JCO 2013;31:2765)

- The kidneys are vulnerable to injury from exogenous toxins d/t to their filtration, concentration, and metabolism; ↓ clearance in CKD may cause ↑ toxicity
- Older adults use OTC (42%), dietary supplements (49%) frequently (JAMA 2008;300:2867)
- 1/12 US adults is taking ≥1 harmful supplement with kidney disease (AJKD 2013;61:739)
- Herbal supplements are not regulated by FDA for content or purity; Side effects may rise from contaminants, such as heavy metals
- Purpose of the medicine may give clues: pain control (analgesic nephropathy, salicylate intoxication), diuretic (salt wasting, hypokalemia, volume depletion)
- Renal toxicity could be from other organ injury: hepatorenal syndrome from hepatotoxic substance, rhabdomyolysis from seizure evoking component
- Lists of herbal supplements to avoid in CKD, hyperkalemia, and hyperphosphatemia: https://www.kidney.org/atoz/content/herbalsupp

HERBAL AND DIETARY SUPPLEMENTARY AGENTS

Aristolochic Acid
- Source: aristolochia plant containing slimming Chinese herbs; flour in Balkan endemic nephropathy (BEN): endemic in Bosnia, Croatia, Bulgaria, and Romania
- pRTA, tubular proteinuria, concentrating capacity impairment, interstitial fibrosis/tubular atrophy, cellular atypia
- Renal insufficiency is a/w cumulative dose; may progress after d/c
- TCC: ↑ lifelong risk; the renal pelvis, ureter > bladder: cystoscopy not sufficient (NEJM 2000;342:1686); 52.9% after txp during 27 mo f/u (Urol Int 2009;83:200)
- Tx: GC may be tried in early nephropathy (AJKD 1996;27:209)
- Cancer surveillance: yearly CT + ureteroscopy
- Bilateral nephroureterectomy prior to LDKT or DDKT listing (Ann IM 2013;158:469)

Herbal, Supplementary, or Nonprescription Agents and Renal Toxicity		
Substance	Used for	Renal Toxicity
Bee pollen	Appetite, stamina	AIN
Cat's claw	Anti-inflammatory	AIN
Chromium picolinate	Glc, lipid, wt control	ATN, AIN
Cranberry	UTI	Oxalate nephropathy/nephrolithiasis
Creatine	Muscle performance	AIN
Djenkol Bean	Meal in Southeast Asia	AKI, needle-like crystals
Ephedra (Ma-Huang)	Allergy, weight loss	HTN, urinary stone
Flavonoid	Vascular disease	ATN
Germanium	Immunity	ATN
Glucosamine	Joint pain	AIN
Glycyrrhiza (Licorice)	Anti-inflammatory, sweet taste	AME (HTN, hypokalemia, metabolic alkalosis)
Larrea tridentata (Chaparral)	Joint pain, weight loss	RCC
Mg trisilicate	Antacids	Silicate calculi
Quinine	Drink (Tonic water), cramp	TMA (NEJM 2017;376:74); 33% of drug-induced TMA (Blood 2015;125:616)
Rough Bark (guaifenesin)	Chest congestion, cough	Urinary stone
Star fruit (carambola)		Oxalate nephropathy (AJKD 2001;37:418) Delirium, hiccups, vomiting, paresis in CKD; dialyzable (NDT 2003;18:120)
Sugar sweetened beverages		↑ CKD (CJASN 2019;14:49)
Triptolide (Thunder God Vine)	Anti-inflammatory	Hypotension, ATN
Vitamin C	Cold	Oxalate nephropathy/nephrolithiasis
Vitamin D		Milk alkali syndrome/hypercalcemia
Willow Bark (salix daphnoides)	Pain	Papillary necrosis
Wormwood	Digestion	AKI, rhabdomyolysis
Yohimbine	Erectile dysfunction	AKI, drug induced lupus

Drugs of Abuse

- IVDU is a/w interstitial inflammation and renal parenchymal calcification (AJKD 2014;63:945)

Tobacco
- Current smoking ↑ risk of CKD (34%) and ESRD (51%) (NDT 2017;32:475)
- a/w nodular glomerulosclerosis (Hum Pathol 2002;33:826), glomerular hyperfiltration & proteinuria (CJASN 2011;6:2462); passive smoking ↑ CKD (CJASN 2019;14:515)

Heroin
- Heroin-associated nephropathy: FSGS, AA amyloidosis (95% used heroin in the Pacific Northwest) (CJASN 2018;13:1030) from recurrent infection and inflammation. Declined with high-purity heroin.
- Possibly a/w ApoL1 nephropathy, HIV, HCV-mediated renal lesions
- Rhabdomyolysis; heroin crystal nephropathy (CKJ 2015;8:339); CKD (Am J Nephrol 2016;44:447)

Oxymorphone
- Injection of reformulated Opana ER®: TMA (MMWR 2013;62:1; AJKD 2014;63:1022), HIV, HCV
- PLEX was tried, but unnecessary (AJH 2014;89:695)

Cocaine
- Rhabdomyolysis, malignant hypertension; hypertensive and ischemic damage (AJKD 2014;63:945), renal infarction (Clin Nephrol 2009;72:234), AIN (CJASN 2008;52:792)
- ANCA GN (very high MPO or MPO and PR3) w/ skin ulcer: contaminated levamisole (CJASN 2011;6:2799); hyponatremia (Clin Nephrol 2011;75:11)

Methylenedioxymethamphetamine (Ecstasy) (CJASN 2008:3:1852; NDT 2013;28:2277)
- Amphetamine derivative: release serotonin, dopamine, norepinephrine
- Hyponatremia: ↑ ADH secretion + polydipsia (thirst, hyperpyrexia, ready availability of fluids and ↓ GI motility → water absorption); common in single, first use in young ♀
- AKI: nontraumatic rhabdomyolysis, liver failure, and vasculitis
- Cerebral edema, pulmonary edema, hypertension, arrhythmia

Anabolic Steroid (JASN 2010;21:163)
- Used by bodybuilders with high-protein diet
- RI, proteinuria (1.3–26.3 g/d), NS (3/10); Can improve w/ d/c and recur with reuse
- Biopsy: FSGS, collapsing or perihilar, 15–95% foot process effacement

Cannabis (Marijuana)
- Cannabinoid hyperemesis syndrome is associated with heavy daily use of marijuana; AKI (mainly prerenal azotemia) has rarely been reported in such pts
- Synthetic ("designer") drugs that do not appear on urine toxicology screen have also been associated with AKI (MMWR 2013;62:93; CJASN 2013;8:523)
- Biopsy: ATN, AIN (CJASN 2014;9:1996); AKI resolved w/o RRT
- Brodifacoum associated ↑ INR, gross hematuria and abdominal pain; renal imaging abnormalities: perinephric stranding, dilatation of collecting system (NEJM 2018;379:1216)
- a/w DKA in T1DM (×1.98) (JAMA IM 2019;179:115)

Synthetic Cathinone (Bath Salts)
- Not detected on toxicology screen
- AKI, rhabdomyolysis, hyperuricemia (AJKD 2012;59:273)
- DIC, liver failure, multiorgan failure, coagulopathy (some contains vitamin K antagonist)

Metals

Aluminum (KDOQI MBD 2003; KDIGO MBD 2009)
- Source: aluminum-containing phosphate binder and antacid, dialysate contamination
- Dementia, osteomalacia, bone and muscle pain, iron-resistant microcytic anemia, hypercalcemia, and neurologic abnormalities
- Rare d/t less use of aluminum hydroxide, improved water purification, high flux dialyzers
- Dx: ✓Serum level; if 20–200 μg/L, ✓deferoxamine stimulation test (+ if increase in serum aluminum of >50 μg/L 2 d after infusion)
- Prevention: avoid aluminum-containing drug and citrate (↑ GI aluminum absorption)
- Tx: daily HD w/ high flux dialyzer if baseline >200 μg/L; deferoxamine if stimulation test+

Cadmium
- Source: battery, metal alloy plants, glass, contaminated rice, cigarette smoke
- Itai-itai disease: osteoporosis, osteomalacia, and kidney damage
- Tubular proteinuria (eg, β2-micoglobulin), pRTA/Fanconi syndrome, hypercalciuria, stone, chronic TIN, glomerular ischemia, HTN
- Occupational exposure is a/w ESRD (×2.3) (AJKD 2001;38:1001)

Lead

- Source: foundry, paint (pre-1978 building), gasoline (removed in 1980s), diet, drinking water, smoking, dust, soil
- Organic cation transport system at PCT reabsorbs lead; mitochondrial damage
- Stored in bones; half-life is decades
- Acute toxicity: pRTA (inclusion body in PT cells)/Fanconi syndrome, hemolytic anemia, peripheral neuropathy
- Chronic toxicity: triad of gout, HTN and CKD (chronic TIN); nephrolithiasis, CKD progression (NEJM 2003;348:277); CVD (Lancet Public Health 2018;3:e177)
- High level is a/w lower kidney function (JAMA IM 2010;170:75; AJKD 2018;72:381)
- Chelation (JAMA 2013;309:1241) controversial; High-dose EDTA is a/w AKI

Other Metals and Renal Toxicity		
Metal	Source	Manifestation
Chromium	Contaminated food and water	CKD esp with lead and cadmium (KI 2017;92:720)
Mercury	Battery, alloy, mirror plants	Chronic TIN, ATN, pRTA, MN
Arsenic	Food, water, mining, pesticide, wood preservatives	TIN, ATN; CKD, proteinuria (AJKD 2017;70:787)
		CVD (Ann IM 2013;159:649)
	Seafood containing organic form is less toxic	Kidney, bladder, lung cancer (JNCI 2018;110:241)
Gold	Medical use (RA)	MN
Platinum	Medical use (cancer)	ATN (apoptosis and necrosis)

ENVIRONMENTAL SUBSTANCE

- Particulate matter air pollution is a/w ↑ CKD and ESRD (JASN 2018;29:218) and ↑ MN; PLA2R was (+) in 83% (JASN 2016;27:3739)
- Pathogenesis: inflammation, oxidation stress, coagulability (Nat Rev Nephrol 2018;14:313)
- Silica exposure is a/w ANCA vasculitis (CJASN 2007;2:290) and CKD (Ren Fail 2012;34:40)

Renal Effects of Environmental Chemicals	(Nat Rev Nephrol 2015;11:610)
Phthalates	↑ Albuminuria, BP; used in IV tubing; level may ↑ ×9 after HD
Bisphenol A	↑ Albuminuria, BP; used in IV tubing; levels high in HD, PD pts
Dioxins	↑ Albuminuria, BP, uric acid, ↓ eGFR
Polychlorinated biphenyls	↑ Albuminuria, BP, uric acid, ↓ eGFR
Perfluorinated chemicals	↑ BP, uric acid, ↓ eGFR (CJASN 2018;13:1479)
Melamine	Radiolucent stone, ↓ eGFR

EXERCISE AND HEAT

- Sweat is hypotonic: ↑ Na (28%) > ↓ Na (5%) (Am J Clin Pathol 2009;132:336)
- Heat stroke: AKI, rhabdomyolysis

Exercise-associated Hyponatremia (EAH) (Clin J Sport Med 2015;25:303)
- Occurs often in endurance events in 6% (PNAS 2005;102:18550)
- Risk factors: high fluid intake w/ weight gain, NSAIDs use, low BMI
- Pathogenesis: excessive water intake with hypotonic fluid >water loss; ADH secretion
- Manifestation: asymptomatic, weakness, headache, N/V, seizure, coma, cerebral edema
- Tx: if mild, oral hypertonic saline; if severe 100 mL 3% (51 mEq) NaCl or 50 mL 8.4% (50 mEq) NaHCO₃ over 10 min; can repeat ×2; avoid hypo- or isotonic fluid
- Prevention: "drink to thirst"

Mesoamerican Nephropathy (CKD of Unknown Etiology, CKDu)
- Endemic in Central America (El Salvador, Nicaragua, Costa Rica) (AJKD 2012;59:531), Sri Lanka (CJASN 2019;14:224), Uddanam in India (AJKD 2016;68:344)
- Potential pathogenesis: recurrent dehydration (hyperosmolarity)-induced aldose reductase (polyol pathway) leading to glucose to sorbitol and fructose, hyperthermia, volume depletion → "Heat stress nephropathy" (CJASN 2016;11:1472)
- Risk factors of rapid GFR decline: outdoor work, agricultural work, lack of shade availability during work break (JASN 2018;29:2200)
- Manifestation: ↓ Na, K, Mg, ↑ uric acid, low-grade proteinuria
- Bx: glomerular ischemic injury, interstitial fibrosis, and tubular atrophy (AJKD 2017;69:626)

PLASMA EXCHANGE (PLEX)

Apheresis

- Extracorporeal treatment that removes blood components
- Therapeutic plasma exchange (PLEX) is a type of apheresis that removes plasma and replaces with allogenic plasma, colloid, or crystalloid. PLEX can be performed using highly permeable filter with standard HD equipment or a centrifugation device.
- Membrane used for apheresis has pore size of 0.2 μm with MW cut-off ~2,000 kDa

Substances Removed by Apheresis

- PLEX: proteins (cryoglobulin, Ig including Ab form drugs), complement components, immune complex, cytokines, drugs w/ Vd <0.2 L/kg and protein binding >80% (*Plasma Ther Transfus Technol* 1984;5:305)

  Rituximab can be given 24–36 hr before PLEX (*Am J Clin Pathol* 2006;125:592)

Drug Removal by PLEX (Pharmacotherapy 2007;11:1529)	
Removed	**Unlikely or Not Removed**
Cisplatin, Vincristine, Propranolol, Verapamil, Diltiazem, Dalteparin, Lepirudin, Ampicillin, Ceftriaxone, Tobramycin, Gentamicin, Vancomycin, Carbamazepine	Prednisone, Prednisolone, Cyclosporine, Tacrolimus, Cyclophosphamide, Azathioprine

- Cytapheresis (hemapheresis): leukocytes (hyperleukemic leukostasis), platelets (severe thrombocytosis), abnormal red cells (sickle cell disease), and parasites
- LDL apheresis: lipoproteins

Indications in Renal Diseases (American Society for Apheresis; J Clin Apher 2016;31:149)	
Should be Considered	**Can be Considered**
ANCA RPGN w/ Cr >6, dialysis dependence or DAH	Catastrophic APLS
Anti-GBM disease w/ DAH or dialysis independence	Symptomatic/severe cryoglobulinemia
Atypical HUS with factor H antibodies, TTP	Myeloma cast nephropathy
Recurrent FSGS after txp, AMR	Severe SLE
Desensitization in LDKT, ABO incompatible in LDKT	

Considerations Prior to Start PLEX

- Ideally, diagnostic lab specimen should be drawn prior to start PLEX: ANCA, anti-GBM Ab, ADAMTS13, CFH Ab, C3 nephritic factor
- Timing of antibody-based medicine: dose eculizumab, rituximab after PLEX session

PLEX Regimen

- Volume: 1–1.5 plasma volume will maximize efficiency
  1 plasma volume = 50 mL/kg of weight or 70 mL/kg of weight × [1-Hct]
  Single 1 plasma volume ↓ plasma macromolecule by 60%; 1.4 plasma vol ↓ 75%
- Replacement fluid (RF): 5% albumin +/– NS +/– FFP
  FFP is given at the end of session to prevent coagulation factor removal
  FFP if (1) repletion of any plasma component is desired: TTP, some forms of aHUS or (2) coagulation factor should be repleted: DAH, recent surgery, kidney bx, ↑ PT
- Cryoprecipitates: for low fibrinogen
- Schedule: daily if life threatening (eg, active DAH) then qod
- Number: not standardized; 7 in ANCA vasculitis (MEPEX JASN 2017;18:2180); can continue until disappearance of target (eg, anti-GBM Ab)
- Access: dialysis catheter, AVF or AVG; anticoagulation: citrate, heparin

Complications and Monitoring

- Albumin RF is a/w less adverse reaction than FFP (1.4 vs 20%) (AJKD 1994;23:817)
- ACEi-associated reaction: flushing, hypotension, abdominal cramping; Kinin mediated; a/w albumin RF (Transfusion 1994;34:891); Withhold ACEi for 24 hr prior
- Coagulation factor def: √PT, fibrinogen; replace w/ FFP, cryoprecipitates, respectively
- Immunoglobulin depletion, infection (including catheter related)
- Metabolic alkalosis: from FFP containing citrate conversion to bicarbonate and reduced renal excretion; Tx: switch to albumin replacement; can be corrected by HD
- Metabolic acidosis: acidic profile of albumin replacement
  Tx: can be partially corrected by 40 mEq NaHCO₃ PO or IV (Transfusion 2015;55:2653)
- Hypokalemia: common with nonplasma RF, dilutional; Hypomagnesemia
- Hypocalcemia: ↓ iCa by citrate chelation; Albumin RF also can cause (J Clin Apher 1999;14:114)
  Can be prevented by 10% calcium gluconate 10–20 mL (1–2 g)
- Potentially rebound antibody production; use as supplementary to antiproliferative therapy in antibody producing conditions
- Anaphylactic reaction, hives, transfusion-related acute lung injury, serum sickness

INTOXICATION AND POISONING

General Management of Drug Intoxication
• Airway, breathing, circulation; volume repletion: prevent AKI, increase toxin elimination
• Dextrose: correct hypoglycemia in ΔMS. Hemoperfusion can cause hypoglycemia. In aspirin intoxication seizure can happen from low CNS glucose w/ nl serum glucose
• Poison Control 800-222-1222; http://www.extrip-workgroup.org

Activated Charcoal
• Dose: 1 g/kg up to 50 g followed by 25 g q2–3 hr or 50 g q4–6 hr
• Contraindications: bowel obstruction, GI perforation, risk of aspiration (unconscious)

Drug Removal by Activated Charcoal	
Effective	**Not Effective**
Aspirin, Phenobarbital, Theophylline, Digoxin, Phenytoin, Carbamazepine	Alcohols, TCA, Boric acid, Corrosives (acids, alkali), Hydrocarbons, Essential oils Heavy metals: arsenic, Lead, Mercury, Iron, Zinc, Cadmium Inorganic ions: Li^+, Na^+, Ca^{2+}, K^+, Mg^{2+}, Fluoride, Iodide

Urine Alkalinization (Goal: Urine pH ≥7.5)
• Facilitate renal excretion of weak acids: aspirin, barbiturates, methotrexate
• $NaHCO_3$ IV 1–2 mEq/kg bolus followed by 150 mEq/L $NaHCO_3$ in 1 L of D_5W
• Complication: hypokalemia, hypocalcemia, volume overload, CaP precipitation

---

EXTRACORPOREAL THERAPY OF INTOXICATION

Characteristics of Drug and Toxin Removed by Hemodialysis (HD)
• Small Vd (<1 L/kg): any noncontinuous extracorporeal methods
  Large Vd: need for continuous therapy; rebound after therapy
• Small solute (MW <500 D) can be removed by HD with diffusive clearance
  5–20 kD: high flux membrane with high Qb and Qd; convective clearance helps
  45–100 kD: only high cut-off membrane (unavailable in USA) can remove
• Lower (<80%) protein bound; high protein bound drug can be removed by PLEX
• Water soluble; less rebound (movement from storage compartments into circulation)

Considerations for HD
• May need high flux (efficiency) dialyzer and long session for maximal clearance
• Dialysate designed for reduced renal function can cause ↓ K, ↓ PO_4, ↓ Mg, and metabolic alkalosis in normal kidney function
• Maximal clearance may cause dialysis disequilibrium in CKD patients
• If significant rebound is expected (lithium, methotrexate, dabigatran, metformin) repeat HD early or initiate CRRT

Hemoperfusion
• The passage of blood through a circuit containing an adsorbent (charcoal, carbon, or polystyrene resin)
• Remove theophylline, disopyramide, phenytoin, phenobarbital, procainamide, carbamazepine, valproic acid, dapsone, methotrexate, Amanita mushrooms
• Can remove large MW, protein-bound, and lipophilic toxins and drugs
• Blood flow (Qb) 250–400 mL/min: can cause hypotension
• Circuit similar to HD; w/o dialysate: no electrolyte/fluid overload correction
• Anticoagulation required
• s/e: charcoal embolization, ↓ Ca, ↓ glc, ↓ BP; leucopenia, thrombocytopenia

Other Extracorporeal Therapies
• CRRT: lower clearance than HD; consider for hemodynamically unstable pts; molecule with rebound; when dialysis disequilibrium risk exceeds benefit of rapid removal
• PD: ineffective, not recommended
• Plasma exchange (PLEX): can remove lipid- or protein-bound substances with small Vd (<0.2 L/kg) regardless of size; rarely used for Amanita mushroom poisoning, snake envenomation, paraquat, digoxin (digoxin-fab complex removal), cisplatin, amitriptyline, natalizumab (Semin Dial 2012;25:201)

Drugs Removed by HD (MW, Vd, Protein Binding)			
Drugs	**Clinical Findings**	**Indication of HD**	**Other Treatments**
Aspirin (138, 0.2 L/kg, 80–90%, lower w/ toxic level)	AGMA, respiratory alkalosis Acidemia ↑ CNS toxicity Seizures d/t low brain glucose w/ NL serum glucose level	>100 mg/dL >80 mg/dL w/ CKD Metabolic acidosis w/ pH ≤7.2 Pulmonary edema Seizures, coma, cerebral edema AKI	Activated charcoal Keep blood pH 7.5– 7.59: avoid acetazolamide Keep glucose ≥80: urine alkalinization
Dabigatran (628, 50–70 L, 35%)	Bleeding (CJASN 2013; 8:1533)	Life-threatening bleeding	Idarucizumab: neutralizing Ab (Lancet 2015;386:680)
Metformin (165, 1–5 L/kg, No)	Lactic acidosis (type B) N/V, abd pain Death 23–30% (Ann Emerg Med 2009;54:818; Crit Care 2008;12:R149)	Lactate >20 mmol/L pH ≤7.0 Shock Failure of supportive measures Decreased level of consciousness	Activated charcoal (acute overdose) NaHCO₃: controversial
Lithium (7, 0.6–1.0 L/kg, 0%)	↓ AG (Li⁺ is cation) N/V/D, leukocytosis ΔMS, ataxia, seizure, irritability, tremor, myoclonus, fasciculations Flat T wave, ↑ QT, bradycardia	>5 mEq/L >4 mEq/L w/ AKI, CKD >2.5 mEq/L with symptoms	IV fluid: ↑ urinary Li excretion Bowel irrigation with SR tab Sodium polystyrene sulfate
Theophylline (180, 0.5 L/kg, 50–60%)	Ventricular arrhythmias, ↓ BP, tremor, seizure, abd pain, N/V, ↓ K, PO₄, ↑ Ca, glc, lactic acidosis	60 µg/mL >50 µg/mL in infants <6 mo or >60 y/o Seizures, shock, arrhythmias	Activated charcoal Hemoperfusion
Methotrexate (454, 0.4–0.8 L/kg, 50%)	Renal intratubular precipitation Liver toxicity, N/V	No consensus Marked rebound	IV fluid, urine alkalinization Leucovorin Glucarpidase

INTOXICATION 3-35

TOXIC ALCOHOLS

- For an AGMA of uncertain cause or clinically suspected toxic ingestion, ✓osmolality, alcohol (methanol, ethanol, ethylene glycol, isopropanol and acetone) level
- Isopropanol ingestion manifests w/o anion gap

Osmolal Gap (OG) = measured serum osmolality − calculated osmolality
- Calculated osmolality = $[2 \times Na] + ([BUN]/2.8) + ([glucose]/18) + ([EtOH (mg/dL)]/4.6)$
  - If unit is mmol/L, $[2 \times Na] + [BUN] + [glucose] + [EtOH]$

Causes of Osmolal Gap (OG) >10 mOsm/kg	
(+) Anion Gap Metabolic Acidosis	**(−) Metabolic Acidosis**
Methanol, ethylene glycol, diethylene glycol, propylene glycol Formaldehyde, paraldehyde Advanced CKD w/o regular dialysis Ketoacidosis (diabetic and alcoholic) Lactic acidosis	Ethanol, isopropanol, diethyl ether Glycine, sorbitol, or mannitol solutions Pseudohyponatremia: severe hyperproteinemia or hyperlipidemia

- Early stage: typically OG >10
- Late stage: metabolites are not active osmoles, but are anions with sodium as the accompanying cation; ↓ OG, ↑ AG *(NEJM 2018;378:270; CJASN 2008;3:208)*

ΔS_{osm} (mOsm/L) per 10 mg/dL Serum Alcohol *(CJASN 2008;3:208)*					
Methanol	3.09	Isopropyl alcohol	1.66	Propylene glycol	1.31
Ethanol	2.12	Ethylene glycol	1.60	Diethylene glycol	0.9

Clinical Manifestations of Toxic Alcohol Ingestion

Manifestations of Toxic Alcohols (AG/OG)			
Alcohol	**Source**	**Metabolism (toxic)**	**Manifestation**
Methanol (↑/↑↑)	Windshield wiper fluid, industrial products	Formaldehyde → <u>formic acid/formate</u> <u>Lactic acid, Ketones</u>	Hemorrhagic/ischemic injury to basal ganglia, Blurred vision, central scotomata, blindness, coma, death
Ethylene glycol (↑/↑)	Antifreeze (fluorescence of urine under UV light), adhesives, pesticides, inks	Glycolaldehyde → <u>Glycolic acid</u> (tubular toxicity) → <u>Oxalic acid/oxalate</u> (crystal can be seen on urine sediment)	CaOx deposition in kidney (AKI, hematuria, oliguria, flank pain), heart (myocardial dysfunction), lung and brain (CN palsies) ↓ Ca (tetany, low BP)
Isopropanol (**NL**/↑↑)	Rubbing alcohol, hand sanitizers	Acetone	CV collapse, coma in massive ingestion (levels >500 mg/dL and osmolal gap >100)
Diethylene glycol (↑/↑ or NL)	Automotive brake fluid, industrial products	2-hydroxyethoxy-acetaldehyde → <u>2-hydroxyethoxyacetic acid</u>	AKI: could be irreversible Hepatitis, pancreatitis ΔMS, peripheral facial diplegia, flaccid tetraparesis
Propylene glycol (NL or ↑/↑)	IV lorazepam, diazepam, phenobarbital, etomidate	Lactaldehyde → <u>D- and L-lactate</u>	Minimal clinical abnormality Rare AKI

General Management of Toxic Alcohol Ingestion
- Acidemia ↑ uncharged toxic metabolite, formic acid that can enter end-organ tissue
- IV NaHCO₃ to correct metabolic acidosis (1–2 mEq/kg for pH <7.3 followed by a continuous infusion to maintain systemic pH >7.35)
- No role for GI decontamination, eg, activated charcoal

Fomepizole (4-Methylpyrazole)
- Inhibits alcohol dehydrogenase and aldehyde dehydrogenase; has ↓ need for HD
- Initiate if alcohol level >20 mg/dL
- Preferred over ethanol that requires level monitoring (>100 mg/dL) and sedative effect
- To ↓ more toxic metabolites: methanol, ethylene glycol, diethylene glycol
- Do not use when metabolites are less toxic: isopropanol (acetone less toxic)
- Dose: IV 15 mg/kg loading followed by 10 mg/kg q12h ×4, then 15 mg/kg q12h (increased dose for alcohol dehydrogenase induction by fomepizole)
- Until alcohol level <20 mg/dL (methanol <6.2 mmole/L or ethylene glycol <3.2 mmole/L)
- Removed by HD; 1–1.5 mg/kg/hr during HD or redose immediately after HD

HD in Toxic Alcohol Ingestion
- All of the alcohols are dialyzable: low MW, little or absent protein binding, low Vd
- General indication: AKI, anion gap metabolic acidosis with pH <7.3

Treatment of Toxic Alcohol (MW, Vd) Ingestion		
Alcohols	Indication of HD	Other Treatment
Methanol (32, 0.6–0.7 L/kg)	>50 mg/dL Blurred vision or blindness, seizures	Fomepizole Folic acid 50 mg IV q6h or leucovorin 50 mg IV q6h to replete tetrahydrofolate: ↑ Formate metabolism
Ethylene glycol (62, 0.5–0.8 L/kg)	>50 (300 if fomepizole given) mg/dL Altered sensorium, coma, seizures	Fomepizole Thiamine 100 mg IV qd and pyridoxine 100 mg IV qd: ↑ Glyoxylate metabolism
Isopropranolol (60, 0.6 L/kg)	>500 mg/dL Hypotension, lactic acidosis	Supportive Do not use fomepizole
Diethylene glycol (106.12, 0.5 L/kg)		Fomepizole
Propylene glycol (76.1)	Lactic acidosis	Stop infusion containing propylene glycol if able

- HD duration (h): **-V ln (5/A)/0.06k** (AJKD 2005;46:509)
  V: Watson estimate of total body water (L), A: the initial alcohol level (mmol/L)
  For mg/dL → mmol/L, ×0.3121 (methanol), 0.1611(ethylene glycol), 0.1644 (isopropanol)
  k: 80% of the dialyzer urea clearance (mL/min) at the observed Qb
- Avoid heparin if methanol ingestion suspected (risk of basal ganglia hemorrhage)

PROXIMAL TUBULE (PT)

Physiology of the Proximal Tubule	
NaCl, water: 60–70% of isotonic reabsorption	Peritubular capillaries pressures ↑ AII and Norepinephrine
Glucose: full reabsorption	Luminal SGLT-1, SGLT-2
AA: full reabsorption	Luminal Na-AA cotransport
HCO₃: reabsorption	Luminal NHE3
PO₄: reabsorption	Luminal NaPi
Reabsorption of K, PO₄, Ca, Mg, urea, urate; ammonia production	
Complete reabsorption and metabolism of LMW proteins	
Secretion of urate, cationic drugs	
Transporters + paracellular transport allow ~70% of ultrafiltrate reabsorption	

Cystinosis
- AR mutation of *CTNS* gene encoding cystinosin, protein that transports cysteine across the lysosomal membrane → accumulation of cystine in lysosome → Cystine ↓ glutathione → ↑ oxidative stress → apoptosis; cystine forms crystals in DT → stone
- 3 clinical presentations depending on the underlying genetic mutation: the infantile (nephropathic) form, the late-onset (juvenile) form, and the adult (benign) form
- Nephropathic cystinosis → PT dysfunction: polyuria/polydipsia, tubular proteinuria, glycosuria, phosphaturia, hypouricemia, and aminoaciduria (symptoms of volume depletion and electrolytes imbalance starting at 3–6 mo). Usually progress to ESRD by mid-teens.
- Extrarenal symptoms: rickets, growth retardation, corneal cysteine deposits/photophobia, hepatomegaly, portal hypertension, hypothyroidism, T1DM, myopathy, hypogonadism, azoospermia, and excessive bone fracture. Patients have normal cognitive function.
- Dx: ↑ cystine content of WBC, cystine corneal crystals, or genetic testing
- Tx: (1) symptomatic treatment for the volume and the electrolyte imbalances; (2) nutrition supplement (some pt require G-tube feeding); (3) cysteamine
- Cysteamine (metabolizes cysteine): preserves kidney function and delays most extrarenal manifestation except for the cornel deposits (treated w/ cysteamine eye drops), it does not reverse the pre-existing organ dysfunction immediate release q4, enteric release form q12h. ✓ WBC cystine level for efficacy. s/e: GI intolerance, unpleasant breath, sweat odor, and bruise-like skin lesions at the elbow and knee.
- Renal txp: successful w/ excellent long-term outcome w/o recurrence in the graft. Continue cysteamine to avoid progression of the extrarenal manifestations.

LOOP OF HENLE

- Urine dilution and sodium reabsorption (15–25%) via NKCC2
- Countercurrent multiplier creates the medullary osmotic gradient: responsible for concentrating the urine in collecting duct
- Basolateral Na-K-ATPase → ↓ intracellular Na → reabsorption of Na, K, Cl via luminal NKCC2 → K secretion via luminal ROMK → electropositive lumen
- Paracellular reabsorption of Ca, Mg via claudin 16, 19, driven by luminal + charge
- CaSR inhibits ROMK and NKCC2 to decrease calcium uptake in hypercalcemia
- Tubuloglomerular feedback: ↓ NaCl delivery to macula densa of ascending limb of Henle → ↑ PGE2 production → ↑ renin release from juxtaglomerular (JG) cells and ↓ adenosine-mediated afferent arteriole vasoconstriction; SGLT-2 inhibitor may inhibit renin release

Bartter Syndrome
- Heterogeneous presentation: childhood onset, MR, growth defects, polyuria/polydipsia

	Types of Bartter Syndrome	
Type	Mutated Protein	Clinical Manifestations
I	Luminal NKCC2	Severe, nephrocalcinosis, ESRD, early onset
II	Luminal ROMK	
III	Basolateral ClCKb	Classic, less severe, later onset; some mutations have hypocalciuria; CKD, nephrocalcinosis
IV	Bartin, β subunit of ClC-Kb	Sensorineural deafness, less nephrocalcinosis, CKD
V	GOF mutation of basolateral CaSR	AD, Milder, later onset, ↓ Ca ↓ Mg, No ↑ PGE2

- Impaired NaCl uptake into macula densa → ↑PGE2 production → ↑RAAS → ↓K
- Bartter-like conditions: polyvalent cations, gentamicin, amikacin, colistin activate the CaSR
- X-linked transient antenatal Bartter: MAGE-D2 affects NKCC2, NCC (*NJEM* 2016;374:1853)
- Tx: NSAIDs, high-dose K-sparing diuretics (spironolactone up to 300 mg/d, eplerenone up to 150 mg/d, amiloride up to 40 mg/d), electrolytes repletion; ACEI/ARBs might help with the electrolytes imbalances but induce hypotension

DISTAL TUBULE

- Reabsorption of NaCl via NCC; last diluting segment of the tubule
- Reabsorption of Ca (TRPV5) and Mg (TRPM6)
- Connecting tubule glomerular feedback: ↑NaCl transport in the connecting tubule (sensed by ENaC → afferent arteriole vasodilatation)

Gitelman Syndrome: Loss of Function of NCC
- AR, late childhood and adulthood presentation, more severe phenotype in ♀
- Polyuria, nocturia, cramping, fatigue, chondrocalcinosis, CPPD disease
- Tx: NaCl *ad libitum*, K/Mg supplements, K-sparing diuretics (can worsen sodium depletion), NSAIDs (*JASN* 2015;26:468), avoid QT prolonging meds

Bartter Syndrome	Gitelman Syndrome
AR, ↓K, metabolic alkalosis, 2° ↑renin (hyperplasia of the JG apparatus) and ↑aldo	
Volume contraction, ↓BP, loss of maximal diluting capacity	
Mimics/bunted response to loop diuretics	Mimics/blunted response to thiazide
Mutations in NKCC in the TAL	Mutations in NCC in the distal tubule
Loss of concentrating capacity	Preservation of the concentrating capacity
Hypercalciuria +/− hypomagnesemia	Hypocalciuria + hypomagnesemia
↑PGE2 → Vasodilation	Normal PG secretion

EAST/SeSAME Syndrome
- Mutations of the basolateral K channel (KCNJ10; Kir4.1) → ↓Na^+-K^+ ATPase activity → ↓Na gradient for NCC → renal salt wasting, ↑renin, hypoK, met alk, and low-nl BP
- **E**pilepsy, **a**taxia, **s**ensorineural deafness, and **t**ubulopathy/seizures, **s**ensorineural deafness, **a**taxia, **m**ental retardation, and **e**lectrolyte imbalance)

Pseudohypoaldosteronism Type 2 (Gordon Syndrome)
- WNK1, 4, Cullin-3, or Kelch-3 mutation → ↑NCC, mirror image of Gitelman/thiazides
- Familial hyperkalemic HTN, metabolic acidosis, ↓renin, ↓aldosterone, low BMD, hypercalciuria d/t ↓Na and Ca reabsorption in PCT
- Tx: low salt diet, thiazides

COLLECTING DUCT

- K secretion via ROMK and BK: ↑by aldo (ROMK, BK), tubular flow (BK), ↓Mg
- Sodium reabsorption via ENaC: ↑by aldo
- Urine concentration via aquaporin: ↑by ADH
- Urea absorption is both passive and UT1: ↑by ADH
- Acid (H^+) secretion at type A intercalated cell via H^+ ATPase
- Base (HCO_3^-) secretion at type B intercalated cell via pendrin, Cl^-/HCO_3^- exchanger

Liddle Syndrome
- AD, GOF mutation of ENaC (inability to bind w/ a ubiquitin protein ligase, Nedd4)
- HTN at young age, ↓K, metabolic alkalosis, ↓PRA, ↓PAC
- Tx: amiloride, triamterene; spironolactone is NOT effective

Pseudohypoaldosteronism Type 1
- AR form: ENaC mutation, miliaria crystallina papular rash d/t high Na in sweat, chest congestion d/t airway expression of EnaC (*NEJM* 1999;341:156)
- AD form: mutation of MR milder salt wasting, improves with age
- Volume depletion, FTT, ↑PRA, ↑PAC (aldosterone resistance)
- Tx: high salt diet, high-dose fludrocortisone (1–2 mg/d), carbenoxolone (↓metabolism of cortisol, as w/ licorice → activate the mineralocorticoid receptor)

Pendred Syndrome
- AR mutation of pendrin; no electrolytes imbalance under normal conditions
- Metabolic alkalosis and hypovolemia with thiazide therapy
- Associated phenotype: sensorineural hearing loss and hypothyroidism with goiter

EVALUATION OF ACID–BASE BALANCE

Background
- Acid–base balance is maintained by renal excretion of noninducible titratable acid ($HPO_4^{2-}/H_2PO_4^-$) and inducible buffers (mainly $NH_3 + H^+ \leftrightarrow NH_4^+$), and pulmonary excretion of CO_2 ($CO_2 + H_2O \leftrightarrow H_2CO_3 \leftrightarrow HCO_3^- + H^+$)
- Henderson–Hasselbalch equation: $pH = 6.10 + \log([HCO_3^-]/[0.03 \times pCO_2])$
- On the ABGs, HCO_3^- is calculated; usually 2 mEq/L less than the measured blood CO_2

	Normal Values of Blood Gas Analysis		
	pH	HCO₃⁻	pCO₂
ABGs	7.36–7.44	21–27	36–44
Peripheral VBGs	↓ 0.02–0.04	↑ 1–2	↑ 3–8
Central VBGs	↓ 0.03–0.05	↔	↑ 4–5

Step 1: Arterial pH Defines the Primary Disorder
- Acidosis (pH <7.36) or alkalosis (pH >7.44)
- VBGs has a good diagnostic accuracy for most acid–base imbalances

Step 2: Metabolic vs Respiratory Disorder
- Acidosis + low HCO_3^- → Metabolic acidosis
- Acidosis + high pCO_2 → Respiratory acidosis
- Alkalosis + high HCO_3^- → Metabolic alkalosis
- Alkalosis + low pCO_2 → Respiratory alkalosis

Step 3: Compensation Assessment
- In a simple disorder, the compensatory changes in the same direction of 1° disorder
- The respiratory compensation of metabolic disorder starts within 30 min and is complete in 12–24 hr
- The metabolic (renal) compensation of respiratory disorder takes 3–5 d to complete, thus the difference in expected compensation for acute (<3 d) and chronic respiratory disorders (>5 d)

	Compensation Assessment		
	Primary	Compensation	Expected Compensation
Metabolic acidosis	↓ HCO₃	↓ PaCO₂ (hyperventilation)	1 mEq/L ↔ 1.25 mmHg PaCO₂ = 1.5 × HCO₃⁻ + 8 ± 2 PaCO₂ = HCO₃⁻ + 15 PaCO₂ = decimal number of the pH Down to 8–12 mmHg
Metabolic alkalosis	↑ HCO₃	↑ PaCO₂ (hypoventilation)	1 mEq/L ↔ 0.7 mmHg Up to 55 mmHg
Respiratory acidosis	↑ pCO₂	↑ HCO₃	10 mmHg ↔ 1 mEq/L (acute) 10 mmHg ↔ 3.5–5 mEq/L (chronic)
Respiratory alkalosis	↓ pCO₂	↓ HCO₃	10 mmHg ↔ 2 mEq/L (acute) 10 mmHg ↔ 4–5 mEq/L (chronic)

Step 4: Assess for Mixed Disorders
- Mixed acid–base is present when:
  1. Greater or lesser than expected respiratory or metabolic compensation
  2. PaCO₂ and HCO₃ change in opposite directions
  3. ↑ AG in other forms of imbalance: additional AG metabolic acidosis
- In metabolic disorder
  - PaCO₂ is higher than expected: additional respiratory acidosis
  - pCO₂ is lower than expected: additional respiratory alkalosis
- In respiratory disorder
  - HCO₃ is higher than expected: additional metabolic alkalosis
  - HCO₃ is lower than expected: additional metabolic acidosis

METABOLIC ACIDOSIS

Background

- Daily acid ingestion (50–100 mEq of H^+) is balanced by reabsorption of HCO_3 at PCT, excretion of H^+ by the distal part of tubule; most of the renal excretion is in the form of titratable acids $H_2PO_4^-$ and NH_4^+
- Renal ammoniagenesis excretes hydrogen ions: $NH_3 + H^+ \rightarrow NH_4^+$
- Stimulus for renal ammoniagenesis is intracellular acidosis secondary to metabolic acidosis or hypokalemia due to exit of intracellular K in exchange with extracellular H^+

Workup

- In pure metabolic acidosis, pH is decreased, serum HCO_3^- is reduced and $PaCO_2$ is reduced as a compensatory mechanism
  - Winters formula: $PaCO_2 = 1.5 \times$ serum $HCO_3 + 8 \pm 2$
- To diagnose mixed acid–base disorders, the degree of $PaCO_2$ compensation needs to be assessed; Mixed disorder, arterial pH may not be decreased:
  1. If $PaCO_2$ is higher than expected: metabolic acidosis + respiratory acidosis
  2. If $PaCO_2$ is lower than expected: metabolic acidosis + respiratory alkalosis
  3. These assumptions are valid as long as HCO_3 is >7 ($PaCO_2$ can be lowered only to the range of 8–12)

Serum Anion Gap (AG, mEg/L) = Na – (Cl + HCO₃) = unmeasured anions (albumin, PO₄, urate, sulfate, IgA) – unmeasured cations (K, Ca, Mg, IgG)	
Normal AG	3–9 (Variation can occur dependent on the lab)
High AG (>9)	Organic metabolic acidosis (ketoacidosis; lactic acidosis; ingestions; pyroglutamic acid)
	Hyperalbuminemia, metabolic alkalosis: ↑ in albumin negative charge
	Hyperphosphatemia, anionic monoclonal IgA
Low AG (<3)	Hypoalbuminemia: expected AG: 2.5 × [albumin]
	Severe NAGMA: ↓ albumin negative charge
	↑ K, ↑ Ca, ↑ Mg, lithium intoxication, cationic monoclonal IgG, bromide (pseudohyperchloremia)
Negative AG	Na underestimation (severe hypernatremia)
	Cl overestimation (hyperlipidemia; salicylate intoxication; Bromide)

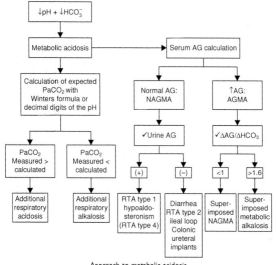

Approach to metabolic acidosis.

- In NAGMA, appropriate (>200) vs inappropriate (<75) urinary NH_4^+ can be estimated by urine anion gap (UAG) and urine osmolar gap (UOG)
- Urine anion gap (UAG, $U_{Na} + U_K - U_{Cl}$) is used as indirect measurement of the urine NH_4 concentration, this relation is disrupted in some disorders: (1) urinary excretion of unmeasured anions (DKA→β-hydroxybutyrate, ketoacetate; toluene inhalation → hippurate; proximal RTA → bicarbonate; D-lactate; acetaminophen → 5-oxoproline); (2) Neonates; (3) CKD
- In the presence of unmeasured anion, the calculated UAG will have a positive value which falsely suggest a low level of NH_4 excretion. In these disorders UOG is used to estimate NH_4 excretion

Urinary Osmolal Gap (UOG) = measured U_{osm} − calculated U_{osm}	
Calculated $U_{osm} = (2 \times [Na + K]) + [Urea\ mg/dL]/2.8 + [Glucose\ mg/dL]/18$	
U_{NH_4} is 50% of UOG	
Normal value if no metabolic acidosis	10–100 mOsmol/kg or NH_4 5–50
Expected values in metabolic acidosis	>200 mOsmol/kg
Abnormal values in metabolic acidosis (↓ U_{NH_4}) (ie, distal RTA)	<150 mOsmol/kg or NH_4 <75 mEq/d
Limited value of UOG	• Mannitol, alcohols • UTI with urease-producing bacteria (formation of NH_4 in the bladder)

ANION GAP METABOLIC ACIDOSIS (AGMA)

- If AG is elevated, ✓$\Delta AG/\Delta HCO_3$ ratio;
  - ΔAG = calculated AG − expected AG; ΔHCO_3 = 24 − measured HCO_3
  - $\Delta AG/\Delta HCO_3$ 1–1.6: anion gap metabolic acidosis (AGMA)
    - In lactic acidosis, due to intracellular H^+ buffering the fall of bicarbonate is not equal to the increase in the AG and the expected $\Delta AG/\Delta HCO_3$ can be up to 1.6
  - $\Delta AG/\Delta HCO_3$ <1: AGMA + hyperchloremic acidosis (NAGMA)
  - $\Delta AG/\Delta HCO_3$ >1.6: AGMA + metabolic alkalosis

Etiologies

Etiologies of AGMA	
Increased Acid Generation	
Ketoacidosis*	Diabetes mellitus, starvation, alcohol
Ingestion	Methanol, Ethylene glycol, Aspirin, Toluene (early phase) Diethylene glycol, Propylene glycol Pyroglutamic acid (5-oxoproline) d/t chronic acetaminophen ingestion (usually malnourished women)
L-Lactic acidosis	Hypoperfusion, aerobic glycolysis
D-Lactic acidosis	Metabolism of carbohydrate by intestinal bacteria in patients with short bowel syndrome Metabolism of propylene glycol (solvent for IV lorazepam, automotive antifreeze)
Decreased Renal Acid Excretion: CKD	

*High acetone level (>100 mg/dL) can falsely elevate sCr (↑ sCr with normal BUN).

Treatment

- Address and treat the underlying process
- Use of IV HCO_3 for the treatment of AGMA is controversial; the common practice is to use IV bicarbonate only when pH <7.1
- Potential benefits of treating chronic metabolic acidosis with alkali (bicarbonate or citrate) are: ↓ dyspnea, improve skeletal growth, ↓ kidney stone and nephrocalcinosis in RTA type 1, slow progression of CKD
- Potential concerns with bicarbonate therapy includes: ↑ pCO_2 and worsening intracellular acidosis, ↑ lactate generation though ↑ phosphofructokinase activity, decrease of ionized Ca, hypernatremia, and hypervolemia
- Bicarbonate is available in 8.4% 1 mEq/mL, 50 mL vials of hypertonic $NaHCO_3$
- Calculation of the HCO_3 deficit:
  - The volume of distribution (Vd) of HCO_3 is 50–55% (↑ up to 70% in severe metabolic acidosis due to high buffering capacity).
  - HCO_3 deficit = 0.7 × Lean body weight × (desired HCO_3 − measured HCO_3)

Pathogenesis

- Lactic acidosis occurs when generation of lactate exceeds consumption
- Anaerobic glycolysis generates Pyruvate which is metabolized by lactate dehydrogenase (LDH) to lactate

$$Pyruvate + NADH + H^+ \leftrightarrow lactate + NAD^+$$

- Lactate is consumed for gluconeogenesis and oxidative phosphorylation
- Hyperlactatemia can occur due to systemic or local tissue hypoxia (type A), the resulting acidemia is autoexacerbated by ↓ of lactate removal by the liver in cases of severe hypoxia and acidemia
- Hyperlactatemia results from aerobic glycolysis (type B) in hyperdynamic states (eg, sepsis, severe asthma, shock, pheochromocytoma)
- Metabolic alkalosis stimulates 6-phosphofructokinase leading to hyperlactatemia from aerobic glycolysis
- Lactic acidosis contributes to cellular dysfunction: ↑ cardiac arrhythmias, ↓ myocardial contractility, and responsiveness to catecholamines
- Hyperkalemia is very common when the etiology is ↓ O_2 delivery; with hyperlactatemia d/t epinephrine stimulation, hypokalemia occurs d/t β_2-adrenergic stimulation

Etiologies of Lactic Acidosis	
Decrease Local or Systemic O_2 Delivery (Type A)	
Shock	Cardiogenic, hypovolemic, septic, severe trauma
Severe hypoxemia	Lung disorders, CO poisoning
Others	Severe anemia, vigorous exercise, seizure, shivering, cocaine
Aerobic Glycolysis (Type B)	
Epinephrine stimulation	Cardiogenic, hypovolemic, septic shock Sepsis, Pheochromocytoma, Cocaine, β_2-agonists
Cancer	Warburg effect: usually in the setting of concomitant liver metastases limiting the lactate clearance by the liver
Others	NRTIs, toxic alcohols (methanol, ethylene glycol), salicylates, cyanide, propofol, thiamine deficiency
Other Mechanisms	
DM	Unknown mechanism
Liver disease	↓ lactate clearance
Metformin	Suppression of hepatic gluconeogenesis
Propylene glycol	Metabolized to D-lactate and L-lactate

Treatment

- Restore tissue perfusion with volume expansion using crystalloids; albumin can be used as alternative for volume expansion, avoid other colloids
- Balanced salt solutions (less chloride content) could prevent dilutional acidosis
- IV bicarbonate is potentially helpful for severe acidemia (pH <7.2). Use with caution (intracellular acidification, ↓ iCa leading to ↓ cardiac contractility)

D-Lactic Acidosis

- Etiologies: short bowel syndrome (carbohydrate metabolism by colonic bacteria), ingestion of propylene glycol (solvent for IV medications notably lorazepam and diazepam) and DKA
- Episodic metabolic acidosis with neurologic symptoms (confusion, ataxia, slurred speech)
- Diagnosis: special enzymatic assay for D-lactate (the commonly used lactic acid assay does not detect D-lactic acid); It cause a combined AGMA and NAGMA (NAGMA is due to excretion of D-lactate with Na and retention of the H^+)
- Treatment: oral antimicrobials, $NaHCO_3$ and addressing the underlying cause

KETOACIDOSIS

Background

- Metabolic acidosis secondary to ketone (acetoacetic acid, β-hydroxybutyric acid, acetone) accumulation: diabetic, alcoholic or fasting ketoacidosis
- Urine dipstick detects acetoacetate and acetone, not β-hydroxybutyric acid (can be measured in the blood)
- Correction of ketoacidosis leads frequently to NAGMA secondary to renal loss of ketone bodies which are considered "potential bicarbonate"

Fasting Ketoacidosis

- β-hydroxybutyrate is the main ketone
- Neonates and pregnant lactating women are at risk d/t ↑ metabolic requirements

Alcoholic Ketoacidosis

- Malnourished alcoholic patients, the severe acidosis occurs after the patient stops alcohol ingestion (alcohol ingestion limits fatty acid lipolysis and decrease generation of acetyl-CoA); plasma levels may be low or undetectable
- Manifestations: hypo- or hyperglycemia, hypokalemia (GI and renal loss), ↓ PO_4 (↓ intake and ↑ renal loss), ↓ Mg, ↑ OG

Diabetic Ketoacidosis

- Ketone bodies are both β-hydroxybutyric and acetoacetic acids
- DKA is the result of insulin deficiency, glucagon excess leading to glucose utilization, increased gluconeogenesis, increased glycogenolysis, and lipolysis
- Treatment:
  - Correction of the hypovolemia with isotonic solution; Insulin administration
  - Correction of the hypokalemia: early and aggressive correction is needed in anticipation of worsening of the ↓ K following insulin therapy and volume expansion

---

METHANOL AND ETHYLENE GLYCOL

Background

- Methanol and ethylene glycol can be ingested as ethanol substitute, accidently (illicit distillation) or to inflict self-harm. It is found in: antifreeze and deicing solutions, windshield wiper fluid, solvents, cleaners, fuels

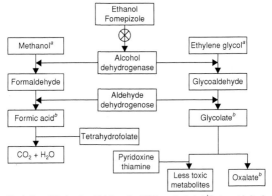

Metabolism of Methanol and Ethylene glycol ([a]Nontoxic alcohol; [b]Toxic metabolites).

Pathogenesis

- Formate causes retinal injury (hyperemia and blindness), basal ganglia hemorrhage
- Glycolate causes tubular injury; oxalate-Ca crystals causes tubular obstruction
- The toxic metabolite causes the ↑ AG; the parent alcohol contributes to the osmotic gap (as the alcohol is metabolized the osmolar gap decrease and the AG increase)
- Folic acid accelerates the metabolism of formic acid
- Ingestion of 1 g/kg is lethal; toxicity can occur with as little as1 tsp of methanol

Clinical Manifestations

- CNS sedation and inebriation similar to ethanol intoxication than can progress to coma, seizure, and hypotension
- Methanol poisoning: visual blurring, central scotomata, and blindness. On eye exam, mydriasis, retinal edema, hyperemia of the optic disc and loss of afferent pupillary reflex
- Ethylene glycol: oliguria, hematuria, flank pain, tetany (hypocalcemia)
- When ethanol is coingested, the clinical manifestation is delayed d/t alcohol dehydrogenase inhibition

Diagnosis

- Advanced degree of AGMA (frequently HCO_3 <8) w/o ↑ lactic acid
- Alcoholic ketoacidosis causes AGMA but with a lesser degree of acidosis
- ↑ Osmolal gap (OG) >10 can be seen during the early phase of the intoxication (before the alcohol is metabolized)

  OG = Measured Posm – Calculated Posm

  Calculated Posm = $(2 \times$ [Na]$)$ + [glucose]/18 + [BUN]/2.8
- Limitation of OG measurement:
  (1) Cannot differentiate among the different alcohols (ethanol, methanol, ethylene glycol, or isopropyl alcohol); (2) a decrease of OG is a sign of metabolism of the alcohol to the toxic metabolites and it is not a correlate of recovery; (3) OG increases in critically ill patients due to idiogenic osmoles
- "Solvent screen" does not measure for ethylene glycol
- Lactate can ↑ in ethylene glycol intoxication (glycolate has similar structure as lactate)
- Oxalate crystal and fluorescence of the urine with UV light in ethylene glycol intoxication

Treatment

- GI decontamination has a limited role since these alcohols are rapidly absorbed
- $NaHCO_3$ to correct systemic acidosis (in an acidic milieu, the toxic metabolic are in their uncharged form and thus easier to penetrate and cause organ damage; goal to keep arterial pH >7.3
- Inhibition of alcohol dehydrogenase: early treatment is important before the formation of the toxic metabolites
  - Fomepizole 15 mg/kg loading then 10 mg /kg q12h; adjust after 2 d; adjust for HD; Continue therapy until pH is normal and serum alcohol concentration <20 mg/dL
  - Ethanol if fomepizole is unavailable; target ethanol level 1/3 of the other alcohol; Loading 10 mL/kg of 10% ethanol with maintenance of 1 mL/kg
- HD remove both the alcohol and the toxic metabolites, it is indicated in any patient with (1) AGMA regardless of the alcohol level or (2) evidence of organ damage or (3) large methanol ingestions
- If a toxic ingestion is suspected but not yet confirm: the threshold to start HD is pH <7.1 (it is unlikely for alcoholic ketoacidosis to cause such an advanced acidosis); a concomitant fomepizole therapy can be started until the diagnosis is confirmed or rule out; treating with ethanol for nonconfirmed intoxication is debatable due to SE profile of the therapy
- ✓ toxic alcohol levels every 2 hr of end of HD to determine the need for additional HD; fomepizole is dialyzable and an additional should be given at the start of HD
- PD and CRRT are inefficient at clearing alcohols
- Treating with cofactors (folic acid, thiamine, and pyridoxine) to optimize nontoxic metabolic pathways: for methanol intoxication folic acid 50 mg IV q6h; thiamine 100 mg IV or pyridoxine 50 mg IV in ethylene glycol

Isopropyl Alcohol

- Isopropyl alcohol is used as disinfectant (rubbing alcohol), antifreeze, and solvent
- Causes CNS inebriation and depression, a fruity breath odor
- It does NOT cause an elevated anion gap acidosis; it is metabolized by alcohol dehydrogenase to a ketone
- Diagnosis: ↑ isopropyl alcohol levels and ↑ OG; Isopropyl alcohol does NOT cause ↑ AGMA nor ↑ β-hydroxybutyrate; ketone in the urine are expected after 2 hr of ingestion (the urine ketone detection can be delayed if the patient receives fomepizole or ethanol)
- Treatment: hydration and supportive care, no role for GI decontamination, no indication for alcohol dehydrogenase inhibitors, HD can help in massive ingestion

Toluene Inhalation (Glue Sniffing)

- Toluene is metabolized to hippuric acid and benzoate leading to AGMA
- With normal renal function these anions will be excreted with Na, NH_4, and K, and the AG is progressively corrected and the patient start developing NAGMA
- Despite an increase in urinary NH_4, U_{Cl} does not increase due to the presence of hippurate leading to a positive UAG. NAGMA + ↑ urine pH + ↑ UAG can be misdiagnosed as type 1 RTA; in this disorder UOG is used to estimate NH_4 excretion
- Hypokalemia is frequently present: (1) volume contraction leading to 2° hyperaldo, (2) high distal Na delivery (Na-hippurate and Na-benzoate)

NONANION GAP (HYPERCHLOREMIC) METABOLIC ACIDOSIS

Causes and Pathogenesis
- Normal anion gap metabolic acidosis is due to $NaHCO_3$ deficit

Mechanisms of NAGMA	
Renal	Reduction of acid excreting capacity: CKD, distal RTA, type 4 RTA Bicarbonate loss: proximal RTA
GI	Bicarbonate loss: diarrhea, pancreatic fistula, ureteric diversion (ileal loop)
Other	Loss of organic anions: recovery phase of AGMA (DKA, toluene ingestion, and D-lactic acidosis); Na and K salt excretion w/ impaired acid excretion Dilutional acidosis: volume expansion with a nonalkali containing fluid; rare unless extraordinarily large volume is given Addition of HCl: TPN

Diarrhea
- Diarrhea-induced NAGMA is frequently associated with hypokalemia, hypokalemia-induced intracellular acidosis, and ↑ NH_4 excretion and elevate urine pH
- The more chronic is the diarrhea and the more profound is the hypokalemia, the higher is the urine pH (can be falsely diagnosed as dRTA or toluene inhalation)

Resolution Phase of an AGMA
- In patients with AGMA and normal kidney function, the renal excretion of ketoacid anions reduces the AG, a NAGMA is generated by loss of the ketoacid anions (potential bicarbonate) with retention of H^+

Ureteral Diversion (Ileal Loop)
- Ureterosigmoidostomy: (1) urine is exposed to colonic mucosa, the U_{Cl} is exchanged for bicarbonate by anion exchanger (SLC26A3) → bicarbonate loss and NAGMA; (2) urea in the colon is metabolized to NH_4 that is reabsorbed in exchange of Na leading to NAGMA
- Ileal conduit: unlikely to cause NAGMA since the urine is not in contact with the epithelium for long before it is drained to an external bag, if NAGMA develops it is sign of malfunctioning of the loop
- Treatment: $NaHCO_3$ administration

DISTAL RENAL TUBULAR ACIDOSIS (dRTA, TYPE 1 RTA)

Causes and Pathogenesis
- Impaired distal acid secretion/urine acidification in the presence of NAGMA
- ↓ Activity of H-ATPase or increase luminal membrane permeability (leading to movement of the H^+ from the urine lumen back to the blood)
- Hypokalemia: due to ↑ K excretion which offsets impaired H^+ secretion needed to maintain electroneutrality from sodium absorption

Etiologies of Distal (Type 1) RTA	
Autoimmune	Sjögren's, rheumatoid arthritis, SLE Autoimmune hepatitis, primary biliary cirrhosis
Medications	Amphotericin B: reversible dRTA; less w/ liposomal formulation Lithium: incomplete RTA (mild to no metabolic acidosis) Ifosfamide, ibuprofen/codeine
Hypercalciuria	Hyperparathyroidism, Vit D intoxication, sarcoidosis, idiopathic hypercalciuria
Hereditary	SLC4A1 encoding Cl/HCO_3 exchanger (AE1 or band3): AD, milder acidosis than AR, presents later in life (young adults). Hypercalciuria, nephrolithiasis, nephrocalcinosis, osteomalacia, and erythrocytosis ATP6V1B1 encoding apical H-ATPase: AR; Sensorineural hearing impairment, nephrocalcinosis ATP6V0A4 encoding apical H-ATPase: AR; No early hearing loss
Other	Obstructive uropathy: ↓ Na entry in the principal cells → ↓ H^+ excretion Medullary sponge kidney, transplant rejection, Wilson disease Idiopathic

Diagnosis
- Urine pH >5.5; U_{Na} >25; positive UAG; ↓ UOG
- Other causes of persistently elevated urine pH >5.5: diarrhea with hypokalemia, toluene inhalation

- Urine osmolal gap <150: dRTA
- Urine osmolal gap >400: chronic diarrhea, toluene

Clinical Manifestations
- Recurrent calcium phosphate kidney stones and nephrocalcinosis, from associated hypercalciuria and hypocitraturia

Treatment
- Correction of the acidosis is indicated in children to restore normal growth, in adults with K wasting, nephrocalcinosis, osteoporosis, and CaP stones
- Goal [HCO_3] 22–24
- $NaHCO_3$ or Na citrate (bicitra) 1–2 mEq/kg/d; K citrate + Na citrate (Polycitra)
- K citrate: for recurrent kidney stones (increases urinary citrate and K moves intra-cellularly → K exit the cell → ↓ intracellular acidosis)
- Avoid Na citrate: may increase stone formation
- Correcting the systemic acidosis will ↑ urinary citrate (acidosis ↑ proximal citrate reabsorption)

Incomplete dRTA
- Impaired urinary acidification and inability to reduce urine pH to less than 5.3 but the net acid excretion is maintained at a rate equal to acid generation by overforma-tion of NH_4. In chronic condition, patients are not acidotic. Some patients progress to complete dRTA
- ↓ Urinary citrate → calcium phosphate stones; osteoporosis
- Pathogenesis: not well understood, it is related to low intracellular pH in the proximal tubule leading to increase formation of NH_4, the acidosis episodes are intermittent
- Diagnosis with acid load (NH_4Cl 0.1 g/kg or 3 d of modified diet) → ↓ serum HCO_3 by at least 3 and urine pH is >5.3

Voltage-dependent RTA
- Defects in distal sodium reabsorption leading to loss of the electronegativity of the lumen leading to ↓ K and H secretion
- Etiology: severe hypovolemia, obstructive uropathy (↓ Na-K-ATPase pump), lupus nephritis, sickle cell disease, amiloride, lithium
- Hyperkalemic RTA

PROXIMAL RENAL TUBULAR ACIDOSIS (pRTA, TYPE 2 RTA)

- **Isolated pRTA**: defect in proximal bicarbonate reabsorption
- **Fanconi syndrome**: a **generalized** proximal tubular dysfunction with impaired reab-sorption of phosphate, glucose, uric acid, and amino acids
- Patients are in chronic acid–base balance and can reduce the urine pH to less than 5.3

Pathogenesis

Etiologies of Proximal (Type 2) RTA	
Paraprotein	Light chain proximal tubulopathy
Drugs, heavy metals	Ifosfamide, tenofovir, aminoglycosides, cisplatin, valproic acid, deferasirox Carbonic anhydrase inhibitors: acetazolamide, dorzolamide, topiramate Lead, cadmium, mercury, copper
Hereditary	Dent disease, cystinosis, tyrosinemia, galactosemia, Wilson disease, Lowe disease, hereditary fructose intolerance, mitochondrial myopathies, glycogen storage disease (type 1) Mutations of: $SLC4A4$ encoding Na-HCO_3 cotransporter (NBCe1): AR, isolated pRTA. Eyes, teeth, and cognitive disorders $SLC9A3$ encoding NHE3: AD pRTA $CA2$ encoding carbonic anhydrase II (CA II)
Other	Renal transplantation, Vit D deficiency, paroxysmal nocturnal hemoglobinuria, Sjögren syndrome

- Variable K excretion dependent on the alkali intake:
  In chronic stable alkali/acid intake, K level is normal
  After alkali therapy → ↑ distal tubule Na delivery → ↑ K excretion → hypokalemia

Diagnosis
- NAGMA, hypophosphatemia, glucosuria, hypouricemia, LMW protein, and aminoaciduria
- Bicarbonate load (0.5–1 mEq/kg/hr of IV $NaHCO_3$) will ↑ urine pH and FE_{HCO_3} >15%:
  $FE_{HCO_3} = 100 \times (U_{HCO_3}/S_{HCO_3})/(U_{Cr}/S_{Cr})$

Treatment
- pRTA requires a higher load of alkali therapy (10–15 mEq/kg/d)
- Alkali therapy increases bicarbonaturia and ↑ K loss; thiazide can help by inducing volume depletion that stimulates proximal Na and bicarbonate reabsorption

Carbonic Anhydrase (CA) Inhibitors
- Acetazolamide, methazolamide, dorzolamide, topiramate
- Inhibits intracellular CA II and intraluminal CA IV in proximal and distal tubules
- pRTA (w/o Fanconi syndrome) + dRTA, ↓ K, nephrocalcinosis, CaP nephrolithiasis

Mixed Renal Tubular Acidosis (Type 3 RTA)
- Mainly in the Middle East and North Africa, Arabic descent
- AR, carbonic anhydrase 2 deficiency, Guibaud–Vainsel syndrome or marble brain disease
- Both pRTA and dRTA, osteopetrosis, cerebral calcification, mental retardation, facial dysmorphism with conductive hearing loss and blindness

---

HYPOALDOSTERONISM (TYPE 4 RTA)

Pathogenesis
- Either decreased aldosterone secretion or aldosterone resistance
- ↓ ENaC activity → ↓ electronegative lumen → ↓ K excretion → hyperkalemia
- NAGMA through multiple mechanisms mainly mediated by hyperkalemia
  1. K enter the proximal tubular cells → H^+ exit the cells → intracellular alkalosis → ↓ NH_4 production from decreased glutaminase
  2. Hyperkalemia ↓ NH_4 medullary reabsorption in the thick ascending limb of Henle
  3. In the collecting duct, K competes with NH_4 at the level of the Na-K ATPase which leads to decrease the amount of intracellular H^+ available for excretion
- In summary, the tubule has the capacity to secrete H^+, but the lack of the luminal buffer prevents excretion of higher load of acid

Etiologies of Hypoaldosteronism	
Hypoaldosteronism, hyporeninemic	Diabetic nephropathy, chronic interstitial nephritis, acute GN
	NSAIDs: ↓ Renin + ↓ All-induced aldosterone release
	Calcineurin inhibitors (75% of transplant patients)
	Pseudohypoaldosteronism type 2
Hypoaldosteronism, hyperreninemic	ACEi/ARBs, Direct renin inhibitor
	Heparin and LMWH: direct adrenal toxicity
	1° adrenal insufficiency: autoimmune, infection, HIV
	Congenital isolated hypoaldosteronism: defect in aldosterone synthase
Resistance to aldosterone	Mineralocorticoid receptor blocker: spironolactone, eplerenone
	Epithelial Na channel (ENaC) blocker: amiloride, triamterene, trimethoprim, pentamidine
	↓ Mineralocorticoid receptor expression: calcineurin inhibitors
	Pseudohypoaldosteronism type 1

- Pseudohypoaldosteronism type 1: mutation of mineralocorticoid receptor (AD form) or ENaC (AR form); resistance to aldosterone
- Pseudohypoaldosteronism type 2, Gordon syndrome, familial hyperkalemic hypertension

Diagnosis
- Mild metabolic acidosis (HCO_3 >17), hyperkalemia
- ✓ Plasma renin activity (PRA), plasma aldosterone concentration (PAC), and serum cortisol after the administration of a loop diuretic or 3 hr in the upright position

Treatment
- d/c offending drugs if possible
- Hypertensive: loop or thiazide diuretics
- Hypotensive: fludrocortisone ± high salt diet or isotonic fluid

METABOLIC ALKALOSIS

- ↑pH caused by ↑[HCO_3]; frequently associated with hypokalemia

Pathogenesis

- Normally the kidney has a high capacity to excrete alkali load in the PT
- Metabolic alkalosis develops as a result of excessive alkali load and/or impaired renal excretion of HCO_3 (eg, effective hypovolemia)

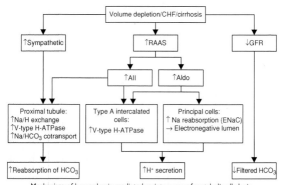

Mechanism of hypovolemia-mediated maintenance of metabolic alkalosis.

- **Hypokalemia** is common occurrence due to several reasons:
  1. Same pathogenic mechanisms contribute to both disturbances: primary or secondary hyperaldosteronism + high distal Na and water delivery
  2. Metabolic alkalosis → ↑$NaHCO_3$ distal delivery (non-Cl anion + high load of Na) → ↑K secretion
  3. Hypokalemia → K^+ exit and H^+ enter the cell → intracellular acidosis → ↑NH_3 renal production, ↑H^+ secretion (↑H/K-ATPase in type A intercalated) and ↑ reabsorption of HCO_3
- 1° hyperaldosteronism: ↑distal Na and water delivery + high Aldo → ↑K and ↑H^+ secretion (distal tubule H/K-ATPase and H-ATPase in the type A intercalated cells)
- Type B intercalated cells express increased luminal pendrin (HCO_3/Cl exchanger) with the net effects being secretion of HCO_3 and reabsorption of Cl
- The compensatory hypoventilation contributes to the maintenance of the metabolic alkalosis: hypoventilation → ↑P_{CO_2} → ↑intracellular acidosis → ↑renal H^+ excretion

Etiologies

- Most of the etiologies combine a process that directly or indirectly generated HCO_3 with a process of ↓renal HCO_3 excretion to maintain the alkalosis

Etiologies of Metabolic Alkalosis	
Etiologies That Help Maintain Metabolic Alkalosis	
Hypovolemia, ↓arterial blood volume (heart failure or cirrhosis)	
Hypochloremia hypokalemia: ↑renal ammoniagenesis	
AKI or CKD, Hyperaldosteronism	
Etiologies that Generate (Directly or Indirectly) HCO_3	
Intracellular H^+ shift	Hypokalemia
GI H^+ loss	N/V, NGT suction
	Gastric H^+ secretion is neutralized by the HCO_3 secreted by the pancreas, liver, and intestine; the loss of H^+ leads to HCO_3 absorption

Exogenous alkali	Antacids in advanced renal failure
	Mg hydroxide, Ca carbonate (when combined with SPS)
	Without SPS, the Mg and Ca recombine with HCO_3 in the distal intestine and does not cause acid–base disturbance
	With SPS, Mg and Ca are chelated by SPS and the net outcome is absorption of HCO_3
	Hypercalcemia, milk- or Ca-alkali syndrome
	Bicarbonate therapy, citrate after blood transfusion, freebase or crack cocaine
Renal H^+ loss: ↑distal Na and water delivery + ↑mineralocorticoid activity	1° hyperaldosteronism: aldosterone-secreting adenoma; Bilateral/unilateral adrenal hyperplasia; familial hyperaldo (type I/glucocorticoid-remediable aldosteronism, type II and III), adrenocortical carcinoma
	2° hyperaldosteronism: CHF, cirrhosis + diuretics
	Bartter and Gittelman syndrome
	Pendred syndrome (Cl/HCO_3 exchanger mutation: AR)
	Posthypercapnic alkalosis
Other	Some diarrhea: villous adenoma, laxative abuse, congenital chloridorrhea (mutation of the Cl/HCO_3 exchanger → high Cl diarrhea)
	Excessive chloride-rich sweat in CF
Contraction alkalosis	↓Extracellular volume with a constant total amount of HCO_3 → ↑$[HCO_3]$, eg, early phase of diuretics

Clinical Manifestations
- Since HCO_3 moves slowly across the different body compartments, specifically the brain, symptoms are uncommon in Met alkalosis
- Muscular spasms, tetany, and paresthesia (due to ↓iCa, ↓Mg)
- Etiology-related symptoms and signs (hypovolemia, CHF, cirrhosis)
- Compensatory hypoventilation → ↑pCO_2

Workup
- ✓ U_{Cl}: help to assess volume status
- U_{Na}: may increase d/t biacarbonaturia

Treatment
- Both the generation and maintenance of HCO_3 should be corrected
- For vomiting and NGT suction, H_2-blockers and PPI ↓ HCl loss
- Correct hypokalemia: K repletion may correct metabolic alkalosis, volume expansion w/o hypokalemia correction would not correct the metabolic alkalosis
- Correct hypovolemia, restoring the blood volume with a Cl-containing solution will correct the alkalosis and allows the kidney to excrete the excessive bicarbonate: type B intercalated cells express luminal Cl/HCO_3 exchanger allowing excretion of HCO_3 after restoring euvolemia
  ↑U_{Cl} is marker of resolution of the hypovolemia; urine pH ↑ to >7 d/t bicarbonaturia
- CHF/cirrhosis (edema + low intra-arterial blood volume): mineralocorticoid blockers (spironolactone and eplerenone) helps with the metabolic alkalosis and corrects the hypervolemia; acetazolamide (carbonic anhydrase inhibitor) can be added to the diuretic regimen (inhibits proximal Na/HCO_3 reabsorption)
- Posthypercapnic metabolic alkalosis: if nonedematous, volume expansion with Cl-containing solutions (0.9% NS) will correct the alkalosis; If edematous (requires additional diuresis), acetazolamide treats acidosis and corrects the hypervolemia
- Dialysis will correct the alkalosis in ESRD or severe AKI
- HCl (only given through a central line) or NH_4Cl is only used in patient with severe alkalosis (pH >7.55) in whom dialysis cannot be done
- Calculation of the HCO_3 excess
  - HCO_3 excess = $0.6 \times LBW \times ([HCO_3] - 24)$ for men
  - HCO_3 excess = $0.5 \times LBW \times ([HCO_3] - 24)$ for women
- When infusing acid frequent assessment of pH and BMP should be done

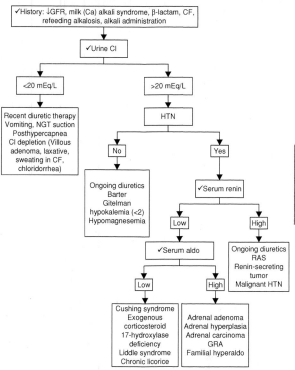

Diagnostic approach for met alkalosis.

RESPIRATORY ALKALOSIS

Background
- Hyperventilation ($\uparrow$ minute ventilation on vent) $\rightarrow \downarrow pCO_2 \rightarrow \uparrow$ pH
- The renal compensation for acute respiratory alkalosis (1–2 d) is $\downarrow HCO_3$ by 2 mEq/L for every $\downarrow pCO_2$ by 10 mmHg, for chronic respiratory alkalosis (>3–5 d) is $\downarrow HCO_3$ by 4–5 mEq/L for $\downarrow pCO_2$ by 10 mmHg

Pathogenesis
- $\uparrow$ Minute ventilation is sec to $\uparrow$ depth and/or rate of ventilation
- Some of the symptoms (eg, tetany, muscle cramps) are due to changes in the binding of Ca to alb: resp alkalosis $\rightarrow \uparrow$ Ca-alb binding $\rightarrow \downarrow$ ionized Ca
- Within 10 min, H^+ is released from body buffers (intracellular protein, Hb, and phosphate). In addition, $\uparrow$ lactate levels possible from hypoxia from peripheral vasoconstriction.
- Renal compensation takes 2–3 d and includes $\downarrow NH_4$ and $\uparrow HCO_3$ excretion

Etiologies
- Hypoxemia ($\downarrow pO_2 \rightarrow \uparrow$ minute ventilation): pneumonia, interstitial lung disease, pulmonary emboli, CHF, hypotension, severe anemia, high altitude
- Stimulation of the resp centers: psychogenic (eg, anxiety), liver cirrhosis, salicylate intoxication, postcorrection of met acidosis, pregnancy, stroke, CNS tumor
- Mechanical ventilation

- Paresthesias, headache, light-headedness, due to local and cerebral vasoconstriction ($\downarrow pCO_2 \rightarrow \downarrow$ cerebral blood flow); Tetany and carpedal spasm due to $\downarrow$ ionized calcium
- Pts are only intermittently aware of hyperventilation (SOB, air hunger), SOB is at rest with frequent sigh (normal 0–3/15 min) exacerbated by anxiety
- $\downarrow PO_4$ through intracellular consumption (intracellular alkalosis $\rightarrow \uparrow$ glycolysis $\rightarrow \uparrow$ formation of phosphorylated compounds), [Phos] as low as 0.5 mg/dL have been reported, severe hypoPhos causes muscle weakness and respiratory muscle weakness

Treatment
- Treat the underlying pulmonary or extrapulmonary etiology (PE, AMI, etc.)
- For anxiety pts: reassurance, benzodiazepine, and breathing into a paper bag leads to improvement of pCO_2 levels and pH

RESPIRATORY ACIDOSIS

Background
- $\downarrow$ pH and $\uparrow pCO_2$; CO_2 is formed through endogenous metabolism and accumulated when alveolar ventilation is $\downarrow$ (hypoventilation); $CO_2 + H_2O \leftrightarrow H_2CO_3 \leftrightarrow H^+ + HCO_3$
- CO_2 is eliminated by alveolar ventilation; stimuli are $\downarrow pO_2$ and $\uparrow pCO_2$

Pathogenesis
- In physiologic conditions, $\uparrow CO_2$ is the major stimulus of the respiratory center
- In chronic hypercapnia, $\downarrow O_2$ becomes the major respiratory stimulus; Treatment of the hypoxemia in chronic hypercapnic pts can lead to $\uparrow pCO_2$ and $\downarrow$ pH
- Renal compensation: $\uparrow H^+$ excretion and retention of HCO_3 and takes 3–5 d

Etiologies
- Inhibition of the CNS respiratory center: medications (opiates, benzodiazepine, sedatives, anesthesia); obesity hypoventilation syndrome; CNS lesion; oxygen therapy for chronic hypercapnia; metabolic alkalosis
- Chest wall and respiratory muscle defect: myasthenia gravis, Guillain–Barré, severe $\downarrow$ K, severe $\downarrow PO_4$, spinal cord injury, ALS, MS, myxedema, kyphoscoliosis, obesity
- Upper airway obstruction: OSA, foreign body aspiration, laryngospasm
- Lower airways disease: COPD, asthma, pneumonia, ARDS, pneumothorax
- $\uparrow CO_2$ production (associated with impaired alveolar ventilation): fever, thyrotoxicosis, sepsis, steroid, overfeeding, exercise and metabolic acidosis

Clinical Manifestations
- Depending on the baseline CO_2 (symptomatic at higher pCO_2 for chronic hypercapnic pts)
- CNS: $\downarrow$ level of consciousness (at advanced stages it $\downarrow$ respiratory drive $\rightarrow CO_2$ retention), $\uparrow$ cerebral blood flow and $\uparrow$ ICP
- Cardiac: $\downarrow$ myocardial and diaphragmatic contractility, cardiac instability, and arrhythmia
- Hyperkalemia due to respiratory acidosis is mild

Treatment
- Treat the underlying etiology; Mechanical ventilation if indicated

POTASSIUM

POTASSIUM REGULATION

Transcellular Shift
- 98% of K is intracellular
- Balance of K between intracellular and extracellular fluid depend on:
  1. Na-K-ATPase pumps 3Na out and 2K into the cell: $\uparrow$ activity by catecholamines, insulin, thyroid hormone; $\downarrow$ by digitalis
  2. Catecholamine: β_2-receptors $\uparrow$; α-receptors $\downarrow$ K cellular entry
  3. Insulin: $\uparrow$ K entry into the liver and skeletal muscle
  4. K load: passive K entry into the cell after high K load
  5. Extracellular pH: metabolic acidosis $\uparrow$ K exit (uncommon with organic acidemia)
  6. Hyperosmolarity: plasma [K] $\uparrow$ by 0.4–0.8 for every $\uparrow$ 10 of P_{osm} (hyperglycemia, hypernatremia, mannitol); solvent drag
  7. Exercise: through skeletal muscle ATP-dependent K channels
     Normokalemia: exercise $\rightarrow$ ATP $\rightarrow$ Open K channels $\rightarrow$ Local $\uparrow$ K $\rightarrow$ Vasodilation
     Hypokalemia: exercise $\rightarrow \downarrow$ Local $\uparrow$ K and vasodilation $\rightarrow$ Rhabdomyolysis

Determinants of Renal Potassium Excretion

- Aldosterone: ↑ secretion in the principal cells by ↑ the number of ENaC allowing Na absorption creating an electronegative lumen favorable for K secretion through ROMK and BK channels (stimulus for ↑ aldosterone includes ↑ K and hypovolemia)
- Plasma [K]: ↑ K secretion (independent from aldosterone)
- Distal flow: ↑ distal flow → ↑ K secretion; GFR

Tubular Potassium Handling		
Proximal Tubule	Both account for >90% of the filtered K is reabsorbed	Passive reabsorption paracellular
Loop of Henle		NKCC
Distal convoluted tubule	K secretion	Basolateral Na$^+$/K$^+$-ATPase → ↓ intracellular Na$^+$ → Na$^+$ entry via NCC → Electroneutral K into tubular lumen via ROMK
Initial and outer medullary CD	Principal cells: K secretion α-intercalated cells: K reabsorption	Basolateral Na$^+$/K$^+$-ATPase → ↑ intracellular K$^+$ → K$^+$ secretion via ROMK H$^+$/K$^+$ ATPase (H$^+$ secretion and K$^+$ reabsorption)
Inner medullary CD	K secretion	? Passive

- K secretion in the distal tubules is dependent on Na$^+$ reabsorption from the lumen into the peritubular capillary creating a negative charged lumen that potentiates K secretion; this potential is continuously dissipated by the paracellular absorption of Cl$^-$. This mechanism explains the hypokalemia in pathologic conditions where Na$^+$ is reaching the distal tubule with an anion other than Cl$^-$ (eg, RTA type 2, carbenicillin-induced or toluene-induced hypokalemia)

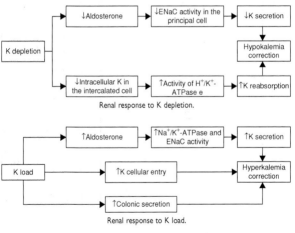

Renal response to K depletion.

Renal response to K load.

HYPERKALEMIA

Pathogenesis

- Potassium adaptation: the efficiency in handling a K load is enhanced if preadapted by a previous K load (the initial smaller load ↑ Na-K-ATPase activity and the density of luminal K channels making the kidney more adapt to handle a higher load)
- Chronic high K intake is unlikely to cause hyperkalemia unless associated with another K balance defect (impaired secretion or cellular entry)

Etiologies of Hyperkalemia

Increased Cell Release	
Pseudohyperkalemia	Blood draw technique (hard venipuncture, repeated fist clenching, tight tourniquet)
	Long specimen storage
	Thrombocytosis (↑ by 0.15/↑ 100K plts): ✓K in a heparinized plasma; nonclotted specimen
	Leukocytosis (WBC >120K) in CLL; ↑K in plasma and serum: ✓K in the serum of clotted specimen before centrifugation
	Hereditary RBC fragility (eg, stomatocytosis)
Red cell breakdown	Transfusion of old PRBC; Intravascular hemolysis
NAGMA	H^+ enter the cell and K exit (Lactic and ketoacid enter the cell with H^+ and do not cause ↑K)
Hyperosmolarity	Solvent drag (eg, hyperglycemia, sucrose after IVIG, radiocontrast)
Insulin deficiency	eg, Fasting in ESRD patients
Respiratory acidosis	Mild effect
Tissue catabolism	TLS, Rhabdomyolysis
Exercise	Level of ↑K depends on the intensity and physical conditioning
Medications	β2-blockers; not with selective β1 blockers
	Digitalis overdose (inhibition of Na^+-K^+-ATPase)
	Succinylcholine, aminocaproic acid (K exit the cell)
	CNI, diazoxide, minoxidil (↑ATP-dep K channels)
Decreased Renal Excretion	
↓ Aldosterone secretion	Hyporeninemic hypoaldosteronism (DN; CNI)
	ACEIs, ARBs, and direct renin inhibitors
	Impaired aldosterone synthesis: chronic heparin therapy, Primary adrenal insufficiency, Severe illness, Inherited disorders (21-hydroxylase deficiency and isolated hypoaldosteronism)
↓ Response to aldosterone	Mineralocorticoid receptor antagonists: spironolactone, eplerenone
	ENaC blockers: amiloride, triamterene, trimethoprim, pentamidine
	Pseudohypoaldosteronism type 1 (AR mutation of the ENaC or AD mutation of the mineralocorticoid receptor)
	Acquired or congenital defects in Na reabsorption by the distal tubule principal cells (voltage RTA): obstructive uropathy, SLE, renal amyloidosis, and sickle cell disease
	Progesterone antagonize aldosterone. Pregnancy improves ↓K, HTN, and metabolic alkalosis in primary aldosteronism. Drospirenone 3 mg ≈ spironolactone 25 mg
↓ Distal Na and water delivery	Volume depletion
	CHF, cirrhosis
Ureterojejunostomy	Urinary K absorption in the jejunum
CKD and AKI	
aka Gordon syndrome	Pseudohypoaldosteronism type 2: mutations causing ↑ NCC → Metabolic acidosis, HTN, ↓K excretion

Workup

- r/o pseudohyperkalemia; review of the history, med; volume status and renal function
- Transtubular K gradient (TTKG), $(U_K/P_K) ÷ (U_{osm}/P_{osm})$ is used to evaluate renal K excretion corrected for the movement of water. The presence of urea recycling in the inner medullary segments of the collecting tubules affects U_{osm} and TTKG is not a valid formula to assess renal K excretion (Curr Opin Nephrol Hypertens 2011;20:547)
- Urinary potassium has limited diagnostic value since it correlates with K intake
- 24-hr urine K >40 mEq/d, spot K/Cr ratio >200 mEq/g, TTKG >11 → ↑ cell release
- 24-hr urine K <30 mEq/d, spot K/Cr ratio <20 mEq/g, TTKG <7 → ↓ renal excretion
- ECG abnormalities: arrhythmias with K >7 or very rapid rise (sinus bradycardia, sinus arrest, slow idioventricular rhythms, VT, VF, and asystole)
  Tall peaked T wave with a shortened QT interval → ↑ PR interval and QRS duration → QRS widens to a sine wave

Treatment

- Assess for emergency: (1) muscle weakness/paralysis; (2) cardiac arrhythmia/conduction abnormalities; (3) K >5.5 with ongoing TLS/rhabdomyolysis; (4) K >6.5
- In emergent case, treat with IV Ca, IV insulin + glucose and start K removal (diuretics, cation exchangers +/- dialysis if refractory); EKG monitoring; K check Q 1-2 hr
- Treat the underlying etiology of hyperkalemia
- Avoid long fasting period for ESRD pts (oral intake ↑ insulin which ↓ K)

Therapy of Hyperkalemia	
Stabilization of the Membrane	
IV calcium	Works within min; action lasts up to 1 hr
	Ca gluconate 3 amp (3 g, 10% 30 mL, 14 mEq Ca) via peripheral line or $CaCl_2$ 1 amp (1 g, 10% 10 mL, 13.6 mEq Ca) via central line over 2-3 min
	Avoid in digitalis toxicity
Drive Extracellular Potassium into the Cells	
Insulin + glucose	Bolus 5-10 units of insulin R + 50 mL of 50% dextrose
	Effect starts in 10-20 min, peaks at 30-60 min, lasts for 4-6 hr
	K drops 0.5-1.2 mEq/L
Albuterol	Lowers the serum potassium concentration by 0.5-1.5 mEq/L
	10-20 mg nebulizer; peak effect in 90 min
	Used as adjuvant to insulin + glucose
Sodium bicarbonate	Beneficial mainly in metabolic acidosis in acute ↑ K; and in chronic ↑ K in CKD
	150 mEq in 1 L of 5% dextrose in water
Removal of Potassium from the Body	
Diuretics	Can be used for both acute and chronic hyperkalemia
	Dosage depends on the renal function
GI cations exchangers	Patiromer (NEJM 2015;372:211)
	8.4-25.2 g qd; give 3-6 hr after or before other po meds
	Exchanges K for Ca in the colon
	s/e: constipation, ↓ Mg
	Sodium zirconium cyclosilicate (NEJM 2015;372:222)
	Sodium polystyrene sulfonate (SPS)
	15-60 g single dose po (+/- sorbitol); 50 g enema (without sorbitol)
	Avoid in postop, ileus or bowel obstruction (s/e: intestinal necrosis)
Dialysis	HD is more efficacious in K removal than PD
	CRRT can be used subsequently in patients with ongoing K release
	Dialysate K <2 a/w sudden cardiac arrest (KI 2011;79:218)
	Rebound ↑ K: K shift to serum after HD. More pronounced after albuterol, insulin and high Na^+ dialysate (JASN 2000;11:2337), post-HD ↓ K should not be corrected unless clinically indicated

HYPOKALEMIA

Pathogenesis

- Decreased intake is rarely a cause of hypokalemia since renal excretion can be lowered to 5 mEq/d; Main hypokalemia etiologies are cell entry and renal excretion
- If lab processing is delayed, pseudohypokalemia occurs in AML (WBC consume K)

Etiologies of Hypokalemia	
Increased Cell Entry	
Insulin mediated	Exogenous insulin in DKA therapy; refeeding syndrome
β2-adrenegic mediated	Endogenous catecholamines: alcohol withdrawal, acute myocardial infarction, head injury, and theophylline intoxication
	Exogenous agonists: albuterol, terbutaline, dobutamine, pseudoephedrine, and ephedrine
Metabolic or respiratory alkalosis	↓ K by <0.4 for every ↑ pH by 0.1
	Hypokalemia maintains the metabolic alkalosis (↑ HCO_3 reabsorption)

Hypokalemic periodic paralysis	Inherited AD or acquired in hyperthyroidism Sudden entry of K into the cell leading to paralysis and resp failure ↓ K (1.5–2.5 mEq/L) precipitated by exercise, high CHO meal Risk of rebound hyperkalemia after therapy
↑ Blood cell production	Vit B₁₂ or folic acid therapy in megaloblastic anemia GM-CSF treatment of neutropenia
Others	Hypothermia, antipsychotic drugs intoxication: chloroquine, Barium (blocks K channels), Cesium
Increased Gastrointestinal Loss	
Diarrhea, villous adenoma	Lower intestinal losses are high in K Acute colonic pseudo-obstruction (Ogilvie syndrome) have high K in the colon lumen due to activation of colonic K secretion
Geophagia	White clay binds K in the GI tract (red clay is high in K and ↑ K)
Increased Urinary Loss	
Vomiting, NGT drainage	Gastric secretions are low in K Metabolic alkalosis → ↑ HCO₃ filtration → ↑ distal flow → ↑ urinary K loss
↑ Mineralocorticoid activity	Diuretics, 1° hyperaldo, renin secreting tumor, RAS Chronic licorice ingestion: inhibition of the 11β-hydroxysteroid dehydrogenase-2 (11-β-HSD2) Apparent mineralocorticoid excess (mutation of 11-β-HSD2)
↑ Distal delivery of Na and water	1° polydipsia, diuretics therapy, primary hyperaldo, Loss of gastric secretions
Nonreabsorbable anions	RTA type 2 (bicarbonate), DKA (β- hydroxybutyrate), toluene use (hippurate) and penicillin derivative Low-calories diet (ketogenesis induces ↑ urinary K loss)
Others	Polyuria, RTA type 1 Hypomagnesemia: K renal loss with open ROMK channels of the DCT Amphotericin B: ↑ K membrane permeability Salt-wasting nephropathies: Bartter, Gittelman, reflux nephropathy, Sjögren Liddle: gain of function mutation of ENaC ↑ Sweat losses (cystic fibrosis) Dialysis, plasmapheresis

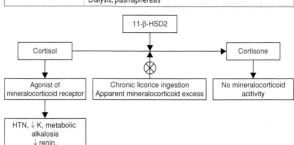

Mechanism of AME and chronic licorice ingestion.

Workup

- Assessment of acid–base status, Mg level
- Urine K >30 mEq/d, spot K/Cr >13 mEq/g, TTKG >7 → renal loss
- Urine K <25 mEq/d, spot K/Cr <13 mEq/g, TTKG <3 → extrarenal loss or cellular entry

Clinical Manifestations

- Dependent on the degree and duration of hypokalemia
- Severe weakness, muscle cramps, and rhabdomyolysis (K <2.5); Resp failure, ileus
- Cardiac arrhythmia: PACs, PVCs, sinus bradycardia, paroxysmal atrial or junctional tachycardia, AVB, VT, VF, Torsade de pointe if ↓ K is a/w ↓ Mg
- Depression of ST segment, ↓ amplitude of the T wave, and ↑ amplitude of U waves

- Risk for arrhythmia ↑ in elderly pts, organic heart disease, or concomitant digoxin
- Can precipitate hepatic encephalopathy in cirrhotic patients

Effects of Hypokalemia on Kidney

- Nephrogenic DI: impaired urinary concentrating ability d/t (1) the resistance to ADH is due to ↓ expression of aquaporin-2 in the collecting tubules; (2) ↓ Activity of Na-K-2Cl cotransporter of the thick ascending loop of Henle leading to defect of the interstitial corticomedullary gradient the driving force for free water reabsorption
- Electrolytes imbalances: ↑ HCO_3 reabsorption (maintenance of metabolic alkalosis), ↑ Na reabsorption (hypertension)
- **Hypokalemic nephropathy:** reversible proximal tubule vacuolar lesions develop after 1 mo of hypokalemia, more prolonged hypokalemia (eg, eating disorders, laxative or diuretics abuse) leads to chronic irreversible interstitial changes with tubular atrophy (more pronounced in the medulla)
- The patient can still maintain the ability to conserve K

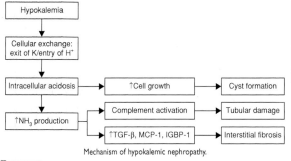

Mechanism of hypokalemic nephropathy.

Treatment

- Repletion of K should be cautious in hypokalemia d/t entry of K into the cell; risk of rebound hyperkalemia in hypokalemic periodic paralysis and thyrotoxic periodic paralysis
- Hypomagnesemia should be corrected to avoid continuous renal wasting
- β-blockers (nonselective) is helpful in hypokalemic thyrotoxic periodic paralysis
- Estimation of K deficit: 200–400 mEq total K deficit ↓ [K] by 1 mEq/L
- The total deficit of K needs to be adjusted with the associated metabolic disorder: in DKA, correction of the hyperosmolarity and the insulin deficiency will drive additional K inside the cell, K supplementation should occur for K <4.5; in diarrhea associated NAGMA, the total K requirement need to be adjusted up since the correction of the acidosis will drive K intracellularly
- K-rich food is less effective since it is under the form of K citrate and K phos which have only a 40% retention
- For chronic hypokalemia from loop diuretic therapy, K-sparing diuretics could be considered as chronic therapy
- Rarely or citrate (RTA, diarrhea), K acetate, K phos (Fanconi Sd) are used

Potassium Supplement	
KCl IV	Should be given in dextrose-free solution to avoid K entry inside the cell Rate 10–20 mEq/hr (max 40 mEq/hr); max IV concentration is 60 mEq/L High concentration is a/w pain and phlebitis
KCl PO	Solid formulation is preferred; good bioavailability Extended release formulations may result in a ghost tablet in the stool s/e: pill-induced esophagitis from osmotic injury Liquid form: 15 mL 10% (1.5 g) ≈ 20 mEq KCl
K citrate	In nephrolithiasis, dRTA with hypocitraturia
KHCO₃	
K phosphate	Used in Fanconi syndrome
Salt substitutes	**1 g** (≈1/6 teaspoon) contains 10–13 mEq KCl (*JAMA* 1977;238:608)

POTASSIUM 4-20

SODIUM AND WATER

Determinants of Serum Sodium Concentration (S_{Na})
- Plasma sodium concentration (P_{Na}): a measure of total body solute concentration; does not correlate with extracellular volume; it does reflect the total body sodium to water ratio, a surrogate for osmolality of the extracellular compartment
- P_{Na} = (total body exchangeable Na + total body exchangeable K)/total body water (TBW)
- Serum sodium concentration (S_{Na}): a reflection of water balance
- Conversely, alteration of sodium balance (high or low intake of salt) leads to changes in extracellular volume
- Urine sodium (U_{Na}): correlates with the extracellular volume (hypovolemia → ↓ U_{Na})
- Dehydration (water loss → ↑ [Na]) ≠ volume depletion
- P_{osm}, and by consequence P_{Na}, is regulated by ADH secretion and thirst

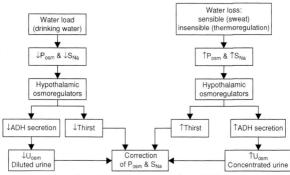

Feedback mechanism to maintain P_{osm} and [Na].

- The urine output varies according to both U_{osm} (adjusted by ADH) and the total solute excretion (exogenous from diet and endogenous for metabolism): V_{urine} = total solute/U_{osm}

HYPONATREMIA

Background
- Definition: [Na] <136
- Usually due to ↓ water excretion and rarely solely from ↑ free water intake
- Classification
  Mild (130–135); moderate (125–130); severe/profound (<125)
  Acute (<24 hr); chronic (>48 hr)
  Symptomatic; asymptomatic
  Hypotonic; pseudohyponatremia (or isotonic); hypertonic
  Hypovolemic; euvolemic; hypervolemic

Clinical Manifestations
- Water movement into the brain leading to brain edema acutely
- Related to the degree and the rapidity of establishment of the hyponatremia
- Symptoms in acute hyponatremia can be nonspecific like malaise, nausea progressing to headache, lethargy, gait imbalance and in extreme cases seizures and coma
- Chronic hyponatremia <130 is associated with subtle neurologic symptoms leading to fall, general malaise, and decrease attention span
- Severe acute hyponatremia can rarely lead to brain edema–induced brain herniation especially in premenopausal women and young children

WORKUP OF HYPONATREMIA (JASN 2017; 28:1340)

Step1: Differentiate Hypotonic from Nonhypotonic Hyponatremia
- Measure P_{osm} to rule out nonhypotonic hyponatremia
- Calculated $P_{osm} = 2 \times [Na] + [Glucose]/18 + BUN/2.8$ (normal: 275–290 mOsmol/Kg)
- Measured P_{osm} (done in the lab) reflects the total of all osmolytes in plasma
  - Hypertonic hyponatremia: osmotically active compounds (eg, glucose, mannitol, alcohols) drawing water out of cells
  - Isotonic hyponatremia: water-insoluble substances (eg, protein and lipid) may interfere with the measurement of sodium. The osmolar gap (Measured-Calculate P_{osm}) is helpful in these circumstances: a difference of more than 10 is in favor of an additional osmolar substance
- Treatment of nonhypotonic hyponatremia is centered around the underlying etiology, eg, hyperglycemia where indicated

Step 2: U_{osm} and GFR to Assess the Role of the Kidney
- U_{osm} is expected to decrease in response to hyponatremia. If hypotonic hyponatremia coexist with low U_{osm} (<100), this can be explained by:
  1. 1° polydipsia (usually >12 L): overwhelming the excretion of dilute urine
  2. Low dietary solute intake (eg, malnutrition, alcoholism): the low total solute excretion limits the amount of maximal daily urinary water excretion due to reduce delivery of fluid in the diluting segment and creates an environment where even a mild increase of hypotonic intake leads to hyponatremia

Step 3: Volume Status Assessment for Patient with High U_{osm} (>100) and U_{Na}
- U_{osm} >100 in a hyponatremia (elevated ADH levels): true hypovolemia, effective hypovolemia, SIADH, hypothyroidism, and Addison disease
- It is sometimes difficult to differentiate clinically hypovolemic hyponatremia from euvolemic hyponatremia (sensitivity and specificity ≈ 50%) (Am J Med 1995;99:348)
- U_{Na} <30 can be used as a supplement to assess volemia (using a cutoff of 30)
- U_{Na} diagnostic value is limited in CKD, recent diuretics use, dietary Na restriction
- ↑ [Na] with isotonic saline infusion trial is favor of hypovolemic hyponatremia (in SIADH with U_{osm} <500, [Na] improves with isotonic saline infusion)
- Since ADH is a uricosuric hormone, fraction of excretion of uric acid (FE_{UA}) is a helpful diagnostic tool: FE_{UA} >12% is sensitive and specific for SIADH

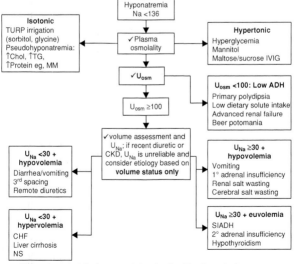

Diagnostic approach for hyponatremia based on P_{osm}, U_{osm}, U_{Na}, and volume status.

- When hypokalemia is concomitant with hyponatremia, the correction of hypokalemia may contribute to the correction of the hyponatremia (the repletion of K helps restore plasma osmolarity by ↑ total body osmoles)
- For acute or severely symptomatic hyponatremia, a bolus of hypertonic saline 3% (100 mL over 10 min ×3 as needed to relieve symptoms or the [Na] increases by 6)
- In hypovolemic hyponatremia, patients will start autocorrecting as soon and the volume is expanded; to avoid rapid correction, it is recommended to combine volume expansion with desmopressin
- The limit for correction is 8 mmol/L/d; Hypotonic fluids and/or DDAVP can be used to relower [Na] if overcorrection occurs
- Restrict fluid intake (both PO and IV) to 500 mL/d below the 24-hr urine volume in low U$_{osm}$ hypervolemic hyponatremia and **Syndrome of Inappropriate Antidiuresis (SIAD)**
- If U$_{osm}$ >300–500, consider furosemide to lower U$_{osm}$
- Urea: induces osmotic diuresis → free water excretion; used as second line to fluid restriction; safe and effective (CJASN 2018;13:1627); Even if overcorrection occurs with urea, the risk of ODS and demyelination lesions is low
- Salt tablets increase urine solute load; Usual doses for NaCl tablets are 6–9 g daily

ADH Antagonist (Vaptans) (NEJM 2015;372:2207)

- Block V2-receptors in collecting duct principal cells → aquaresis
- Tolvaptan (PO): start with 15 mg qd; up to 60 mg, 30 days
- Conivaptan (IV): start with 20 mg over 30 min then 20 mg/24 hr; up to 40 mg/24 hr, 4 days
- NOT indicated in the treatment of acute or severely symptomatic hyponatremia
- s/e: overcorrection, liver toxicity
- On initiation, fluid restriction should be stopped and patient should be allowed access to free water intake to avoid overcorrection; if the target Na is not achieved after 24 hr of vaptan initiation, fluid restriction will be resumed

Treatment of Hyponatremia		
Correction limit	8–10 mEq/L/24 hr	
Correction rate	4–6 mEq/L/24 hr	
Overcorrection	Hypotonic solution DDAVP 2–4 µg IV	Only if baseline <120 mEq/L
Treatment of ODS	Hypotonic solution DDAVP 2–4 µg IV	Lower [Na] by 16 mEq/L
Severe symptomatic hyponatremia	NaCl 3% (100 mL over 10 min) ×3 as needed	Symptoms improve or ↑ Na by 6 mEq/L
SIAD	1st line: address the stimulus of ADH secretion + Fluid restriction^a 2nd line: urea, salt tablets 3rd line: lithium, demeclocycline	Fluid restriction calculation (U$_{Na}$ + U$_K$)/S$_{Na}$ >1 → <500 mL/d ≈1 → 500–700 mL/d <1 → <1 L/d
Hypovolemic hyponatremia	Isotonic volume expansion	DDAVP concomitant in patients with high risk of ODS (hypokalemic, alcoholic, malnutrition) 4–8 µg IV q6-8h
Hypervolemic hyponatremia	1st line: fluid restriction 2nd line: vaptan^b or hypertonic saline + loop diuretics	High risk of overcorrection with Vaptan

^{a}Risk of nonresponders: U$_{Na}$ ≥130 mmol/L; U$_{osm}$ ≥500 mOsm/kg; UOP <1,500 mL/d
^{b}Avoid Vaptan in patients with liver disease

Hyponatremia Formulas
- Effective P$_{osm}$ = 2 × [Na] + [glucose]/18; (normal value: 270–285 mOsmol/kg)
- Since Na and K is the main extracellular and intracellular solutes, respectively:

$$Plasma\ [Na] = (total\ body\ Na + total\ body\ K)/TBW$$

This formula explain why correcting hypokalemia could improve hyponatremia
- Plasma volume: 93% aqueous (water), 7% nonaqueous (fat and protein)
Physiologic [Na] = reported [Na]/0.93 (eg, 143/0.93 ≈ 154 [Na] in 0.9% isotonic saline fluid)

Brain Adaptation to Hyponatremia
- Hyponatremia and $\downarrow P_{osm}$ → water flow across the blood–brain barrier → $\uparrow$ ICP → loss of Na and water into the CSF → improving ICP within min (acute adaptation)
- Chronic adaptation starts within hours through intracellular K loss (cell swelling sensitive cationic channels) followed by loss of brain organic osmolytes (glutamine, glutamate, taurine, and myoinositol) that needs up to 72 hr to be complete

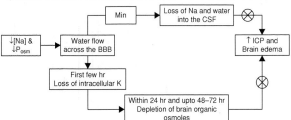

Brain adaptation to hyponatremia.

- The rate of correction of hyponatremia is important whenever the brain has adapted to hypotonicity (after 48–72 hr of established hyponatremia)

Osmotic Demyelination Syndrome (ODS)
- a/w rapid correction of hyponatremia (>8 mEq/L in 24 hr; >16 mEq/L in 48 hr)
- The hourly rate is not a risk factor of ODS unless the daily rate threshold is exceeded
- Prevention: target a rate of correction of 4–6 mEq/L/d in chronic "asymptomatic" hyponatremia

Risk Factors for ODS	
Admission plasma Na	• [Na] ≤120 mEq/L (mainly for ≤105 mEq/L) • [Na] >120 postliver transplant or CDI after dDAVP discontinuation
Therapy	• Hypertonic saline • Vasopressin antagonists
Autocorrection following therapy (rapid renal free water loss)	• Hypovolemic hyponatremia treated with volume expansion • Adrenal insufficiency treated with glucocorticoids • Holding DDAVP in overtreated Central DI; Holding thiazide diuretics • ESRD on HD
Patient related	• Alcoholism; malnutrition; liver disease; pregnancy • Hypokalemia

- In hyponatremic ESRD, during dialysis, the rapid $\uparrow P_{osm}$ induced by the correction of hyponatremia is counterbalanced by HD-induced $\downarrow$ of potassium, uremic toxins including urea (urea does not cross the BBB as fast as water and act as an effective osmole relative to the brain compartment)

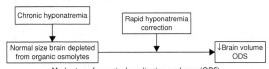

Mechanism of osmotic demyelination syndrome (ODS).

- Clinical manifestation are delayed (2–6 d), irreversible, or partially reversible: dysarthria, dysphagia, paraparesis, quadriparesis, and locked in Sd; behavioral disturbances, tremors, catatonia and seizures; lethargy, confusion, disorientation, obtundation, and coma
- MRI could show the demyelination lesions (delayed finding up to 4 wk) which can affect any part of the brain and spinal cord
- Some proposed preventive measures:
  - In pts likely to overcorrect (hypovolemic hyponatremia): DDAVP (1–2 μg IV or SC q6–8h) is given at the start of onset volume expansion (NS or hypertonic saline)
  - In pts on therapy where the goal is likely to be exceeded or overcorrected → stop therapy + D5W (6 mL/kg) or dDAVP

- Relowering [Na] to the daily correction limit of 8 mEq/L can ↓ the severity of ODS and even after the onset of neurologic, it is recommended to relower [Na] by 16 mEq/L
- For patient with baseline [Na] ≥120, it is probably unnecessary to relower Na in case of overcorrection, slowing the correction rate is enough in these cases

---

SPECIFIC ETIOLOGIES OF HYPONATREMIA

Diuretics-induced Hyponatremia
- More common with thiazides than loop diuretics because loop diuretics prevent the generation of a corticomedullary interstitial osmotic gradient which limits the ability of the collecting tubule to reabsorb free water even if ADH is elevated
- Thiazide-induced hyponatremia is due to several mechanisms: (1) reduction in diluting function of the distal tubule; (2) an underlying tendency to increased water intake (polydipsia); (3) impaired urea-mediated water excretion

Hypervolemic Hyponatremia
- Hyponatremia is an important prognostic factor in CHF and cirrhosis

Syndrome of Inappropriate Antidiuresis (SIAD) (NEJM 2007;356:2064)
- Desalination: since volume expansion does not affect U_{osm} in SIAD, an expansion with isotonic solution results in a net electrolyte-free water gain in patients with SIAD (especially if U_{osm} >500) leading to worsening of the hyponatremia
- Etiologies: drugs, cancer (small cell lung cancer), pulmonary disorders, CNS disorders, hereditary nephrogenic SIAD (GOF mtation of V2 receptor; treated with urea; vaptan are ineffective therapy), idiopathic and transient (nausea, pain, anesthesia)
- Copeptin is produced during the cleavage of the vasopressin prohormone, it can be used as an indirect measurement tool for vasopressin levels
- U_{osm} is an indirect measurement for the ADH concentration, using copeptin in hyponatremia is of limited utility (beyond distinguishing primary polydipsia from the other etiologies of hyponatremia) (Endocrine 2018;60:384)
- SIAD has 5 subtypes:
  Type A: vasopressin/copeptin secretion is not related to S_{osm}; erratic ADH secretion
  Type B: relationship between S_{osm} and Vasopressin/copeptin is intact but lower threshold (reset osmostat)
  Type C: vasopressin/copeptin secretion is not related to S_{osm}; constant ADH secretion
  Type D: undetectable vasopressin/copeptin (nephrogenic SIAD)
  Type E: reverse relationship between S_{osm} and copeptin/vasopressin (barostat reset) due to increased sensitivity of baroreceptors to increased vasopressin release

Cerebral (or Renal) Salt Wasting
- The same lab profile as SIAD (hyponatremia, concentrated urine, high U_{Na}, hypouricemia, and ↑ FE_{UA} >11%). The FE_{UA} does not decrease after correction of the hyponatremia: stays >11%; in SIAD the FE_{UA} decreases to less than 11% with the correction of the hyponatremia (Am J Med Sci 2016;352:385)

Adrenal Insufficiency
- Cortisol deficiency disrupts the negative feedback loop that inhibits ADH release. The increase of corticotropin-releasing hormone production in response to cortisol deficiency promotes hypothalamic ADH release leading to hyponatremia (PNAS 2000;97:483)

Acute Hyponatremia
- Etiologies always involve a high free water intake with additional pathogenesis: postop, exercise, the use of 3,4-methylenedioxymethamphetamine (MDMA, "Ecstasy"), haloperidol, thiazide diuretics, desmopressin, oxytocin, TURP/hysterectomy irrigants (glycine, sorbitol, mannitol, and IV cyclophosphamide)
- Glycine and sorbitol cause cerebral edema; mannitol does not cause cerebral edema (hypertonic hyponatremia)
- MDMA ↑ ADH release and free water intake in an effort to prevent hyperthermia
- Hypertonic saline 3% is an effective and life-saving for hyponatremia-induced cerebral edema

Mild Chronic Hyponatremia (CJASN 2015;10:2268)
- Asymptomatic, >72 hr and [Na] between 125 and 135 mEq/L
- Hyponatremia is a/w higher mortality and morbidities in outpatient, inpatient, and ICU settings (neurocognitive deficits, gait disturbances, falls, bone fractures, osteoporosis)
- It is not clear if correction of hyponatremia improves outcomes

HYPERNATREMIA

Pathogenesis

- Thirst reflex tend to correct hypernatremia/hypertonicity for patients with access to free water. For hypernatremia to occur, in addition to the free water loss, the patient has to lose access to free water (eg, ΔMS, infants, loss of thirst)

Etiologies

- For the etiologies of hypernatremia, the pathogenesis is a combination of electrolyte-free water loss combined with impaired thirst or limited access to free water
- Not all fluid loss will induce hypernatremia, the Na + K content in the fluid should be lower than the plasma [Na] to induced a net fluid loss and ↑ plasma [Na]
  - Secretory diarrhea: Na + K loss in the stools ≈ plasma [Na] → no effect on [Na]
  - Osmotic diarrhea, lactulose, vomiting, osmotic diuresis, sweating: Na + K loss < plasma [Na] → ↑ plasma [Na]
- Hyperglycemia and mannitol therapy initially lead to hyponatremia from ↑ P_{osm} and ↑ water exit from the cells → Osmotic diuresis → free water loss and hypernatremia

Etiologies of Hypernatremia	
Unreplaced Water Loss	
Skin	Insensible (transepidermal loss) Sensible: sweat (sweat is hypotonic to plasma)
GI	Vomiting, NGT suction Nonsecretory diarrhea
Urinary	Central and nephrogenic DI Osmotic diuresis
Decreased Water Intake	
1° hypodipsia	Defect in thirst; patient should be encouraged to ↑ water intake
Adipsic DI	Congenital and acquired CNS lesions Mild volume expansion → suppression of ADH Treatment by adjusting water intake based on body weight
Reset Osmostat	Primary mineralocorticoid excess Mild hypernatremia (high 140s)
Water Loss into Cells	
Severe exercise, seizure (transient hyperNa for 5–15 min)	
Na Overload	
Intake or administration of hypertonic sodium solutions eg, infusion of hypertonic Na bicarbonate solution, hypertonic saline for traumatic brain injury, hypertonic saline during procedures (hydatic cyst irrigation, abortion), salt poisoning (child abuse, accidental)	

Clinical Manifestations

- Acute hypernatremia (<24 hr) can cause irreversible brain damage (osmotic demyelination and cerebral hemorrhage); since the brain did not have time to adapt to hypernatremia, [Na] should be acutely corrected to normal level by giving the entire water deficit volume within 24 hr
- The clinical symptoms are mainly neurologic
- Acute hypernatremia: lethargy, weakness, irritability, seizures, and coma
- Chronic hypernatremia (>48 hr): it is difficult to attribute the symptoms to hyperNa itself or to the underlying etiology causing the impaired mental status

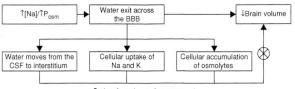

Brain adaptation to hypernatremia.

TREATMENT OF HYPERNATREMIA

General Approach
- Administration of dilute fluid to correct the free water deficit and the ongoing loss
- In DI, desmopressin is the main therapy (review polyuria)
- Free water deficit + electrolyte-free water clearance at

Free Water Deficit = TBW × ([Na]/140 − 1)
- Total Body Water (TBW) = Lean Body Weight (LBW)* × 0.6 (young male), 0.5 (young female, elderly male), or 0.45 (elderly female)
- Another way to estimate: 1 mEq/L of ↑ [Na] ≈ Water deficit of 3 mL/kg
  eg, To correct [Na] by 10 point in a 50-kg female patient with a sodium of 150
  Using the formula: water deficit = 50 × 0.5 (150/140 − 1) = 1,700 mL
  Using the estimation: water deficit = 3 × 10 × 50 = 1,500 mL
- Calculation does not estimate the ongoing free water loss

*Fat has lower water content than muscle: TBW is lower in obese and elderly

Free Water Clearance (C_{H_2O}) = V_{urine} × (1 − U_{osm}/P_{osm})
- If (+): the amount of free water that is lost in the urine; ADH absent or ineffective (NDI or CDI)
- If (−): the amount of free water retained by the kidney; ADH present and effective (osmotic diuresis)
- The cell membrane is permeable to urea: urea does not contribute to the effective P_{osm}
- Since the medullary collecting tubules are not permeable to urea and NH_3, urea does contribute to the effective U_{osm}
- This discrepancy in the handling of urea between the kidney and the other organs limits the value of C_{H_2O} in predicting the effect of urine output on serum [Na] especially if solute diuresis is suspected (postobstructive, hyperalimentation, high catabolic state) and $C_{electrolyte-free\ H_2O}$ is used in solute diuresis to measure the ongoing renal water loss

Electrolyte-free Water Clearance ($C^e_{H_2O}$) = V_{urine} × [1 − ($U_{Na} + U_K$)/P_{Na}]
- The absolute value of free water volume needed to avoid worsening of the hyperNa
- Estimates the contribution of free urinary loss on P_{osm} and plasma [Na]
- If (+): the amount of electrolyte-free water that is loss in the urine; should be added to total volume of free water deficit calculation
- If (−): the amount of electrolyte-free water retained by the kidney (kidneys are correcting the hypernatremia); this amount should be subtracted from the total volume of free water deficit

Repletion Solution
- Oral or NG or PEG tube free water tube boluses are the preferable repletion access
- D5W: preferred IV solution. Can cause hyperglycemia especially in DM, leading to osmotic diuresis worsening hypernatremia. Tx: D2.5W or insulin therapy
- Na (for hypovolemia) or K (for hypokalemia) added ↓ free water amount in IVF
  - 1 L of 0.45% saline (≈154 mOsm): 500 mL of free water
  - 1 L of 0.45% saline + 40 mEq of KCl (≈234 mOsm): 250 mL of free water

The Rate of Correction
- Chronic hypernatremia (>48 hr): lower Na by 10 in 24 hr; max is 12/d
- Acute hypernatremia (<48 hr): lower [Na] by 1–2 mEq/L/hr until [Na] of 140
  - (Initial rate of D5W is 3–6 mL/kg/hr until [Na] reaches 145 and then 1 mL/kg/hr until [Na] 140)
- Rapid correction of the of chronic hypernatremia may cause brain edema, but evidence is not strong (CJASN 2019;14:656)
- Chronic hypernatremia causes accumulation of intracellular osmoles as chronic adaptation to avoid ↓ of brain volume; rapid correction of hypernatremia creates a hypo-osmolar serum compared to the brain and leads to brain swelling mainly in children
- Slow correction rate (<6 mEq/L/d) are associated with higher mortality
- ✓ [Na] q2–4 hr initially, then adjust depending on correction rate

CALCIUM

CALCIUM REGULATION

- Role: bone structure, muscle contraction, coagulation; cell signaling, secretion, and adhesion
- Daily intake ~1,000 mg, net intestinal absorption ~200 mg
- Bone contains 1,000–1,300 g Ca (>99%) by weight as hydroxyapatite: $Ca_{10}(PO_4)_6(OH)_2$
- ECF Ca content is <0.1% of total body stores

Hormones Regulating Ca and PO₄			
Regulator	Stimulus	Net Effects	Major Site of Action
PTH	↓ Ca, ↑ PO₄	↑ Ca, ↓ PO₄	Kidney, Bone
1,25(OH)₂D₃ (Calcitriol)	↓ Ca, ↓ PO₄	↑ Ca, ↑ PO₄	Intestine
Calcitonin	↑ Ca	↓ Ca	Bone
FGF-23	Dietary ↑ PO₄	↓ PO₄	Kidney

- CaSR in parathyroid gland senses ionized Ca (iCa) and controls PTH secretion
- Vitamin D₃ (cholecalciferol, from UV light-mediated skin production, animal) and vitamin D₂ (ergocalciferol, from fish, plants) are converted to 25-(OH)D₂ (calcidiol) in liver; converted to 1,25(OH)₂D₃ (calcitriol) by 1-α hydroxylase in kidney: activated by PTH; inhibited by FGF-23

Serum Calcium Regulating Mechanisms (CJASN 2015;10:1257)		
Site	Increasing Serum Ca	Decreasing Serum Ca
Intestine	Calcitriol: calbindin, TRPV6 mediated	Excreted in the bile
Bone	PTH: ↑ RANKL → osteoclast-mediated resorption → ↑ Ca, PO₄ release Metabolic acidosis: Ca, PO₄ released from bone (NEJM 1979; 301:535)	Calcitonin: ↓ osteoclast activity → ↓ bone resorption (Am J Physiol 1996;271:F216)
Kidney	PTH: reabsorption in TAL, DCT; ↑ calcitriol synthesis Volume depletion, thiazide Metabolic alkalosis: ↑ TRPV5 → ↑ renal reabsorption (JASN 2010;21:1440)	Calcitonin: ↓ reabsorption ↑ Ca: CaSR → ↓ reabsorption Volume expansion, loop diuretics Metabolic acidosis: ↓ TRPV5 → ↓ renal reabsorption (JASN 2006;17:617)
Serum	Acidosis: ↓ albumin binding (↑ iCa)	Alkalosis: ↑ albumin binding (↓ iCa)

- Kidney filters ~10 g/d; reabsorbs 97–99%; excretes 100–300 mg/d; 24-hr FE_{Ca} 1–3%

Renal Reabsorption of Filtered Calcium (CJASN 2015;10:1257)	
PCT (60–70%)	Passive solvent drag by sodium transport; ↑ by volume depletion, thiazide; ↓ by acetazolamide, osmotic diuretics Minor active transport regulated by PTH and calcitonin
TAL (20–25%)	Paracellular via claudin-16/19, driven by (+) lumen from ROMK/NKCC2: inhibited by loop diuretics Basolateral CaSR inhibits claudin-16/19 via claudin-14: ↓ reabsorption PTH inhibits claudin-14: ↑ reabsorption (PNAS 2017;114:E3344)
DCT (10%) and CD (~5%)	Apical TRPV5, intracellular calbindin-D28K: ↑ by PTH Basolateral NCX moves Ca to blood: ↑ by thiazides

Calcium Measurement

- Ionized Ca (iCa): preferred measurement, unbound, physiologically active form
  ΔpH by 0.1 ≈ 0.08 mmol/L ΔiCa in opposite direction (d/t ΔH⁺ albumin binding)
- Serum protein (albumin and Ig) level changes serum total Ca level to maintain iCa level
  - Adjusted Ca = Ca + {0.8 × (4 − albumin in g/dL)}
  - If ↓ GFR, unadjusted value may be more accurate (BMJ Open 2018;8:e017703)
- Pseudohypocalcemia: gadodiamide, gadoversetamide interfere w/ total Ca assay

Calcium Balance in CKD

- KDOQI target: 8.4–9.5; both below and above range are a/w ↑ mortality (NDT 2011;26:1948)
- Hypercalcemia: a/w extraskeletal calcification and cardiovascular morbidity
- Hypocalcemia: common in CKD; a/w ↑ PTH secretion

Pathogenesis and Causes of Hypercalcemia	
PTH	1° hyperparathyroidism (HPT), 3° HPT s/p kidney transplantation Parathyroid cancer; MEN 1/2A (pituitary/thyroid cancer FHx), lithium
PTH-related peptide (PTHrp)	SCC, RCC, breast, ovarian, bladder cancer > leukemia, lymphoma Pregnancy, tends to be mild (Endocr J 2008;55:95)
Calcitriol	Vit D excess, granuloma (TB, sarcoidosis, ANCA, Crohn's), lymphoma Sarcoidosis + vit D ($\times$2) or renal dysfunction ($\times$4.1) (Am J Med Sci 2016;352:252) Idiopathic (Arch IM 1997;157:2142)
Osteolysis, ↑ Bone turnover	Multiple myeloma, metastasis, hypervitaminosis A Paget disease, hyperthyroidism (Endocr Pract 2003;9;517)
Renal retention	Thiazide, milk (or $CaCO_3$)-alkali syndrome: vomiting or volume depletion worsen metabolic alkalosis → ↑ renal Ca reabsorption Familial hypocalciuric hypercalcemia (FHH): AD CaSR inactivating mutation → ↑ Mg, Ca reabsorption; ↑ PTH Acquired form: Ab against CaSR (NEJM 2004;351:362)
Immobilization	Usually <11, possibly resorptive mechanism (NEJM 1982;306:1136)

- Malignancy: m/c cause (35%) of hypercalcemia at ED (Am J Emerg Med 2013;31:657)
  - Humoral hypercalcemia of malignancy (PTHrp >> PTH) > osteolysis > calcitriol mediated

Clinical Manifestations and Workup
- AKI (vasoconstriction), constipation, weakness, fatigue, memory loss, confusion
- NDI: ↓ aquaporin-2 & ↑ medullary Ca deposition → osmotic gradient impairment
- Chronic hypercalciuria (1° HPT, sarcoidosis) → nephrolithiasis, nephrocalcinosis → CKD
- EKG: Short QT interval, prolonged QRS, bradycardia, U waves
- Hypomagnesemia: d/t CaSR activation → ↓ renal reabsorption

Typical Calcium Level (g/dL) by Causes	
>12	Malignancy, calcitriol production, ingestion
<12	1° HPT, immobilization, FHH, thiazide, lithium

- If PTH inappropriately normal (not suppressed) in hypercalcemia, 1° HPT possible

PTH and PO_4 Changes in Hypercalcemia					
PTH	PO_4	Possible Causes	PTH	PO_4	Possible Causes
↓	↓	Thiazide, milk-alkali syndrome	↑	↓	1° HPT, FHH
↓	↑	↑ Calcitriol, ↑ bone turnover	↑	↑	3° HPT
↓	Var.	Malignancy: ✓ PTHrp, 1,25-Vit D, SIFE/UIFE, FLC			

- Renal retention: 24-hr FE_{Ca} <1%, Ca <100–200 mg/d; random Ca/Cr <0.01 (less reliable)

Treatment
- Fluid: PO; IV if symptomatic or Ca >13; goal UOP 1–2 mL/kg/hr; NS to avoid alkalosis
- Loop diuretics: after volume repletion; little effect solely (Ann IM 2008;149:259); may ↑ alkalosis
- Restrict Vitamin D and dietary Ca (<400 mg/d) in calcitriol mediated
  - Supplement if 1° HPT: deficiency may ↑ PTH
- Bisphosphonates: inhibit osteoclast activity; onset of action is 2–4 d after administration

Bisphosphonate Use in Hypercalcemia (KI 2008;74;1385; Nat Clin Pract Nephrol 2006;2:459)			
Drug	Side Effects	CrCl <30	CrCl >30
Pamidronate	Rare collapsing FSGS (JASN 2001;12:1164)	60–90 mg over 4–6 hr HD: 30 mg qd × 3 d	90 mg over 2–3 hr
Zoledronic acid: superior in malignancy (J Clin Onc 2001;19:558)	Dose and infusion rate dependent ATN (KI 2003;64:281)	Avoid	>60: 4 mg 50–60: 3.5 mg 40–49: 3.3 mg 30–39: 3 mg over 15 min

- 1α-hydroxylase inhibition in ↑ calcitriol: hydrocortisone 100–300 mg/d, prednisone: 10–60 mg/d, ketoconazole, hydroxychloroquine 400 mg qd (CMAJ 2019;191:E390)
- Calcitonin: 4 IU/kg q6–12hr × 2 d, not dosed >48 hr d/t tachyphylaxis

- **Denosumab**: anti-RANKL monoclonal Ab; inhibits osteoclasts and bone resorption
  - s/e: prolonged ↓ Ca; common in CKD. Low dose, eg, 0.3 mg/kg w/ vitamin D may be safe *(Clin Lymphoma Myeloma Leuk 2014;14:e207)*
- **Gallium nitrate**: ↓ osteoclast activity; AKI reported. Not recommended if Cr >2.5
- **Cinacalcet**: start at 30 mg bid, titrate up to 90 mg bid; in 1° and 2° HPT
- **HD/CRRT**: in volume overloaded CKD or severe symptoms; low Ca bath; <2.5 mEq/L bath a/w arrest *(KI 2011;79:218)*
- **Parathyroidectomy**: in 1° HPT with Ca >1.0 or more above the ULN *(JCEM 2014;99:3561)*

HYPOCALCEMIA

CALCIUM 4-30

Pathogenesis and Causes of Hypocalcemia

PTH-Related Mechanisms	
Hypoparathyroidism *(JCEM 2016;101:2273; JCEM 2016;101:2300)*	Neck surgery (75%), neck radiation, DiGeorge syndrome CaSR-activating Ab and mutation (AD), Idiopathic Infiltrative: Wilson's, hemochromatosis, metastasis Pseudohypoparathyroidism: ↑ PTH (resistance), ↑ Ca, ↑ PO₄
Hungry bone syndrome *(Am J Med 1988;84:654)*	Abrupt ↓ PTH after parathyroidectomy → ↑ bone uptake of Ca, PO₄, and Mg, ↓ renal reabsorption of Ca, ↓ intestinal reabsorption of Ca, PO₄ Nadir Ca typically 2–4 d postop; ↓ Ca may last mo
Hypomagnesemia	PTH deficiency and receptor resistance *(JASN 1999;10:1616)*
CaSR-Related Mechanisms	
Hypermagnesemia	CaSR-mediated PTH suppression
AD hypocalcemia/ hypoparathyroidism	CaSR activating mutation *(NEJM 1996;335:1115)* → ↓ PTH secretion; inhibition of ROMK/NKCC2 → type V Bartter syndrome w/ ↓ K, metabolic alkalosis; ↓ Ca, Mg
Calcimimetics (cinacalcet, etelcalcetide)	↑ CaSR sensitivity to Ca → ↓ PTH ↓ Ca in 69% and 60%, respectively *(JAMA 2017;317:156)*
Vitamin D Related Mechanisms	
Vit D deficiency	↓ Sun exposure, diet, aging, postmenopause, malabsorption
CKD	↑ FGF-23 inhibits calcitriol synthesis
Nephrotic syndrome	Loss of calcidiol bound to vitamin D-binding protein
CYP inducers	Phenytoin, phenobarbital, rifampin, INH; metabolize calcidiol
Other Mechanisms	
Sequestration	Pancreatitis, foscarnet, acute respiratory alkalosis Citrate: used in blood transfusion and CRRT; a/w liver dysfunction: ↓ conversion to HCO₃, nl total Ca, ↓ iCa ↑ PO₄: CKD, AKI, rhabdomyolysis, TLS Osteoblastic metastases: breast, prostate cancer
↓ Bone resorption	Bisphosphonates, denosumab
Spurious hypocalcemia	Assay interference of gadodiamide, gadoversetamide

Clinical Manifestations and Workup
- ↓ BP, irritability, spasms, oral/distal paresthesia → papilledema, seizure, tetany
- Chvostek sign: facial nerve tapping → facial muscle contraction; low specificity
- Trousseau sign: BP cuff inflation 3–5 min → carpal spasm; high specificity *(NEJM 2012;367)*
- EKG: ΔQT length ∝ Δ Ca level from baseline; narrow T, heart block → TdP

PTH and PO₄ Changes in Hypocalcemia

PTH	PO₄	Common Causes	PTH	PO₄	Common Causes
↓	↓	↓ Mg	↑	↓	Vit D deficiency
↓	↑	Hypoparathyroidism	↑	↑	CKD Pseudohypoparathyroidism

- Hypoparathyroidism: ↑ CKD 3–5 (41%, ×2–17), ↑ renal calcification (31%) *(JCEM 2012;97:4507)*, ↑ kidney stone (×4.22) *(JBMR 2013;28:2277)* d/t Ca supplement, ↓ PTH-mediated Ca reabsorption

Treatment
- Correct low Mg: IV or PO Mg depending on severity, PO access
- Correct high PO₄: ↑ Ca-PO₄ product may cause AKI; still need IV Ca if symptoms

- Correct respiratory alkalosis
- Vitamin D: if deficient; ↓ Ca requirement by ↑ intestinal absorption
  - Ergocalciferol 50,000 IU weekly ×8 wk (BMJ 2008;336:1298) or active vitamin D if ESRD
- In postsurgical hypoparathyroidism, maintain Ca 8–8.5, 24-hr urine Ca <300 mg to prevent hypercalciuria induced nephrocalcinosis and nephrolithiasis d/t absence of PTH-mediated Ca reabsorption (Endocr Pract 2011;17 suppl1:18)

Calcium Supplementation		
IV: if symptomatic, EKG Δ, iCa <1.0 mmol/L or total Ca <7.5 Ca gluconate 1–2 g over 10–20 min; if iCa in 30 min <1.0 mmol/L, drip + PO calcium ✓ Ionized Ca, BMP, Mg, PO$_4$ q6h Do **NOT** mix w/ HCO$_3$ or PO$_4$ to avoid insoluble Ca salts; IV Ca can worsen digoxin toxicity		
Ca gluconate	1 g (1 ampule, 10% 10 mL) ≈ 93 mg (4.65 mEq) elemental Ca Start drip with 0.5–1 mg/kg/hr of elemental Ca (5.4–10.8 mg/kg/hr Ca gluconate) and adjust to maintain total Ca 9, iCa 1.2 mmol/L 1 mg/mL elemental Ca solution: 11 g (≈1,023 mg elemental Ca) + 890 mL or 12 g (≈1,116 mg elemental Ca) + 1,000 mL of NS or D5W	
Ca chloride	1 g (1 ampule, 10% 10 mL) ≈ 272 mg (13.6 mEq) elemental Ca Use only in unstable patients; s/e: infusion site reactions	
PO: if mild, asymptomatic; between meals if PO$_4$ is normal or low; with meals if PO$_4$ is high s/e: constipation, ↓ PO$_4$, (+) Ca balance; kidney stone (NEJM 2006;354:669)		
Ca carbonate	Elemental Ca 40% by weight, give tid up to 2–4 g/d	
Ca citrate	Elemental Ca 21% by weight; avoid in CKD (↑ Aluminum absorption)	

- HD in advanced CKD: 3–3.5 mEq/L Ca bath; avoid high HCO$_3$ dialysate: can ↓ iCa rapidly

PHOSPHATE

PHOSPHATE REGULATION (Curr Opin Nephrol Hypertens 2013;22:481)

- Phosphorus (P): chemical element, always in combo w/ other elements
- Organic phosphate (PO$_4^{3-}$): phosphoric ester; component of ATP, DNA, RNA; intracellular
- Inorganic phosphate (Pi): measured in ECF; HPO$_4^{2-}$/H$_2$PO$_4^-$ = 4:1 at pH 7.4
- Typical American diet contains 1,000–1,500 mg/d; recommended minimum 700 mg/d
- GI absorption: nonsaturable, constant, 60–80% of dietary load; by calcitriol-dependent type IIb Na PO$_4$ cotransporter (Npt2b) + calcitriol-independent paracellular transport
- Total body stores ~900 g: ~85% in bone, ~15% in soft tissues, ~0.01% in ECF
- ECF is reservoir for all Pi exchange, tightly regulated (CJASN 2015;10:1257)

Serum Phosphate Regulating Mechanisms (Ann Rev Phys 2013;75:535; ACKD 2011;18:77)		
Site	Increasing PO$_4$	Decreasing PO$_4$
Intestine	Calcitriol, ↓ PO$_4$	FGF-23 via ↓ calcitriol; nicotinamide
Bone	Calcitriol, PTH	
Kidney	Calcitriol, ↓ PO$_4$, Thyroid hormone, IGF-1, Etidronate, Alkalosis	PTH, FGF-23, ↑ PO$_4$ → ↓ reabsorption FGF-23 also ↓ calcitriol synthesis Steroids, estrogens (KI 2008;73:1141) Acidosis (CJASN 2014;9:1627)

- Kidney filters 6–9 g/d; Tubular reabsorption of PO$_4$ is 75–95% = 1 − FE$_{PO_4}$ (5–25%)
- PCT is a major site (80–85%) of phosphate reabsorption via apical Npt2a, Npt2c, and Na-dependent PO$_4$ transporter 2 (PiT-2)
- PTH and FGF-23/Klotho ↑ endocytosis of Npt2a (Mol Cell Endocrinol 2016;436:224) → phosphaturia
- Nicotinamide: metabolite of niacin; ↓ intestinal Npt2b and renal Npt2a, Npt2c

ACUTE PHOSPHATE NEPHROPATHY

- Acute PO$_4$ load from tumor lysis syndrome (TLS), sodium phosphate PO (JASN 2005;16:3389; KI 2009;76:1027) or enema (Arch IM 2012;172:263) → AKI
- Kidney biopsy: CaP deposition in tubular lumen and tubular cells with (+) von Kossa stain
- Prevention: avoid sodium phosphate agent in high risk patients (CKD, volume depletion); PO$_4$ binder in established or high risk TLS

Causes of Hyperphosphatemia	
Nonrenal Origin (FE$_{PO_4}$ >15%)	**Renal Retention (FE$_{PO_4}$ <15%)**
Acute load: Na-PO$_4$ bowel prep (JASN 2005;16:3389), high dose fosphenytoin Transcellular shift: rhabdo, TLS, (rarely) hemolysis ECF shift: severe metabolic acidosis, hyperglycemia	Renal dysfunction: inadequate renal excretion ± 2° HPT ↑ bone release in CKD Hypoparathyroidism Pseudohypoparathyroidism: PTH resistance Vit D toxicity: ↑ Ca →↓ PTH Familial tumoral calcinosis: mutations ↓ FGF-23 or action, soft tissue calcified masses Acromegaly, etidronate

Clinical Implication in CKD
- Hyperphosphatemia is a/w ↑ PTH, ↑ FGF-23, ↓ calcitriol (directly and indirectly from ↑ FGF-23), ↑ vascular injury: oxidative stress and calcification
- Sequence in CKD: ↑ FGF-23 → ↓ Calcitriol → ↑ PTH → ↑ PO$_4$ (JASN 2010;21:1427)
- In HD pts, PO$_4$ >5.5 a/w ↑ mortality by 20% c/t 3.5–4.5 (NEJM 2008;359:584)
- In nondialysis CKD pts, PO$_4$ 3.5–4.0 a/w ↑ mortality by 32% c/t 2.5–3 (JASN 2005;16:520)
- ↑ FGF23: a/w mortality in HD (NEJM 2008;359:584), ESRD and mortality in CKD (JAMA 2011;305:2432)

Clinical Manifestations and Workup
- Hypocalcemia: skeletal and extraskeletal CaP precipitation
- Rarely symptomatic from accompanied hypocalcemia: could be life threatening
- Pseudohyperphosphatemia: lab error d/t high level of Ig, lipids, bilirubin, liposomal amphotericin B

Treatment of Acute Hyperphosphatemia
- IV fluid in volume depleted AKI and nondialysis-dependent CKD
- HD:AKI/TLS with symptomatic hypocalcemia or Ca × PO$_4$ ≥70 mg^2/dL^2 or advanced CKD

Treatment of Chronic Hyperphosphatemia
- Diet restrict <1 g/d (JAMA 2009;301:629), then use PO$_4$ binders
- Goal in CKD: 3.5–5.5 (KDOQI AJKD 2003;42:S1); "normal range" (KDIGO MBD KI 2017;92:26)
- Phosphate binders: 29%↓ all-cause mortality, 22%↓ CV mortality in CKD5 (KI 2013;84:998)

Phosphate Binders	
Drugs	**Comments**
Calcium-based binders	Affordable; help control of metabolic acidosis and ↓ Ca s/e: ↑ Ca and Ca × PO$_4$, constipation, metabolic alkalosis
Ca acetate, Ca carbonate	
Ca citrate	↑ GI aluminum absorption (KI 1990;38:937) → toxicity
Noncalcium-based binders	↓ Mortality in CKD (RR 0.54) (CJASN 2016;11:232) ↓ Mortality overall (Lancet 2013;382:1268)
Sevelamer carbonate (Renvela®), Sevelamer hydrochloride (Renagel®)	↓ Mortality, hypercalcemia, ↓ LDL c/w Ca-based binders (CJASN 2012;7:487; AJKD 2013;62:771; CJASN 2016;11:232) s/e: metabolic acidosis (sevelamer hydrochloride)
Lanthanum carbonate	↓ Pill burden (CJASN 2008;3:1437); s/e: diarrhea; ↑ bone turnover; in rats, accumulates in the liver (KI 2005;68:2809)
Nicotinamide	↑ HDL (CJASN 2008;3:1131)
Ferric citrate	↑ Tsat, Hb (JASN 2015;26:493)
Sucroferric oxyhydroxide	↓ Pill burden (NDT 2015;30:1037), ↑ Tsat, Hb (NDT 2017;32:1330)
Aluminum hydroxide	Potent PO$_4$ lowering effect; s/e: aluminum toxicity: dementia, osteomalacia; should be limited to a few days

- HD: removes 800–900 mg/session; significant rebound after HD (mobilization of PO$_4$ occurs more slowly than K, Ca, BUN); can be used in non-CKD (AJKD 2018;72:457)
- Cinacalcet: in 2° HPT/CKD, more pts achieve <5.5 (CJASN 2008;3:36)
  - ↓ PTH-mediated bone resorption, ↓ requirement of active vitamin D may ↓ GI absorption
- Parathyroidectomy: ↓ bone resorption; consider if refractory
- Acetazolamide in familial tumoral calcinosis: ↑ renal excretion of PO$_4$

Causes of Hypophosphatemia	
Nonrenal Origin	**Renal Wasting**
FE_{PO_4} <5%, 24-hr urine PO_4 <100 mg	FE_{PO_4} >5%, 24-hr urine PO_4 >100 mg
Transcellular shifts: insulin, glucose, refeeding syndrome, hungry bone, respiratory alkalosis (head injury)	Fanconi syndrome
	1° or 2° HPT, Vit D deficiency
↓ Absorption: GI resections, diarrhea, PO_4 binders, aluminum, Mg	↑ FGF-23: genetic hypophosphatemic rickets, oncogenic osteomalacia
CRRT, immediately after HD	Hepatectomy *(JASN 2014;25:761)*
	Chronic alcohol use *(NEJM 2017;377:1368)*

- Vitamin D deficiency: ↓ intestine absorption and ↑ renal wasting; ↓ Ca → 2° HPT → ↑ FE_{PO_4}
- Nutritional phosphate deficiency: low FE_{PO_4}, low/normal PTH, ↑ calcitriol
- Fanconi syndrome: PCT damage→ renal wasting of glc, UA, AA, PO_4; from light chain (LCPT), heavy metals, NRTIs, tenofovir, ifosfamide, cystinosis, Wilson disease
- Genetic hypophosphatemic rickets: x-linked *(PHEX)*, AD *(FGF23)*, AR *(DMP1, ENPP1)*

Oncogenic Osteomalacia (Tumor-induced Osteomalacia)
- Mesenchymal tumor secreting FGF-23; rarely osteosarcoma, SCLC, colon ca *(JCEM 2013;98:887)*
- Labs: ↑ FE_{PO_4}, ↑ FGF-23, ↓ or inappropriately nl calcitriol, nl or ↑ (by ↓ calcitriol) PTH, nl Ca, ↑ Aφ
- Imaging: skeletal survey (fractures, osteomalacia), 68Ga-DOTATATE PET/CT
- Manifestations: weakness, bone pain, recurrent fractures; Tx: tumor resection

Clinical Manifestations
- Symptomatic if <1: myopathy, seizure, confusion, ↓ myocardial contractility *(NEJM 1977;297:901)*
- ↓ diaphragmatic contractility *(NEJM 1985;313:420)*, rhabdomyolysis

Treatment
- Correct any existing vitamin D deficiency: ↑ intestinal absorption, ↓ renal wasting
- PO if asymptomatic: 1–1.3 mmol/kg/d divided ×3; can add skim milk (15 mmol PO_4/480 mL)
  - Phos-NaK powder: 250 mg elemental P (8 mmol), Na 6.9 mEq, K 7.1 mEq/packet
  - Phos-NaK tablet: 250 mg elemental P (8 mmol), Na 13 mEq, K 1.1 mEq/tablet
- IV if symptomatic: Na- or K-PO_4; max 80 mmol within 12 hr
  - if PO_4 <1.5, 0.64–1 mmol/kg; if PO_4 1.6–2.2, 0.32–0.64 mmol/kg
  - s/e: precipitation of Ca × PO_4 can cause hypocalcemia w/ tetany
- Dipyridamole: ↑ renal reabsorption

MAGNESIUM

- Intake ~350 mg/d; absorption in small bowel via saturable TRPM6, passive diffusion
- Total body stores: ~26 g; ~60% in bone, ~40% in soft tissues, <1% in ECF
- 70% of total plasma Mg is not protein-bound: filtered in kidney; 95% reabsorbed

Renal Magnesium Reabsorption *(CJASN 2015;10:1257)*	
PCT (20–30%)	Passive
TAL (50–70%)	Paracellular via claudin-16/19, driven by (+) lumen from ROMK/NKCC2. Inhibited by basolateral CaSR via claudin-14 *(JASN 2015;26:11)*.
DCT (5–10%)	Apical TRPM6: mediated by epidermal growth factor receptor (EGFR)

Causes of Hypermagnesemia	
Nonrenal Origin	**Renal Retention**
IV for preeclampsia (mother and neonate)	↓ Renal excretion: AKI, CKD
Mg-containing laxatives/enemas, Epsom salt (=$MgSO_4$) *(J Acute Med 2015;5:80)*	Familial hypocalciuric hypercalcemia: AD CaSR inactivating mutation; ↑ Mg, ↑ Ca reabsorption
Transcellular release: tumor lysis, rhabdo	

Clinical Manifestation

- Symptomatic if >5, progressive neurologic silencing effect: loss of DTR, nausea, lethargy, confusion, paralysis; AV block, arrest
- ↓ Ca: by CaSR-mediated suppression of PTH

Treatment

- d/c administration; if ↓ renal function IV fluid and/or loop diuretic; HD if severe
- If symptomatic, Ca gluconate IV 2 g over 10–20 min to stabilize membrane; dialysis

HYPOMAGNESEMIA

Causes of Hypomagnesemia	
Nonrenal Origin	**Renal Wasting**
FE$_{Mg}$ <2%, 24-hr urine <10 mg/d	FE$_{Mg}$ >2%, 24-hr urine >10–30 mg/d
↓ GI absorption: PPI (*NEJM* 2006;355:1834), patiromer, large bowel resection, chronic diarrhea ↑ Bone uptake: hungry bone Alcohol, poor nutrition Complexation: pancreatitis, transfusion Intracellular shift: insulin, refeeding (*Diabetologia* 1986;29:644); β-agonist, acute alkalosis, severe burns	Metabolic acidosis: ↑ filterable Mg Loop and thiazide diuretics, Bartter, Gitelman Post-ATN, postobstruction, uncontrolled DM Cisplatin, amphotericin, foscarnet Basolateral CaSR activation: ↑ Ca, aminoglycosides (poly-cation) → inhibits ROMK and claudin 16/19 → ↓ Mg, Ca reabsorption Familial hypomagnesemia w/ hypercalciuria and nephrocalcinosis: AR claudin-19 mutation ↓ TRPM6: tac (*JASN* 2004;15:549), CsA, EGFR Abs: cetuximab, panitumumab, matuzumab; AR mutation (*Nat Genet* 2002;31:171)

- Chronic alcohol abuse: poor nutrition + renal tubular wasting (*NEJM* 1993;329:1927)
- If unclear w/ history, ✓ FE$_{Mg}$ = [(U_{Mg} × P_{Cr})/(0.7 × P_{Mg}) × U_{Cr}] × 100%

Clinical Manifestation

- Tetany and seizure (similar to ↓ Ca), nystagmus, apathy, depression, athetosis
- QRS widening, peaked T waves, prolonged PR (similar to ↑ K), torsade de pointes
- ↓ K: ↑ ROMK-mediated K secretion in DCT from ↓ intracellular Mg (*JASN* 2007;18:2649)
- ↓ Ca: PTH deficiency and resistance
- ↑ NODAT (*JASN* 2016;27:1793), ↑ mortality in HD (*AJKD* 2015;66:1047)

Treatment

- PO if asymptomatic: use sustained-release or small frequent doses to ↑ absorption
  Elemental Mg content: oxide (60%) > OH (41%) > SO$_4$ (10%) > gluconate (5%): least diarrhea;
  s/e: diarrhea, GI discomfort, ↑ Mg; Half dose for eGFR <30
- IV if symptomatic or <1 mg/dL: 2 g MgSO$_4$ (192 mg, 16 mEq elemental Mg) over 15 min; if symptoms persist infuse up to 8 g over 24 hr; monitor telemetry, DTRs
- For patients with arrhythmias (esp. ventricular), maintain Mg >2 mg/dL
- Amiloride, triamterene, and spironolactone: for renal wasting or medical conditions requiring diuresis despite hypomagnesemia

Background
- ATN and prerenal azotemia are the leading causes of acute kidney injury (AKI)
- ATN causes 38% of AKI in hospitalized pts, 76% of AKI in ICU (Ann IM 2002;137:744)

Causes
- **Main causes of ATN:** ischemia, sepsis, and nephrotoxins
- Ischemia includes any cause of renal hypoperfusion and prolonged prerenal state
  Hemorrhagic, cardiogenic, hypovolemic, anaphylactic shock
  Renal artery occlusion (eg, embolic, renal artery dissection)
  Surgery (especially cardiac, intra-abdominal)
- Nephrotoxins: numerous medications, iodinated contrast media, pigment (hemoglobin/myoglobin from hemolysis/rhabdomyolysis), ethylene glycol, synthetic cannabinoids
- Less frequent causes: nephrotic syndrome (especially MCD), hyperbilirubinemia, hypercalcemia

Pathogenesis of Ischemic ATN (Nat Rev Nephrol 2011;7:189)
- Decreased effective arterial volume in prerenal azotemia leads to activation of neuro-hormonal cascade including ↑ sympathetics, RAAS, and vasopressin
- ↑ Angiotensin II during hypovolemia leads to preferential efferent arteriolar vasoconstriction, which attempts to preserve GFR despite ↓ renal blood flow; eventually afferent arteriole vasoconstricts and overall renal blood flow and GFR drop
- To prevent excessive vasoconstriction, kidney produces vasodilatory NO and prostaglandins, but this counter-regulatory system has its limits
- Ischemia → tubular cell apoptosis/necrosis, esp in PT b/c high metabolic demands and susceptible microcirculation; leakage/dysfunction of PT cells → ↑ afferent arteriole vasoconstriction, inflammation, endothelial damage
- Ischemia also injures endothelium causing deranged coagulation and permeability → ischemic microcirculation, extending AKI damage
- ATN may cause dysfunction in other organs; animal models show increase in pulmonary vascular permeability and cardiac inflammation

Pathogenesis of Septic ATN (Curr Opin Crit Care 2014;20:588)
- Occurs even in setting of preserved or increased renal blood flow
- Sepsis triggers dysfunction in renal microcirculation involving endothelium, vascular tone, abnormal coagulation, oxidative stress, and inflammation

Clinical Manifestations and Workup
- As with other causes of AKI, presents with rising creatinine +/− oliguria (see AKI definition)
- Nonoliguric ATN with better prognosis than oliguric
- FE_{Na} >1%, FE_{Urea} >35%, Urine sodium >20–40, BUN:Cr ratio <20:1
  FE_{Na} can be <1% if ATN occurs in cirrhosis or CHF
- Urinalysis: usually acellular with <1 g proteinuria, sediment can have "muddy brown" casts and renal tubular epithelial casts
- Kidney Bx: PT simplification/flattening, loss of PAS+ brush border, vacuolization

Management
- Correct ischemia and sepsis; discontinue nephrotoxins

ATN FOLLOWING CARDIAC SURGERY
- 18% incidence of AKI, 2–6% requiring HD (CJASN 2015;10:500)
- Similar pathogenesis as for other ischemic ATN; also mechanical trauma, embolization
- Risk factors: usual ATN risk factors; also: multiple cardiac surgeries in one operation, prolonged bypass time cardiogenic shock (CJASN 2015;10:500)
- Off pump surgery did not improve rates of AKI requiring dialysis (NEJM 2013;368:1179)
- Cleveland score may predict need for RRT after cardiac surgery (JASN 2005;16:162)
  5 points for preop Cr > = 2.1; 2 points for preop Cr 1.2–2.09
  2 points for preop balloon pump, emergency surgery, CABG +valve
  1 point for female, CHF, EF <35%, COPD, IDDM, prior cardiac surgery
  1 point for valve only surgery, 2 points if other cardiac surgery
  Risk of AKI requiring RRT: (0–2 pts 0.4%; 3–5 pts 1.8%; 6–8 pts 7.8%; 9–13 pts 21.5%)

PIGMENT NEPHROPATHY

HEMOLYSIS

Causes (AJKD 2008;52:1010) **and Pathogenesis** (JASN 2007;18:414)

- **Mechanical:** cardiopulmonary bypass, ECMO, LVAD/RVAD, Impella, mechanical heart valves, perivalvular leaks
- **Other:** ABO-incompatible blood transfusions, Auto-immune hemolytic anemia, Drug-mediated (N.B. cephalosporins), G6PD deficiency, PNH, Malaria, Envenomation (Snake and Insect venom), poisoning, hypotonic IVFs
- Hb: poorly filtered d/t large size (tetramer 69K, dimer 34K) and binding to hapto
- Only once amount of free Hb has fully saturated haptoglobin will dimeric form be filtered (then same pathogenesis as Rhabdomyolysis)

Clinical Manifestations and Diagnosis

- Asymptomatic; Red or brown urine, +/– oligoanuria (only late, no volume depletion like in rhabdomyolysis), red plasma (free hemoglobin)
- U/A w/ +Heme but no RBCs, +/– AKI (FE$_{Na}$ often <1%), ↓ hapto (Se 83%, Sp 96%) (JAMA 1980; 243:1909), ↑ LDH, ↑ RDW (smear w/ schistocytes, reticulocytes, or spherocytes), n AST/ALT

RHABDOMYOLYSIS

Causes (NEJM 2009;361:62) **and Pathogenesis** (NEJM 2009;361:62; KI 1996;49:314)

Category	Examples
Trauma	Crush injuries, exercise, seizures, electrocution, thermal (hypothermia, hyperthermia, NMS), limb compression from LOC, compartment syndrome, iatrogenic occlusion in OR, thrombosis, embolism
Infections	Bacterial (Strep, Staph, Clostridium, Legionella, Tularemia), Viral (Influenza A & B, EBV, HIV, Coxsackie), Malaria
Electrolytes	↑ [Na], ↓ [Na], ↓ [K], ↓ [Ca], ↓ [PO₄], hyperosmolar states
Endocrine	Hyperaldosteronism, hypothyroidism, ketoacidosis
Drugs and Toxins	Statins, fibrates, antipsychotics, antidepressants, antihistamines Recreational: alcohol, heroin, cocaine, amphetamines, LSD, toluene Environmental: heavy metals, insect venom, snake venom, CO
Genetic and Metabolic	Disorders of: glycolysis, glycogenolysis, lipid metabolism, mitochondria, pentose phosphate pathway, purine nucleotide cycle
Autoimmune	Polymyositis, dermatomyositis

- Imbalance of cellular ATP causes K/Na-ATPase and Ca-ATPase dysfunction → ↑ [Ca]$_{in}$
- Myocyte breakdown releases Myoglobin, CPK, K, PO₄, purines
- Massive fluid sequestration in damaged muscles, CaP precipitation and deposition
- Myoglobin is rapidly filtered (MW 17.8 kDa and not protein bound)
- Endocytosed by PCT and causes cytotoxicity via hydroxyl radical
- Precipitates w/ Tamm–Horsfall protein (promoted by acidic urine) forming obstructive casts
- Vasoconstriction from sequestration → RAAS activation and local inflammatory mediators

Clinical Manifestations and Diagnosis

- May be asymptomatic; Myalgias, red or brown urine, +/– oligoanuria
- **Labs:** U/A with +Heme but no RBCs (Sens. 80%), +/– pigmented granular casts, +/– AKI (FE$_{Na}$ often <1%), ↑ CPK (mostly MM isoform, >5–10K to cause AKI, rises within 12 hr of injury and T$_{1/2}$ of 1.5 d), ↑ uric acid, ↑ AST/ALT, ↑ LDH, ↑ [K], ↑ [P], ↓ [Ca], later can see ↑ [Ca] (leaches from muscle). Do not ✓ serum or urinary myoglobin (insensitive).

Treatment of Pigment Nephropathy (Intensive Care Med 2001;27:803; NEJM 2009;361:62)

- **Address the underlying cause** of rhabdomyolysis and hemolysis
- **Aggressive IVF:** (1) volume resuscitate in rhabdomyolysis d/t sequestration (1–2 L/hr initially); (2) ↑ urinary tubular flow rate to prevent pigment casts (target UOP >300 mL/hr). Continue until CPK <5K or hemolysis improved & able to take PO.
- **Consider urinary alkalinization** (pH >6.5) but no clear benefit. Monitor iCa and pH
- If oliguric or volume overload, loop diuretics. No clear benefit from mannitol, and potential for harm (if used, restrict <200 g/d and OG <55).
- **Medically manage electrolyte complications:** avoid repleting Ca unless severe or symptomatic. Allopurinol if uric acid >8 mg/dL
- HD or CRRT only for renal failure indications. **No role** for preventive myoglobin clearance with CVVHDF (Acta Anesthesiol Scand 2005;49:859) or plasmapheresis
- Risks of poorer prognosis (AKI, need for RRT, mortality) include: age >50, female, Cr >1.4, CPK >40K, PO₄ >4, Ca <7.5, Bicarb <19, and uncommon cause (JAMA 2013;173:1821)

CRYSTAL NEPHROPATHY

- Crystal nephropathy: acute or chronic kidney injury caused by crystal precipitation; Uric acid nephropathy is m/c
- Nephrocalcinosis: generalized calcium deposition in the kidney parenchyma and tubules
- Nephrolithiasis/Urolithiasis: condition a/w renal intratubular/urinary stones, formed from crystals precipitating from the urine

Pathogenesis

- Crystallization is determined by supersaturation (SS) of constituent molecules
- SS: depends on the product of the free ion activities of components, promoter, inhibitor (citrate, Mg, pyrophosphate), and urine pH

Urine pH Favoring Crystal/Stone Formation	
Acidic Urine	Uric acid, cysteine, MTX, triamterene, sulfadiazine, djenkolic acid Alkalinization (citrate, HCO_3) might be preventive and therapeutic
Alkaline Urine	CaP, indinavir, atazanavir, ciprofloxacin
pH independent	CaOx

- Interstitial inflammatory reaction contributes to kidney injury

Clinical Manifestation and Workup

- AKI, hematuria, pyuria, renal colic (flank pain, N/V), precipitation can cause turbid urine
- Crystals on urine sediment: not sensitive/specific
- Renal U/S: KUB, US or CT; may need 2 studies (Nephron Clin Pract 2007;106:c119)
- Kidney biopsy: definitive diagnosis

Manifestations Based on Type of Crystals			
Crystals	Crystal Nephropathy	Nephrolithiasis	Nephrocalcinosis
CaOx	+	+	+
CaP	+	+	++
Uric acid	++	+	−
Cystine	+	+	−

OXALATE NEPHROPATHY

- Source of oxalate: dietary (30–60%), liver; Excretion: >90% into the urine, 10–40 mg/d
- Intestinal *Oxalobacter formigenes* breaks down oxalate
- Intestinal oxalate secretion via SLC26A6 and CFTR (JASN 2017;28:242)
- Obesity associated inflammation ↓ intestinal secretion (KI 2018;93:1098)
- Kidney bx: CaOx deposits w/ birefringence under polarized light; interstitial inflammation

Primary Hyperoxaluria

- ↑ oxalate production of liver caused by mutations of genes encoding: hepatic alanine glyoxylate aminotransferase (AGT, type 1), glyoxylate reductase/hydroxypyruvate reductase (type 2), 4-hydroxy-2-oxoglutarate aldolase (type 3)
- Severe hyperoxaluria (usually >80 mg/d)
- Manifest during childhood or adolescence; ESRD at median 33 y/o (Am J Nephrol 2005;25:290)
- Systemic deposition → flecked retina, arrhythmias, cardiomyopathy, arthropathy, fracture
- Tx: pyridoxine (vit B_6; cofactor of AGT) and PO_4 (NEJM 1994;331:1553), combined liver and kidney txp in type 1; very high recurrence rate w/o liver txp

Enteric Hyperoxaluria

- Causes: pancreatic insufficiency, CF, IBD (CD > UC), small bowel resection, jejunoileal or gastric bypass, orlistat (lipase inhibitor) (Arch IM 2011;171:703)
- Mechanism:
  1. Fat malabsorption → Ca binds to fatty acids → ↓ free Ca → ↑ free oxalate → ↑ oxalate absorption → ↑ CaOx crystal formation in kidney
  2. Diarrhea → metabolic acidosis → hypocitraturia → ↑ CaOx crystal formation
- Impairment of SLC26A6-mediated intestinal secretion may contribute (AJKD 2012;60:662)
- Mean urine oxalate 85.4 mg/d; >50% require RRT (KI Rep 2018;3:1363)
- Tx: low-oxalate diet, ↑ fluid intake, K citrate for metabolic acidosis or hypocitraturia, PO Ca; reversal of gastric bypass may improve renal function (Case Rep Nephrol Dial 2016;6:114)

Oxalate Loading

- Causes: ethylene glycol, Vit C (*Int J Nephrol* 2011;2011:146927), laxative containing ascorbic acid (*KJ* 2017;91:989), methoxyflurane, rhubarb leaves, star fruit (carambola), nuts, cocoa, parsley, potato, spinach (*KJ* 2016;90:711), beetroot, almond, chocolate, yellow dock, sorrel, cranberry concentrate tablets (*Urology* 2001;57:26)
- Tx: d/c oxalate; HD for ethylene glycol, large amount of ascorbic acid (*Urolithiasis* 2016;44:289)

ACUTE PHOSPHATE NEPHROPATHY

- Causes: hyperphosphaturia/hyperphosphatemia from sodium phosphate PO (*Hum Pathol* 2004;35:675), TLS, enema a/w ↓ eGFR (*AJKD* 2016;67:609)
- CaxP >60 mg^2/dL^2 ↑ risk of precipitation in the renal tubule
- Kidney bx: intraluminal tubular and tubular intracellular CaP deposition
- Tx: d/c offending drug, IVF, avoid urine alkalinization; RRT if CaxP ≥70 mg^2/dL^2

CALCIUM PHOSPHATE STONE AND NEPHROCALCINOSIS

- Apatite (crystal) >brushite (calcium hydrogen phosphate CaHPO$_4$ • 2H$_2$O)

Causes of Calcium Phosphate Crystals (*AJKD* 2018;71(4):A12)	
Hypercalciuria w/ hypercalcemia	**Hypercalciuria w/o hypercalcemia**
Systemic excess ± renal handling	Dysregulation of renal handling of calcium
1° HPT, sarcoidosis, vitamin D overdose, Milk-alkali syndrome	dRTA, medullary sponge kidney, Dent disease, Bartter syndrome, chronic hypokalemia

Primary Hyperparathyroidism (1° HPT)

- 24% of hypercalcemia on thiazide has 1° HPT (*JCEM* 2016;101:1166)
- If normal serum Ca, hypercalciuria and high PTH, ✓ thiazide challenge (HCTZ 25 mg po bid × 2 wk); PTH remaining high may suggest 1° HPT (*J Endourol* 2009;23:191)

Distal RTA (dRTA)

- Causes: CAI (acetazolamide, topiramate, zonisamide), Sjögren syndrome
- Pathogenesis: (1) Chronic metabolic acidosis → ↑ Ca, P release from bone; (2) intracellular acidosis → ↑ mitochondrial citrate uptake → ↑ citrate reabsorption in PCT → ↓ urinary citrate
- Manifestation: CaP stone/nephrocalcinosis, osteomalacia
- Hypokalemic NAGMA, severe hypocitraturia, (+) urine AG, constant urine pH >5.8
- Incomplete dRTA: w/o systemic NAGMA; could be difficult to diagnose
- K >3.8 + second morning fasting urinary pH <5.3 excludes dRTA (*CJASN* 2017;12:1507)
- Urinary acidification test: NH$_4$Cl 100 mg/kg ×1 or PO furosemide 40 mg + fludrocortisone 1 mg (*KJ* 2007;71:1310) and ✓ urine pH hourly × 8 hr; failure to ↓ urine pH <5.3 is diagnostic

Medullary Sponge Kidney

- Congenital malformation of pericalyceal terminal collecting duct
- Asymptomatic, dRTA, CaP ± mixed CaOx stone and nephrocalcinosis, UTI, rare ESRD
- IVP: paintbrush appearance; CT: calcium stones at calyceal area
- Tx: K citrate to ↑ urine citrate >450 mg/d provided urine pH <7.5 ↓ stone despite pH ↑ from 6.4–6.9 (*CJASN* 2010;5:1663)

Diagnosis

- Stone analysis; kidney bx: tubular, interstitial, and intracellular basophilic calcification

Characterization of Crystals		
Crystals	**von Kossa Stain**	**Birefringence Under Polarized Light**
CaP	+	–
CaOx, 2,8-dihydroxyadenine	–	+

Treatment

- Correct risk factors: low urine vol, hypercalciuria, hypocitraturia, hyperphosphaturia
- Correct dRTA w/ K citrate: ↓ Ca, P release from bone, ↓ urine Ca, P, ↑ urine citrate ↑ Urine pH w/ citrate may augment CaP crystal formation
- Parathyroidectomy in 1° HPT with nephrolithiasis/nephrocalcinosis, CrCl <60 or 24-hr urine Ca >400 mg with increased stone risk (*JCEM* 2014;99:3561)

URATE STONE AND NEPHROPATHY

Pathogenesis and Causes

- pH decides the form: insoluble uric acid in low pH; soluble urate in high pH
- Urine pH is more important than hyperuricosuria

- Tumor lysis syndrome in hematologic malignancy > solid tumor, seizure
- Exercise-induced AKI in familial renal hypouricemia (URAT1 mutation ↓ uric acid reabsorption)

Clinical Manifestation
- Usually asymptomatic AKI, random urine uric acid/cr >1 mg/mg; radiolucent stone

Prevention and Treatment
- Acute management: volume repletion, rasburicase for high risk for TLS
- Chronic management: urine alkalinization with K citrate with goal pH 6.5 or above, ↓ animal protein and salt intake

CYSTINURIA

- AR mutation of SLC3A1, SLC7A9-encoding PT apical amino acid transporter, rBAT
- ≠ Cystinosis causing Fanconi syndrome and tubular proteinuria
- 1st stone 24 y/o, 21% after 40 y/o; 20% staghorn; CKD (70%), ESRD (9%) (CJASN 2015;10:1235)
- Cystinuria may be a/w Ca calculi (JASN 2015;26:543); may present w/ staghorn calculi
- Dx: family history, stone analysis, hexagonal crystals on urine sediment
- Cyanide-nitroprusside test: screening; purple color suggest cystine >75 mg/L
- √ urine cysteine level for diagnosis (>400 mg/d) and estimation of required fluid intake
- Bx: rarely done; intratubular cystine crystals (KI 2006;69:2227)
- Tx: ↑ fluid intake to keep urine cystine <1 mmol/L (243 mg/L), urine alkalinization >7.5, low protein, sodium diet, Tiopronin (2-mercaptopropionylglycine), D-penicillamine (can cause MN, crescentic GN)

ADENINE PHOSPHORIBOSYLTRANSFERASE (APRT) DEFICIENCY

- AR mutation of ARRT, purine metabolism enzyme → ↑ insoluble 2,8-dihydroxyadenine (DHA) crystals in urine → CKD, radiolucent stone (can be misdiagnosed as uric acid)
- Urine crystals with Maltese cross-like pattern under polarized microscopy
- Kidney Bx: tubular, interstitial deposits with strong birefringence (can be misdiagnosed as oxalate) (NDT 2010;25:1909)
- Tx: allopurinol ↓ eGFR decline (AJKD 2016;67:431), low purine diet, high fluid intake
- Txp: recurrence is common; frequently diagnosed by graft biopsy

DRUG FORMING CRYSTALS AND STONES

- Common risk factors: volumed depletion, high dose use, reduced kidney function
- Clinical manifestation: AKI with resolution of d/c of drg; frequently radiolucent

Drugs Forming Crystals	
Antivirals	
Acyclovir	a/w high dose IV, volume depletion; ganciclovir has lower risk
Atazanavir	In alkaline urine. Crystalluria, Stone (AJKD 2017;70:576)
Foscarnet	AKI, crystal nephropathies (AJKD 2015;65:152)
Indinavir	In alkaline urine. 8% developed urologic symptoms: renal colic flank pain dysuria plate-like rectangles and fan-shaped or starburst forms (Ann IM 1997;127:119)
Antibacterials	
Ciprofloxacin	In alkaline urine.
Sulfonamides	In acidic urine, esp. sulfadiazine
Other Drugs	
Sulfasalazine	Anti-inflammatory agent used in RA and IBD can form crystals and stones (AJKD 2017;70:869)
Triamterene	
Methotrexate (MTX)	In acidic urine. MTX precipitate in the tubules (NEJM 2015;373:2691)
Ephedrine	Ma huang containing ephedrine (AJKD 1998;32:153)
Pseudoephedrine	Urolithiasis (NDT 2004;19:263)
Djenkol Bean	Meal in Southeast Asia; djenkolic acid forms needle-like crystal in acidic urine; AKI, needle-like crystals
Mg trisilicate	Silicate urolithiasis (J Urol 1984;132:739)

- Tx: d/c offending drug, volume repletion ± loop diuretics, urine alkalinization with goal pH 7 in sulfadiazine, MTX. Urine acidification is not recommended

URINARY STONE DISEASE

Epidemiology
- Prevalence 8.8%; Increasing w/ climate change (PNAS 2008;105:9841)
- Risk factors: male, obesity, DM, white (NHANES Eur Urol 2012;62:160), Southeastern (J Urol 1994;151:838), oral antibiotics (JASN 2018;29:1731)
- Recurrence is common, esp after ≥2 episodes (J Nephrol 2017;30:227)
- CKD 3b-5 (×1.74); ESRD (×2.16) (BMJ 2012;345:e5287)
- Composition: Ca (CaOx > CaP) > Urate ≈ Struvite > Cysteine
- Inherited disease ~2% (NDT 2013;28:811)

Conditions Associated with Urinary Stone	
1° HPT	CaOx > CaP (BJU Int 2009;103:670); consider parathyroidectomy
Sarcoidosis	CaOx > CaP
dRTA	CaP; nephrocalcinosis common
CF	CaOx; microscopic nephrocalcinosis 92% (NEJM 1988;319:263)
ADPKD	Uric acid > CaOx (AJKD 1993;22:513)
Dent disease	CaP
Horseshoe kidneys	CaOx
Metabolic syndrome	Uric acid > CaOx

Clinical Manifestations
- Acute, colicky flank pain radiating to the groin; CVA tenderness may be present
- Hematuria (90%): absence does not r/o; Presence w/ flank pain is not diagnostic of stone
- 26% of pts has persistent ureteral stone after cessation of pain (J Urol 2018;199:1011)

Workup
- r/o medication-induced stone: triamterene, indinavir, atazanavir, sulfonamides, CAI (topiramate), cipro, Mg Trisilicate antacids abuse, guaifenesin, and ephedrine
- CT: preferred if urological intervention is planned; low dose CT may miss small stone
- Dual energy multidetector CT may characterize stone composition (Radiology 2010;257:394)
- U/S: low sensitivity, no difference in important missed Dx c/w CT (NEJM 2014;371:1100)
- MRI if pregnant; KUB for f/u; IVP: less sensitivity/specificity
- Strain urine to type stone; urine culture
- 24-hr urine at home before dietary modification and after

Precipitating Factors of Crystals and Stones			
Precipitating Factor (Goal)	Type	Related Condition	Management
Low urine vol (>2–2.5 L/d)	Any type	AKI, CKD	↑ Fluid intake >2 L/d
Hypercalciuria (♂ <250 mg/d ♀ <200 mg/d)	CaOx, CaP	1° HPT, Vit D excess, sarcoidosis, dRTA, hyperthyroidism, cancer, Dent disease ↑ Na, animal protein intake	↓ Na/protein intake, Thiazide (CJASN 2010;5:1893; JCEM 2017;102:1270) Amiloride, d/c excessive Ca, parathyroidectomy
Hyperoxaluria (<40 mg/d)	CaOx	↑ Ox intake, ↓ Ca intake 1° hyperoxaluria Pyridoxine (vit B6) def. Small bowl disease or surgery	↓ Ox, Vit C intake ↑ Dairy/nondairy Ca intake (J Urol 2013;190:1255) Cholestyramine in case of prior bowel surgery
Hyperuricosuria (♂ <0.8 ♀ <0.75 g/d)	CaOx, Uric acid	↑ Purine intake, cell lysis, uricosuric agent (probenecid, fenofibrate, losartan)	↓ Purine intake, weight loss, K citrate, allopurinol
Hypocitraturia (♂ >450 mg/d ♀ >550 mg/d)	CaOx, CaP	↑ Nondairy animal protein, Na intake, dRTA, hypoK, UTI, bowel disease, CKD	↓ Nondairy animal protein/ Na intake, Citrate, watching SS CaP and pH (caution urine pH >6.5)
Hypercystinuria	Cysteine	Genetic mutation	Tiopronin, Penicillamine
Urea splitting bacteria	Mg ammonium phosphate	UTI (Proteus, Pseudomonas, Klebsiella)	Treat UTI

High sodium (<100 mEq/d)	CaOx, CaP	High sodium diet	↓ Sodium intake
Acidic urine (>6.5)	Uric acid, Cysteine, MTX, Sulfadiazine, Triamterene	High protein diet	Alkalinization (citrate, bicarb) ↓ Protein intake
Basic urine	CaP, Xanthine	dRTA, CAI, urea splitting organism (>8)	Antibiotic in urea splitting organism UTI

MANAGEMENT

Acute Management
- IVF: ↑ UOP; no Δ pain, rate of passage (*J Endourol* 2006;20:713)
- Analgesics: ketorolac > meperidine (*Ann Emerg Med* 1996;28:151)
- Passage of stone: small and distal stone
- α blockers: ↑ passage of ureteric stones ≥5 mm (*BMJ* 2016;355:i6112); no difference in small stone with mean diameter of 3.8 mm (*JAMA IM* 2018;178:1051)
- Nifedipine: ↑ passage of ureteric stones (*Ann Emerg Med* 2007;50:552)
- Urologic intervention: >10 mm, infection, obstruction >4 d, uncontrolled pain
- Extracorporeal shock wave lithotripsy (proximal, <2 cm), ureteroscopic removal, percutaneous nephrolithotomy, open surgery

Long-term Management
- PO fluid >2–2.5 L/d (*J Urol* 1996;155:839)
- Low Na diet: high Na → hypercalciuria; monitor w/ 24 hr
- High K diet: ↑ urine citrate, pH, volume, ↓ SS CaOx and SS Uric acid (*CJASN* 2016;11:1834)
- Low protein diet: monitor urine sulfate, PCR
  Sulfur containing animal protein → ↑ urine acid loading → ↓ urine citrate
  Dairy protein is beneficial ↑ urine citrate, ↓ oxalate (*CJASN* 2016;11:1834)
- Low ox diet: avoid nuts, chocolate, dark green leafy vegetables, rhubarb, okra, beets
- High Ca diet: low calcium → ↑ oxalate absorption (*J Urol* 2012;187:1645)
- Avoid excessive vitamin D: high 1,25(OH)₂D is a/w stone (*CJASN* 2015;10:667)
- Diuretics with hypocalciuric effects: thiazide, amiloride

Citrate Supplementations
- Used for inhibition of calcium stone formation and urine alkalinization in uric acid stone
- Plasma alkalinization ↑ renal Ca reabsorption
- ↓ stone size, ↓ new stone (*Cochrane Database Syst Rev* 2015;CD010057)
- K citrate: start 30 (urine citrate >150 mg/d) – 60 (urine citrate <150 mg/d) mEq/d
- Compliance can be monitored with 24-hr urine K amount (should be > than prescribed amount; should ↓ ammonia)
- It is normal to see K citrate tablet remnant in the stool
- Side effect: metabolic alkalosis (keep urine pH <7.5 in CaP stone), ↑ K, N/V/D

Citrate and Bicarbonate Regimens	
Lemon juice	120 mL (4 oz) contains 5.9 g (≈90 mEq) citric acid: ↑ urine citric acid by 142 mg/d (*J Urol* 1996;156:907)
K citrate tab (Urocit-K®)	5 mEq (540 mg), 10 mEq (1,080 mg)
K citrate-citric acid powder (Cytra-K®)	1 packet: K citrate monohydrate 3,300 mg, citric acid monohydrate 1,002 mg = K 30 mEq, bicarb 30 mEq
K citrate-citric acid (Cytra-K®, Virtrate-K®)	Solution: 1,100–334 mg/5 mL = K 10 mEq, bicarb 10 mEq
Na citrate-citric acid (Bicitra®, Cytra-2®)	Solution: 500–334 mg/5 mL = Na 5 mEq, bicarb 5 mEq
Na citrate-K citrate-Citric acid (Virtrate-3®, Cytra-3®)	Solution: 500–550–334 mg/5 mL = Na 5 mEq, K 5 mEq, bicarb 2 mEq
K bicarbonate (Effer-K®, Klor-Con/EF®)	1 g = 10 mEq; 2.5 g = 25 mEq

INTERSTITIAL DISEASES

ACUTE INTERSTITIAL NEPHRITIS (AIN)

- Interstitial nephritis may be acute, subacute, or chronic. Characterized by ↓ renal function and an inflammatory infiltrate limited to the tubulointerstitial compartment.
- AIN accounts for 12.9% of AKI; prevalence is increasing (NDT 2013;28:112)

Causes of AIN (AJKD 2014;64:558; KI 2010;77:956)
- Drugs (~70%): antibiotics (35%, PCN, FQ, cephalosporins, sulfonamides, vancomycin), PPI (10%), NSAIDs (7%), 5-aminosalicylates; checkpoint inhibitors (KI 2016;90:638), thiazide, allopurinol, lamotrigine
- Autoimmune (~20%): sarcoidosis, Sjögren's, TINU, IgG4-related disease, ANCA-vasculitis, MCTD, Sweet syndrome
- Others (~10%): infection eg, E. coli, TB, leprosy, histoplasma, candida, cryptococcus (KI 2009;76:453), BK virus, Hantavirus; CLL, mantle cell lymphoma, idiopathic
- In 65 ≥y/o drug (87%) especially PPI (18%) and antibiotic are more common (KI 2015;87:458)
- Antibrush border antibody disease: immune complex TIN d/t antibrush border antibody (JASN 2016;27:380) against (JASN 2018;29:644)

Clinical Manifestations
- Drug-induced AIN may show triad (fever, eosinophilia, and rash) in 10% (NDT 2004;19:8)
- Usually asymptomatic; N/V, malaise, arthritis
- Oliguric or nonoliguric, gross hematuria (5%), Dialysis requirement (40%) (KI 2010;77:956)

Laboratory Manifestations
- Azotemia, pRTA, eosinophilia
- Urine: WBC ± WBC casts, eosinophiluria, occasionally bland sediment; microhematuria common; RBC casts not typically seen. High FENa. Isosthenuria (SG 1.008–1.012).
- Tubular proteinuria. Nephrotic-range proteinuria in NSAID induced MCD or MN
- Serology: ANA, anti-DSDNA, anti-Ro/SSA, anti-La/SSb, C3, C4, ANCA, IgG4. Other systemic disease based on clinical manifestations (eg, chest imaging for TB, sarcoid)
- ↑ IgG4 levels, hypocomplementemia in IgG4-RD; Renal and abdominal masses may be seen

Diagnosis
- Kidney biopsy is diagnostic: interstitial edema, infiltrate of T lymphocytes and monocytes > eosinophils, plasma cells and neutrophils, tubulitis; Interstitial fibrosis can be seen w/i 7–10 d after inflammation initiation (KI 2010;77:956)
- IF: occasionally linear or granular tubular basement membrane (TBM) staining

Pathologic Clues in Tubulointerstitial Nephritis	
Plasma cell rich infiltrate	IgG4-RD, Sjögren's, SLE, chronic pyelonephritis, HIV, BK virus, chronic T-cell–mediated rejection
Non-necrozing granuloma	Drugs: NSAIDs, antibiotics, thiazide, lamotrigine, intravesical BCG (NDT 2006;21:1427), adalimumab (AJKD 2010;56:e17) Sarcoidosis, ANCA GPA, Crohn disease, TINU, infections
Necrotizing granuloma	TB (AJKD 2008;51:524), fungal infections
Linear TBM IgG staining	Anti-GBM disease and MIDD: w/ GBM linear staining NSAIDs, allopurinol, phenytoin, methicillin
Granular or semilinear TBM IgG staining	IgG4-RD, MN, cryoglobulinemic GN, Hantavirus, autoimmune (SLE, Sjögren), antibrush border antibody disease, Idiopathic hypocomplementemic TIN (AJKD 2001;37:388)

- Gallium-67 scan: Gallium binds to lactoferrin on WBC; not sensitive/specific

Treatment
- d/c of inciting drug; Treatment of underlying infection eg, TB, fungus
- Glucocorticoids: prednisone 1 mg/kg daily or 2 mg/kg qod for 3–12 wk; long duration is not a/w improved outcome (CJASN 2018;13:1851). Poor response with tx delay, severe tubular atrophy/interstitial fibrosis and small kidneys (AJKD 2014;64:558).
- MMF: ↓ Cr in steroid intolerant/relapsing cases (CJASN 2006;1:718)

Prognosis
- Most recover after d/c of causative drug; median recovery time 3 wk in fluoroquinolone-associated AIN (Mayo Clin Proc 2018;93:25)
- Poor prognostic factors: higher degree of interstitial fibrosis/tubular atrophy, small kidneys, longer duration of drug exposure, longer time from AKI onset or bx to steroid treatment (AJKD 2014;64:558). The majority of patients do no reach ESRD.

- Early steroid treatment may improve recovery in drug-induced AIN. Chronic dialysis in 44.4 (w/ steroid) vs 3.8% (w/o steroid) (KI 2008;73:940)

TINU SYNDROME

- Subset of patients with tubulointerstitial nephritis have uveitis (TINU)
- HLA-DQA1*01, HLA-DQB1*05, and HLA-DQB1*01 may be associated
- Monomeric CRP may be pathologically implicated

Clinical and Laboratory Features

- Median onset 15 yr (9–74); female preponderance (Surv Opthalmol 2001;46:195)
- Systemic symptoms: fever, wt loss, fatigue may be present
- Uveitis: typically bilateral (unilateral or alternating may occur). Timing: 2 mo before, concurrently, and up to 14 mo after TINU. Slit lamp examination to confirm diagnosis.
- TIN: usually AIN. Signs of proximal tubular dysfunction may be seen. On renal biopsy nonspecific interstitial infiltrate, sometimes granulomas present

Treatment

- Renal disease is thought to be self-limited (AJKD 1999;34:1016)
- For progressive renal disease, prednisone 1 mg/kg/d (40–60 mg) for 3–6 mo followed by a taper (based on response). Limited experience with steroid-sparing agents.

CHRONIC TUBULOINTERSTITIAL DISEASE

- Chronic tubulointerstitial injury can cause interstitial fibrosis, tubular atrophy (IF/TA), and macrophage and lymphocytic infiltration
- It can happen from primary tubulointerstitial injury or secondary to glomerular injury
- The degree of IF/TA predicts renal prognosis in all type of renal injury

Causes

- Drugs: lithium, cyclosporine, tacrolimus, cisplatin, indinavir (crystal nephropathy)
- Toxins: aristolochic acid, heavy metals (lead, cadmium, arsenic, mercury, gold, uranium)
- Analgesic nephropathy, radiation, obstruction
- Chronic pyelonephritis, xanthogranulomatous pyelonephritis, malakoplakia
- Vascular: ischemia, renovascular disease
- Metabolic: hyperuricemia, hypokalemia, hypercalcemia, hyperoxaluria, nephrocalcinosis
- Mesoamerican nephropathy, Balkan nephropathy
- Progression of AIN and primary glomerular disease

Clinical Manifestations and Diagnosis

- CKD, salt wasting, salt sensitive HTN; RTA: pRTA, dRTA, type 4 all possible
- Nephrogenic DI: decreased concentration ability d/t medullary dysfunction
- Tubular proteinuria unless secondary to glomerular disease, bland urine sediment
- Anemia: relatively early stage CKD d/t ↓ interstitial erythropoietin production
- Imaging: small kidneys w/ indented or irregular contour; papillary calcification in analgesic nephropathy; cystic changes in lithium nephropathy; nephrocalcinosis on U/S or CT

Treatment

- Identify and stop insult if possible; manage CKD; prepare RRT

Hereditary Tubulointerstitial Diseases

- Autosomal dominant tubulointerstitial kidney disease (ADTKD, aka medullary cystic kidney disease), nephronophthisis (NPHP), and cystinosis can manifest with CKD

Hereditary Tubulointerstitial Disease (KDIGO KI 2015;88:676)		
Disease	Gene	Pathogenesis and Manifestation
ADTKD-UMOD	UMOD	↓ NKCC2 expression → water, sodium loss → ↑ PT uric acid absorption, FEurate <5% ↓ Urine uromodulin excretion Hyperuricemia, gout, and ESRD at median age 24, 40, and 56, respectively (CJASN 2013;8:1349)
ADTKD-MUC1	Mucin-1	Intracellular accumulation of mucin-1 frameshift protein in distal tubule
ADTKD-REN	REN	Childhood anemia, hypotension, frequent AKI, ↑ K Tx: avoid NSAIDs, low sodium diet
ADTKD-HNF1B	HNF1B	Maturity onset diabetes of the young type 5, renal cysts, renal Mg wasting, pancreatic atrophy, genital abnormalities
NPHP (AR)	NPHP 1-10	Retinal degeneration
Cystinosis (AR)	CTNS	Fanconi syndrome, photophobia (corneal cystine crystals), CKD/ESRD (CJASN 2008;3:27)

IMMUNOGLOBULIN G4-RELATED DISEASE

- IgG4: higher rate of dissociation than other IgG, does not fix complement by the classical pathway; may bind other Igs and form immune complexes
- Immunoglobulin G4-related disease (IgG4-RD): autoimmune infiltrative condition that involves multiple organs including the kidney with ↑ serum concentrations of IgG4
- Virtually any organ may be involved including pancreas, biliary tree (sclerosing cholangitis), aorta, lung, salivary and lacrimal glands, thyroid, pachymeninges, and kidney

Clinical Manifestation

- Common in older, male, Asian, and Caucasian
- Asthenia (26%), weight loss (21%), fever (4%) (Mayo Clin Proc 2015;90:927)
- From a renal standpoint pts present with worsening renal function, or kidney masses
- Occasionally, NS from concomitant PLA2R Ab (−) MN (KI 2013;83:455)
- Obstructive uropathy from retroperitoneal fibrosis; IgG4-RD was 54% (Medicine 2013;92:82)

Workup

- Azotemia, hypocomplementemia (~60%, C3 and C4), eosinophilia (~40%)
- Variable proteinuria, hematuria, and pyuria
- ↑ IgG4 levels (typically 6–8-fold ULN) in most patients
- Typically needs a biopsy to confirm the diagnosis (Mod Pathol 2012;25:1181). The 3 major histologic criteria are: (1) dense lymphoplasmacytic infiltrate; (2) Fibrosis, arranged at least focally in a storiform pattern; (3) Obliterative phlebitis
- IF: TBM immune complex deposits (80%)
- Not all features are present simultaneously and some of the features predominate in some organs (eg, storiform fibrosis in pancreas, not commonly seen in kidney). Further the number of IgG4 cells may vary.

Diagnostic Criteria for IgG4-related Kidney Disease (Clin Exp Nephrol 2011;15:615)	
1. Kidney damage	Abnormal urinalysis or urine marker(s) or decreased kidney function with either elevated serum IgG level, hypocomplementemia, or elevated serum IgE level
2. Renal imaging (CT scan is the best)	a. Multiple low-density lesions on enhanced CT b. Diffuse kidney enlargement c. Hypovascular solitary mass in the kidney d. Hypertrophic lesion of the renal pelvic wall without irregularity of the renal pelvic surface
3. Serum IgG4	>135 mg/dL
4. Renal histology	a. Dense lymphoplasmacytic infiltration with infiltrating IgG4-positive plasma cells >10/high power field (HPF) and/or ratio of IgG4-positive plasma cells/IgG positive plasma cells >40% b. Characteristic "storiform" fibrosis surrounding nests of lymphocytes and/or plasma cells
5. Extrarenal histology	Dense lymphoplasmacytic infiltration with infiltrating IgG4-positive plasma cells >10/HPF and/or ratio of IgG4-positive plasma cells/IgG-positive plasma cells >40%
Definite	1+3+4a,b; 2+3+4a,b; 2+3+5
Probable	1+4a,b; 2+4a,b; 2+5; 3+4a,b
Possible	1+3; 2+3; 1+4a, 2+4a

Treatment

- The optimal therapy is unknown (no RCT)
- CS: 1st line; prednisone 0.6 mg/kg daily for 2–4 wk, tapered over 3–6 mo. Most authors favor maintenance 2.5–5 mg/d for up to 3 yr (Curr Opin Rheumatol 2011;23:67)
- Azathioprine and MMF: steroid-intolerant/relapsing pts (Gastroenterology 2008;134:706)
- Rituximab in glucocorticoid-refractory or relapsing pts (Arthritis Rheum 2010;62:1755)
- Unclear whether renal masses without symptoms need treatment

Prognosis

- In glucocorticoid-treated pts, despite improvement in eGFR, there was progression of renal atrophy on imaging (KI 2013;84:826)
- Relapses occur in ~20% pts

SPORADIC CYSTIC DISEASES

Simple Renal Cysts

- Benign renal cysts are rare in children, but occur commonly in advanced age
- Most often simple cysts are asymptomatic and detected as incidental findings during abdominal imaging studies; usually of no clinical significance
- U/S: smooth walls, good sound transmission, and no intracystic debris
- If U/S is indeterminate, ✓ CT. On CT, benign cysts have homogenous attenuation, no contrast enhancement, and smooth walls without calcifications.

The Bosniak Category Classification on CT Imaging (Urology 2005;66:484)		
	Features w/o Contrast	Features w/ Contrast	Management
I	Water density (0–20 HU), thin margins, sharp delineation with the renal parenchyma, thin and smooth walls, homogeneous	No contrast enhancement	No further workup or an ultrasonogram in 6–12 mo
II	Presence of one or few thin septations, small and fine calcifications; hyperdense cysts measuring up to 3.0 cm (60–70 HU)	No contrast enhancement, or no measurable or perceptible enhancement of septa	
IIF	More complex lesions which cannot be included in category II or III. Multiple septa. Walls or septa with nodular or irregular calcifications. Hyperdense cysts >3.0 cm or with only 25% of their walls visible (exophytic)	Absent, dubious, or hair-like enhancement	Continued surveillance
III	Thick-walled cystic lesion, septum irregularity and heterogeneous septum and wall and/or contents; Gross and irregular calcifications	Wall or septum enhancement	Continued surveillance, fine needle biopsy, partial nephrectomy
IV	Lesions with all the findings of category III, and solid component, soft parts, independent of finding of wall or septa	Enhancement of wall and/or solid component(s)	Require surgery (malignancy in 85–100%)

Acquired Cystic Kidney Disease (ACKD)

- Occurs in individuals with advanced CKD or ESRD
- The occurrence of acquired renal cystic disease increases with the number of years on dialysis, the majority of patients develop cysts after 5–10 yr on dialysis
- The cysts in ACKD are more numerous than benign simple renal cysts, but share similar radiographic features
- ACKD is associated with increased risk of malignancy

Hypokalemia-related Cystic Kidney Disease

- Prolonged hypokalemia due to urinary K^+ wasting (such as in primary hyperaldosteronism) predisposes to kidney cyst formation

Medullary Sponge Kidney

- A congenital disorder; malformation of the terminal collecting ducts in the pericalyceal region of the renal pyramids; Usually bilateral
- Etiology: unknown; not clear if the disorder has genetic basis
- Clinical presentation: mostly asymptomatic. Incomplete or overt dRTA in >80% of pts. Recurrent **calcium kidney stones**, gross or microscopic hematuria w/ or w/o stones, UTI, flank pain w/ or w/o an obstructing stone or UTI.
- Usually remains undiagnosed or is discovered incidentally by a radiographic study. The diagnosis can be made by IVP or noncontrast CT.
- Prognosis: renal function remains nl in most cases. However, there is a risk of renal injury d/t recurrent stone-induced episodes of obstruction and/or infections.
- Treatment: manage UTIs and recurrent stones

HEREDITARY CYSTIC DISEASES

AUTOSOMAL DOMINANT POLYCYSTIC KIDNEY DISEASE (ADPKD)

- The m/c inherited renal disease affecting 1 in 500–1,000 individuals
- Accounts for ~5% of ESRD population in the US
- The penetrance is incomplete; family history is positive in only about 60% of cases

Clinical Manifestation

- The clinical onset typically occurs from the third through the fifth decades of life
- Massive enlargement of the kidneys due to the gradual development of cysts that arise from the distal nephron segments and gradually replace normal renal parenchyma, ultimately leading to progressive functional impairment
- Hypertension: the earliest and most prevalent manifestation; frequently predates the onset of renal dysfunction; Likely caused by activation of the renin–angiotensin–aldosterone
- Flank or abdominal pain (compression by enlarged kidneys)
- Macroscopic hematuria (cyst hemorrhage), low-grade proteinuria (tubular dysfunction)
- Fever and abdominal pain (cyst infection), kidney stones (stagnant urinary flow)
- Decreased concentrating ability (distorted anatomy of the medulla)
- Extra-renal manifestations:
  Gastrointestinal system: hepatic cysts and colonic diverticula
  Cerebral aneurysms: relatively rare (<10%)
  Heart: patent foramen ovale (PFO), mitral valve prolapse (MVP)
  Abdominal wall and inguinal hernia
  Subcutaneous, ovarian, testicular, seminal vesicle, pancreatic, and pulmonary cysts

Diagnosis

- The preferred diagnostic procedure is renal ultrasound: multiple bilateral kidney cysts in the setting of a positive family history are typically diagnostic

Diagnostic Criteria of ADPKD (near 100% specificity, 100% PPV, 82–100% sensitivity depending on the age group) (JASN 2009;20:205)	
Age	Diagnostic Number of Cysts
15–39 y/o	At least three unilateral or bilateral kidney cysts
40–59 y/o	At least two cysts in each kidney
>60 y/o	At least four cysts in each kidney

- 10-yr ESRD risk can be calculated by total kidney volume (TKV) or kidney dimensions (Available at QxMD app; JASN 2015;26:160)

Genetics and Pathogenesis

- ADPKD is caused by mutations in PKD1 (75–85%) or PKD2 (15–25%)
- The proteins encoded by PKD1 and PKD2, polycystin-1 and polycystin-2, are components of a multifunctional signaling pathway that regulates key cellular processes including growth, differentiation, and orientation of tubular epithelial cells; polycystins form signaling heterodimers that localize to primary cilia of all epithelial cells
- Direct sequencing: because of high cost, primarily used for the evaluation of at-risk individuals with equivocal imaging results, younger at-risk individuals being evaluated for living kidney donation, and individuals with atypical cystic disease
- Sanger sequencing of all exons and splice junctions of the PKD1 and PKD2 genes is the method of choice. Mutation screening of PKD2 is straightforward, but PKD1 is challenging because it is a large gene with its first 33 exons duplicated in six pseudogenes. Current diagnostic sequencing protocols exploit rare mismatches between PKD1 gene and its six pseudogenes. If Sanger sequencing is (–), one should test for structural rearrangements, which occur in <5% of the cases. These can be detected by additional MLPA testing.
- NextGen sequencing panels are gaining popularity and will likely replace Sanger sequencing given their declining costs
- Patients w/ PKD1 mutations have earlier disease onset and ↑ progression to ESRD

Treatment

- No curative treatment, ~50% of patients reach ESRD before the age of 60
- Primarily directed toward complications: HTN, infections, pain, and hematuria
- Dietary salt restriction: may slow eGFR decline (KI 2017;91:493)
- HTN: control w/ RAAS inhibitor

- In eGFR >60, intensive BP control (95/60–110/75) ↓ KTV increase and urine albumin excretion w/o ∆eGFR *(HALT-PKD NEJM 2014;371:2255)*
- In eGFR 25–60, addition of ARB to ACEi did not alter ∆eGFR *(HALT-PKD NEJM 2014;371:2267)*
- Vasopressin suppression to inhibit cyst growth
  - ↑ Fluid intake: >3 L/d *(CJASN 2010;5:693)*; difficult to achieve daily for many patients
- Tolvaptan vs placebo ↓ renal function decline in eCrCl >60 *(TEMPO NEJM 2012;367:2407)*
- Tolvaptan vs placebo ↓ renal function decline in eGFR 25–65
  - ↑ Liver enzymes (>3× baseline) in 5.6% of the tolvaptan vs 1.2% in the placebo group. These changes normalize after d/c of tolvaptan. Up to 6.8% of patients do not tolerate aquaretic side effects (polyuria, nocturia, thirst) *(REPRISE NEJM 2017;377:1930)*
- Long-acting octreotide: not statistically significant ↓ ∆KTV *(Lancet 2013;382:1485)*
- Everolimus: ↓ ∆KTV w/o effect on renal progression *(NEJM 2010;363:830)*

AUTOSOMAL RECESSIVE POLYCYSTIC KIDNEY DISEASE (ARPKD)

- ARPKD is a rare AR disorder that usually presents in early childhood
- The prevalence is approximately 1 in 20,000 individuals
- ARPKD is invariably associated with liver fibrosis and portal hypertension
- Both kidneys are enlarged w/ a cystic dilatation of the renal collecting ducts

Clinical Manifestation: Bimodal
- Newborns can be diagnosed by prenatal US and present with severe renal failure, oligohydramnios, and lung hypoplasia (30% of infants die of respiratory failure)
- Older children and adolescents may present with complications of portal hypertension, such as hepatosplenomegaly and bleeding from esophageal varices. Severe systemic hypertension in the setting of renal dysfunction is also common.

Genetics
- ARPKD is caused by mutations in the *PKHD* gene encoding fibrocystin, a large ciliary protein found in renal and biliary epithelial cells
- Dysfunction of fibrocystin leads to altered ciliary signaling, which is normally required for regulation of proliferation and differentiation of renal and biliary epithelial cells

Treatment
- There is no curative treatment for ARKD
- Infants surviving the newborn period should be monitored closely for decreased renal function, hypertension, infections, and dehydration
- Most cases progress to ESRD requiring dialysis or kidney transplantation

---

NEPHRONOPHTHISIS (NPHP)

- NPHP is a rare AR disease that presents as severe chronic tubulointerstitial nephritis
- The incidence is less than 1 in 50,000 individuals

Clinical Manifestations
- Low urinary osmolarity (<300 mOsm/kg) d/t reduction in the ability to concentrate urine in early childhood causing polyuria and polydipsia
- Urinary sodium wasting is also present and may cause hypovolemia
- Progressive renal failure manifests as poor growth and anemia
- ESRD develops at a mean age of about 13 yr but can also occur during adulthood
- The most frequent extrarenal manifestation is retinal degeneration causing early blindness, with an incidence between 10% and 30%

Diagnosis
- Renal ultrasonography is useful only in the advanced stages of the disease, when renal cysts are visible. Kidneys are typically highly echogenic.
- Although biopsy findings combined with clinical presentation can be suggestive of NPHP, genetic testing is the only definitive diagnostic modality

Genetics
- Mutations in several genes (NPHP1 through NPHP10 and likely many more encoding various ciliary proteins) are responsible for NPHP
- The presence of the NPHP gene products in cilia of various organs (photoreceptor, tubular cells, cholangiocytes) explains extrarenal manifestations in some patients
- Molecular testing by sequencing is now available, NPHP genes are included on several kidney disease NextGen sequencing panels

Treatment
- No curative tx; Most cases progress to ESRD requiring dialysis or kidney transplantation

AUTOSOMAL DOMINANT TUBULOINTERSTITIAL KIDNEY DISEASE (ADTKD)

- ADTKD, aka Medullary Cystic Kidney Disease (MCKD), presents as severe chronic tubulointerstitial nephritis, similar to NPHP
- Distinct from NPHP by its AD inheritance and by the late onset of renal failure

Clinical Manifestation

- Typically present after the third decade of life with advanced CKD
- Extrarenal manifestations include hyperuricemia and gout
- The kidneys have ↑ echotexture, but there are no visible cysts by u/s
- Kidney biopsy: chronic tubulointerstitial nephritis, tubular atrophy, and microscopic cysts in the medulla or at the corticomedullary junction (similar findings to NPHP)

Genetic

- Mutations in 2 genes encoding proteins produced by the renal tubular epithelium
- *MUC1* gene: encoding mucin-1, a transmembrane protein expressed on the apical surface of most epithelial cells. Among other functions, mucin provides a protective barrier to prevent pathogens from accessing the cell. In the kidney, mucin-1 is strongly expressed in the loop of Henle, DCT, and the collecting duct. A single cytosine insertion into one variable-number tandem repeat sequence within the MUC1 gene cause ADTKD. Not detectable by standard genetic tests and can only be tested in a research setting.
- *UMOD* gene: encoding uromodulin (Tamm–Horsfall protein). This protein is produced and secreted by TALH. Sanger sequencing-based mutational analysis of the UMOD gene is commercially available and can be used to establish a molecular diagnosis.

Treatment

- No curative treatment for ADTKD
- Xanthine oxidase inhibitors (allopurinol or febuxostat) should be used for prevention in pts with recurrent gout. There may be a role for these drugs in slowing CKD progression in asymptomatic pts if started early (QJM 2002;95:597)

	Summary of Inherited Cystic Disorders			
	ADPKD (AD)	**ARPKD (AR)**	**NPHP (AR)**	**ADTKD (AD)**
Gene (Protein)	PKD1, PKD2 (Polycystins-1 and 2)	PKHD1 (Fibrocystin)	NPHP1–12+ (Nephrocystins, other ciliary proteins)	MUC1 (Mucin-1), UMOD (Uromodulin)
Localization	Tubules (cilia)	Tubules (cilia)	Tubules (cilia)	Tubules (apical)
Onset	Adults >30 y/o	Newborns and children	Children and adolescents	Adults >30 y/o
Imaging	Massively enlarged kidneys, multiple large cysts easily visible	Enlarged kidneys, cysts visible only in advanced disease	Normal-sized kidneys without cysts, increased echotexture	Normal-sized kidneys without cysts, increased echotexture
Pathology	Massive cysts that replace normal renal parenchyma	Cystic dilatation of the renal CDs	Chronic tubulointerstitial nephritis	Chronic tubulointerstitial nephritis
Clinical Features	HTN, flank pain, cyst infection, nephrolithiasis, hematuria, low-grade proteinuria, renal failure, hepatic cysts, cerebral aneurysms, PFO, MVP, colonic diverticula	Potter syndrome, respiratory failure, hepatosplenomegaly, variceal bleeding, hematuria, low-grade proteinuria, renal failure, lung hypoplasia, liver fibrosis, portal HTN	Urinary concentrating defect, renal failure w/o hematuria or proteinuria, growth failure, retinal degeneration (retinitis pigmentosa), blindness	Urinary concentrating defect, renal failure w/o hematuria or proteinuria, hyperuricemia, gouty arthritis

RENAL CELL CARCINOMA (RCC)

Background
- Renal mass is frequently found with imaging during AKI/CKD w/u
- 26% of RCC pts had CKD before tumor nephrectomy (Lancet Oncol 2006;7:735)

Risk Factors and Pathogenesis
- Smoking, HTN, CKD, obesity, M:F 1.6:1
- Acquired cystic kidney disease (CJASN 2007;2:750): ↑ w/ dialysis duration (AJT 2011;11:86)

Type of Renal Cell Carcinoma		
Type (%)	Origin	Associated Genes and Pathway
Clear cell (75–90)	PT	VHL, TSC1/TSC2 BAP1 (Mol Cancer Res 2013;11:1061)
Papillary (10–20)	PT	Type 1: MET Type 2: NRF2-ARE pathway (NEJM 2016;374:135)
Chromophobe (5)	DT	Folliculin (FLCN): Birt–Hogg–Dube syndrome
Collecting duct (<1)	CD	
Medullary (<1)	Medullary	Sickle cell trait > SCD

- von Hippel–Lindau (VHL) gene: encodes VHL protein, E3 ubiquitin ligase; proteasome degradation of a hypoxia-inducible factor (HIF), transcription factor of erythropoietin gene
- VHL syndrome: AD VHL mutation causing constitutive activation of HIF
  Other malignancies: hemangioblastoma (CNS, retina), pheochromocytoma, pancreatic serous cystadenomas and neuroendocrine tumor, middle ear endolymphatic sac tumors
- VHL somatic mutation is found in 91% of clear cell RCC (Clin Cancer Res 2008;14:4726)
- Tuberous sclerosis: angiomyolipomas > benign cysts, RCC, lymphangioma
  Skin: forehead papules, plaques, lower trunk, angiofibroma
- Birt–Hogg–Dube syndrome: mutation of folliculin gene; bilateral multifocal RCC

Clinical Manifestations
- Hematuria, flank pain, HTN, fever, fatigue, weight loss, anemia, hepatic dysfunction
- ↑ Ca: osteolytic metastasis, IL-6 mediated PTHrp, PG mediated bone resorption
- Erythrocytosis: erythropoietin production
- NS with AA amyloidosis, IgAN
- 1/3 of diagnosed with metastasis

Diagnosis
- U/S: simple vs complex cyst
- Contrast CT: standard imaging test; required for Bosniak classification of cystic disease

Surveillance of Complex Renal Cysts

Bosniak Classification (J Urol 2017;198:12)		
Category: Imagining Features	Intervention	RCC Risk
I: simple cyst	None	–
II: complex cyst with thin septations	None	–
IIF: complex cyst with multiple thin or minimal thickening septations w/o measurable enhancement	F/U	6–18%
III: complex cyst with thickened irregular or smooth walls, contrast enhancing (>15 HU)	Surgery or close F/U	51–55%
IV: III + solid component, enhancing soft tissue	Surgery	89–91%

- 80% continued surveillance and 20% (5% of Bosniak IIF, 30% of III, 62% of IV) underwent surgery; metastasis, death rare, suggesting surveillance is safe (J Urol 2018;199:633)

Renal Mass Biopsy (J Urol 2017;198:520)
- ~14% nondiagnostic; very high sensitivity, specificity, and PPV
- Consider to rule out hematologic, metastatic, inflammatory, or infectious mass
- US or CT-guided multiple core biopsies
- Not required if it would not Δ management: (1) young pts who are unwilling to accept the uncertainties; (2) older/frail patients who will be managed conservatively
- No reported cases of tumor seeding in the contemporary literature

RCC Staging and Primary Treatment		
Stage	TNM	Treatment
I	T1 (≤7 cm, limited to the kidney) N0	
	T1a (≤4 cm)	PN
	T1b (>4, (≤7 cm)	PN (or RN)
II	T2 (>7 cm, limited to the kidney) N0	RN (or PN if clinically indicated) + adjuvant treatment
III	T1 or 2, N1 (regional LN) T3 (major veins or perinephric tissues)	
IV (advanced)	T4 (beyond Gerota fascia) or M1 (distant metastasis)	Nephrectomy + metastasectomy or Systemic therapy ± cytoreductive nephrectomy

Nephrectomy

Partial Nephrectomy (PN) vs Radical Nephrectomy (RN) (AUA J Urol 2017;198:520)	
PN Preferred	**RN Preferred**
cT1a (≤4 cm) renal mass Anatomic or functionally solitary kidney bilateral tumors, familial RCC Pre-existing CKD, or proteinuria Young, have multifocal masses, or comorbidities that are likely to impact renal function in the future	High tumor complexity No pre-existing CKD or proteinuria Normal contralateral kidney and new baseline eGFR will likely be >45

- Split radionuclide renal scan can be done to predict postnephrectomy dialysis requirement
- CKD incidence after nephrectomy (JASN 2018;29:207): 7.9% (CKD4-5), 14.2% (CKD3b-5)
  PN (vs RN) was a/w ↓ CKD 4–5 (×0.34), ↓ CKD 3b–5 (×0.15), ↓ mortality (×0.55);
  CKD Risk factors: preop renal function, tumor >7 cm, old age
  Renal function decline occurs within 12 mo after surgery
- PN was a/w less eGFR fall than RN by 10.5 (CJASN 2017;12:1057)
- AKI postsurgery: increasing to 10.4%. a/w male, RN, older age, black race, higher
  comorbidities, preoperative CKD stage (Urol Oncol 2016;34:293.e1)
- Concurrent RN and IVC thrombectomy a/w higher incidence of AKI and CKD
- Surgically induced CKD has less annual renal function decline than pre-op CKD (4.7
  vs 0.7%). Postop mortality was higher in pre-op CKD ×1.8 (CKD3), ×3.5 (CKD4),
  and ×4.4 (CKD5) (J Urol 2013;189:1649)
- Kidney biopsy review of nontumor tissue by medical renal pathologist in all pts with
  preop CKD and proteinuria: 15% had renal disease; severe vascular sclerosis (>50%
  luminal narrowing), global sclerosis >5% and IF/TA >10% was a/w postoperative creatinine elevation (Arch Pathol Lab Med 2013;137:531)

Systemic Therapy

Renal Toxicity of Systemic Therapy for Advanced RCC	
IFNα-2a (Lancet 2007;370:2103)	Collapsing FSGS, TMA
Antiangiogenic VEGF/tyrosine kinase inhibitors Bevacizumab (Lancet 2007;370:2103) Sorafenib (NEJM 2007;357:203) Sunitinib (NEJM 2007;356:115; NEJM 2016;375:2246) Sunitinib alone not inferior to nephrectomy + Sunitinib (NEJM 2018;379:417) Pazopanib (J Clin Oncol 2010;28:1061) Axitinib (Lancet 2011;378:1931) Cabozantinib (NEJM 2015;373:1814), Lenvatinib	TMA (proteinuria and HTN) HTN could be a biomarker of efficacy (JNCI 2011;103:763)
Checkpoint inhibitors Nivolumab + ipilimumab (NEJM 2018;378:1277) Avelumab w/ axitinib (NEJM 2019;380:1103) Pembrolizumab w/ axitinib (NEJM 2019;380:1116)	Tubulointerstitial nephritis (KI 2016;90:638)
mTOR inhibitors Everolimus Temsirolimus	AKI (BMC Cancer 2014;14:906) ATN (Ann Oncol 2013;24:2421)
IL-2	Capillary leak, AIN

Transplantation
- RCC risk: KTR >other organ txp recipient > general population (*JAMA* 2011;306:1891)
- a/w graft failure: kidney function associated >immunosuppression effect (*JASN* 2016;27:1495)
- Risk factors: black, prolonged dialysis predicting KT; 89% in native kidney; papillary RCC risk is esp high (*AJT* 2016;16:3479)

Transmission Risks of Donor RCC (*AJT* 2011;11:1140)	
Minimal (0.1%)	Resected solitary RCC ≤1.0 cm, well differentiated
Low (0.1–1%)	Resected solitary RCC 1.0–2.5 cm, well differentiated
Intermediate (1–10%)	Resected solitary RCC T1b 4–7 cm, well differentiated
High (>10%)	RCC >7 cm or stage II–IV

- Screening: U/S w/i 1 mo of txp, then q5y w/o cysts; q2y w/ cysts (*AJT* 2011;11:86)

URINARY TRACT OBSTRUCTION (UTO)

Background
- Common cause of CKD in children with CAKUT (Pediatr Nephrol 2016;31:1411)
- In adults, more common in men due to prostatic enlargement

Pathogenesis
- UTO can occur anywhere in the urinary tract system
- Renal tubular injury is the consequence of mechanical stretching, hypoxia, and exposure to oxygen-free radicals that result (Biomed Res Int 2014;2014:303298)

Causes of Acute UTO
- Outflow obstruction: mechanical (narrow urethra) vs dynamic (↑ muscle tone)
- Neurologic impairment: in sensory or motor nerve supply to detrusor muscle
- Inefficient detrusor muscle, following anesthesia
- Medications, particularly anticholinergics and sympathomimetic drugs
- Trauma; Urinary tract infection (UTI)

Causes of Chronic UTO
- Children: posterior urethral valves, ureterovesical, or ureteropelvic junction obstruction
- Young adults: nephrolithiasis
- Older adults: BPH, malignancy, nephrolithiasis, retroperitoneal fibrosis

Clinical Manifestations
- Acute UTO: hematuria, AKI, +/− pain, abdominal distention, hypertension, UTI
- Nondilated obstructive uropathy: happen with volume depletion, hypotension, infiltrative metastatic cancer and retroperitoneal fibrosis; Percutaneous nephrostomy tube placement and resolution of AKI is diagnostic (Ren Fail 2010;32:1226)
- Chronic UTO: may be asymptomatic. Overflow incontinence sometimes, nocturia. Discovered during workup of renal insufficiency.

Workup
- Renal U/S: false (+) rate of mild hydronephrosis w/o UTO is 26%, NPV of 98%
- Color duplex Doppler: intrarenal artery resistive index >0.7 in obstruction due to vasoconstriction
- Bladder ultrasound: can aid in evaluating for trabeculation of bladder wall and postvoid residual, as well as bladder wall mass or bladder stone
- Noncontrast CT scan: recommended for nephrolithiasis when presenting with signs of renal colic (severe flank or groin pain, emesis, gross hematuria) or risk factors (family history or prior renal stone) or in patients with polycystic kidney disease
- Cystoscopy/retrograde pyelography: if U/S (−) and obstruction is suspected
- Renography: Tc 99m-MAG3 scan with IV furosemide to differentiate collecting system dilatation from obstruction
- Cystoscopy and urodynamics in patients with suspected outflow obstruction

Differential Diagnosis of Hydronephrosis
- Peripelvic cysts, extrarenal pelvis, dilated renal veins
- Hydronephrosis without obstruction: notable in pregnancy

Obstructive Nephropathy (NEJM 1981;304:373)
- ↑ intratubular pressure → renal vasoconstriction, rapid ↓ in renal blood flow and GFR, with interstitial fibrosis and nephron dropout if obstruction is prolonged
- Chronic obstructive uropathy a/w hyperkalemia and dRTA

Treatment
- Dependent on location and etiology of obstruction
- Outflow obstruction: clean intermittent catheterization and bladder management
- Nephrolithiasis: stone and urine analysis for mineral solubility. Increase urine flow >2 L daily and low salt diet
- Mass or obstructing stone: nephrostomy until obstruction removed
- If bilateral chronic renal obstruction is relieved, may experience postobstruction diuresis, monitor for hemodynamic instability if unable to keep up with urine output

Prognosis
- If acute urinary retention is addressed <72 hr, likely complete renal recovery
- If obstruction remains >2 wk, recovery less likely if not achieved at 12 wk
- Risk factors for worse prognosis include recurrent obstructive renal disease, hypertension, diabetes, obesity, and albuminuria

REFLUX NEPHROPATHY

Background and Pathogenesis (*Lancet* 2015;385:371)
- VUR: the retrograde passage of urine from bladder into the upper urinary tract
- 1° VUR: incompetent closure of ureterovesical junction (UVJ), which contains a segment of the ureter within the bladder wall. Reflux is prevented by bladder contraction compressing the intravesical ureter and sealing it off with bladder muscle. Congenital short intravesical ureter. Low-grade VUR may improve with pt growth.
- 2° VUR: abnormally high voiding pressure in the bladder results in failure of closure of the UVJ during bladder contraction
  Anatomic (posterior urethral valve) vs functional obstruction (neurogenic bladder)

Epidemiology
- 1° VUR occurs in 1% of newborns, incidence higher in neonates with prenatal hydronephrosis, and in children with febrile urinary tract infections
- White children are 3× (than black children); ♀ : ♂ = 2 : 1
- Genetics: familial rate is higher for milder forms of 1° VUR. Although no single gene mutations have been identified certain syndromes may be a/w VUR, eg, renal coloboma syndrome (*Curr Genomics* 2016;17:70)

Clinical Manifestations and Workup
- Prenatal hydronephrosis, with prevalence rate of VUR of 16.2%; Febrile w/ UTI
- Renal and bladder U/S; Lab: serum creatinine, urinalysis, urine culture
- Voiding cystourethrogram is the diagnostic procedure of choice. Radionuclide cystography is an alternative method and may be used to monitor pts.
- Dimercaptosuccinic acid (DMSA) renal scan to detect renal cortical abnormalities

Grading of VUR (International Reflux Study Group)		
Grade I	Reflux fills ureter w/o dilatation	Mild
Grade II	Reflux fills ureter and collecting system w/o dilatation	
Grade III	Reflux fills/mildly dilates ureter and collecting system w/ mild blunting of calices	Moderate
Grade IV	Reflux fills/grossly dilates ureter and collecting system w/ blunting of calices; + Tortuosity of ureter	
Grade V	Reflux dilates collecting system, calices are blunted w/ a loss of papillary impression; + Ureteral dilation and tortuosity	Severe

Prognosis (*J Urol* 1997;157:1846)
- 1° VUR usually spontaneously resolve when age of diagnosis is <2 y/o, unilateral
  I and II resolves in 80% of children by age 5
  III with bilateral involvement at age 5–10 yr had lowest spontaneous resolution (20%) vs children presenting at 1–2 yr with unilateral disease (70%)
  IV: 60% (unilateral) and <10% (bilateral) resolution despite age at presentation
  V: spontaneous resolution rare, except in ♂ infants (30% resolve in 1st year of life)
- Recurrent UTI: grade III and IV (23%) vs grade I and II (14%) (*JAMA Pediatr* 2014;168:893)

General Treatment
- Surveillance is recommended for mild Grade I–II VUR as these usually self-resolve
- Monitor for symptoms, best in children who are verbal and toilet-trained

Prophylactic Antibiotics for Recurrent Pyelonephritis and UTI
- Indications: not toilet-trained or have bladder and bowel dysfunction, with any grade; moderate to severe VUR (III–V); recurrent febrile UTIs regardless of grade of VUR
- TMP-SMX or co-trimoxazole, nitrofurantoin, cephalexin, ampicillin, and amoxicillin, although resistance to E. coli UTIs do arise (*Lancet* 2015;385:371)
- Stopping antibiotic: re-evaluation of VUR as child grows or after correction of VUR

Prevention of Renal Damage: VUR Correction
- Indications: IV–V beyond age 2–3; medical therapy failure w/ breakthrough infections
- Open surgical reimplantation (ureteroneocystostomy, UNC); permanently correct VUR vs endoscopic injection (EI) of a biodegradable polymer (can have recurrent VUR)
  Repeat imaging: routine to f/u endoscopic correction, and in setting of recurrent UTI
  UNC more likely to have higher 30-d GU-related readmissions compared to EI
  (4.8% vs 1.1%, OR = 4.76); however, EI demonstrated increased odds of repeating antireflux procedures (OR = 7.13) (*J Pediatr Urol* 2017;13:507.e1)

URINARY TRACT INFECTION (UTI)

Definition (Infect Dis Clin North Am 2014;28:1)
- Asymptomatic bacteriuria (ASB): positive urinalysis and culture without symptoms
- Acute uncomplicated cystitis: urine culture + with symptoms, UTI confined to bladder
- Complicated UTI: special populations with acute cystitis; urologic abnormalities, immunocompromise, poorly controlled DM, kidney transplant, or pregnant women
- Pyelonephritis: inflammation of renal parenchyma +/– systemic illness

Common Micro-organisms Causing UTI	
Immune competent	Immunosuppressed or immunocompromised
• Enterobacteriaceae: *Escherichia coli* (m/c), *Klebsiella, Proteus* spp • *Pseudomonas* • Enterococci and staphylococci (MSSA, MRSA) • *Staphylococcus saprophyticus*	• *Candida* spp and mold Recent broad-spectrum antimicrobial use • Extended-Spectrum Beta-Lactamase (ESBL)-producing Enterobacteriaceae • Carbapenemase-producing gram-negative bacilli

Clinical Manifestations
- Cystitis: frequency, urgency, dysuria
- Pyelonephritis: fever (>37.7°C); Chills/rigors, malaise or significant fatigue; costovertebral angle tenderness; pelvic or perineal pain in men
- AKI is rare; reported with solitary kidney and NSAID use (Clin Infect Dis 1992;14:243)

Complications of Acute Pyelonephritis (Infect Dis Clin North Am 1997;11:663)
- Renal cortical abscess/carbuncle: result from hematogenous spread of bacteria from a primary focus of infection (bacteremia, osteomyelitis, endovascular infections)
- Renal corticomedullary abscess: a/w underlying urinary tract abnormality, such as vesicoureteral reflux or urinary tract obstruction
- Emphysematous pyelonephritis: suspect if DM + septic shock, worsening clinical status despite aggressive medical therapy, known or suspected UTO (NEJM 2018;378:48)
- Xanthogranulomatous pyelonephritis: a/w obstruction by struvite stone causing destruction of kidney tissue by granulomatous changes w/ lipid laden macrophages; frequently require surgical removal of infected tissue – nephrectomy
- Perinephric abscess: abscess between renal capsule and renal fascia, usually a/w rupture of an intrarenal abscess, renal cortical abscess, chronic/recurrent pyelonephritis, +/– obstruction, xanthogranulomatous pyelonephritis, or renal carbuncle

Risk Factors
- Urinary catheter use, UTO/VUR, DM, pregnancy, immunocompromised, ADPKD

Imaging: CT Scan with or without Contrast
- Indicated for recurrent symptoms, acute pyelonephritis with sepsis, septic shock, known or suspected urolithiasis, urine pH ≥7.0, new GFR ≤40 (NEJM 2018;378:48)

Management (IDSA; Clin Infect Dis 2011;52:e103)
- Empiric antibiotics based on severity of illness, risk factors for resistant pathogens, previous susceptibility to antibiotics, local community resistance prevalence
- Screen and treat all pregnant ♀ w/ ASB (IDSA Clin Infect Dis 2019; PMID 30895288)
- Acute uncomplicated cystitis: nitrofurantoin 100 mg bid × 5 d: superior to fosfomycin (JAMA 2018;319:1781), TMP-SMX DS bid × 3 d, or fosfomycin 3 g ×1
  Fluoroquinolones × 3 d are efficacious but can have secondary effects
  β-Lactams should be reserved if no other options due to their lower efficacy
- Pyelonephritis: oral fluoroquinolone (bid or extended release daily) × 7 d (+/– IV initial dose). IV ceftriaxone 1 g q24h dose or IV aminoglycoside q24h in lieu of IV fluoroquinolone depending on community resistance patterns.

UTI in CKD (CJASN 2006;1:327)
- Nitrofurantoin: absent in urine if CrCl <20; FDA recommends against use if CrCl <60
- Sulfamethoxazole: urine level is subtherapeutic if CrCl <50
- Ciprofloxacin, levofloxacin, and trimethoprim: therapeutic level achieved in CKD

UTI in ADPKD (AJP Renal 2017;313:F1077)
- ↑ UTI, infected renal cysts, pyelonephritis; 30–60% of ADPKD pts experience UTI
- Prevention through "flushing" of kidneys and preventing stasis through increasing urine volume, vitamin C rich cranberry juice, and usual hygiene measures
- Treatment targeted to penetrate renal cysts, empiric IV fluoroquinolone or cefotaxime or ampicillin plus gentamicin based on resistance panels

MINIMAL CHANGE DISEASE (MCD)

- Most common cause of nephrotic syndrome in pediatric population (2–7 cases/100,000, accounting for ~90% of nephrotic syndrome under age 10)
- Third most common cause of nephrotic syndrome in adults (~10% of cases)
- Usually idiopathic, but secondary MCD associated with:
  - Neoplasms: Hodgkin disease, NHL, leukemia, renal cell carcinoma
  - Medications: NSAIDs, interferon, gold, mercury, methimazole, penicillamine
  - Infections: syphilis, HIV, mycoplasma
  - Autoimmune disorders: sclerosing cholangitis, sarcoidosis
  - Other renal disorders: IgAN (CJASN 2014;9:1033), lupus nephritis (CJASN 2016;11:547)

Pathogenesis
- Pathologic T-cell–mediated circulating factor ("Shalhoub hypothesis") (Lancet 1974;7880:556)
- Activation of T-cell costimulatory CD80 (B7-1) on podocytes is a/w proteinuria in MCD, and may be stimulated by cytokines such as IL-13 (Semin Nephrol 2011;3:320; Ped Nephrol 2015;30:469). ↑ urinary CD80 during relapses of MCD, but not FSGS (KI 2010;78:296).
- Role of B cells implied by effectiveness of B-cell depleting agents (rituximab) and associations with lymphoid malignancies. IL-4–mediated mechanism (JCI Insight 2017;2:81836).

Pathology
- **LM:** normal appearance; **IF:** no staining (unless secondary to other GN); **EM:** ≥80% foot process effacement, no electron dense deposits (unless secondary to other GN)
- Mesangial deposits of IgM (Ped Nephrol 2009;24:1187) or C1q may be seen in both MCD and FSGS, and are associated with worse prognosis in MCD

Clinical Manifestations
- Acute onset edema (LE periorbital, ascites); GI distress common in children (diarrhea, nausea, pain; attributed to intestinal edema); often follows viral infection or atopic episode
- Complications: AKI/ATN, thrombosis

Workup
- Labs: proteinuria >3.5 G/24 hr, ↓ serum albumin, ↑ cholesterol (especially triglycerides), hematuria in 10–30% of adults (JASN 2013;24:702). May present with AKI.
- Rule out secondary causes, as above
- Consider genetic testing if age <1 yr, significant FHx, or steroid resistant disease

Treatment
- Prednisone 1 mg/kg (up to 80 mg) QD or 2 mg/kg QOD (up to 120 mg) for 4–16 wk; if responding, taper over 3–6 mo
- If unable to tolerate CS or FR/SD, use CNI: CsA (3–5 mg/kg/d divided bid, goal trough 100–150) or Tac (0.05–0.1 mg/kg/d divided bid goal trough 5–7) ×1–2 yr, then taper

Definitions of Steroid Responsiveness	
Steroid resistant (SR)	Failed to achieve remission with 16 wk of steroid
Steroid dependent (SD)	Relapses ≥2 during steroid taper or w/i 2 wk of d/c of steroid
Frequently relapsing (FR)	Relapses ≥2 w/i 6 mo or ≥4 w/i 1 yr of achieving remission

- For FR/SD patients unable to tolerate CNI, older guidelines suggest cyclophosphamide (2–2.5 mg/kg PO daily) for 8 wk or MMF (1,000 mg bid) for 1–2 yr (KDIGO GN 2012)
- Rituximab: effective for FR/SD MCD (NEMO JASN 2014;25:850; CJASN 2016;11:710)

Prognosis
- In pediatric population, 90% of cases are steroid responsive, but 60% develop FR/SD state (J Pediatr 1981;98:561; Lancet 1988;8582:380; J Pediatr 2005;147:202)
- 20–30% of pediatric FR/SD patients continue to have relapses into adulthood (J Pediatr 2005;147:202; CJASN 2009;4:1593)
- 88% of adult onset MCD respond to CS, w/ 56% having relapsing course (AJKD 2017;69:637)
- Most FR/SD patients have good renal prognosis but high risk of treatment-related complications (osteoporosis, cataracts, infertility) (CJASN 2009;4:1593). Few will progress to ESRD (AJKD 2017;69:637)

FOCAL SEGMENTAL GLOMERULOSCLEROSIS

- FSGS is a pathologic lesion that can be caused by a diverse set of diseases
- **Idiopathic FSGS** also called "primary," usually presents with nephrotic syndrome (NS)
- **Secondary FSGS:** should be interpreted cautiously. It may refer to FSGS with cause (KDIGO GN 2012), nonprimary podocyte injury excluding genetic FSGS (AJKD 2013;62:403), or non-nephrotic syndrome w/ foot process effacement <80% (NDT 2015;30:375)
- Most common biopsy diagnosis in US, incidence rising (AJKD 2016;68:533)
- Most common glomerular cause of ESRD (AJKD 2016;68:533)
- Male:female incidence 1.5:1 (CJASN 2017;12:502)
- Accounts for 20% of pediatric and 40% of adult cases of NS

Conditions Associated With FSGS	
Infections	HIV, Parvovirus B19, CMV, Malaria, SV40 virus, Schistosomiasis, Strongyloidiasis (KI Rep 2018;3:14)
Malignancies	Hodgkin and Non-Hodgkin lymphoma
Drugs	Interferon, Pamidronate, Lithium, Heroin, Anabolic steroids, HCV DAA (Hepatology 2017;66:658)
Hemodynamic maladaptation	↓ nephron endowment (unilateral kidney agenesis, ↓ birth weight) Nephron loss (reflux nephropathy, nephrectomy/ablation, cortical necrosis, residual sclerosis from proliferative nephritis) Hyperfiltration (obesity, chronic allograft nephropathy, sickle cell, cyanotic congenital heart disease, HTN, diabetes mellitus)
Inflammatory disease	SLE, HLH, MCTD, giant cell arteritis, adult onset Still disease, sarcoidosis, systemic sclerosis
Genetic mutations	Mostly monogenic mutations of critical podocyte genes
Genetic syndromes	Charcot–Marie–Tooth, Alport, Type I glycogen storage disease, Branchio-oto-renal syndrome, Partial lecithin-cholesterol acyltransferase deficiency, Spondylometaphyseal dysplasia

Pathogenesis
- Podocyte injury leads to detachment from GBM; parietal epithelial cells (PEC) migrate from Bowman capsule, forming cellular bridges to the capillary tuft, eventually causing tuft adhesion, loop obliteration, and segmental sclerosis (ACKD 2014;21:408)
- Idiopathic: podocytes injured by circulating permeability factor of uncertain identity, likely produced by immune cells, analogous to minimal change disease (Nat Rev Nephrol 2016;12:768). Evidence: (1) improvement of proteinuria w/ PLEX; (2) resolution of FSGS lesions upon retransplant to non-FSGS recipient (NEJM 2012;366:1648)
- Adaptive hyperfiltration: nephron loss leads to distention of individual glomerular capillaries and increased glomerular pressure, causing GBM adaptation, slit diaphragm widening, and podocyte detachment (Pedatr Nephrol 2017;3293:405; KI 2017;91:1283)

Apolipoprotein 1 (APOL1) and the Kidney
APOL1 is a minor component of HDL synthesized in the liver and found in the kidney, endothelium, pancreas, liver, brain, and heart
APOL1 variants G1 and G2, compared to reference variant G0, confer resistance against trypanosomal species and are more common in sub-Saharan Africa (JASN 2015;22:2098)
>50% of African Americans carry 1 APOL1 risk variant and 13% have 2 risk variants (Semin Nephrol 2015;35:222)
The occurrence of homozygosity or double heterozygotes for G1/G2 ↑ renal disease in people of African heritage: 18% of FSGS and 35% of HIVAN (JASN 2011;22:2129)
Also a/w HTN associated ESRD and sickle cell disease (ACKD 2014;21:426; BJH 2017;179:323)

Pathology
- **LM:** at least 1 glomerulus with lesion of segmental (partial) sclerosis, may see tubular microcysts (esp in collapsing variant)
- **IF:** typically no staining. Mesangial IgM may be seen, associated with worse prognosis. C1q staining raises concern for C1q nephropathy, a rare variant of FSGS
- **EM:** FP effacement typically diffuse (>80%), may be patchy in adaptive FSGS. Mesangial EDD and tubuloreticular inclusions may be seen in secondary FSGS, especially immune complex-mediated disease. GBM wrinkling seen in collapsing variant
- Histologic subtypes help differentiate primary from secondary lesions and may help prognosticate disease course (ACKD 2014;21:400)

Histologic Subtypes of FSGS (ACKD 2014;21:400; KI 2011;80:868)

FSGS NOS (68%)	≥1 glomerulus with segmental increase in matrix obliterating the capillary lumina. There may be segmental glomerular capillary wall collapse without overlying podocyte hyperplasia.
Collapsing variant (12%)	≥1 segmental or global collapse of the glomerular tuft with overlying podocyte hyperplasia or hypertrophy. Most likely to progress to ESRD.
Tip lesion variant (10%)	≥1 segmental lesion involving tip domain of glomerulus. Often steroid-sensitive. Best prognosis even if SR (CJASN 2013;8:399)
Perihilar variant (7%)	≥1 glomerulus with perihilar hyalinosis, more common in adaptive/hyperfiltration mediated FSGS
Cellular variant (3%)	≥1 glomerulus with endocapillary hypercellularity without foam cells or karyorrhexis

Clinical Manifestations
- Proteinuria, typically nephrotic range (>3.5 g/d); Idiopathic FSGS usually presents as full nephrotic syndrome; Adaptive FSGS less likely to have full nephrotic syndrome
- May present as subnephrotic in collapsing and TRPC6-related FSGS

Workup
- Urine protein excretion, serum albumin, lipid panel
- Rule out potential infectious causes (HIV, Parvovirus B19, CMV), inflammatory diseases (SLE, MCTD, HLH, giant cell arteritis, adult onset Still disease), drug-related causes (interferon, pamidronate, anabolic steroids, lithium, heroin)
- Consider genetic evaluation in patients with significant family hx, steroid-resistant (SR) NS, pediatric onset disease

Renal-Limited Genetic FSGS

Gene	Product	Gene	Product
NHPS1 (AR)	Nephrin	CD2AP (AD)	CD2-associated protein
NHPS2[a] (AR)	Podocin	ACTN4 (AD)	Alpha actinin 4
PLCE1 (AR)	Phospholipase Cε1	TRPC6 (AD)	Transient receptor potential cation channel 6

Genetic FSGS With Possible Extrarenal Manifestations

Gene	Product	Associated Conditions
INF2[b] (AD)	Inverted formin 2	Charcot–Marie–Tooth: motor and sensory nerve manifestations with distal leg weakness, foot deformities (pes cavus, hammer toes)
WT1 (AD)	Wilms tumor 1	Denys–Drash syndrome: Wilms tumor, male pseudohermaphroditism Frasier syndrome: gonadoblastoma, male pseudohermaphroditism
MTTL1, MTTL2, MTTY (mito-chondrial)	Mitochondrial tRNA	MELAS syndrome: mitochondrial myopathy, encephalopathy, lactic acidosis, stroke-like episode
LMX1b (AD)	LIMHboxTF1	Nail–patella syndrome: hypoplastic patella, dystrophic nails, dysplasia of elbows Collagenofibrotic glomerulopathy
LAMB2 (AR)	Laminin beta 2	Pierson syndrome: microcoria, NM junction defects
ITGB4 (AR)	Beta 4 integrin	Epidermolysis bullosa
CD151 (AR)	Tetraspanin CD151	Epidermolysis bullosa, sensorineural deafness, nail dystrophy
SCARB2 (AR)	Scavenger receptor class B member 2	Action myoclonus-renal failure syndrome: ataxia, myoclonus
MYH9 (AD)	Nonmuscle myosin 11a	Bleeding diathesis, macrothrombocytopenia, progressive sensorineural deafness, ↑ liver enzyme, cataract

[a]Most common cause of genetic SRNS in childhood
[b]Most common cause of familial FSGS in adults, often subnephrotic (NDT 2012;27:882)

Treatment of Idiopathic FSGS

- Prednisone 1 mg/kg (up to 80 mg) QD or 2 mg/kg QOD (up to 120 mg) for 4–16 wk or complete remission; if responding, taper over 6 mo
- If intolerant of or resistant to CS, CNI: CsA (3–5 mg/kg/d divided bid w/ goal trough 125–175) or Tac (0.05–0.1 mg/kg/d divided bid w/ goal trough 5–10) for at least 12 mo if responding by 6 mo
- SR FSGS unable to tolerate CNI: dexamethasone and MMF (KI 2011;80:868)
- Rituximab generally not recommended for treatment-resistant FSGS, but has been used in small trials to treat resistant FSGS with improvement in proteinuria, relapse rate, and need for IS (JASN 2014;25:850; Am J Nephrol 2014;39:322)
- Conservative care with RAS inhibition, dietary sodium restriction, and BP control particularly important if incomplete response to immunosuppression

Treatment of FSGS With Identifiable Cause

- Treat underlying disease: eg, ART for HIVAN

Treatment of Adaptive/Hyperfiltration-mediated and Genetic FSGS

- No role for immunosuppression
- RAS inhibition, dietary sodium restriction, optimize BP control

Prognosis

- Patients with subnephrotic proteinuria are unlikely to progress to ESRD but are at increased risk of cardiovascular morbidity and mortality
- Patients with nephrotic range proteinuria are more likely to progress to ESRD
- Tip-lesion FSGS associated with best outcomes and most steroid-responsive, more similar to minimal change disease
- Collapsing FSGS associated with worst outcomes and ESRD
- Steroid resistance is most important predictor of poor outcome, regardless of histology (JASN 2004;15:2169; 2017;28:3055)

Transplantation

- Idiopathic FSGS has high rate (~40%) of recurrence after transplant and can recur within 48–72 hr (Transplant Proc 2017;49:2256; CJASN 2016;11:2041)
- Risk factors for recurrence include younger age, non-African American race, heavier proteinuria and low serum albumin pretransplant, and more rapid progression to ESRD
- Surveillance for recurrence necessary with frequent ✓ urine protein excretion
- Prompt initiation of plasmapheresis ± rituximab may improve outcomes for recurrent FSGS; prophylactic treatment may not be effective (Transplantation 2018;102:e115)

MEMBRANOUS NEPHROPATHY (MN)

- Most common cause of nephrotic syndrome in nondiabetic Caucasian pts
- Primary MN (PMN) (60–70%) vs secondary MN (30–40%)

Pathogenesis

- PMN is an autoimmune disease in which antibodies (usually IgG4) are produced against a podocyte antigen, most commonly the phospholipase A2 receptor (PLA2R)
- Abs may also form against Ag trapped in the GBM (eg, bovine serum albumin), or preformed Ag-Ab complexes may in theory deposit from the circulation (not proven in human disease). Complement activation then contributes to podocyte injury.

Identified Antigens of PMN	
M-Type Phospholipase A2 Receptor (PLA2R) (NEJM 2009;361:11)	70–80% of PMN, rare in HBV, malignancy-associated MN
Thrombospondin type-1 domain-containing 7A (THSD7A) (NEJM 2014;371:2277)	2–5% of PMN, 10% of PLA2R Ab (–) PMN Expressed in GB cancer & LN metastasis; 7/25 had malignancy (NEJM 2016;374:1995)
Neutral endopeptidase (NEJM 2002;346:2053)	Rare; antenatal MN in fetuses of mothers with deficiency of neutral endopeptidase
Bovine serum albumin (NEJM 2011;364:2101)	Rare cause of childhood MN
Recombinant arylsulfatase B (JASN 2014;25:675)	Enzyme replacement for Pompe disease

Causes of Secondary MN	
Drugs	NSAIDs, gold, mercury
Autoimmune	SLE, RA, Sjögren's
Alloimmunity	Kidney allograft rejection, GVHD (NDT 2011;26:2025)
Infection	HBV (HBeAg, anti-HBeAb present on immune deposit) Syphilis, malaria, ? HCV (dubious causal relationship)
Malignancy	Solid organ tumors (lung, GI, breast, prostate, uterus) Hematologic (Hodgkin and Non-Hodgkin, CLL)

Clinical Manifestations
- Classically NS (80%), less commonly with subnephrotic-range proteinuria (<3.5 g/d). Onset of NS may be gradual compared to the rapid onset seen with MCD.
- If AKI is present, consider renal vein thrombosis or rare crescentic MN
- CKD may be present after years of persistent high-grade proteinuria
- Thrombosis is more common in MN (7%) vs other causes of NS. Hypoalbuminemia <2.8 g/dL is a significant independent predictor of thrombotic risk (CJASN 2012;7:43)

Diagnosis: Kidney Biopsy Is Gold Standard
- **LM:** thickened glomerular capillary wall with spikes
- **IF:** IgG and C3 granular staining
- **EM:** subepithelial deposits, foot process effacement
- In PMN 15% of patients will have glomerular antigen-positive PLA2R staining despite negative serum anti-PLA2R antibodies

Suggestive Pathologic Features of Primary vs Secondary MN		
Features	Primary MN	Secondary MN
LM		Leukocyte infiltration in malignancy (KI 2006;70:1510)
IgG subtype	IgG4: dominant in PLA2R, THSD7A	IgG1, 3 in LN IgG1, 2 in malignancy
Tubular basement (TBM) IgG staining	(−)	(+) in LN; can have anti-TBM ab with tubulointerstitial nephritis
Other Ig, C1q	(−)	(+) in class V LN
Electron dense deposits	Subepithelial, Intramembranous	Additional mesangial, subendothelial in LN
Endothelial tubuloreticular inclusion	(−)	(+) in class V LN

- Serum anti-PLA2R antibodies: the presence of has 96–100% specificity for PMN; diagnostic, esp biopsy is contraindicated and renal function is preserved (PLoS One 2014;9:e104936; KI 2019;95:429)

Evaluation
- Serum anti-PLA2R level; if negative consider anti-THSD7A testing where available
- If history and biopsy are suggestive of secondary MN: age and risk-appropriate cancer screening, especially in older adults (age >65 yr) and those who are anti-PLA2R negative

Recommended Cancer Screening (USPSTF)	
Colorectal	50–75 y/o
Breast	Biennial mammography 50–74 y/o
Cervical	Pap smear q3y 21–65 y/o
Lung	Annual low dose CT for 55–80 y/o adults who have a 30 pack-yr smoking history and currently smoke or have quit within the past 15 yr

- Serologic testing for autoimmune disease, including ANA and complement levels
- Hepatitis B and C serologies, HIV, RPR
- Consider GVHD in patients who have had a bone marrow transplant
- If nephrotic: high index of suspicion for RVT, DVT, or PE
  - RVT prevalence ~30% in nephrotic MN (Am J Med 1980;69:819)
  - RVT usually asymptomatic, but if acute may present with abdominal/flank pain and if bilateral may present as AKI. Renal venography is gold standard to diagnose but rarely done. No consensus on best radiologic test to use for diagnosis if suspected (CT angio, Doppler ultrasound MRI), depends on local expertise but all have false-negatives.

Treatment

- Antiproteinuric tx w/ ACE-I or ARB; If secondary MN, treat underlying disease
- If complications of the NS are present then initiate **immunosuppression (IS)**
- If proteinuria >4 g/d persists after 6 mo of ACE-I or ARB, **consider IS**
- If eGFR <30, KDIGO 2012 suggests against IS (recommendation not graded)
- Among immunosuppressive regimens, glucocorticoid monotherapy should not be used

Immunosuppressive Regimens for MN			
Treatment Dosing		**Duration**	**Efficacy**
Alternating Cyclophosphamide (CYC) and glucocorticoids (aka modified "Ponticelli" protocol) (NEJM 1989;320:8; JASN 1998;9:444; 2007;18:1899)	Glucocorticoids (mo 1, 3, 5) IV methylprednisolone 1 g on d 1, 2, 3 followed by PO prednisone 0.5 mg/kg daily × 27 d CYC (mo 2, 4, 6) 2.0–2.5 mg/kg PO daily	6 mo	72–93% PR/CR *Relapse:* 10–25% by 3–4 yr
Continuous Cyclophosphamide and glucocorticoids (NDT 2004;1:1142)	CYC 1.5–2.0 mg/kg PO daily × 12 mo Glucocorticoids for first 6 mo: prednisone 0.5 mg/kg daily × 6 mo with methylprednisolone 1 g IV on day 1, 2, 3 of mo 1, 3, 5	12 mo	92% PR/CR, 36% CR *Relapse:* 28% by 5 yr
Cyclosporine (CsA) (MENTOR NEJM 2019;381:36; KI 2001;59;1484)	CsA: 3.5–5.0 mg/kg/d divided bid, trough 120–200 ± prednison 5–10 mg QD or QOD	12–18 mo (stop if no response by 6 mo)	52–75% PR/CR *Relapse:* 36% by 1.5 yr
Tacrolimus (Tac) (KI 2007;71;924)	Tac: 0.05–0.075 mg/kg/d divided bid, trough 3–5 ± prednisone 5–10 mg QD or QOD	12–18 mo (stop if no response by 6 mo)	76% PR/CR *Relapse:* 47% by 2.5 yr
Rituximab (MENTOR NEJM 2019;381:36; JASN 2012;23:1416)	Rituximab IV 375 mg/kg Qwk × 4, or 1 g Q14d × 2	May repeat at 6 mo	60–65% PR/CR, 27% CR *Relapse:* 28% by 5 yr

PR, partial remission; CR complete remission

- Anticoagulation for patients with known thrombosis. Prophylactic anticoagulation should be considered for patients with albumin <2.8. Decision analysis tool can be found at http://www.unckidneycenter.org/gntools

Prognosis

- Approximately 1/3 of patients have spontaneous remission, usually within the first 6–9 mo. Spontaneous remission is more likely in those with preserved kidney function and subnephrotic range proteinuria, but has been reported in pts with high-grade proteinuria
- Complete remission (<300 mg/d proteinuria) and partial remission (<3.5 g/d proteinuria) is associated with a 10-yr kidney survival of 100% and 90%
- 50% have persistent NS; of these, 30–40% progress to ESRD within 5–15 yr
- Proteinuria >8 g/d is a risk factor for progression regardless of GFR (KI 1997;51:901)
- Anti-PLA2R Ab titers may predict disease course: low and falling titers are associated with spontaneous remission, while high titers are associated with development of persistent proteinuria (JASN 2014;24:1357; Am J Nephrol 2015;42:70)
- Anti-PLA2R Ab titers may be used to monitor response to therapy. Immunologic remission typically precedes fall in proteinuria

Transplantation

- Recurrence: 40–50%.
  - Risk factors: higher pre-txp proteinuria, (+) PLA2R Ab (Transplantation 2016;100:2710)
  - Tx: rituximab (AJT 2009;9:2800)
- De novo disease is rare and may be a/w DSA and antibody-mediated rejection

Membranous-Like Glomerulopathy With Masked IgG
Kappa Deposits (MGMID)
- Rare secondary form of MN where subepi deposits show C3-predominant staining on routine immunofluorescence of fresh tissue (may be misdiagnosed as C3 glomerulopathy), but reveal strong IgG-k staining after pronase digestion (KI 2014;86:154)
- Most commonly found in young women with positive autoimmune serologies. At least one case recurred post-transplant (KI Rep 2016;1:299)

MALIGNANCY-ASSOCIATED MN

- The m/c glomerular disease in patients with cancer
- Incidence of cancer in MN: ×2.25 (AJKD 2007;50:396) – 9.8 (KI 2006;70:1510)
- Reported case numbers: lung > stomach > kidney > prostate > colon, breast cancer (Nat Rev Nephrol 2011;7:85)
- Other reported cancer: bladder, pancreas, head and neck, Wilms tumor, teratoma, ovarian, cervical, endometrial, skin (melanoma, SCC, BCC), pheochromocytoma, hematologic malignancy (Hodgkin disease, NHL, CLL, AML, CML); s/p HCT
- 10% of MN; 52% had symptoms of cancer at time of biopsy (KI 2006;70:1510)
- Risk factors: age over 65 yr and history of smoking >20 p.y. (KI 2006;70:1510)
- Biopsy: leukocyte infiltration (KI 2006;70:1510), IgG1, 2 dominance (NDT 2004;19:574)
- THSD7A expressed in GB carcinoma and LN metastasis and serum Ab disappeared with treatment (NEJM 2016;374:1995); 8 of 40 pts with THSD7A-associated MN was diagnosed with malignancy w/i 3 mo from the MN diagnosis (JASN 2017;28:520)
- Cancer surveillance in PLA2R (−), THSD7A (+), or non-IgG4 MN (JASN 2017;28:421):
  - At least age and risk factor appropriate screening; may need upper endoscopy, colposcopy and PSA/prostate biopsy (CJASN 2014;9:609)
- Remission with cancer removal or remission; relapse with cancer recurrence

PAUCI-IMMUNE GLOMERULONEPHRITIS

- Most common type of crescentic glomerulonephritis
- Small vessel vasculitis distinguished from other vasculitides by the absence of immune deposits. ANCA present in ~85% of cases (J Rheumatol 2001;28:1584)
- Predominantly affects older adults; m/c renal biopsy diagnosis in >80 (CJASN 2009;4:1073)
- Incidence 20 cases per million annually, slight male predominance (Sem Nephrol 2017;37:418)
- Clinical subtypes are defined histologically in the Table below (Chapel ill Consensus Conference Arthritis Rheum 2013;65:1). However, there is substantial overlap between MPA and GPA.
- Prognosis, genetics, epidemiology, and treatment response are better associated with the specific ANCA antigen rather than histology (Nat Rev Rheumatol 2016;12:570)

Clinical Subtypes of Pauci-immune GN (Arthritis Rheum 2013;65:1; AJKD 2006;47:770)		
Disease	Histologic Features	ANCA
Microscopic Polyangiitis (MPA)	Necrotizing vasculitis without granulomatous inflammation, Often renal-limited	60% +MPO or p-ANCA
Granulomatosis with Polyangiitis (GPA), formerly "Wegener's"	Necrotizing granulomatous inflammation, Often involves kidneys, upper and lower respiratory tract	75% +PR3 or c-ANCA
Eosinophilic Granulomatosis with Polyangiitis (EGPA), formerly "Churg-Strauss"	Eosinophil rich necrotizing granulomatous inflammation, Usually involves respiratory tract, about half of cases involve kidney, a/w asthma and circulating eosinophilia	75% +ANCA (mostly MPO/p-ANCA) if renal disease present 26% +ANCA if no renal disease present

Antineutrophilic Cytoplasmic Antibody (ANCA)
- Presence of ANCA was traditionally diagnosed by performing IF on ethanol-fixed human neutrophils incubated with pt's serum (indirect immunofluorescence, IIF). Cytoplasmic (C) ANCA pattern is usually seen with ab against serum proteinase 3 (PR3) and Perinuclear (P) ANCA is usually seen with ab against myeloperoxidase (MPO).
- Elevated P-ANCA/MPO ab can been seen with other autoimmune diseases such as SLE or inflammatory bowel disease

Pathogenesis

- Distinct genetic associations exist for PR3 vs MPO disease (NEJM 2012;367:214)
- Formation of ANCA may be potentially triggered through the following:
  Environmental stimuli: silica, asbestos (JASN 2001;12:134; Ren Fail 2005;27:605)
  Drugs: hydralazine, propylthiouracil (Arthritis Rheum 2000;43:405)
  Infection (NDT 2010;25:31119; Clin Rheumatol 2010;29:893)
  Molecular mimicry (Nat Med 2008;14:1088), **Epigenetic dysregulation** (JCI 2010;120:3209)
  Loss of T cell regulation (Immunology 2010;130:64)
- ANCA causes the development of vasculitis through several proposed mechanisms: activation of neutrophils via Fc receptors (J Immunol 1994;153:1271)
  Release of neutrophil extracellular traps (NETS) containing chromatin and granule proteins that trigger damage to endothelial cells and ANCA antigen presentation to immune system (Nat Med 2009;15:623)
  Activation of the alternative complement pathway and generation of C5a, a neutrophil chemoattractant and activator (KI 2007;71:646; JASN 2009;20:289)

Pathology

- **LM:** fibrinoid necrosis of glomerular tufts +/− rupture of GBM, proliferation of epithelial cells forming crescents
- **IF:** no staining for Ig, no or mild complement staining (Pauci Immune)
- **EM:** no electron dense deposits
- Affected nonrenal tissue shows leukocytoclastic vasculitis

Clinical Manifestations

- Constitutional: malaise, fatigue, fever, weight loss, night sweats, anorexia
- Renal: rapidly progressive glomerulonephritis (AKI, hypertension, edema, microscopic hematuria, subnephrotic proteinuria over wk to mo)
- Pulmonary: hemoptysis (from alveolar hemorrhage), cough, dyspnea on exertion, alveolar infiltrates on CXR
- Sinonasal: sinusitis, otitis media, "saddle-nose" deformity (particularly GPA)
- Dermatologic: palpable purpura (usually in lower extremities), petechiae, ulcers, nodules, urticaria, ecchymoses, bullae
- Ocular: iritis, uveitis, episcleritis
- GI: bleeding or perforation due to vasculitic ulcers
- Cardiovascular: pericarditis, myocarditis
- Neurologic: mononeuritis multiplex, cranial nerve abnormalities

Comparison of PR-3 vs MPO ANCA Disease		
	PR-3 Disease	**MPO Disease**
Clinical manifestation (Arthritis Rheum 2012;64:3452)	Saddle nose, nasal ulcer/crusting, bone destruction Epistaxis, hearing loss, Subglottic stenosis Lung with cavities	Renal limited GN Lung involvement w/o nodules Lung involvement w/o ENT disease
Pathology (AJKD 2003;41:539)	Focal GN, Necrosis	Global sclerosis, Interstitial fibrosis
Recurrence	More frequent	Less frequent

Workup

- Lab: elevated Cr, hematuria (including dysmorphic RBCs and red cell casts), proteinuria, normal complement levels, eosinophilia (in EGPA), elevated MPO or PR3 ab (or both), positive P-ANCA or C-ANCA (or both)
- Rule out drug-induced causes, esp if dual MPO and PR3 positivity or concomitant ANA positivity. Common culprits are propylthiouracil, hydralazine, levamisole, allopurinol, anti-TNF-alpha agents (CJASN 2015;10:1300)

Induction Therapy

- CYC w/ CS (3-d pulse of methylprednisolone 500 mg IV, then 1 mg/kg daily prednisone up to 60 mg for 1 mo, then taper off by 6 mo)
- CYC: in monthly IV doses (0.5–1 g/m²) or dosed orally (1–2 mg/kg/d). Dose should be adjusted for age >60, eGFR <20, and to avoid neutropenia (KDIGO GN). IV regimen has lower cumulative dose and may be equally effective (CJASN 2013;8:219)
- Rituximab (RTX) 375 mg/m² weekly ×4 is an acceptable alternative (NEJM 2010;363:211; 2010;363:221; 2013;369:417; Ann Rheum Dis 2016;75:1166; KDIGO GN 2012)
- Plasmapheresis ×7 over 14 d for rapidly rising Cr, severe renal impairment (Cr >5.8 mg/dL OR oliguria), AKI requiring dialysis, pulmonary hemorrhage, or concomitant anti-GBM disease (MEPEX JASN 2007;18:2180; KDIGO GN 2012)

RCTs of Rituximab (RTX) vs Cyclophosphamide (CYC) Induction		
Trial	**RAVE**	**RITUXVAS**
RTX group	RTX 375 mg/m^2 weekly ×4 w/o maintenance therapy	RTX 375 mg/m^2 weekly ×4 + CYC 15 mg/kg IV w/ 1st & 3rd RTX
CYC group	CYC 2 mg/kg PO QD followed by AZA	CYC IV for 3–6 mo followed by AZA
Results	RTX noninferior in inducing remission by 6 mo (64 vs 53%), 12 mo (48 vs 39%), and 18 mo (39 vs 33%) *(NEJM 2010;363:221; 2013;369:417)* PR-3 group respond better to RTX *(Ann Rheum Dis 2016;75:1166)*	RTX not superior in sustained remission at 12 mo and severe adverse events *(NEJM 2010;363:211)* No difference in death, ESRD and relapse at 24 mo *(Ann Rheum Dis 2015;74:1178)*
All RAVE and RITUXVAS groups received corticosteroids		

- MMF: 2~3 g/d noninferior to CYC w/ more relapse esp in PR-3 in non-RPGN, non-life threatening vasclitis with eGFR >15 *(Ann Rheum Dis 2019;78:399)*

Maintenance Therapy
- 18 mo of maintenance therapy in patients who achieve remission. No further therapy in patients who progress to ESRD without extrarenal disease *(KDIGO GN 2012)*
- Azathioprine (AZA) 1–2 mg/kg/d or Mycophenolate mofetil (MMF) 1 g BID in patients unable to tolerate AZA *(KDIGO GN 2012)*. MMF has been associated with a higher rate of relapse in a single study *(Arthritis Rheum 2004;51:278)*
- Rituximab 500 mg on d 0 and 14, mo 6, 12, and 18: more effective than AZA (AZA group had HR 6.61 for major relapse) (MAINRITSAN *NEJM 2014;371:1771*)
- Trimethoprim–Sulfamethoxazole (TMP-SMX) should be considered in addition to immunosuppression in patients with upper respiratory tract disease *(KDIGO GN 2012)*

Relapse
- Rate 30–50% by 5 yr. Higher with PR3 disease, respiratory involvement, and nasal carriage of S. aureus (in GPA) *(Ann IM 2005;8:1709; NEJM 1996;335:16; Arthritis Rheumatol 2016;68:690)*
- Reappearance or ↑ of ANCA correlates strongly with renal relapse. Persistently elevated titer is a/w relapse *(KI 2009;63:1079; JASN 2015;26:537; Arthritis Rheum 2004;51:269)*
- Persistent hematuria >6 mo (×3.99), but not proteinuria is a/w relapse *(CJASN 2018;13:251)*
- RTX appears more effective than CYC in recurrent disease *(NEJM 2013;369:417)*

Transplantation
- Wait until 1 yr after remission of extrarenal disease before transplant. Presence of circulating ANCA ab does not increase the risk of recurrence *(KDIGO GN 2012)*
- Risk of recurrence after transplant is estimated 10% and responds well to repetition of induction therapy *(KI 2007;71:1296)*
- Recurrence after transplant may be more likely in PR3 disease *(J Nephrol 2017;30:147)*
- Patient and graft survival 92% and 88% at 5 yr, and 68% and 67% at 10 yr, similar to other nondiabetic kidney diseases *(Curr Opin Rheum 2014;26:37)*

Prognosis
- Complete remission is attained in the majority (70–90%) of treated patients
- Untreated disease is associated with 80% mortality at 1 yr. Estimated 1- and 5-yr patient survival 84% and 76% *(AJKD 2003;41:776)*
- Presence of pulmonary hemorrhage is most important determinant of patient survival *(KDIGO GN 2012)*
- 20–25% patients will progress to ESRD *(NDT 2004;19:1964)*
- Single most important prognostic marker for long-term renal outcome is Cr *(NDT 2004;19:1964)*
- Biopsy predictors of poor prognosis include degree of glomerulosclerosis, interstitial fibrosis, and tubular atrophy *(KI 2002;62:1732)*

ANTI-GBM DISEASE

Definitions and Pathogenesis

- Characterized by ab against a glomerular basement membrane (GBM) antigen, often cross-reactive w/ alveolar basement membrane, causing RPGN +/− alveolar hemorrhage
- **Anti-GBM disease:** kidney involvement alone
- **Goodpasture syndrome:** kidney and lung involvement ("pulmonary-renal syndrome")
- **Goodpasture disease:** kidney and lung involvement + anti-GBM serology
- Principal antigen: $\alpha 3$ noncollagenous (NC1) region of type IV collagen
- Trigger for autoantibody production is unclear, but may involve a conformational change (eg, induced by airborne irritants such as cigarette smoke) that unmasks EA and EB epitopes (KI 2003;64:2108)
- Antibody binding linearly along GBM induces crescentic glomerulonephritis
- HLA-DRB1 alleles strongly associated with disease susceptibility (KI 1999;56:1638)

Epidemiology

- Incidence: 0.5–2 cases/million/yr, significantly lower than other RPGNs, eg, ANCA GN
- Two peaks of incidence: (1) young adult males; (2) elderly women
- A/w cigarette smoking, hydrocarbon, viral URI, alemtuzumab (NEJM 2008;359:768)

Clinical Manifestations

- **Kidney:** hematuria +/− proteinuria usually with rapidly progressive glomerulonephritis. Symptoms include tea-colored urine, and those related to kidney failure
- **Lung:** hemoptysis due to diffuse alveolar hemorrhage (DAH); Other symptoms include cough, shortness of breath, tachypnea
- Constitutional symptoms (eg, fevers, fatigue, nausea, weight loss) are largely absent
- Younger patients may present with more fulminant disease when compared to older adults
- Pulmonary involvement a/w pulmonary irritants, eg, cigarette smoke (Lancet 1983;8364:1390)

Diagnosis

- **Kidney biopsy:** crescentic GN w/ linear IgG (usually IgG1 and 3, rarely IgA, IgM) by IF
- **Bronchoscopy** (gold standard to identify DAH); **Chest CT:** ground glass opacities
- **Anti-GBM Ab:** diagnosis and for tracking disease activity. Reasonably sensitive (63–93%) and specific (92–97%) (Biochem Mol Med 1996;59:52). In a severely ill patient, the clinical manifestations plus (+) Anti-GBM ab may be enough to make the diagnosis.
- **ANCA ab:** in 15–50%, usu. MPO, more common in the elderly

Disease Variants

- **Dual (+) anti-GBM + ANCA disease:** 47% of anti-GBM disease, 6.1% of ANCA disease; similar prognosis and clinical features of anti-GBM disease, though may be a/w clinical features of vasculitis and higher chance of relapse and renal recovery (KI 2017;92:693)
- **Atypical anti-GBM disease:** rare; (−) serum anti-GBM antibody; usually milder, non-fulminant kidney disease; biopsy shows linear anti-GBM staining (may be a monoclonal Ig), without crescents. Thought to be caused by antibodies to an alternative GBM protein (ie, not α3 NC1 type IV collagen). Clinical course more indolent (KI 2016;89:897)

Treatment

- If kidney-limited, dialysis dependent on presentation and 100% cellular crescents or >50% globally sclerotic glomeruli, **chance of kidney recovery is exceedingly low** and IS may be deferred (Ann IM 2001;134:1033)
- **Cyclophosphamide:** 2–3 mg/kg/d PO ×3 mo, consider dose reduction in the elderly
- **Corticosteroids:** methylprednisolone pulse (0.5–1 g/d ×3) followed by oral prednisone 1 mg/kg/d (max 80 mg/d) tapered to 20 mg by 11–12 wk
- **Plasma exchange:** daily for 14 d or until anti-GBM ab undetectable
- **Alternative immunosuppressives:** insufficient data to recommend; case reports using azathioprine, mycophenolate, and rituximab
- **Maintenance therapy:** not required unless ANCA (+)

Prognosis

- **Outcomes** in patients who receive appropriate therapy (Ann IM 2001;134:1033): 5-yr kidney survival 94% if Cr <5.7 on presentation; 50% if Cr >5.7 but not on dialysis
- **Predictors of ESRD:** dialysis on presentation, % interstitial infiltrate, % normal glomeruli (CJASN 2018;13:63)

Transplantation

- Require (−) anti-GBM ab for 6 mo; Recurrence ~50% if anti-GBM ab (+) at time of txp
- Low recurrence (3–14%), lower rates in current era likely d/t better txp immuno-suppression (KI 2013;83:503; Clin Transplant 2009;23:132)
- Alport syndrome w/ large deletions in the COL4A5 gene: at risk of developing de novo anti-GBM disease after KT, since the wild-type COL4A5 in the allograft will be immu-nologically foreign. "Autoimmune conformeropathy" (NEJM 2010;363:343)

IMMUNOGLOBULIN A NEPHROPATHY

Epidemiology
- Immunoglobulin A nephropathy (IgAN) is the m/c glomerular disease (NDT 2011;26:414)
- Disease prevalence varies by ancestry: highest in Asians and northern Europeans, lowest in those with sub-Saharan African ancestry (PLoS Genet 2012;8:e1002765)
- In Whites, the disease is more common in men than in women

Pathogenesis
- **Primary IgAN:** immune complexes of **galactose-deficient IgA1** deposit in the mesangium (JCI 2009;119:1668)
  - Galactose-deficient IgA1 is a heritable trait (KI 2001;80:79)
  - GWAS have identified multiple susceptibility loci (Nat Genet 2014;46:1187)
  - Up to 5% of patients with IgAN have a relative with IgAN
- Subclinical IgA deposits common in healthy individuals in high-prevalence countries, eg, up to 16% in Japanese (KI 2003;63:2286)
- **Secondary IgAN** associated with liver ds, HIV, seronegative arthritis (esp ankylosing spondylitis), inflammatory bowel ds, and celiac ds (Sem Neph 2008;28:27)
  - Liver dysfunction ↓ clearance of circulating IgA, → deposits in mesangium
  - Other causal relationships in secondary disease largely uncertain

Clinical Manifestations
- Classically presents with hematuria (macro or micro), subnephrotic-range proteinuria and hypertension. Nephrotic syndrome is less common
- Complements (C3 and C4) usually within normal limits; rarely C3 may be low
- Recurrent gross hematuria, especially with URIs ("synpharyngitic") may be present
- AKI during episodes of gross hematuria usually due to pigment nephropathy and resolves once hematuria clears (3–5 d); if no resolution of AKI after 5 d, then consider kidney biopsy to evaluate for crescentic disease vs other cause

Kidney Biopsy
- The gold standard for diagnosis; reserved for those with hematuria and one of the following: (1) proteinuria >0.5–1 g/d; (2) ↓ GFR; and/or (3) new-onset HTN

Pathology
- The pathognomonic finding is mesangial deposits of IgA, most commonly polymeric IgA1
- Oxford Classification of IgAN developed to identify prognostically important, reproducible features across biopsies: used to generate "MEST-C" score

Oxford Classification of IgAN (NDT 2017;91:1014)		
Feature	Score	Clinical Implications
Mesangial hypercellularity	0 = <50% 1 = >50% gloms	M1 predicts worse outcomes (vs M0)
Endocapillary proliferation	0 = None 1 = Any	E1 independently a/w worse renal survival (vs E0) only in studies where patients did not receive IS E1 NOT predictive of outcomes in studies that included immunosuppressed patients E1 a/w improved outcome in those treated with corticosteroids
Segmental glomerulosclerosis	0 = None 1 = Any	S1 predictive of worse outcomes (vs S0) Podocytopathic features a/w ↑ proteinuria, faster ↓ GFR, but better survival with IS
Tubulo-Interstitial fibrosis	0 = <25% 1 = 25–50% 2 = >50%	Strongest independent predictor of adverse renal outcomes
Crescents, cellular/fibrocellular	0 = None 1 = at least 1 2 = ≥25% gloms	C1 predictive of worse outcomes if no IS C1 NOT predictive if IS used C2 predictive of worse outcomes regardless of IS

Disease Variants
- IgA-dominant infection-related GN: staph infection in elderly diabetics (JASN 2011;22:187)
- IgAN with minimal change disease: clinically similar to MCD, presents with nephrotic syndrome and usually steroid sensitive, likely reflects dual disease (CJASN 2014;29:1033)
- IgAN with ANCA vasculitis: ✓ MPO and PR3-ANCA in crescentic disease
- "Crescentic" IgAN variably defined: range from >10% to >50% crescents

Treatment (Recommendation Grade Based on KDIGO GN 2012 Guidelines)

- ACE-I or ARBs: for BP control (goal <130/80) and proteinuria reduction
- Corticosteroids (CS): for patients who do not achieve proteinuria of <1 g/d with first-line therapy over 3–6 mo and have eGFR >50 (2C)
- Cyclophosphamide (CYC): considered for patients with rapidly progressive renal failure, usually characterized by crescentic GN or nephrotic proteinuria (NDT 2003;18:1321)
- Large RCTs of CS w/ or w/o alkylating agents and antimetabolites have not shown consistent benefit

Key RCTs of Immunosuppression (IS) in IgAN			
Study	**Patients Characteristics**	**IS Protocol vs Placebo**	**Outcomes**
STOP IgAN (NEJM 2015; 373:2225)	• >750 mg/24 hr proteinuria despite ACEI or ARB, statin, BP <125/75 • NS and RPGN excluded • N = 162 randomized to IS vs placebo	Determined by GFR: • eGFR ≥60: prednisone QOD × 6 mo + methylpred 3 g IV at mo 1, 3, 5 • eGFR 30–60: PO CYC + pred ×3 mo then AZA/pred × 3 yr	• No difference in number experiencing 15 loss of eGFR • ↑ clinical remissions in IS group (UPCR <0.2 with stable GFR) • ↑ severe infections in IS group
TESTING (JAMA 2017;318:432)	• Proteinuria >1 g/d • eGFR 20–120 • N = 262 randomized to IS vs placebo	Methylprednisolone 0.6–0.8 mg/kg/d PO × 2 mo then tapered over 6–8 mo	• Study terminated early due to serious infections in CS group (8.1% including 2 fatal) • Fewer composite renal endpoints (5.9% vs 15.9%), slower rate of GFR decline and ↓ proteinuria in CS group (1.31 g/d vs 2.19 g/d)

- Fish Oils: inconsistent benefit. Studied doses range between 3.3 and 12 g/d. KDIGO 2012 suggests 3.3 g/d for those with proteinuria >1 g/d despite supportive care (2D)
- Tonsillectomy: a/w improved outcomes in observational studies (particularly from Japan); not superior to CS in randomized controlled trial (NDT 2014;29:1546)
- MMF: several negative trials despite one Chinese study suggesting benefit (KI 2010;77:543)
- RTX: in eGFR 30–90 did not improve eGFR and proteinuria (JASN 2017;28:1306)
- Supportive care: for AKI in IgAN with gross hematuria and kidney biopsy showing ATN and intratubular erythrocyte casts (2C)

Prognosis
- 35–40% reach ESRD by 30 yr from diagnosis
- Prognosis, from better to worse: episodic microscopic hematuria > episodic gross hematuria > persistent hematuria > hematuria + proteinuria less than 1 g/d at dx > hematuria + proteinuria greater than 1 g/d on treatment
- Most important prognostic indicators: time-averaged proteinuria, ↑ BP, and T-score
- Spontaneous remission may occur in patients with minor glomerular abnormalities. In a retrospective study of children with IgAN who did not receive IS, 60% achieved spontaneous remission (Pediat Nephrol 2013;28:71)

Transplantation
- Post-transplant recurrence of IgAN up to 30% of patients 10 yr post-transplant. Graft loss due to IgAN only 3–4%.
- Predictors of recurrence post-transplant include pre-transplant high levels of galactose-deficient IgA1, earlier age of disease onset, and crescents (Am J Nephrol 2017;45:99)
- Maintenance CS a/w ↓ recurrence in some, but not all series (AJT 2011;11:1645)
- For post-transplant recurrence, high-dose CS may be considered

IgA VASCULITIS (IgAV) (Arthritis Rheumatol 2017;69:1862)

- IgAV is preferred term of Henoch–Schönlein Purpura (HSP) and anaphylactoid purpura
- Small vessel vasculitis affecting skin (100%, palpable purpura), kidney (70%, hematuria, proteinuria, AKI), joints (61%), and GI tract (53%, bowel angina, bleeding, ischemia)

- Some IgAN progress to IgAV in 5 mo–14 yr (Pediatr Nephrol 2016;31:779)
- Adult IgAV: cause CKD, unlike self-limiting pediatric IgAV (Semin Arthritis Rheum 2002;32:149)
- Kidney biopsy: indistinguishable from IgAN; extracapillary hypercellularity (crescents) 41%; fibrinoid necrosis 32%
- Skin biopsy: leukocytoclastic vasculitis (LCV) with IgA deposition; 30% of all LCV (Mayo Clin Proc 2014;89:1515)
- Tx: CS;+ CYC w/o benefit (KI 2010;78:495); possible role in severe (crescent >50%) disease (NDT 2004;19:858); MMF may be used as CS sparing agent (Am J Nephrol 2012;36:271)

LUPUS NEPHRITIS

- Renal involvement: 50% of SLE; most important predictor of death (Rheumatology 2009;48:542)
- SLICC included LN as a standalone diagnostic criteria for SLE (Arthritis Rheum 2012;64:2677)

Pathogenesis
- Risk genes (J Autoimmun 2013;41:25) and environmental factors (eg, infections, hormones, UV light, drugs) → cell death → delay in dead cell clearance → activation of viral recognition receptors of the innate immune system, IFN-inducible genes and autoreactive B and T cells (Semin Immunopathol 2014;36:443)
- Nonspecific trapping of circulating immune complexes, in situ formation, or by interaction with negatively charged components of the glomerular capillary wall → formation and deposition of immune complexes → the binding and activation of complement → the ensuing inflammatory cascade
- TMA w/ or w/o APL ab can coexist and worsens prognosis
- Lupus podocytopathies a/w heavy proteinuria but no active inflammatory lesions
- Interstitial or vascular renal disease

Clinical Manifestations
- Variable: asymptomatic hematuria, proteinuria, NS, RPGN

Workup
- ↑ ESR, ↑ CRP, ↑ anti-dsDNA Ab, ↓ C3, C4, CH50; APLA
- Lab do not always correlate w/ LN class; Bx is frequently necessary
- Bx if: ↑ Cr w/o alternative explanation, proteinuria >1 g/d, proteinuria >0.5 g/d with active urine sediment (dysmorphic RBCs or cellular casts) (Arthritis Care Res 2012;64:797)

Pathology
- **IF:** IgG dominant full, house pattern (glomerular stain IgA, IgM, C3, and C1q codominance).
- **EM:** endothelial tubuloreticular inclusion (TRI), subendothelial and subepithelial deposits; extraglomerular immune-type deposits within TBM, the interstitium, and blood vessels

Lupus Nephritis Classification (ISN/RPS KI 2004;65:521; JASN 2004;15:241)
- I (**minimal mesangial LN**): nl LM, w/ mesangial immune deposition on IF and/or EM
- II (**mesangial proliferative LN**): mesangial hypercellularity w/ immune deposition
- III (**focal LN**): inflammatory injury affecting <50% of the glomeruli by LM w/ crescents, fibrinoid necrosis, and/or subendothelial immune deposition
  - Classes III and IV are subclassified as **A** with active lesions of proliferation and necrosis, **C** with chronic lesions of sclerosis and fibrosis, or **A/C** with a combination of these lesions
- IV (**diffuse LN**): inflammatory injury affecting >50% of the glomeruli, again classified as A, C, or A/C. This class is further divided into segmental (**S**) or global (**G**) depending on the extent of injury to the individual glomerular tuft, greater than 50% in the latter category
- V (**lupus membranous nephritis**): glomerular capillary thickening on LM w/ subepithelial immune deposition on EM/IF
- VI (**advanced sclerosing LN**): ≥90% global glomerulosclerosis w/o residual activity
- Upcoming proposed changes to ISN/RPS (KI 2018;93:789)
  Elimination of IV-S and IV-G subdivisions
  Replacing the A/C subclasses w/ a modified NIH lupus activity/chronicity scoring

Modified NIH Lupus Activity and Chronicity Scoring System (KI 2018;93:789)		
Activity Index (0–24)	Endocapillary hypercellularity	(0–3)
	Neutrophils/karyorrhexis	(0–3)
	Fibrinoid necrosis	(0–3) ×2
	Hyaline deposits: wire loop lesions and/or hyaline thrombi	(0–3)
	Cellular/fibrocellular crescents	(0–3) ×2
	Interstitial Inflammation	(0–3)
Chronicity Index (0–12)	Glomerulosclerosis	(0–3)
	Fibrous crescents	(0–3)
	Tubular atrophy	(0–3)
	Interstitial fibrosis	(0–3)

General Treatment

- RAAS inhibition for all proteinuria >0.5 g/g cr
- Hydroxychloroquine (HCQ) for all LN: ↓ renal disease and severity (Medicine 2016;95:e2891) Max 6–6.5 mg/kg IBW (lipophobic); s/e: retinopathy (✓ophthalmologic exam q12m)
- Crescents, interstitial and vascular lesions: a/w renal progression, mortality (Lupus 2016;25:1532)
- Classes III and IV: consider activity and chronicity index for IS decision
- Class VI: prepare for RRT

Treatment of Classes III and IV

- Contraception in active classes III and IV LN

Induction Treatment of Classes III and IV LN	
Corticosteroid (CS)	Give CS plus any of below regimen unless otherwise specified IV methylprednisolone 250–1,000 mg/d × 3 d → prednisone 1 mg/kg qd with taper >70% remain on CS 10 yr after (Ann Rheum Dis 2010;69:61)
NIH CYC	0.5–1 g/m² BSA qm × 6, q3m × 4, q6m × 2 (NEJM 1986;314:614)
Low-dose IV CYC	500 mg q2w × 6 w/ AZA maintenance ≈ NIH dose (ELNT Arthritis Rheum 2002;46:2121). Remain same after 10 yr (Ann Rheum Dis 2010;69:61) Works on African American (ACCESS Arthritis Rheum 2014;66:3096)
PO CYC	2.5 mg/kg/d ≈ MMF (NEJM 2000;343:1156)
MMF	MMF w/ target 3 g/d × 6 m ≈ NIH CYC (ALMS JASN 2009;20:1103)
AZA	≈ CYC > CS only (NEJM 1984;311:1528); Option for pregnancy
Multitarget	CS + Tac + MMF superior to CS + NIH CYC at 24 wk in class V+ (III or IV) (Ann IM 2015;162:18)
Rituximab 2 g: 1 g ×2, 2 wk apart	2 g, ×2 cycles addition to MMF and CS not superior (LUNAR Arthritis Rheum 2012;64:1215) Induces remission in refractory cases (NDT 2013;28:106) 2 g + MMF w/o PO CS achieved CR in 52%, PR in 34% (RITUXILUP Ann Rheum Dis 2013;72:1280)

- If CYC doesn't induce remission, MMF and vice versa (ACR Arthritis Care Res 2012;64:797)
- Once remission has been achieved, maintenance treatment should be continued

Maintenance Treatment of Classes III and IV LN	
CS	Prednisone ≤10 mg/d with one of below
MMF	2 g/d superior to AZA (ALMS NEJM 2011;365:1886)
AZA	2 mg/kg/d
CYC	↑ Death, Cr doubling and s/e (NEJM 2004;350:971); not recommended

- Relapse: treat with induction agent

Treatment of Class V

- If class III or IV is accompanied, treat as in class III or IV
- IS if proteinuria >3–3.5 g/d despite RAASi: CS + MMF or CYC or CNI or AZA

Treatment of Class V	
CS	CS monotheraphy is not recommended (*JASN 2009;20:901*)
MMF	≈ NIH CYC in efficacy and side effect profiles (*KI 2010;77:152*)
CYC	Low-dose CYC is preferred
CNI	Remission 83% vs NIH CYC 60%, relapse is common. Proteinuria >5 g/d a/w no remission (*JASN 2009;20:901*).
Rituximab	2 g w/o PO CS induced CR in 38% PR in 24% by 12 mo (*Ann Rheum Dis 2013;72:1280*)

OTHER FORMS OF GLOMERULAR LESION IN SLE

Renal-limited Lupus-Like Nephritis (*NDT 2012;27:2337*)
- Renal biopsy with lupus nephritis features w/o systemic SLE
- Some patients may develop SLE later; needs monitoring
- Tx: corresponding LN classification

Necrotizing and Crescentic LN with ANCA (*CJASN 2008;3:682*)
- Necrosis and crescents exceeding the degree of endocapillary proliferation & subendo deposits
- ✓ ANCA ELISA; Tx: d/c hydralazine if taking; CYC

Lupus Podocytopathy (*CJASN 2016;11:547*)
- SLE + MCD or FSGS, mesangial proliferation w/o endocapillary proliferation, necrosis, and/or crescents. Extensive foot process effacement w/o GCW deposits on EM.
- Tx: 94% responded to CS w/i 4–8 wk. Frequent relapse (56%) (*CJASN 2016;11:585*)

Collapsing Glomerulopathy in SLE (*CJASN 2012;7:914*)
- CG and SLE (positive serologies +/- lupus sx at time of Bx)
- Common in female (79%) and African descent (89%)
- Genetics: strongly a/w APOL1 risk allele in AA with SLE (*JASN 2013;24:722*)
- Clinical: massive proteinuria with rapid progression of renal dysfunction
- Pathology: global or segmental collapse of glomerular capillary tuft, with wrinkling and retraction of the capillary walls, overlaid by epithelial cell proliferation in Bowman space (*KI 1996;50:1734*)
- Tx: variable in series, irrespective of concomitant LN on histology: CS, MMF, IVIG, and AZA
- Prognosis: poor, 7/13 went onto ESRD within 2 yr time

INFECTION-RELATED GLOMERULONEPHRITIS

POSTINFECTIOUS GLOMERULONEPHRITIS (PIGN)

Background
- **Post-streptococcal GN (PSGN),** the prototype of PIGN is increasingly uncommon in the developed world
- PSGN is more common in children; highest incidence between 4–15 yr old
- PIGN formally implies *antecedent* infection and latent period of d–wk after infection has cleared (10–14 d for PSGN). Particularly for adults with non-strep infections, GN often occurs *during* ongoing infection: thus the preferred term is Infection-related GN (IRGN).
- m/c organisms: *Streptococcus* (pharyngeal/skin infections), *Staphylococcus* (skin infections), and rare gram-negative organisms (*Pseudomonas, Escherichia, Yersinia, Pseudomonas*)

Pathogenesis
- Nephritogenic antigens produced by pathogens stimulate an initial immune response. Two streptococcal antigens have been implicated in the development of PSGN, the streptococcal pyrogenic exotoxin B (SPE B) and the plasmin receptor, a glyceraldehyde phosphate dehydrogenase (GAPDH/NAPlr) (*KI 2005;68:1120*)
- Immune complexes formed in circulation or in situ induce local activation of alternative complement and coagulation pathways and recruitment of neutrophils to glomeruli

Pathology
- **LM:** diffuse endocapillary proliferative GN w/ intracapillary neutrophils ("exudative")
- **IF:** coarse, granular GBM and mesangial staining of C3 alone or Ig with C3 dominance ("starry sky appearance")
- **EM:** large, scattered subepithelial electron dense deposits ("humps")

Clinical Manifestations and Workup
- Acute GN including RPGN (with HTN), edema (80–90%), dark urine/hematuria
- In PSGN, typically occurs 10–14 d following infection (pharyngitis, cellulitis, pneumonia)

- ↑ Cr, ↓ CH50, C3 (90%), C4 (rare), ↑ ASO (in PSGN), red cell casts, proteinuria (usually subnephrotic)

Treatment and Prognosis

- Supportive care of AKI, HTN, and edema
- Elimination of any ongoing active infection. Patients with PSGN should be treated with antibiotics to prevent carrier status, though limited evidence that this affects the course of PSGN. Antibiotics are indicated for *prevention* of PSGN when used to treat streptococcal infections in children.
- Antibiotics should be used prophylactically for close household contacts of PSGN patients and in epidemics of streptococcal infections (*JASN* 2008;10:1855)
- No clear role for immunosuppression, though there are reports of success with corticosteroids or cyclophosphamide in individual cases of severe/progressive disease
- In children, complete renal recovery is likely within 2–3 wk. Persistence of low C3 should raise concern for C3 glomerulopathy. In adults, prognosis is guarded.

STAPHYLOCOCCAL ASSOCIATED GN/IgA DOMINANT IRGN

Background and Pathogenesis

- Risk factors: >50 y/o, diabetes, malignancy, IVDU, and alcoholism (*JASN* 2011;22:187)
- Common site: skin, respiratory, heart, deep tissue/bone, urinary tract (*Am J Nephrol* 2015;41:98)
- Causative organisms: MRSA >> MSSA >> *S. epidermidis/S. haemolyticus* >> Enterobacter species, Escherichia species
- Typically during active infection (often chronic) w/o latency period (*AKJD* 2015;65:826)
- Proposed mechanism: bacterial toxin (eg, *S. aureus* enterotoxin) acts as super-antigen, bind to MHC molecules → T cell activation, cytokine release (*Nephron Clin Pract* 2011;119:c18)

Pathology

- **LM:** proliferative GN with endocapillary and mesangial proliferation +/– crescents
- **IF:** mesangial C3 dominant or codominant staining with IgA +/– IgG
- **EM:** subepithelial "hump"-like electron dense deposits

Clinical Manifestations

- Renal: AKI, acute GN with elevated Cr, hematuria (including macroscopic), subnephrotic proteinuria and HTN; up to 1/3 have nephrotic syndrome
- Extrarenal: purpuric rash, signs of active infection

Workup

- ↑ Cr, hematuria, subnephrotic proteinuria
- ✓ C3, C4 (hypocomplementemia less common than with PIGN), ANCA (a/w crescentic GN)
- Evaluate for active infection (blood cx, urine cx, sputum cx)

Treatment and Prognosis

- Treatment of underlying infection and supportive care of AKI, HTN, edema
- Retrospective studies suggest no benefit from immunosuppression (*CJASN* 2006;1:1179)
- Guarded prognosis; many patients have persistent renal dysfunction and up to 33% of elderly patients remain dialysis dependent
- Risk factors for progression to ESRD and death: age and diabetic nephropathy (*JASN* 2011;22:187; *Medicine* 2008;87:21; *Am J Nephrol* 2015;41:98)

INFECTIOUS ENDOCARDITIS (IE)-RELATED GN (*KI* 2015;87:1241)

Background and Pathogenesis

- ♂:♀ 3.5:1, mean age at biopsy 48
- Associated comorbidities: valve disease, IVDU, HCV, HIV, DM
- Affected valves: tricuspid > mitral > aortic > pulmonic
- Staphylococcus > Streptococcus > Bartonella, Coxiella, Cardiobacterium, Gemella
- Up to 18–24% of IE pts have ANCA (+) (*Arthritis Rheum* 2014;66:1672; *Medicine* 2016;95:e2564)
- Mechanisms: (1) circulating and in situ IC formation; (2) bacterial toxin activation of alternative complement pathway; (3) bacterial toxin activation of ANCA leading to activation of alternative complement pathway via activation of C5a (*KI* 2015;87:1241; 2014;86:905; 2013;83:792)

Pathology

- **LM:** necrotizing/crescentic > endocapillary proliferative > mesangial proliferative GN
- **IF:** C3 dominant (or isolated) staining, may have (+) IgG, IgM, IgA staining
- **EM:** subendothelial and mesangial EDD

Clinical Manifestations

- Renal: most common is AKI, may also see hematuria and signs of RPGN
- Extrarenal: septic pulmonary infarcts (in tricuspid endocarditis), splinter hemorrhages, fevers, weight loss, murmur, Osler nodes, Janeway lesions, Roth spots

Workup
- ↑ Cr, hematuria, proteinuria, ↓ C3 ± C4 (nl in 44%), may have (+) ANCA/ANA
- Check blood cultures and echocardiogram for evidence of endocarditis

Treatment and Prognosis
- Treatment of underlying infection and supportive care of AKI
- Immunosuppression: ANCA (+) and/or persistent GN despite antibiotics *(CID 1999;28:1057; Case Rep Nephrol Urol 2012;2:25; Indian J Nephrol 2013;23:368; Clin Nephrol Case Stud 2017;5:32)*
- Risk of ESRD correlates with elevated serum Cr at diagnosis

---

SHUNT NEPHRITIS

Background and Pathogenesis
- Complication of chronically infected ventriculoatrial (VA) or ventriculojugular (VV) shunts for hydrocephalus. Rarely seen in ventriculoperitoneal (VP) shunts
- Organisms: S. epidermidis/P. acnes >> S. aureus >> Pseudomonas, Serratia species
- IC formation to circulating bacteria/biofilm activating complement pathway *(NDT 1997;12:1143)*

Pathology
- **LM:** MPGN or mesangioproliferative GN, may have ATN and red cell casts
- **IF:** mesangial IgM, C1q, C3 deposition in 2/3 of cases *(Case Rep Nephrol 2017;2017:1867349)*
- **EM:** subendothelial EDD

Clinical Manifestations
- Renal: elevated Cr, hematuria, red cell casts, proteinuria, HTN, edema; may be subacute
- Weight loss, fever, arthralgia, hepatosplenomegaly, rash, sx of ↑ intracranial pressure

Workup
- ↑ Cr, hematuria, proteinuria, hypocomplementemia, elevated ESR and CRP, anemia
- May have (+) ANCA/Cryo/RF *(NDT 1997;12:1143)*
- Infection identification may be delayed d/t to poor growth of S. epidermidis and P. acne

Treatment and Prognosis
- Treat infection; removal of infected hardware is frequently necessary *(NDT 1997;12:1143)*
- Early dx, shunt removal a/w better prognosis *(NDT 1997;12:1143; Case Rep Nephrol 2017;2017:1867349)*

IMMUNE COMPLEX–MEDIATED MPGN

Background
- Accounts for 7–10% of renal biopsies of GN in developed countries
- Among the leading causes of ESRD from primary glomerulopathies *(NEJM 2012;366:119)*
- Commonly presents in childhood and young adulthood
- 2° causes of immune complex (IC) MPGN include chronic infection (esp HCV), hematologic disease (eg, CLL, MGRS), and autoimmune disease. True idiopathic is rare

Pathogenesis
- Ag-Ab ICs form in glomeruli, either after forming in the circulation or forming in situ following glomerular antigen trapping. ICs trigger an inflammatory response and activate complement, leading to disruption of the GBM and endocapillary proliferation.

Pathology
- **LM:** endocapillary and mesangial proliferation, leading to lobular appearance. Duplication of basement membrane over deposits leads to "tram track" appearance of capillary walls.
- **IF:** granular deposition of Ig and complement in GBM, often mesangium. Chronic TMA can mimic MPGN but will have no Ig staining. C3G will have almost exclusively C3 staining.
- **EM:** GBM thickening and separation by electron dense immune complex deposits

Clinical Manifestations
- Acute or chronic GN: hypertension, edema, microscopic hematuria, subnephrotic proteinuria with CKD. Severe cases present as nephrotic syndrome.

Workup
- **Lab:** elevated Cr, hematuria, subnephrotic proteinuria, low complement levels C3 or C4
- Seek out secondary causes:
  - *Chronic infection:* HCV, HBV, HIV, endocarditis, shunt infection, visceral abscess, mycoplasma, parasitic infections
  - *Autoimmune disease:* Sjögren's, SLE, RA, MCTD
  - *Hematologic disease:* lymphoproliferative disorders, monoclonal gammopathy, plasma cell dyscrasia (especially if MPGN with masked deposits present) *(KI 2015;88:867)*

Treatment

- BP control and **RAAS blockade** as tolerated for all affected patients
- 2° MPGN: treat underlying causes
- Idiopathic MPGN: immunosuppression if substantial proteinuria (eg, >1 g/d) or falling GFR
- Extended courses of **corticosteroids** have been used in pediatric patients; has not been replicated in adults (*Ped Nephrol* 1992;6:123; 1995;9:268)
- **RTX** (*Clin Nephrol* 2012;77:290; *NDT* 2004;19:3160; 2007;22:1351; *Clin Nephrol* 2010;73:354)
- Rapidly progressive course: **cyclophosphamide + corticosteroids** (KDIGO GN 2012)

Prognosis

- Progressive renal disease with renal survival <50% at 10 yr from dx. Risk factors for progression: GFR, proteinuria, HTN, age, severity of IF/TA, crescents (*KI* 2006;69:504; *NDT* 2002;17:1603)
- High rate of recurrence after transplant (19–48%), confounded by studies grouping different categories of MPGN (*Transplantation* 1997;63:1628; *CJASN* 2010;5:2363; *KI* 2010;77:712)

C3 GLOMERULOPATHY (C3G)

Background

- Glomerulonephritis associated with dysregulation of alternative complement pathway
- Defined on the basis of immunofluorescence: dominant C3 staining

Categorization of GN With Dominant C3 Staining (*KI* 2013;84:1079)

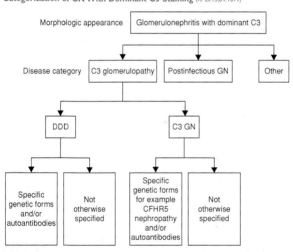

- C3G may present as a nonresolving postinfectious GN. (PIGN may show C3 deposits beyond the acute stage; C3G should be suspected in such cases when clinical resolution is incomplete.) Infection (including with streptococcus) may precipitate C3G.

Pathogenesis

- Hyperactivity of the alternative complement pathway (normally constitutively active at a low level) through hereditary or acquired defects (see table)
- C3G is commonly associated with a circulating autoantibody called C3 nephritic factor which binds to and stabilizes activated C3. Other abnormalities of complement activation may occur including genetic mutations of complement regulatory proteins and other autoantibodies (see table)
- Disease presentation and/or flares may be triggered by acute infection

Mechanisms of Complement Pathway Disruption in C3G	
Abnormality	**Description**
Genetic mutations or risk variants	Implicated genes of the complement pathway include *CFH, CFI, CFB, CFHR5, C3,* and *MCP/CD46*
	Mutations of *CFHR5* cause highly penetrant familial Cypriot nephropathy (NDT 2013;28:282)
	Risk variants found in <20% of cases of C3G (KI 2013;84:1079)
C3 Nephritic factors	Auto-Ab stabilizing C3bBb, alternative pathway C3 convertase (~50% of cases, DDD > C3GN)
C4 Nephritic factors	Auto-Ab stabilizing C4b2a, classical pathway C3 convertase
C5 Nephritic factors	Auto-Ab stabilizing C5 convertase
Factor H auto-Ab	Prevent CFH from downregulating activity of C3 convertase
Factor B auto-Ab	Stabilizes C3 convertase; prevents intrinsic and FH-mediated decay
Monoclonal gammopathies	Likely act via auto-Ab activity; eg, one case documented a monoclonal λ light chain dimer acting as a "miniautoantibody" to FH (J Immunol 1999;163:4590)

Pathology
- **LM:** proliferative GN (MPGN endocapillary, mesangioproliferative, or diffuse proliferative)
- **IF:** C3 dominance and minimal or absent Ig (KI 2014;85:450)
- **EM:** presence (DDD) or absence (C3GN) of intramembranous highly EDD

Clinical Manifestations
- May range from nephrotic syndrome (hypoalbuminemia, proteinuria >3.5 g/d, edema) to chronic or acute GN (HTN, AKI, hematuria, proteinuria <3.5 g/d) or even crescentic GN
- Synpharyngitic hematuria (as seen with PIGN) may be seen reflecting increased activity of the complement system during infectious episodes
- May present as a nonresolving postinfectious GN
- Retinal drusen (yellow granules on optic disc containing complement), partial lipodystrophy

Complement Cascade Schematic

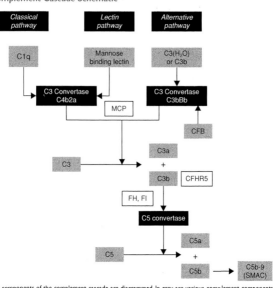

Key components of the complement cascade are diagrammed. In grey are various complement components, in black are convertases that split C3 or C5 into their activated forms, and in white are regulatory molecules.

Workup

- **Labs:** low C3 (40% of cases), normal C4, hematuria, proteinuria, +/- elevated creatinine
- ✓ **Complement pathway abnormalities:** C3Nef, Factor H ab, Factor B level, Factor I level, soluble membrane attack complex (SMAC) level
- ✓ **Monoclonal gammopathy screen:** SPEP/IFE, serum free light chains
- Consider **genetic mutation analysis:** does not currently change treatment but may affect prognosis and risk stratification for post-transplant recurrence

Treatment

- **Immunosuppression** controversial: combination of steroids and MMF may favor clinical remission (KI 2015;88:1153; CJASN 2018;13:406)
- **Eculizumab** (anti-C5 mAb preventing its cleavage): may be effective especially in aggressive forms with elevated SMAC levels (CJASN 2012;7:748) or crescents (AJKD 2018;72:84)
- **Plasma (FFP) therapy** useful in case reports, eg, FH deficiency (KI 2006;70:42)

Prognosis

- >50% progress to ESRD within first two decades of diagnosis (Nat Rev Nephrol 2012;8: 634)
- **Risk factors for progression:** baseline eGFR and degree of interstitial fibrosis/tubular atrophy on biopsy (KI 2012;82:454; KI 2018;93;977)
- **Post-transplant:** 2/3 recur, and 1/2 have allograft failure (JASN 2014;25:1110). Another cohort showed higher recurrence (10/12 in C3GN, 6/7 in DDD) and allograft failure (3/12 in C3GN, 6/7 in DDD) (AJKD 2019;PMID 30413277)

CRYOGLOBULINEMIA

Background/Pathogenesis

- **Cryoglobulins:** Igs that precipitate at <37°C and redissolve upon rewarming
- **Cryoglobulinemia:** the presence of circulating cryoglobulins in serum
- **Mixed cryoglobulinemia (MC):** cryoglobulin with ≥2 Ig clones
- Pathogenesis of MC: antigen (eg, HCV) stimulation → B cell clonal expansion → non-neoplastic B cell lymphoproliferative process → Ab against Fc portion of IgG (RF activity) → IC formation in vessel walls activate complement → leukocytoclastic vasculitis
- **Cryoglobulinemic vasculitis** (10–15% of MC): predominantly involves the small vessels, affecting the skin, joints, peripheral nerves, and the kidneys (Am J Med 2015;128:950)

Classification and Features of Cryoglobulinemia			
Types	**Components**	**Clinical Features**	**Associated Diseases**
Type I (simple)	Monoclonal Ig, most often IgM > IgG or IgA	Hyperviscosity, acrocyanosis, Raynaud's, gangrene, arthralgias rarely	Waldenström macroglobulinemia Multiple myeloma B-cell lymphoma, MGUS
Type II (mixed)	Monoclonal IgMκ w/ RF activity against IgG	Weakness (>80%) Purpura (>75%) Arthralgias (60–90%) Neuropathy (20–80%) Nephritis (20–50%) Cutaneous ulcers (10–20%) Sicca (5–50%) "Meltzer triad"	**Infection** • HCV, HBV, HIV • IE, Lyme • Rickettsia, syphillis **Autoimmunity** • Sjögren's syndrome • SLE, RA **Lymphoproliferative dz** Idiopathic ("essential")
Type III (mixed)	Polyclonal IgM against IgG		
Types II–III (mixed)	Both monoclonal and oligo- or polyclonal IgM against IgG		

Renal Manifestations

- AKI/RPGN, subnephrotic or nephrotic proteinuria w/ microscopic hematuria, NS, HTN
- Renal injury is the most morbid manifestation of cryo vasculitis, typically manifested as immune complex MPGN. However, only a minority of cryo patents with MC show renal manifestations at presentation w/ at least half developing them over followup.

Extrarenal Manifestations

- Meltzer triad: purpura, arthralgia (MCPs, PIPs, ankles and feet), and weakness in 25–80%
- Skin: purpura, ulcers, Raynaud's and acrocyanosis, livedo (exacerbated by cold exposure)
- Neuromusc: myalgias, peripheral neuropathy with paresthesia, mononeuritis multiplex
- Pulmonary: rare; include dyspnea, cough, pleuris, rarely diffuse alveolar hemorrhage
- A smoldering lymphoproliferative process can evolve into NHL (World J Hepatol 2016;8:107)

Diagnosis

- Serum cryoglobulins: measurable cryocrit or protein concentration
- **Cryocrit:** volume percentage of packed cryoglobulins in blood after centrifugation at 4°C; Quantity of cryocrit can correlate with disease severity
- Draw in prewarmed syringe, transported and centrifuged at 37–40°C, serum then stored at 4°C for up to 7 d as cryoglobulins precipitate out (hr to d)
- False (–): common because of technical collection; repeat assays required if high suspicion
- False (+): polyclonal cryoglobulins can be transient during infections
- Immunofixation employed to identify type of cryoprecipitate
- MC: ↑ RF and cryoglobulins, and ↓↓ C4, more variably ↓ C3 and ↓ CH50
- Kidney biopsy: typically MPGN +/– microthrombi (cryoglobulins appear as "pseudo-thrombi"). EM: subendothelial deposits w/ fingerprint pattern substructure

Treatment

- MC a/w HCV: DAA (Hepatology 2016;63:408; Gastroenterology 2017;153:408). Can recur despite HCV eradication d/t ongoing ab production by B-cells (AJKD 2017;70:301)
- Type 1 or 2 a/w lymphoproliferative disorder: treat it based on the type
- IS: for organ-threatening MC to ↓ inflammation and cryoglobulin production
  - CS: acute anti-inflammatory benefit. Relapses are common upon withdrawal.
  - Rituximab: sustained response. Can be used before or after failure of HCV treatment (always screen for HBV coinfection first) (Arthritis Rheum 2012;64:843); Cyclophosphamide
- Plasmapheresis: for severe vasculitis, RPGN, or hyperviscosity (J Clin Apher 2016;31:149)

Prognosis

- Prognosis depends on associated underlying disease and degree of organ involvement
- Renal involvement carries particularly elevated morbidity
- Overall survival 80% at 10 yr; renal failure 11% over 5 yr (AJKD 2007;49:69)
- MC: 10-yr survival rate <60% (Clin Exp Rheumatol 2008;26:S105)

AMYLOIDOSIS

Background

- Amyloid: extracellular deposition of insoluble fibrils resulting from abnormal folding of proteins; >25 precursor proteins of amyloid found
- Overall incidence: 1.3–4% of renal biopsies (Am J Surg Pathol 2009;33:1198)

Clinical Manifestations of Amyloidosis: Depending on Involved Organ	
Kidney	Proteinuria (NS common), CKD, NDI, type 4 RTA
Heart	Nonischemic HF (nl or low LVEF, restrictive or dilated CMP, Afib)
Nerves	Peripheral neuropathy, carpal tunnel, orthostatic hypotension
Coagulation	Easy bruisability, Raccoon eyes, Factor X def
GI	Malabsorption, ulcer, macroglossia
Joint	Arthralgia

Diagnosis

- Biopsy fat pad or involved organ; kidney, liver, and heart are commonly involved
- Congo red stain under polarized light: apple-green birefringence
- LM in kidney biopsy: diffuse glomerular deposition of amorphous hyaline material
- EM: randomly arranged fibrils, measuring 8–12 nm diameter
- Amyloid typing: IF staining of monoclonal light chains (AL) and amyloid A (AA) is diagnostic. M protein in serum/urine is not (NEJM 2002;346:1786). Mass spectrometry: gold standard (KI 2012;82:226)

Renal Amyloidosis (CJASN 2013;8:1515)			
Type	Frequency	Cr > 2	NS
AL, AH, AHL	85.9%	26%	68%
AA	7.0%	63%	54%
ALECT2	2.7%	77%	17%
AFib	1.3%	67%	17%
AApoAI, AApoAII, or AApoAIV	0.6%	–	–

- Other rarer forms are derived from following precursors: apolipoprotein CII (AApoCII) (JASN 2017;28:439), lysozyme (ALys) (JASN 2017;28:431), gelsolin (Agel) (KI 2017;91:964)

AL Amyloidosis

- Precursor: monoclonal κ (20%) or λ (80%) LC produced by a monoclonal plasma cell clone in the BM. Rarely heavy (AH) and heavy and LC (AHL)
- Only about 10% of patients have concomitant multiple myeloma at presentation
- **Localized** form: 12%. Produced by a local, self-limited plasma cell clone, w/ (−) SIFE/UIFE. m/c sites: GU tract, larynx, skin, and upper respiratory tract. Tx is local excision, RT. No systemic progression but recur locally, esp in the GU tract *(Mayo Clin Proc 2017;92:908)*
- **Systemic** form: affects the heart, kidney, liver, and nerves (autonomic/peripheral)
- Manifestations: NS, fatigue, weight loss, bleeding tendency, orthostasis, CHF symptoms

Renal Stage and Prognosis of Renal AL Amyloidosis *(Blood 2014;124:2325)*		
Stage	Definition	Dialysis Dependence 3 yr after dx
I	Proteinuria ≤5 g/24 hr and eGFR ≥50	0%
II	Proteinuria >5 g/24 hr or eGFR <50	7%
III	Proteinuria >5 g/24 hr and eGFR <50	60%

Treatment

- Auto-HSCT eligible (low risk) pts: auto-HSCT w/ high-dose melphalan *(Annals IM 2004;140:85)* or standard dose melphalan plus dexamethasone *(NEJM 2007;357:1083)*
  - Criteria: physiologic age <70, troponin T <0.06 ng/mL, NT-proBNP <5,000 ng/L, CrCl >30, NYHA functional class 1 or 2, ≤2 organs involved, not oxygen dependent
- Auto-HSCT ineligible (intermediate or high risk) pts: combination chemotherapy, eg, melphalan + dexamethasone or CyBorD (CYC, bortezomib, dexamethasone). CyBorD achieved renal response in 25% *(Blood 2015;126:612)*.
- Daratumumab: human mAb against CD38 on plasma cells, if refractory *(Blood 2017;130:900)*

Prognosis of AL Amyloidosis by Treatment Response *(Blood 2014;124:2325)*		
Criteria	Definition	ESRD Risk
Renal Progression	↓ eGFR ≥25%	HR 4.56
Renal Response	↓ Proteinuria ≥30% or <0.5 g/24 hr w/o renal progression	HR 0.15
Hematologic Very Good Partial Response (VGPR)	Difference between involved and uninvolved fLC (dfLC) <4 mg/dL w/ baseline dfLC ≥5 mg/dL	HR 0.47
Hematologic Complete Response (CR)	(−) SIFE, UIFE, nl FLC ratio	

- Goal is to achieve renal response, VGPR, or CR

Transplantation

- 15/19 survived after median f/u 41.4 mo *(NDT 2011;26:2032)*
- Median graft survival 5.8 yr; Pt survival was 8.9 yr if CR (- SIFE, UIFE, nl FLC ratio) or PR (dFLC <50% of pretx) vs 5.2 yr in NR (dFLC >50% of pretx) *(AJT 2013;13:433)*

AA Amyloidosis

- Precursor: serum amyloid apolipoprotein A (SAA) produced by the liver, vascular endothelial cells, monocytes, macrophages. It is induced by pro-inflammatory cytokines including IL-1, IL-6, and TNF-α *(Mod Rheum 2014;24:405)*
- Reactive amyloidosis to:
  Chronic **inflammation**: RA, juvenile idiopathic arthritis, spondyloarthropathies, IBD, FMF, hidradenitis suppurativa, IgG4-related disease *(NEJM 2017;376:599)*
  Chronic **infection**: bronchiectasis, IV drug abuse, infected pressure sores, osteomyelitis
  Neoplasm: RCC, lymphoma
- Organs involved: kidneys, GI tract (including liver), heart, autonomic nerves
- Tx: treat underlying disease
- Tocilizumab: humanized anti-IL6 receptor Ab, inhibits SAA production. Approved for RA. ↓ Amyloid load by SAP scintigraphy, ↓ SAA, proteinuria *(Clin Exp Rheum 2015;33:S46)* In FMF AA amyloid, ↓ proteinuria, ESR, CRP *(Orphanet J Rare Dis 2017;12:105)*
- Canakinumab: humanized anti-IL1 mAb ↓ proteinuria in children *(Pediatric Nephrol 2016;31:633)*
- Txp: median graft survival 10.3 yr; recurrence 19.5% *(AJT 2013;13:433)*

ALECT2 AMYLOIDOSIS (KI 2014;86:370; 2014;86:378)

- Precursor: leukocyte chemotactic factor 2, a cytokine produced by the liver
- Etiology of the hepatic upregulation of this protein's production is unclear
- Strong ethnic associations: Mexican Hispanics, Punjabis, Arabs, Israelis, Native Americans
- Organs involved: kidney, liver, heart (rare); DM, HTN common
- CKD, proteinuria (33% nephrotic range), ESRD (39%) over f/u of 22 mo
- Concurrent renal disease on bx: DN (21%), MN (5%)
- Monoclonal protein in 9.6%: monoclonal protein + amyloid ≠ AL amyloid
- Tx: no specific treatment; Txp: recurrence 1/5 w/o graft demise

AFib AMYLOIDOSIS (CJASN 2013;8:1515; JASN 2009;20:444)

- Precursor: fibrinogen α chain, synthesized by the liver
- AD mutations with variable penetrance. Family history absent in 46%
- Poor prognosis: presenting creatinine 4.1. 62% reached ESRD in 4 yr.
- Txp: 7/12 graft failure in 5.8 yr including 3 recurrence. Combination liver–kidney txp appears to be more effective (QJM 2000;93:269)

ATTR AMYLOIDOSIS

- Precursor: transthyretin, transport tetramer protein that carries T4 and retinol-binding protein; 90% produced by the liver
- Accounted for 1.4% of renal amyloid cases submitted to Nephrocor (KI 2014;86:378)
- The most common form of hereditary amyloidosis
- Mutant forms (>100 known) destabilize the native TTR quaternary structure, leading to misfolding/aggregation of the protein, resulting in amyloidosis
- WT (nonmutant) form: affects the heart in elderly men. Endemic in Portugal and Sweden
- Organ involvement: nervous system, heart, kidney, and GI tract
- Manifestation: neuropathy 3–5 yr later → microalbuminuria 2–3 yr later → overt nephropathy 2–3 yr later → ESRD about 10 yr after neuropathy (CJASN 2012;7:1337)
- Tx: liver or liver/kidney txp; tafamidis, a TTR stabilizer, offers possible improvement cardiovascular outcome (NEJM 2018;379:1007)

Aβ2M AMYLOIDOSIS

- Precursor: β2 microglobulin, LC of the MHC class 1 molecule, excreted by the kidneys
- Clinically affects the osteoarticular structures, ie, scapulohumeral periarthritis and carpal tunnel syndrome (Semin Dial 2017;30:193). Occurs in long-term dialysis patients.
- Cleared by high flux HD membranes along with convection (J Lab Clin Med 1991;118:153)
- Also helpful: use biocompatible HD membranes and ultra-pure dialysate to minimize pro-inflammatory state (JASN 2004;13:972)
- Treatment time is important: slow intercompartmental mass transfer limits β2 microglobulin removal (KI 2006;69:1431)
- Higher prevalence with longer dialysis vintage
- Overall decline in disease prevalence in Europe (KI 1997;52:1077) and Asia (NDT 2016;31:595)
- Tx: renal transplantation is the best prevention and treatment

NONAMYLOID DEPOSITION DISEASES

Fibrillary GN and Immunotactoid GN (KI 2003;63:1450; CJASN 2011;6:775; NDT 2012;27:4137)		
	Fibrillary GN (FGN)	**Immunotactoid GN (ITGN)**
Prevalence	<1% of native bx	0.06% of native bx
Manifestation	HTN, proteinuria (NS –50% in FGN, –69% in ITGN), hematuria, CKD	
MG, low C'	15–17%, 2%	63–66%, 46%
Associated conditions	Cancer, MM Autoimmune: Crohn's, Graves, SLE, ITP, PBC, Sjögren's, ankylosing spondylitis, scleroderma Infection: HCV (AJN 2017;45:248), TB, osteomyelitis	Lymphoproliferative disease (esp CLL) HIV +/– hep C (Clin Nephrol 2011;75:80)
LM	Diffuse proliferative, membranous, Mesangio/membranoproliferative, diffuse sclerosing, crescentic (rare)	Membranoproliferative, diffuse proliferative, and membranous pattern injury
IF	IgG (esp IgG1 and 4), κ and λ light chains (mostly polyclonal) and complement	Deposits contain IgG or IgM, monoclonal κ or λ and complement
EM	Randomly arranged fibrillary deposits; **16–24 nm** in diameter in the mesangium and capillary walls	Microtubules; **30–50 nm** in diameter in parallel arrangement, in the subepi- and subendothelial space Cryo deposits can be indistinguishable from ITGN
ESRD	44–45%	17%
Transplantation	5/14 recurred, 2/5 became ESRD again (CJASN 2011;6:775) 1/13 recurred (AJN 2015;42:177) w/ MG: 5/7 recurred, 3 re-txp, 1 recurred again, 2 died w/ hematologic malignancy w/o MG: 0/5 recurred (KI 2009;75:420)	Recurrence 25% (AJN 2015;42:177) – 50% (Am J Med 1990;89:91)

DnaJ Heat Shock Protein Family B Member 9 (DNAJB9) in FGN
- A heat shock protein; detected by immunohistochemistry (KI rep 2018;3:56) and mass spectrometry (JASN 2018;29:51) in glomeruli with high sensitivity/specificity
- May be used for diagnosis, particularly if EM is not available

Treatment of FGN: Treat Underlying Disorder
- Various IS agents have been tried with suboptimal response
- In group w/ mean Cr of 3.1, IS (CS, CYC, CsA) was not a/w outcome (KI 2003;63:1450)
- In group w/ mean Cr of 2.1, IS use resulted in PR in 10%, persistent renal dysfunction in 38%, ESRD in 52% (CJASN 2011;6:775)
- 6 (5 RTX, 1 CYC)/13 had ↓ proteinuria by >50% w/ stable GFR (AJKD 2013;62:679)
- RTX use was a/w nonprogression in 4/12; nonprogress had lower Cr (NDT 2014;29:1925)
- In crescentic FGN treated w/ CS, CYC, 6/8 went on to ESRD (Indian J Nephrol 2017;27:157)

Treatment of ITGN: Treat Underlying Disorder
- 7/14 (Cr 1.5) had B cell disorder. Chemo+/–HSCT led to NS remission in 5 (KI 2002;62:1764)
- A PR of the hematologic disease led to complete renal remission (Ann Hematol 2007;86,927)
- 7/12 w/o MG were treated w/ CS+/– CYC. 3 achieved PR (NDT 2012;27:4137)

Rare Nonamyloid Deposition Diseases		
Disease	**Pathology**	**Clinical Manifestations**
Fibronectin GP	Mes, subendo fibronectin deposition	AD, proteinuria, HTN, ESRD Can recur (Clin Transplant 2012;26:58)
Collagenofibrotic GP	Mes, subendo type III collagen deposition	AR, proteinuria, ESRD
Nail–patella	Type III collagen deposition in lamina densa	AD, proteinuria, <5% ESRD nail and patella abnormality
Lipoprotein GP	Lipoprotein thrombi w/i glomerular capillary lumina	Proteinuria, ↑ VLDL, LDL, apo E

HEREDITARY GLOMERULAR DISEASES

Background

- Mutations of genes encoding proteins involved in glomerular filtration barrier can directly cause glomerular diseases
- Genetic systemic disease (eg, sickle cell disease, genetic aHUS) may indirectly cause glomerular injury
- Monogenic causes identified in 30% of steroid-resistant NS in <25 y/o (JASN 2015;26:1279)
- Relatively common genetic causes in 19–25 y/o: INF2, TRPC6, NPHS2 (JASN 2015;26:1279)
- Clinical manifestations: proteinuria ± steroid-resistant NS ± hematuria ± CKD
- Pathology of congenital NS in children: FSGS (56%), MCD (21%), mesangioproliferative GN (12%), diffuse mesangial sclerosis (3%) (CJASN 2015;10:592)
- Immunosuppression is generally ineffective in genetic podocytopathy-mediated glomerular disease (JASN 2015;26:230)

FABRY DISEASE

Pathogenesis

- Deficiency of the enzyme α-galactosidase A (α-GalA), encoded by GLA on Xq22
- Accumulation of globotriaosylceramide (Gb3) within lysosomes in a wide variety of cells

Renal Manifestations

- Proteinuria: nephrotic range uncommon; a/w renal progression (CJASN 2010;5:2220)
- pRTA/Fanconi; polyuria and concentrating defect in distal nephron involvement
- ESRD in 14% of ♂, 2% of ♀ at 38 y/o; a/w cardiac event and stroke (NDT 2010;25:769)
- Multiple renal sinus cysts
- Renal variant: later onset, renal limited w/o other organ manifestation (KI 2003;64:801)
- Heterozygous female: asymptomatic carrier ~ all manifestations including renal manifestations; eGFR <60 (19%), proteinuria >1 g/day (22%) (Mol Genet Metab 2008;93:112)

Extrarenal Manifestations

- Cardiovascular: m/c cause of death; premature CAD, LVH, arrhythmia, mimic hypertrophic cardiomyopathy
- Angiokeratomas: tiny painless papules, esp bathing suit area, telangiectasia
- Hypo- or anhidrosis, heat intolerance, acroparesthesia in hands and feet
- Cornea verticillata (vortex keratopathy)
- TIA, stroke, neuropathic pain

Diagnosis

- ✓ Leukocyte α-GalA activity in ♂: <3% diagnostic, 3–35% requires GLA mutation analysis;
  - Not recommended for ♀; low to normal regardless of disease manifestation
- GLA mutation analysis: diagnostic if known mutation
- Tissue diagnosis: if genetic test nondiagnostic

Kidney Biopsy

- **LM:** vacuolization of podocytes, DT cells > PT cells, endothelial cells; glomerulosclerosis
- **EM:** Zebra or myeloid body: osmiophilic inclusions in lamellated membrane structures (enlarged secondary lysosomes)
- Other causes of Zebra body: silicosis, amiodarone (KI 2008;74:1354), gentamicin (PT cells), chloroquine, hydroxychloroquine (AJKD 2006;48:844)

Enzyme Replacement

- Recombinant α-GalA: agalsidase β (Fabrazyme®) 1 mg/kg or agalsidase α (Replagal®, available in Europe) 0.2 mg/kg IV q2wk
- Indicated for all males and symptomatic females even with ESRD
- ↓ Gb3 deposition in most cell types including podocytes (JASN 2013;24:137; CJASN 2017;12:1470)
- Maximal impact if eGFR >55 (Ann IM 2007;146:77); ↓ severe clinical events (J Med Genet 2016;53:495)
- s/e: neutralizing antidrug antibodies development; may need dose adjustment and immunosuppression (JASN 2018;29:2265)

Other Treatments

- RAASi to treat HTN and proteinuria
- Migalastat: pharmacologic chaperone, ↑ trafficking of α-GalA to lysosomes → ↑ α-GalA activity; ↓ kidney and plasma Gb3; improved LV mass index (NEJM 2016;375:545)

Transplantation

- 5-yr graft survival similar, ↑ death (×2.15) *(Transplantation 2009;87:280)*
- Recurrent deposit is common *(JASN 2002;13:S134)*

COL4A-ASSOCIATED NEPHROPATHY

Background

- Hereditary diseases caused by mutation of COL4A genes encoding type IV collagen
- COL4A-associated nephropathy includes benign familial hematuria, thin basement membrane nephropathy, Alport syndrome, COL4A associated FSGS *(KI 2014;86:1253)*
- 62% of patients with COL4A mutations were clinically not diagnosed with Alport syndrome or thin basement membrane nephropathy *(NEJM 2019;380:142)*

Genetics

- Type IV collagen: component of basement membrane (BM) in glomerulus, tubules, and skin
- 6 genes are located at chromosome 13 (COL4A1 & 2), 2 (3 & 4), and X (5 & 6)
- COL4A5 (classic XL) mutation in male or heterozygous female >> COL4A3, COL4A4 (heterozygous AD or homozygous AR)

Expression Collagen IV		
Location	Normal	XL Alport
Immature GBM, BC, TBM	$\alpha 1\alpha 1\alpha 2 + \alpha 1\alpha 1\alpha 2$	$\alpha 1\alpha 1\alpha 2 + \alpha 1\alpha 1\alpha 2$
Mature GBM, dTBM	$\alpha 3\alpha 4\alpha 5 + \alpha 3\alpha 4\alpha 5$	$\alpha 1\alpha 1\alpha 2 + \alpha 1\alpha 1\alpha 2$
BC, dTBM, skin BM	$\alpha 1\alpha 1\alpha 2 + \alpha 5\alpha 5\alpha 6$	$\alpha 1\alpha 1\alpha 2 + \alpha 1\alpha 1\alpha 2$

BC, Bowman Capsule; GBM, Glomerular BM; TBM, Tubular BM; dTBM, distal TBM

- Large deletions and nonsense mutations: progress to ESRD faster (90% at age 30), more frequent hearing loss and eye abnormalities
- Missense mutations: variable course (50% reach ESRD at age 30)
- De novo mutations: ~15%
- Mutation of Laminin β2, component of GBM modify Alport phenotypes *(JASN 2018;29:949)*

Clinical Manifestations

- Hematuria, proteinuria; ESRD before 40 y/o: 90% in male; 12% in female *(JASN 2003;14:2603)*. Age of ESRD a/w type of mutation in male *(JASN 2010;21:876)*
- Risk factors of renal progression in X-linked female: gross hematuria, proteinuria
- Bilateral **anterior lenticonus** is pathognomonic; dot-and-fleck retinopathy; spherophakia, corneal erosion
- High-frequency sensorineural hearing loss

Skin and Kidney Biopsy

- Skin epidermal basement membrane α5 stain:
  (−) In male XL disease; segmental (−) in female is c/w COL4A5 mutation
  (+) In COL4A3, COL4A4 mutation
- **LM:** normal or FSGS; interstitial foam cells (nonspecific, present in other proteinuria)
- **IF:** of collagen: mosaic, skipped α5 in female
- **EM:** GBM thinning (early); thickening, lamination/basket weaving (late), electrolucent zone
- Can have normal GBM appearance in early stage *(Hum Pathol 2018;81:229)*

Treatment

- RAASi: ↓ progression, ESRD *(Pediatr Nephrol 2017;32:131)*. Start early *(KI 2012;81:494)*

Transplantation

- No recurrence. LRKT is possible *(NDT 2009;24:1626)*
- De novo anti-GBM antibody against α5 or α3 detected in 5–10% *(CJASN 2017;12:1162)*
  - Associated with crescentic GN and subsequent graft failure
  - Commercially available anti-GBM α3 NC1 region Ab does not always detect this Ab
  - Retransplantation: high risk for graft loss *(KI 2004;65:675)*

Thin Basement Membrane Nephropathy (Benign Familial Hematuria)

- Mutations of COL4A3 and 4; benign side of the spectrum of Alport *(KI 2014;86:1081)*
- None or minimal proteinuria unless concurrent FSGS
- Rare ear/eye involvement
- Biopsy: diffusely thin GBM 150–225 nM; indistinguishable from early Alport
- Tx: RAASi especially for proteinuria

ANTIPHOSPHOLIPID SYNDROME (APS)

- Antiphospholipid syndrome (APS): an autoimmune disease resulting from the presence of antiphospholipid antibody (APLA) which exert a pathogenic role resulting in arterial and/or venous thrombosis +/– pregnancy morbidity (Nat Rev Rheumatol 2011;7:330)
- Causes of transient APLA: infection, medications (hydralazine, amoxicillin, minocycline, and propranolol) (Curr Rheumatol Rep 2012;14:71; Lupus 2017;28592198)
- a/w autoimmune disease, SLE: APLA is found in about 1/3 of SLE and is an independent risk factor of premature death and progressive renal disease (AJKD 2004;43:28)
- APLA present in 9% of pregnancy losses, 14% of strokes, 11% of MI, and 10% of DVT (Arthritis Care Res 2013;65:1869)
- The common final pathway is that of endothelial injury, exposing phospholipid binding protein, attachment of APLA and the initiation of an inflammatory cascade that activates complement (Blood 2016;127:365), leading to vascular thrombosis and organ dysfunction
- APLA chronically upregulates mTOR in vascular smooth muscle leading to proliferation and obliterative vasculopathy (NEJM 2014;371:303)

Clinical Manifestation and Diagnosis

Diagnostic Criteria of APS: ≥1 Clinical + ≥1 Laboratory (J Thromb Haemost 2006;4:295)	
Clinical Criteria	
Vascular thrombosis	≥1 arterial, venous, or small vessel thrombosis (imaging or histopathology)
Pregnancy morbidity	≥1 unexplained fetal death (at or beyond 10th wk of gestation) ≥1 premature birth (before 34 wk) due to eclampsia, severe preeclampsia, or placental insufficiency ≥3 consecutive miscarriages (before 10th wk of gestation)
Laboratory Criteria: ≥2 tests, 12 wk apart	
Lupus anticoagulant	Positivity
Anticardiolipin Ab	IgG and/or IgM >40 U or >99th percentile
Anti-β2 GP-1 Ab	IgG and/or IgM in medium or high titer (ie, >99th percentile)

- Renal manifestation: depending on the vessel caliber that is affected
  - **Large** renal artery/vein thrombosis/infarction: sudden flank pain, hematuria, and AKI
  - **Small** vessel thrombi in the interstitium: subacute AKI/ CKD with mild proteinuria
  - **Glomerulus:** proteinuria, active sediment +/– renal dysfunction (Clin Nephrol 2005;63:471)
- Biopsy: acutely, TMA, and in chronic stages obliterative arteriopathy, fibrosis and FSGS
- Other lab: thrombocytopenia, AIHA, hypocomplementemia (Case Rep Med 2017;2017:5797041)
- 10-yr survival probability was 90.7%. The top causes of death: severe thrombosis, infection, and catastrophic APS (Ann Rheum Dis 2015;74:1011)

Treatment

- Anticoagulation; heparin/warfarin to maintain INR 2–3 (NEJM 2003;349:1133)
- Rivaroxaban (factor Xa inhibitor) if intolerant of warfarin (Lancet Haematol 2016;3:e426)
- In SLE w/ APS, hydroxychloroquine ↓ secondary thrombosis (Arthritis Rheum 2010;62:863)

Transplantation

- Anticoagulation during the perioperative period in renal txp to ↓ the risk of post-txp thrombosis and graft failure (Transplantation 2000;69:1348)
- mTOR inhibitor: ↓ recurrence of APS-associated vascular lesion (NEJM 2014;371:303)

CATASTROPHIC ANTIPHOSPHOLIPID SYNDROME (CAPS)

Diagnostic Criteria of CAPS: Definite if all 4 (Lupus 2003;12:530)	
1. ≥3 organs, systems, and/or tissue involvement: clinical assessment +/– imaging. Renal involvement: a 50% cr rise, HTN >180/100 and/or proteinuria >500 mg/d.	
2. Development of manifestations simultaneously or in <1 wk	
3. Histopathologic confirmation of small vessel occlusion in ≥1 organ or tissue	
4. APLA (+) ×2 ≥6 wk apart	
Probable	2 organ involvement + 2 + 3 + 4 1 + 2 + 3 + absence of lab confirmation death to the early death 1 + 2 + 4 1 + 3 + 4 + 3rd event in >1 wk, <1 mo, despite anticoagulation

- Widespread thrombosis and multiorgan failure, very high mortality. In a cohort of 1,000 APS patients followed for a decade, 9 developed CAPS and 5 died. *(Ann Rheum Dis 2015;74:1011)*
- Tx: anticoagulation, corticosteroids, plasma exchange +/– IVIG *(Lupus 2014;23:1283)*
- For resistant cases, consider the addition of rituximab *(Autoimmune Rev 2013;12:1085; Eur J Rheumatol 2017;4:145)* or eculizumab *(Arthritis Rheum 2012;64:2719; Case Rep Hematol 2014;704371)*

HUS AND TTP

HEMOLYTIC UREMIC SYNDROME (HUS)

Background
Pathogenesis: Shiga Toxin
- Caused by shiga toxin producing bacteria: enterohemorrhagic *E. coli* 0157:H7 (m/c), many more Shiga toxin-producing *E. coli* (STEC) and *Shigella dysenteriae* serotype 1
- Complicates 6–9% of STEC cases
- Food source: beef (cattle GI tract), spinach, lettuce, sprouts, fruit, raw milk *(CID 2010;51:1411)*, cookie dough *(CID 2012;54:511)*, flour *(NEJM 2017;377:2036)*
- Shiga toxin is absorbed by the gut epithelium → The toxin binding to the glycoprotein receptor globotriaosylceramide (Gb3), expressed in the kidney and brain → the toxin entrance into the tissues → inflammation, lysis, and destruction
- Gb3 is also expressed in platelets, causing activation/aggregation (microthrombi) and thrombocytopenia *(Appl Microbiol Biotechnol 2016;100:1597)*
- Upregulated complement activity *(CJASN 2009;12:1920)* → ↑ membrane attack complex (MAC) → endothelial injury and microthrombi formation *(Blood 2015;125:3253)*

Clinical Manifestation and Workup
- Mainly children w/ abd pain, N/V, diarrhea that precedes HUS by 5–10 d *(NEJM 1995;333:364)*
- End organ involvement: kidney and CNS
- Labs: anemia, schistocytes and helmet cells on peripheral smear, ↑ indirect bilirubin, ↓ haptoglobin, ↑ LDH, thrombocytopenia, renal dysfunction
- Stool culture (selective media required for 0157:H7 and non 0157 serotypes), ELISA/PCR of stool for shiga toxin, also serology against the most frequent STEC serotypes
- Kidney Bx: TMA; cannot distinguish from other causes; not required for Dx
- Prognosis: in pediatric cases w/ 43% of non-0157 serotype, temporary HD needed in 61%, CNS effects (seizures) seen in 25% and mortality rate of about 4% *(JID 2002;186:493)*

Treatment
- Supportive Treatment: IVF, pRBC if severely anemic or symptomatic, transfuse platelets if clinically significant bleeding occurs, BP control (CCB) if HTN, dialysis as needed
- Antibiotics (ciprofloxacin, TMP/SMX) have the potential to ↑ production of shiga toxin. Although azithromycin and meropenem ↓ toxin production *(NEJM 2000;342:1930)*
- Plasma exchange (PLEX): no benefit
- Eculizumab: a mAb against C5 that ↓ production of MAC; In STEC related HUS w/ severe renal (requiring dialysis) and neurologic impairment, early use may improve neurological outcome *(NEJM 2011;364:2561; Medicine 2015;94:e1000)*

THROMBOTIC THROMBOCYTOPENIC PURPURA (TTP)

Pathogenesis: ADAMTS13 Deficiency
- Functional ↓ ADAMTS13 (A Disintegrin And Metalloprotease with a Thrombospondin type 1 motif, member 13) activity. This enzyme cleaves large vWF multimers on the endothelial surface. Accumulation of these structures cause TMA.
- Hereditary disease (<5%): genetic mutation of the ADAMTS13 gene
- Acquired disease (most): Auto-Ab against ADAMTS13

Clinical Manifestation and Workup
- Rare, 3/1 million adults/yr *(Pediatr Blood Canc 2013;60:1676)*
- Diagnosis: ↓ ADAMTS13 activity (<5%), (+) inhibitor before any plasma transfusion
- Only 5% have all components of the pentad: MAHA, thrombocytopenia <20K, renal impairment, CNS involvement and fever *(Blood 2010;116:4060)*
- **Rare** severe renal injury: 4% AKI requiring dialysis, 6% CKD, no ESRD *(Blood Adv 2017;1:590)*
- Kidney Bx: TMA; cannot distinguish from other TMA; not required for Dx
- Untreated, a progressive course of neurologic and cardiac deterioration → death

Treatment

- PLEX: immediately; daily until plt >150K and hemolysis markers normalize; removal of a potential inhibitor and replacing ADAMTS13 from the donor plasma
- Plasma infusion: in case of delay in plasma exchange
- Concomitant CS (IV/PO) (NEJM 1991;325:398)
- Add Rituximab (RTX), if severe disease or no improvement after a few days of PLEX and CS or in relapsing disease (Blood 2015;125,1526); ofatumumab (NEJM 2018;378:92)
- Cyclophosphamide: for disease refractory to PLEX, CS, and RTX (Int J Hematol 2004;80:94)
- Bortezomib: for refractory disease to all of the above (NEJM 2013;368:90)
- Caplacizumab, humanized variable domain of Ig against vWF: faster platelet recovery, ↓ TTP related death, recurrence, and thromboembolic event (NEJM 2019;380:335)

COMPLEMENT-MEDIATED HUS

- Atypical HUS (aHUS): HUS not mediated by Shiga toxin; aka diarrhea (−) HUS
- >50% of aHUS are complement-mediated HUS (KI 2017;91:539)
- Other forms of aHUS include coagulation-mediated TMA, eg, DGKE mutations

Pathogenesis

- The complement system is part of our innate immunity that defends us against infection and maintains internal inflammatory homeostasis. The 3 arms to the system (classic, alternative, lectin) are each tightly controlled by regulatory proteins.
- In complement-mediated HUS, there is disturbance of this balance in the **alternative pathway**, → pathologic overactivation and ultimately tissue destruction and injury

Types

- Hereditary: gene mutation of the regulatory complement factor(s); complement factor H (CFH, m/c), complement factors I, B, C3, thrombomodulin (THBD), and CD46 (MCP). Often require another "hit," eg, infection, pregnancy (CJASN 2007;2:591).
- Acquired: Abs to CFH (<10% of aHUS), CFB. Many pts have concurrent mutation(s).

Epidemiology and Clinical Manifestations

- Incidence: 7/million in children (BJH 2010;148:37). Can occur sporadically w/o FHx.
- Age of onset: variable from <1 to >20 y/o. ~60% were adult onset. Adults progressed to ESRD (46%), death (6.7%) w/i the 1st year of disease, regardless of the type of complement dysregulation (CJASN 2013;8:554).
- Ischemic injury to organs: renal (m/c), gangrene of fingers and toes, heart, lung, GI, death (Nat Rev Nephrol 2014;10:174)

Workup

- Labs: TMA (MAHA, thrombocytopenia). Complement mutation and Ab in select labs; nl complement levels do not exclude complement-mediated HUS
- Diagnosis of exclusion: r/o STEC, TTP (normal ADAMTS13), other causes of TMA
- Kidney Bx: TMA. Cannot distinguish from other causes
  - **LM:** mesangiolysis, GCW duplication, vascular onion skinning, ± fibrin thrombi
  - **IF:** fibrin staining thrombi; no immunoglobulin (Ig) and C3 staining
  - **EM:** endothelial cell swelling, subendothelial electron lucent space

Eculizumab

- Anti-C5 monoclonal Ab. FDA approved. Efficacious in 80% of pts that were either PLEX dependent or refractory; genetic testing not performed (NEJM 2013;368:2169)
- C5 blockade with eculizumab can predispose to encapsulated bacterial infection. Pts should be given meningococcal (both quadrivalent ×2 and serogroup B), pneumococcal (PCV13 and PPSV23), and Haemophilus influenzae type b vaccine. Penicillin VK 500 mg bid or erythromycin until 2–4 wk after last meningococcal vaccine
- Optimal duration therapy is unclear. Attempts to d/c the drug can lead to relapse.
- d/c can be considered in seroconversion of CFH Ab (KDIGO KI 2017;93:519)
- When stopped after 18 mo therapy, 31% (72% of CFH, 50% of MCP, none of no variant) relapsed during 22 mo f/u. Restart w/i 2 day of drug was therapeutic (CJASN 2017;12:50)

Other Treatments

- Immunosuppression if Ab (+): cyclophosphamide (AJKD 2010;55:923; KDIGO KI 2017;93:519)
- Plasma exchange (PLEX): use if eculizumab not available. About half respond (completely/ partially). Pts w/ CD46 mutation do not benefit from PEx whether 90% of episodes resolve whether they received plasmatherapy or not (CJASN 2010;5:1844). Pts w/ ab to CFH do better with the addition of immunosuppression (CS w/ cyclophosphamide or RTX) (AJKD 2010;55:923; NDT Plus 2009;2:458).

Transplantation

- Before eculizumab use, recurrence was ~80%, esp w/ CFH mutation (*Blood* 2006;108:1267)
- Eculizumab +/− PLEX: prevention and tx of recurrence in allograft. Treatment may have to be lifelong (*CJASN* 2011;6:1488; *AJT* 2012;12:3337).
- Combined liver–kidney Txp (rarely done): liver produces modulating proteins. Perioperatively, there is an intense upregulation of the complement system, often leading to allograft demise with widespread microvascular thrombi in the liver sinusoids and kidney graft (*AJT* 2005;5:1146). Perioperative PEx +/− eculizumab may circumvent this problem (*Pediatr Nephrol* 2014;29:477).

GENERAL HYPERTENSION

- About 103 million US adults have HTN (ACC/AHA JACC 2018;71:e127)
- 45.6% prevalence of HTN among US adults >18 yr; pharmacologic treatment is recommended for 36.2% of US adults; 53.4% of Pts receiving treatment for HTN have BP above goal (Circulation 2018;137:109)
- As of 2010, 80.7% are aware of the diagnosis of HTN (JAMA 2010;303:2043)
- Prevalence increases with age: >two-thirds of US adults >60 yr of age have HTN
- HTN is prevalent in 80–85% of pts with CKD; prevalence of HTN ↑ inversely with GFR
- Risk of CVD doubles for every 20/10 rise in BP above 115/75 (Lancet 2002;360:1903)
- Risk factors for primary HTN: age, obesity, family history, black race, excessive dietary sodium intake, heavy alcohol intake, physical inactivity, reduced nephron mass
- HTN in black pts is more common, develops earlier in life, is more severe, and is associated with greater risk of CV complications in comparison with whites
- Complications: LVH, HF w/ reduced EF, HF w/ preserved EF, ischemic heart disease, ischemic stroke, intracerebral hemorrhage, CKD, ESRD

2017 ACC/AHA Definitions of Hypertension (JACC 2018;71:e127)	
Normal BP	SBP <120 and DBP <80
Elevated BP	SBP 120–129 and DBP <80
Stage 1 HTN	SBP 130–139 or DBP 80–89
Stage 2 HTN	SBP ≥140 or DBP ≥90
Isolated systolic HTN	SBP ≥130 and DBP <80
Isolated diastolic HTN	SBP <130 and DBP ≥80

Pathogenesis
- Hundreds of genetic risk variants have been identified; number of risk alleles correlates with likelihood of developing primary → HTN; effect on BP is modulated by environmental factors
- High sodium intake leads to ↑ intravascular fluid volume, cardiac output, peripheral vascular resistance, and BP; elevation in BP leads to ↑ renal perfusion pressure and ↑ excretion of excess sodium and fluid ("pressure natriuresis"). If sodium excretion is impaired (aging, obesity, kidney disease) → HTN
- Other factors: reduced compliance of large conduit arteries, impaired endothelium-mediated vasodilation (↑ PVR), ↑ activation of local renin–angiotensin systems (heart, kidney, adrenals, vasculature), ↑ activity of sympathetic nervous system

Evaluation
- Ensure proper measurement technique: patient sitting with back supported for >5 min and arm supported at level of heart; length of BP cuff bladder >80% and width >40% of circumference of upper arm; take average of ≥2 readings (additional if readings vary by >5); measure BP in both arms; assess for postural hypotension
- Exam: optic fundi, thyroid, heart, lung, kidneys, peripheral pulses, neurologic system
- Testing: electrolytes, Cr, glc, Hb, lipid profile, U/A, UACR, ECG, echocardiogram
- Evaluate for causes of secondary hypertension

BP Measurement		
Strategy	Comments	Criteria
Ambulatory blood pressure monitoring (ABPM)	Device takes BP measurements at regular intervals over 12- or 24-hr period (15–30 min during daytime and 30–60 min during sleep) Predicts CV outcomes independently of office BP; stronger predictor of all-cause and CV mortality than office BP (NEJM 2018;378:1509) Reference standard for confirming diagnosis of HTN (Ann IM 2015;163:778)	Daytime average ≥130/80 OR night-time average ≥110/65 OR 24-hr average ≥125/≥75
Home BP monitoring (HBPM)	May predict CV outcomes as well as ABPM Multiple morning and evening measurements should be taken over a period ≥1 wk Alternative method of confirmation if ABPM not available	Repeated readings ≥130/80

Office-based BP measurements (OBPM)	Can be done routinely (manual or semi-automated) or via automated oscillometric BP (AOBP) device (takes multiple consecutive readings while pt is sitting and resting alone, better approximates daytime ABPM)	See above; based upon average of ≥2 readings at ≥2 office visits

Secondary Causes of HTN *(Circulation 2008;117:e510)*	
Lifestyle factors	Obesity, excessive dietary sodium intake, heavy alcohol intake
Medications	NSAIDs, sympathomimetic agents (decongestants, cocaine), amphetamine-like stimulants, oral contraceptives, glucocorticoids, herbals (ephedra), licorice (↓ metabolism of cortisol), CNIs, ESAs, VEGF ligand inhibitors, antiangiogenic TKIs
Renal disease	CKD, acute GN, vasculitis, HUS
Renovascular dz	Renal artery stenosis
Endocrine disorders	Primary hyperaldosteronism, pheochromocytoma, Cushing syndrome, hyperparathyroidism, renin-secreting tumors
Monogenic HTN syndromes	Glucocorticoid-remediable aldosteronism (GRA), Liddle's, pseudohypoaldosteronism type 2 (Gordon's), syndrome of apparent MC excess (AME), congenital adrenal hyperplasia (CAH)
Other	OSA (discussed below), aortic coarctation, intracranial tumors

Evaluation of HTN in CKD	
Masked HTN	Elevated ambulatory but normal clinic BP ("isolated ambulatory HTN") a/w ↑ long-term risk of sustained HTN and higher risk of all-cause (HR 2.83 vs 1.80) and CV (HR 2.85 vs 1.94) mortality than in Pts w/ sustained HTN in large registry-based study *(NEJM 2018;378:1509)* Occurs in 15–30% of US adults with normal office BP More common among pts w/ CKD; 70% of pts w/ controlled clinic BP in the AASK Cohort had masked HTN; masked HTN was a/w LVH and proteinuria and lower eGFR *(Hypertension 2008;53:20)*
Nondipping	Absence of the normal (10–20%) nocturnal decline in BP; may be related to impaired ability to excrete sodium during daytime Up to 80% of pts with CKD are nondippers Risk factor for LVH, HF, proteinuria, CKD progression Independent predictor of CV events and CV and all-cause mortality in Pts w/ resistant HTN Chronotherapy can restore normal dipping (discussed below)

HYPERTENSION 8-2

Treatment

- Lifestyle Δs: wt loss (maintain BMI 18.5–24.9 kg/m²), dietary sodium restriction (<2.4 g/d or 104 mmol/d Na⁺ or 6 g/d NaCl), DASH diet (rich in fruits, vegetables, and low-fat dairy products), ↑ physical activity (≥30 min/d, 5 d/wk), moderation of alcohol intake
- DASH diet + dietary sodium restriction: high sodium (3.5 g or 150 mmol/d) → low sodium (1.2 g or 50 mmol/d) DASH diet a/w ↓ 7 in SBP; high sodium control → low sodium DASH diet a/w ↓15 in SBP *(NEJM 2010;362:2102)*
- Pharmacologic therapy: in ~2/3 of HTN, ≥2 drugs are required to achieve target BP

Treatment and Followup *(JACC 2018;71:e127)*	
Normal BP	Encourage healthy lifestyle Δs to maintain normal BP, reassess in 1 yr
Elevated BP	Recommend healthy lifestyle Δs, reassess in 3–6 mo
Stage 1 HTN	If 10-yr ASCVD risk <10%: healthy lifestyle Δs, reassess in 3–6 mo If clinical ASCVD or DM or CKD or 10-yr CVD risk >10%: start 1 BP-lowering medication, monthly followup until goal achieved
Stage 2 HTN	Recommend healthy lifestyle Δs and 2 BP-lowering medications of different classes, monthly followup until goal achieved

Background
- 2nd m/c cause of ESRD; usually a/w long-standing HTN ("HTN-attributed nephropathy")
- In black pts, there is a high incidence of renal disease progression despite intensive antihypertensive therapy (3-fold ↑ risk in incidence of ESRD among African Americans with HTN-attributed nephropathy c/w European Americans)

Pathogenesis
- Apolipoprotein L1 (APOL1) risk variants are significantly associated with kidney disease (FSGS and HTN-attributed nephropathy) in black Pts, OR 2.57 (KI 2013;83:114)
- Chronic HTN → medial thickening and intimal thickening → luminal narrowing of large and small arteries and glomerular arterioles; ischemic injury → global glomerulosclerosis → nephron loss; compensatory glomerular hypertrophy and hyperfiltration → rise in intracapillary pressure → FSGS; ischemic injury → severe interstitial nephritis

	BP Targets and Choice of Antihypertensive Agent	
Population	**Goal BP and Benefit**	**Choice of Agent**
CKD and others with known CVD or 10-yr ASCVD risk ≥10%	Target <130/80 (ACC/AHA JACC 2018;71:e127) In ≥50 y/o w/ ↑ CV risk (excluding Pts w/ DM, overt HF, stroke, or ≥1 g/d proteinuria), intensive treatment (SBP <120) is a/w ↓ in all-cause mortality (HR 0.73) and MI, ACS, stroke, HF, CV death (HR 0.75) c/w standard treatment (SBP <140) (SPRINT NEJM 2015;373:2103) In CKD subgroup (eGFR 20–59): intensive BP control is a/w ↓ in all-cause mortality (HR 0.72) and CV outcome (HR 0.81). No Δ in kidney outcome (≥50% ↓ in eGFR or ESRD) (SPRINT JASN 2017;28:2812) In pts w/o baseline CKD: ↑ incident CKD (HR 3.5) and AKI (HR 1.64) but early ↓ eGFR may be reversible hemodynamic effect (CJASN 2018;13:1575) In meta-analysis of RCTs: intensive BP lowering is a/w 14% ↓ risk of all-cause mortality in Pts with CKD stages 3–5 (JAMA IM 2017;177:1498)	In pts who require 2 drugs: Benazepril–amlodipine ↓ CV morbidity, mortality (9.6 vs 11.8%, HR 0.80) and ↓ CKD progression (HR 0.52) c/w benazepril-HCTZ (ACCOMPLISH NEJM 2008;359:2417) Chlorthalidone ↓ rate of HF and CVD outcomes, but no Δ in primary outcome (fatal CHD, nonfatal MI) or mortality c/w lisinopril, amlodipine ALLHAT (JAMA 2002;288:2981)
CKD with proteinuria	More intensive BP control a/w ↓ risk of CKD progression in pts with: >1 g/d proteinuria in long-term f/u of the MDRD study (Ann IM 2005;142:342) >300 mg/d proteinuria among black pts in cohort phase AASK (NEJM 2010;363:918) and in long-term f/u ↓ ESRD in pts w/ >1 g/d proteinuria (JASN 2017;28:671)	ACEi or ARB ↓ rate of progression to ESRD in Pts w/ >500–1,000 mg/d proteinuria; benefit extends to Pts w/ advanced CKD; no benefit and ↑ adverse effects w/ combination ACEi/ARB (ONTARGET NEJM 2008;358:1547)
Diabetes (with and without CKD)	Target <130/80 (ACC/AHA JACC 2018;71:e127) In type 2 DM + CVD or ≥2 additional risk factors for CVD: intensive control (SBP <120) a/w no Δ in CV morbidity/ mortality or all-cause mortality but significant ↓ in total (HR 0.59) and nonfatal stroke (HR 0.63) c/w standard therapy (<140) (ACCORD-BP NEJM 2010;362:1575) Intensive BP control ↓ incidence of microalbuminuria (HR 0.84) but no Δ in renal failure or retinopathy (KI 2012;81:586)	In pts w/ albuminuria ACEi or ARB In pts w/o albuminuria: ACEi, ARB, thiazide, or CCB In pts who require >1 drug: ACEi or ARB + long-acting CCB

| ADPKD | Target ≤130/80; in young pts w/ intact kidney fxn, target <110/75 may ↓ CV events and rate of cyst growth
In pts 15–49 yr w/ eGFR >60, low BP goal (95/60–110/75) a/w ↓ Δ in total kidney volume, LVMI, urinary albumin excretion, no overall Δ in eGFR c/w standard (120/70–130/80) (HALT-PKD NEJM 2014;371:2255) | ACEi as initial agent; ARB if intolerance of ACEi; no additional benefit of combination Rx w/ ACEi + ARB |
| General population w/o above conditions | ACC/AHA: clinical trial evidence strongest for <140/90, but <130/80 may be reasonable (JACC 2018;71:e127)
JNC8: <150/<90 in ≥60 y/o, SBP <140 in <60 y/o (JAMA 2014;311:507)
Isolated systolic HTN: may need to accept SBP >140 to keep DBP >60 | Black and elderly respond better to thiazide-type diuretics or long-acting CCB than to ACEi or ARBs |

HYPERTENSION IN ESRD

Background

- Prevalence of HTN in dialysis Pts is high: >50% and up to 86% (Am J Med 2003;115:291); the majority are treated with antihypertensive agents but not controlled
- Definitions: 1-wk average predialysis SBP >150 or DBP >90 OR 44-hr interdialytic ambulatory BP ≥135/85 OR use of any antihypertensive medications
- In 10–15% of Pts, BP paradoxically increases during dialysis ("intradialytic hypertension"); this a/w volume overload, interdialytic hypertension, and increased short-term mortality

Pathophysiology

- Volume overload is the major cause of HTN in dialysis Pts; ↑ activity of RAAS and SNS; arteriosclerosis; ↑ in intracellular Ca^{2+}, ↑ in endothelium-derived vasoactive substances
- ESAs: incidence of HTN correlates w/ dose but not RBC mass or viscosity; may involve ↑ in vasoactive substances such as endothelin; more likely w/ IV than SC

Evaluation

- There is uncertainty about how to accurately measure BP in dialysis Pts

BP Measurement Strategies	
Predialysis and postdialysis BP measurements	Highly variable in a pt over time; agree poorly with interdialytic ambulatory BP; predialysis BP may be ↑ but predialysis BP ↓ depending on the degree and rate of ultrafiltration
Ambulatory BP monitoring (ABPM)	Gold standard for diagnosis but generally not used clinically Measurements taken over the 44-hr interdialytic interval Amb. BP ↑ by ~2.5 for every 10 hr elapsed after HD
Home BP monitoring (HBPM)	Correlates more closely with ABPM and better predicts long-term outcomes (CVD, all-cause mortality) Home BP ↑ by ~4 for every 10 hr elapsed after dialysis

Treatment

- Guidelines are scarce: target predialysis BP <140/90 and postdialysis BP <130/80 (KDOQI AJKD 2005;45:S1); no recommendations made by KDIGO (KI 2013;83:377); using interdialytic home BP to target BP <135/85 may be more reasonable
- No double-blind RCTs evaluating the target BP or optimal agent in dialysis pts
- Giving antihypertensive drugs at night may ↓ occurrence of intradialytic hypotension

Treatment Strategies	
Nonpharmacologic	
Dietary Na^+ restriction	<1.5–2 g/d Na^+ to target interdialytic wt gain (IDWG) <2–3 kg
Optimizing the dialysis prescription	(1) Individualize dialysate Na^+; Hypertonic dialysate may allow ↑ fluid removal and improve hemodynamic stability BUT leads to ↑ thirst and ↑ interdialytic wt gain (2) Increase length and/or frequency of dialysis; Δ from conventional to frequent/nocturnal HD is a/w ↓ BP, number of antihypertensive medications, and LV mass

Optimizing the management of dry weight	"Dry weight" should be achieved via gradual reduction in post-dialysis weight (0.2–0.5 kg/session) to the lowest tolerated weight that ↓ s/s of hypo- or hypervolemia
	Reducing EDW can improve BP in majority of Pts
	Probing EDW can ↓ ambulatory BP even in Pts w/o overt s/s of volume overload (Hypertension 2009;53:500)
Pharmacologic	
ACEi or ARB	Well tolerated but may ↑ risk of hyperkalemia and anemia
	↓ In LV mass; no large RCT has demonstrated benefit on CV events or mortality
	Lisinopril, enalapril, benazepril are dialyzable and should be given after dialysis; other ACEi and ARBs are not
Dihydropyridine (DHP) CCB	Effective and well tolerated; not dialyzable and do not require supplemental medication
β-blocker	Open-label RCT showed ↓ CV events with atenolol vs lisinopril (NDT 2014;29:672); Atenolol is moderately dialyzable; can be given TIW after HD (25–100 mg)
MR antagonist (MRA)	36-wk RCT showed SPL well-tolerated at ≤25 mg daily, ↑ rate of K >6.5 mEq/L at 50 mg daily (KI 2018;doi:10.1016)
	Meta-analysis suggests benefit on CV- and all-cause mortality but low-quality evidence (AJKD 2016;68:591)

RESISTANT HYPERTENSION

Background
- Defined as BP that remains above goal despite adherence to treatment with ≥3 anti-hypertensive agents of different classes prescribed at optimal doses, ideally including a diuretic, OR BP at goal but requiring ≥4 agents (Circulation 2008;117:510)

Epidemiology (Hypertension 2011;57:1076)
- Using data from NHANES from 2003 to 2008: (1) 8.9% of US adults with hypertension and 12.8% of US adults on treatment with antihypertensive drugs met criteria for resistant HTN; (2) 72.4% of all drug-treated adults with uncontrolled HTN were taking drugs from <3 classes; (3) 85.6% of adults with resistant HTN used a diuretic but 64.4% of those used the weak thiazide diuretic HCTZ
- Prevalence of resistant HTN in nephrology clinics may rise to >50%
- Adults with resistant HTN are more likely to be older, non-Hispanic black, and have higher BMI, albuminuria, CKD, CAD, HF, stroke, and DM

Pathogenesis
- Factors that ↑ prevalence of resistant HTN in CKD: impaired Na handling, chronic fluid overload, ↑ activity of RAAS and sympathetic systems, impaired NO synthesis and endothelium-mediated vasodilation, ↑arterial stiffness, inflammation, renovascular ds

Definitions of Resistant Hypertension	
Apparent resistant HTN	Uncontrolled BP despite being prescribed ≥3 antihypertensive agents or controlled BP despite being prescribed ≥4 agents
True resistant HTN	Uncontrolled BP despite adherence with ≥3 antihypertensive agents at optimal doses or controlled BP despite adherence with ≥4 agents
Pseudoresistant HTN	Appearance of treatment resistance
	Causes: poor adherence to therapy, complicated dosing regimens; suboptimal dosing of medications, inappropriate combinations of agents, physician inertia; improper BP measurement technique, difficult to compress calcified arteries in elderly; white coat HTN
White coat HTN	Elevated BP during clinic visits with normal BP in nonclinic settings and absence of target organ damage ("isolated clinic HTN")
	Pts are at lower cardiovascular risk compared with persistent HTN but white coat HTN may not be benign, a/w HR 1.79 for all-cause mortality in large registry-based study (NEJM 2018;378:1509)
	Occurs in 15–30% of pts with elevated office BP
	More common among patients with resistant HTN
Refractory HTN	BP unable to be controlled despite optimal medical therapy under the care of a hypertension specialist

Evaluation

- Accurate measurement of office BP: attention to environment, body and arm position, and appropriate cuff size; obtain average of multiple measurements at least 1 min apart
- Confirmation with ABPM or HBPM
- Identify contributing lifestyle factors: age, obesity, family history, black race, excess dietary sodium intake, heavy alcohol intake, reduced nephron mass
- Identify substances that interfere with BP control: NSAIDs, sympathomimetics, stimulants, alcohol, oral contraceptives, glucocorticoids, natural licorice, herbal substances
- Screen for secondary causes of HTN

Treatment	
Optimize volume status	Dietary sodium restriction and use of appropriate diuretics: Chlorthalidone 25 mg/d is ~twice as potent as HCTZ 25 mg/d, has a much longer duration of action, and is effective at a lower GFR Use of loop diuretics in advanced CKD Combining loop diuretic with thiazide or low-dose K$^+$-sparing diuretic
Adequate RAAS blockade	Use of mineralocorticoid receptor blockers (MRBs, spironolactone and eplerenone) as add-on therapy: Addition of spironolactone 25–50 mg/d is superior c/w placebo (–8.7 ↓ in home SBP), doxazosin (–4.03 ↓), and bisoprolol (–4.48 ↓) esp. in Pts w/ low plasma renin; low incidence of hyperkalemia though Pts had GFR >45 (PATHWAY-2 Lancet 2015;386:2059)
Chronotherapy	Bedtime dosing of BP medications can restore the normal dipping pattern, improve nocturnal and 24-hr ambulatory BP control, reduce proteinuria, and may be a/w ↓ risk of CV morbidity and mortality (JASN 2011;22:2313)

HYPERTENSIVE EMERGENCIES

Background

- Hypertensive emergency: significantly ↑BP (SBP ≥180 and/or DBP ≥120) with s/s of acute, ongoing, end-organ injury; requires immediate BP reduction
- Severe asymptomatic HTN ("hypertensive urgency"): BP can be lowered within hr to d
- BP usually severely elevated in pts with chronic HTN but can develop at lower BPs in Pts without pre-existing HTN if there is an acute rise in BP (ie, acute GN or pre-eclampsia)

Pathophysiology

- Release of vasoconstricting substances (angiotensin II, norepinephrine) → abrupt rise in vascular resistance → endothelium releases vasodilator molecules but this compensatory response is overwhelmed → endothelial damage and further rise in BP
- As MAP increases (esp >180), cerebral vascular autoregulation is overwhelmed → cerebral vasodilation and edema → hypertensive encephalopathy

Clinical Manifestations and Evaluation

- Symptoms: chest pain (MI or aortic dissection); back pain (aortic dissection); dyspnea (pulmonary edema or HF); neurologic sx, seizure, or AMS (hypertensive encephalopathy)
- Exam: ✓ for BP Δ between arms (aortic dissection); ↑ JVP, S3 (HF); flame hemorrhages, exudates, or papilledema on funduscopic exam (hypertensive retinopathy)
- Causes: renal (acute GN, vasculitis, HUS, renal artery stenosis); endocrine (pheochromocytoma, Cushing's); CNS (head injury, cerebral infarction, cerebral hemorrhage); drugs (cocaine, sympathomimetics, CNIs, ESAs, sudden withdrawal of antihypertensive medications); other (pre-eclampsia/eclampsia, TTP)

Reversible Posterior Leukoencephalopathy Syndrome (RPLS or PRES)

- Associations: HTN, TTP, HUS, eclampsia, vasculitis, immunosuppressive drugs (CyA, Tac)
- Imaging: MRI shows symmetric white matter edema in posterior cerebral hemispheres

Treatment

- Hypertensive emergency: admission to ICU for monitoring and parenteral therapy
- MAP should be ↓ by 10–20% in the first hr and addt'l 5–15% over next 23 hr; after ~24 hr of BP at target levels, oral medications can be started and IV medications tapered off

Treatment Approach for Clinical Scenarios	
Acute ischemic stroke	Labetalol and nicardipine (first-line), Nitroprusside (second-line) Lower BP if ≥220/120 (or ≥185/110 if tPA candidate)
Hypertensive encephalopathy	Nicardipine, clevidipine, fenoldopam, nitroprusside, labetalol, enalapril, hydralazine

Acute HF	Loop diuretics, vasodilators (nitroprusside, nitroglycerin) Avoid hydralazine (↑ cardiac work), β-blockers (↓ contractility)
Acute MI	Nitroglycerin, nicardipine, esmolol (↑ coronary perfusion, ↓ MVO_2)
Acute aortic dissection	First: β-blocker to ↓ HR and wall shear stress (esmolol, labetalol) then vasodilator (nitroprusside or clevidipine) SBP should be rapidly ↓ to 100–120 (within 20 min)
Pregnancy (pre-eclampsia, eclampsia)	Methyldopa, hydralazine, labetalol, fenoldopam, nicardipine IV magnesium sulfate for prevention of eclampsia Delivery of baby and placenta
AKI (acute hypertensive nephrosclerosis)	Calcium channels blockers and α-blockers (preserve renal blood flow); fenoldopam (causes renal arterial dilation → maintains or increases renal perfusion)

Drug Treatment			
Drug	Mechanism	Dose	Adverse Effects
Sodium nitroprusside	Arterial and venous dilator	Start at 0.25–0.5 → max 8–10 µg/kg/min	Cyanide toxicity if Rx prolonged >24–48 hr
Nitroglycerin	Venous > arterial dilator	5–100 µg/min	Headache, reflex tachycardia
Clevidipine	Short-acting CCB	1–21 mg/hr	Reflex tachycardia
Nicardipine	CCB	5–15 mg/hr	Reflex tachycardia
Labetalol	β- and α-blocker	20–80 mg bolus or 0.5–2 mg/min infusion	Bradycardia, bronchospasm
Fenoldopam	Dopamine-1 receptor agonist	0.1–1.6 µg/kg/min	Headache, flushing, ↑ IOP
Hydralazine	Vasodilator	10–20 mg IV bolus	Reflex tachycardia

ANTIHYPERTENSIVES

Features and Dose of Antihypertensives		
Class	Features	Dose
ACEi and ARBs	Beneficial effects in proteinuric CKD, HF, post-MI Synergistic effect with diuretics Remains beneficial in advanced CKD (NEJM 2006;354:131) Contraindicated during pregnancy s/e: ↑ K	
ACEi	↓ formation of angiotensin II (AII), vasodilation (d/t ↑ kinin levels) s/e: cough, angioedema (rare) due to ↑ kinin levels	Lisinopril: 10–40 mg (1×/d) Benazepril: 10–40 mg (1–2×/d) Fosinopril: 10–40 mg (1–2×/d) Ramipril: 2.5–20 mg (1–2×/d) Quinapril: 10–40 mg (1–2×/d)
ARBs	Impair binding of AII to AT1 receptor Losartan: less effective at BP lowering than other ARBs, ↑ uric acid excretion and ↓ plasma uric acid levels	Losartan: 50–100 mg (1–2×/d) Valsartan: 80–320 mg (1×/d) Irbesartan: 150–300 mg Telmisartan: 40–80 mg Candesartan: 8–32 mg Azilsartan: 40–80 mg
Thiazides (NEJM 2009;361:2153)	Inhibit apical NCC in DCT s/e: ↓ K, ↓ Na, ↑ Ca, ↓ uric acid, glucose intolerance	
HCTZ (thiazide-type)	Most effective at GFR >50; $t_{1/2}$ ~10 hr; reasonable choice in frail older Pts <10 above goal BP	Start at 25 mg/d and titrate to 50–100 mg/d; can be given 1–2 ×/d

Chlorthalidone (thiazide-like)	Can be effective to GFR of 30–40; $t_{1/2}$ 50–60 hr; ~2× more potent than HCTZ; greater ↓ in nighttime and 24-hr BP; ↓ HF, CVD (ALLHAT JAMA 2002;288:2981)	Start at 12.5–25 mg/d and titrate to 50 mg/d
Metolazone (thiazide-like)	Retains effectiveness at GFR <30 mL/min; $t_{1/2}$ 14 hr	Start at 2.5–5 mg/d, titrate to 10–20 mg/d; can give TIW
Loop diuretic (NEJM 1998;339:387)	Inhibit apical NKCC in THAL s/e: ↓ K, rash, AIN, ototoxicity at high doses	Normal renal fxn: Bum. 1 mg = furos. 40 mg = tors. 20 mg Severe CKD: Bum. 1 mg = furos. 20 mg = tors. 20 mg
Furosemide	Bioavailability ~50%; $t_{1/2}$ ~2 hr	Maximal response in severe CKD: 160–200 mg IV. Should be given 2–3×/d
Torsemide	Bioavailability ~100%; $t_{1/2}$ ~3–4 hr	Maximal response in severe CKD: 50–100 mg IV/PO; Can be given 1–2×/d
Bumetanide	Bioavailability ~100%; $t_{1/2}$ ~1 hr	Maximal response in severe CKD: 8–10 mg IV/PO
Ethacrynic acid	Only non-sulfa diuretic but ↑ ototoxicity	
K^+-sparing diuretics	Act in the principal cells of the CCD	
Spironolactone (SPL)	Competitively inhibits MR. $t_{1/2}$ >15 hr (active metabolite). s/e: gynecomastia, ↓ libido d/t nonselective binding to steroid receptor	25–100 mg/d; risk of hyperkalemia is predicted by baseline eGFR ≤45 mL/min and baseline K^+ >4.5 mEq/L
Eplerenone (EPL)	Competitively inhibits MR. $t_{1/2}$ 3–6 hr; ↑ specificity for MR, ↓ incidence of s/e but more expensive and may be less effective than SPL	Start at 25 mg/d, titrate to 50–100 mg/d in daily or divided doses; risk of hyperkalemia as above
Triamterene	Inhibits ENaC. s/e: crystalluria, stones, AKI	37.5–75 mg/d in combination pills w/ HCTZ
Amiloride	Inhibits ENaC; prolonged $t_{1/2}$ (~100 hr) in CKD; few side effects	Start at 5 mg daily and titrate to 10 mg daily
Calcium channel blockers	Inhibit L-type Ca^{2+} channel s/e: peripheral edema, constipation, gingival hyperplasia (dose-dependent)	
DHP (amlodipine, nifedipine)	Potent vasodilators. s/e: as above plus headache and flushing; edema is more common. Amlodipine: longer $t_{1/2}$ (30–50 hr vs 2–7 hr); studied in ALLHAT and ACCOMPLISH trials	Amlodipine: start at 5 mg/d (2.5 mg in small pts), titrate to 10 mg/d after 7–14 d. Nifedipine: Start 30–60 mg/d, titrate to 90–120 mg/d, may need to be given twice daily
Non-DHP (diltiazem, verapamil)	Negative inotropes, less potent vasodilators. May ↓ proteinuria. s/e: as above plus ↓ CO, HR. Cause ↑ levels of CYP3A4 substrates (incl. CNI)	Diltiazem: 120–360 mg/d Verapamil: 120–480 mg/d
β-blockers	s/e: hyperkalemia, ↑ Glc and TG, bradycardia, ischemic sx w/ acute withdrawal, depression, ↑ weight	
Selective (β-1) (atenolol, bisoprolol, metoprolol, nebivolol)	Atenolol: excreted by kidney; $t_{1/2}$ prolonged in CKD Atenolol and metoprolol are water-soluble and dialyzable; should be administered postdialysis Nebivolol produces NO-dependent vasodilation	Atenolol: 25–100 mg/d (max 50 mg/d if CrCl 15–35, max 25 m/d if CrCl <15); Metoprolol succinate: 50–300 mg/d Nebivolol: 5–10 mg/d (start at 2.5 mg/d if CrCl <30)

Combined α, β (carvedilol, labetalol)	Vasodilating properties. Carvedilol: no impact on glycemic control, may ↓ renal vascular resistance and ↑ renal blood flow and GFR	Carvedilol: 12.5–50 mg/d (2×/d) Labetalol: 200–1,200 mg/d (2–3×/d)
α-blockers	↑ HDL and insulin sensitivity	
Peripheral α-blockers (doxazosin, prazosin, terazosin)	May have benefit in men w/ BPH. s/e: postural hypotension, dizziness. In ALLHAT, doxazosin a/w ↑ risk of CHF (*JAMA* 2002;288:2981)	Doxazosin: 1–16 mg qhs Prazosin: 2–20 mg/d (2–3×/d) Terazosin: 1–20 mg qhs
Central α-blockers (clonidine, guanfacine, methyldopa)	s/e: sedation, dry mouth, sexual dysfunction, withdrawal hypertension (esp w/ clonidine). Methyldopa is safe in pregnancy but rarely used in other settings	Clonidine: 0.2–1.2 mg/d (2–3×/d) Guanfacine: 1–3 mg daily Methyldopa: 250–500 mg twice daily
Directly acting vasodilators	s/e: headaches, fluid retention, reflex tachycardia	
Hydralazine	s/e: as above plus drug-induced lupus and ANCA-positive vasculitis	25–100 mg/dose (2–3×/d)
Minoxidil	s/e: as above plus hirsutism	5–10 mg daily

Indications for Specific Drug Classes	
Indication	**Drug Class**
HF	ACEi, ARB, diuretic, β-blocker, MRA
Post-MI	ACEi, β-blocker, MRA
Atrial fibrillation	β-blocker, non-DHP CCB
DM	ACEi, ARB, diuretic, β-blocker, CCB
Proteinuric CKD	ACEi, ARB, non-DHP CCB
Fluid overload	Thiazide diuretic, loop diuretic, K⁺-sparing diuretic
BPH	α-blocker
Osteoporosis	Thiazide diuretic

OBSTRUCTIVE SLEEP APNEA (OSA)

Background

- A sleep-related breathing disorder characterized by repetitive partial (hypopnea) or complete (apnea) cessation of airflow caused by collapse of the pharynx during sleep → repeated arousals and hypoxemia
- Common but frequently undiagnosed disorder
- An independent risk factor for HTN; in general, the more severe the OSA, the more prevalent and severe the HTN
- Moderate/severe OSA is a/w with nearly 3-fold ↑ risk of incident HTN (*NEJM* 2000;342:1378)
- OSA may be present in >70% of Pts w/ resistant HTN

Epidemiology

- Prevalence is ~10% in middle-aged individuals (~5% in women, ~15% in men)
- Risk factors: obesity, craniofacial or upper airway soft tissue abnormalities, age, male gender, smoking, + family history
- Prevalence ↑ w/ ↑ BMI and markers of obesity (neck circumference, waist-to-hip ratio)

Presentation

- Common presenting complaints: daytime sleepiness, fatigue, snoring, restless sleep, poor concentration, morning headaches, nocturia
- Common exam findings: obesity, crowded oropharyngeal airway, HTN
- Frequent apneic and/or hypopneic episodes can end with arousals with spikes in BP lasting several seconds → ↑ the risk for "nondipping" HTN, a strong predictor of CV risk; nearly 90% of Pts w/ nondipping HTN patterns may have OSA
- Complications: ↑ mortality, sustained HTN, pulmonary artery HTN, HF, stroke, insulin resistance, impaired daytime functioning, impaired cognition, depression

Diagnosis

- Screening in Pts w/: Excessive daytime sleepiness; snoring + ≥2 additional clinical features of OSA; resistant HTN; unexplained pulmonary HTN; secondary polycythemia
- The STOP-Bang questionnaire can help identify Pts w/ OSA

	STOP-Bang Questionnaire (BJA 2012;108:768)
S	Do you snore loudly?
T	Do you often feel tired, fatigued, or sleepy during daytime?
O	Has anyone observed you stop breathing during your sleep?
P	Do you have or are you being treated for high blood pressure?
B	BMI >35 kg/m^2
a	Age >50 yr old
n	Neck circumference >40 cm
g	Gender: Male?

0–1 pos. responses = low risk, 3–4 pos. responses = intermediate risk, 5–8 pos. responses = high risk of OSA; probability of moderate/severe OSA = 36% for score ≥3, 60% for score ≥7

- Polysomnography (sleep study) evaluation performed in a sleep disorders unit is the gold standard for an accurate diagnosis of OSA
- Criteria: ≥5 obstructive respiratory events per hr of sleep in a Pt w/ ≥1 associated symptom or comorbidity OR ≥15 events/hr regardless of symptoms or comorbidities
- Apnea-hypopnea index (AHI) 5–15 events/hr = mild, 15–30 events/hr = moderate, >30 events/hr of sleep or O_2 saturation <90% for >20% of total sleep time = severe OSA

Treatment

- Behavior modification: Weight loss, exercise, and avoidance of the supine sleep position, alcohol, and medications that can worsen daytime sleepiness or cause weight gain
- CPAP to stabilize the airway and prevent hypopnea and apnea events due upper airway collapse is the mainstay of therapy
- Surgical procedures to relieve nasal obstruction (turbinate reduction, septoplasty, rhinoplasty), upper airway obstruction (uvulopalatopharyngoplasty [UPPP], tonsillectomy, adenoidectomy), and lower airway obstruction (somnoplasty)
- Successful treatment of OSA can lead to a modest but clinically significant ↓ in BP and reduction (rather complete elimination) of the need for antihypertensive medications
- Among Pts w/ OSA and resistant HTN, use of CPAP is a/w greater ↓ in 24-hr mean BP (3.1) and 24-hr DBP (3.2) c/w no CPAP and ↑ percentage of Pts displaying a "dipper" pattern at 12 wk (35.9 vs 21.6%, adjusted OR 2.4) (JAMA 2013;310:2407)
- Number of hours of CPAP use a/w greater ↓ in 24-hr mean BP; ≥4 hr/night likely needed
- Predictors of a greater BP response to treatment with CPAP: OSA severity, presence of excessive daytime sleepiness, presence of uncontrolled HTN

RENAL ARTERY STENOSIS (RAS)

Background

- RAS: narrowing of one or both main renal arteries or their branches
- Renovascular HTN: ↑ BP resulting from renal arterial compromise, often due to occlusive lesions in the main renal arteries
- Ischemic nephropathy: CKD that results from atherosclerotic RAS due to diminished renal blood flow to the poststenotic kidney
- RAS is an anatomical descriptor; the presence of lesion(s) does not necessarily translate to the lesion(s) being responsible for BP ↑ or renal dysfunction
- If systemic hypertension is related directly to an arterial lesion, then relief of the obstruction, presumably, should lead to reversal or improvement of the hypertension

Epidemiology

- Atherosclerosis accounts for ~90% of cases of renal artery stenosis (discussed in this section); fibromuscular dysplasia (FMD) accounts for ~10% (discussed below)
- Risk factors for renovascular atherosclerotic lesions: DM, HLD, aortoiliac occlusive disease, CAD, and HTN
- Prevalence of atherosclerotic renal artery stenosis ↑ w/ age; may rise as high as 30% among Pts with CAD and to 50% among elderly Pts or those w/ diffuse atherosclerotic vascular diseases; ~10–15% among patients with end-stage kidney disease

Pathophysiology

- Decrease in renal perfusion pressure → activation of the RAS, impaired sodium excretion, activation of the sympathetic nervous system, ↑ intrarenal prostaglandin concentrations, ↓ nitric oxide production → renovascular HTN
- Initially, plasma renin activity ↑ due to activation of the RAS; but when HTN is sustained, plasma renin activity ↓
- Advanced vascular occlusion (>70–80% stenosis) → hypoxia within the renal cortex → activation of inflammatory and oxidative pathways → irreversible interstitial fibrosis and loss of renal function ("ischemic nephropathy")

Presentation

- Renovascular disease is more likely to accelerate or impair control of preexisting HTN than to cause new-onset HTN
- Features that suggest renovascular hypertension: resistant HTN, onset of HTN (>160/100) in a Pt ≥50 yr, presence of diffuse atherosclerosis, atrophic kidney or asymmetry in kidney size, absence of family history of HTN, recurrent flash pulmonary edema, unexplained refractory HF, acute rise in serum creatinine (≥50%) after the administration of ACEi or ARB, presence of abdominal bruit
- Atherosclerosis usually involves the ostium and proximal 1/3 of the main renal artery and perirenal aorta; segmental and diffuse intrarenal disease may also be seen
- Stenosis is progressive in the majority of patients

Diagnosis

- Testing is indicated in pts w/ clinical findings suggestive of renovascular disease who have a high likelihood of benefiting from an intervention should a clinically significant stenotic lesion be found
- Renal arteriography is the gold standard but less invasive options are available

Diagnosis of Renal Artery Stenosis	
Modality	**Features**
Duplex Doppler ultrasonography	Provides both anatomic (direct visualization of the main renal arteries) and functional assessment (systolic flow velocity via Doppler) of the severity of stenosis
	Noninvasive and relatively inexpensive; but time consuming, may be technically difficult, operator dependent
CT or MR angiography	Accurate and noninvasive; better for proximal disease
	May be limited by pt-related factors (presence of calcium or stents)
	Toxicity associated with use of contrast media in pts with CKD
Captopril renography	Oral captopril is given 1 hr before a marker of glomerular filtration, such as DTPA is injected → ACE inhibitor-induced decline in GFR in the stenotic kidney and equivalent increase in GFR in the contralateral kidney → Δ between kidneys is enhanced
	Functional test to compare RBF, GFR between the two kidneys
	Low predictive accuracy for renovascular hypertension
	Can be unreliable when baseline kidney function is abnormal as asymmetries in renal flow and function can be present for reasons other than renovascular disease
Measurement of peripheral plasma renin activity (PRA)	PRA measured 1 hr after the administration of oral captopril → Pts w/ a functional lesion should have an exaggerated ↑ in PRA
	Low predictive accuracy for renovascular hypertension
	PRA is ↑ in only 50–80% of pts w/ renovascular hypertension
	PRA may be suppressed by high dietary Na⁺ intake, bilateral renal artery disease, volume expansion, various medications

Treatment

- Treatment goals include: blood pressure control (rather than reversal), preservation or salvage of kidney function, and prevention of flash pulmonary edema
- Options include (1) medical therapy with ACEi or ARB + other agents as needed, (2) percutaneous angioplasty +/- stent placement), (3) surgical revascularization
- Revascularization vs medical therapy alone
  (1) In ~1,000 Pts w/ atherosclerotic renal artery stenosis with ≥60% narrowing and systolic HTN despite ≥2 antihypertensive medications and/or eGFR <60 → no Δ in primary outcome (composite of death from CV or renal causes, CVA, MI, hospitalization for CHF, progressive renal insufficiency, or the need for permanent RRT) between those randomized to medical therapy alone vs medical therapy plus stent (*CORAL NEJM* 2014;370:13)

(2) In ~800 Pts w/ average 76% stenotic occlusion of the renal arteries and entry serum creatinine >2.0 mg/dL, randomized to medical therapy with or without stenting → no Δ in blood pressure control, kidney function, heart failure hospitalizations, or mortality over a median followup period >2 yr (ASTRAL *NEJM* 2009;361:1953)
- Features that suggest benefit from revascularization: short duration of BP elevation; inability of optimal medical therapy to control BP; intolerance of optimal medical therapy, including ACEi or ARB; progressive CKD in a pt with bilateral renal artery stenosis or unilateral stenosis to a solitary kidney; recurrent flash pulmonary edema; refractory HF
- Risks of revascularization: renal artery dissection, thrombosis, perforation; restenosis; AKI due to atheroembolic disease; reaction to radiocontrast agent
- Calculation of the renal resistive index (RI) may help predict the outcome after revascularization; ↑ RI is a/w greater degree of intrinsic renal damage. RI ([1 − (end-diastolic velocity ÷ maximal systolic velocity)] × 100) ≥80 identifies pts w/ renal artery stenosis in whom angioplasty or surgery is not likely to improve renal function, blood pressure, or kidney survival (*NEJM* 2001;344:410).

FIBROMUSCULAR DYSPLASIA (FMD)

Background
- FMD is much rarer than atherosclerotic disease; accounts for <10% of cases of RAS
- Classically, this disease has been described as a cause of HTN in younger females, sometimes first presenting during pregnancy
- Prevalence drops markedly with age: among pts with renovascular HTN, FMD accounts for up to 50% of cases in children but <15% of cases in adults
- Among adults, FMD is far more common among females (10-fold higher prevalence)

Presentation
- FMD typically affects the distal 2/3 of the renal artery and its branches ("string of beads")
- Extracranial cerebrovascular (carotid, vertebral arties) involvement is common
- Only rarely does FMD lead to complete or segmental occlusion of the renal arteries, with most individuals presenting w/ normal kidney function but significantly elevated BP

Diagnosis
- Duplex ultrasonography, CTA, and MRA (less preferred) are noninvasive options
- Renal arteriography (digital subtraction angiography [DSA]) should be the first diagnostic test for Pts at high risk for FMD-associated renovascular hypertension, as this imaging modality allows for simultaneous treatment with percutaneous transluminal angioplasty

Treatment
- FMD and uncontrolled HTN: conventional balloon angioplasty
- Rate of restenosis following angioplasty ranges from 12–34% over followup intervals of 6 mo–2 yr, but restenosis does not always lead to recurrent hypertension
- Likelihood of cure of HTN is more likely in Pts w/ FMD than in those w/ atherosclerotic renal artery stenosis (60% vs <30%)

HYPERALDOSTERONISM

Background
- Aldosterone: hormone primarily involved in the regulation of extracellular volume and potassium homeostasis
  Sites of action: epithelial cells in distal nephron > colon, salivary glands, and sweat glands
  Regulators of secretion: plasma K+, AII, ACTH
- Binds to cytosolic mineralocorticoid receptors → ↑ number of open ENaC channels in apical membrane of CCD principal cells → ↑ sodium reabsorption → electronegative lumen creates a favorable gradient for potassium secretion via ROMK, BK channels
- Primary aldosteronism (PA): renin-independent hypersecretion of aldosterone, nonsuppressible by sodium loading

Epidemiology
- Prevalence of PA: ~4% in primary care clinics, ~10% among Pts referred to HTN specialty clinics; ~13% among Pts w/ severe HTN. Prevalence of elevated aldosterone to renin ratio (ARR): ~16% in primary care clinics, ~20% in specialty clinics (*JCEM* 2016;101:1889)
- Causes of PA: bilateral idiopathic adrenal hyperplasia (IHA; 60–70%), unilateral aldosterone-producing adenoma (APA; 30–40%), less common: Unilateral hyperplasia; familial hyperaldosteronism type I (GRA), type II, and type III; and adrenocortical carcinoma

- Somatic mutations cause aldosterone hypersecretion in ~50% of APAs: *KCNJ5* (most common, ~40% of APAs), *ATP 1A 1*, *ATP2B3*, *CACNA 1D*, *CTNNB 1*

- Persistent volume expansion, severe & resistant HTN, hypokalemia (in <50% of pts), metabolic alkalosis, hypernatremia (mild), hypomagnesemia (mild)
- ↑ CV morbidity/mortality c/w pts w/ same degree of BP elevation: ↑ LV mass and myocardial fibrosis, ↓ LV function, ↑ risk of arrhythmias, MI, stroke, CV death
- Renal effects: ↑ GFR due to glomerular hyperfiltration, ↑ urine albumin excretion
- Pts with APA: usually younger (<50 yr), ↑ aldosterone secretion rates, ↑ plasma and urinary aldosterone concentrations, more severe HTN and hypokalemia

Evaluation
- Case-detection testing w/ plasma aldosterone to renin ratio (ARR = PAC/PRA) should be performed in Pts with: severe HTN (SBP >150 or DBP >100), resistant HTN, HTN and spontaneous or low-dose diuretic-induced hypokalemia, HTN and adrenal incidentaloma, HTN and sleep apnea, HTN and family history of early-onset HTN or CVA at <40 yr, and HTN with first-degree relative w/ PA
- Screening for PA should be done in all Pts w/ resistant HTN, regardless of K level, although the likelihood of positive results ↑ in pts w/ hypokalemia
- PAC and PRA should be measured in a morning blood sample while seated
- Definition of abnormal ARR is assay dependent: PRA is generally undetectable (usually <1 ng/mL/hr); PAC is >15 ng/dL in most pts w/ PA; ARR >20 is suggestive of PA; ARR >30 is the most commonly used cutoff
- Antihypertensive medications can be continued during testing as long as pt has been on stable doses for >3 wk
  (1) EXCEPT mineralocorticoid receptor blockers (MRBs, spironolactone, and eplerenone) which should be stopped for ≥6 wk unless Pt is hypokalemic and PRA is suppressed
  (2) ACE inhibitors and ARBs can ↑ PRA thus a detectable PRA or low ARR does not exclude PA; undetectable PRA will be strongly suggestive of PA
  (3) β-blockers can ↓ PRA and ↑ ARR but PAC >15 still suggestive of PA
  (4) Drugs with minimal effects on PRA and PAC: verapamil, hydralazine, α-blockers

Diagnosis of PA	
Findings	Diagnosis
↓ PRA, ↑ PAC, ↑ ARR	Suspect primary hyperaldosteronism Proceed to confirmatory testing (see below) If spontaneous hypokalemia, undetectable PRA, and PAC >20 mg/dL, confirmatory testing may not be required
↑ PRA, ↑ PAC, ARR <10	Suspect secondary hyperaldosteronism (renovascular disease, diuretic use, malignant HTN, renin-secreting tumor [rare])
↓ PRA and ↓ PAC w/ HTN and hypokalemia	Suspect Liddle syndrome OR nonaldosterone mineralocorticoid excess (syndrome of apparent MC excess [AME], Cushing syndrome, chronic licorice root ingestion, congenital adrenal hyperplasia)

- Confirmatory testing to demonstrate inappropriate aldosterone secretion:
  (1) After consumption of a high sodium diet for 3 d, if 24-hr urine collection shows UU_{Na} >200 mmol/d, then urine aldosterone >12 μg/24 hr is confirmatory (modern practice); (2) IV saline suppression test or fludrocortisone suppression test (cumbersome, difficult to implement); (3) captopril challenge test (high false-negative result)
- Subtype classification is the next step once primary hyperaldosteronism is confirmed, to distinguish a unilateral APA from bilateral hyperplasia and to exclude adrenal carcinoma

Studies for Subtype Classification	
Adrenal CT	Preferred imaging modality Superior spatial resolution c/w MR with contrast Imaging findings: APAs usually appear as small hypodense nodules (<3 mm diameter); in bilateral hyperplasia, adrenal gland may appear normal or nodular; adrenal carcinomas usually >4 cm in diameter and have suspicious imaging phenotype Limitations: imaging findings may be misleading; absence of a mass does not exclude adenoma (can be missed if lesion <1 cm); solitary unilateral adenomas may be nonfunctioning and cannot be distinguished from APAs
Adrenal vein sampling (AVS)	Gold standard test to distinguish whether excess aldosterone production is unilateral (ie, APA that is a candidate for adrenalectomy) or bilateral (ie, IHA that should be treated medically) Sensitivity and specificity (95 and 100%) superior to adrenal CT Indications: pts with PA who are candidates for surgical management and have adrenal CT showing: normal findings or bilateral abnormalities or unilateral abnormalities in pts >35 yr; may not be needed in pts <35 yr w/ spontaneous hypokalemia, marked hyperaldosteronism, and unilateral lesion c/w adenoma on CT Limitations: expensive, invasive, technically difficult Method: ✓ cortisol to confirm successful cannulation of both adrenal veins; w/ cosyntropin infusion, the adrenal vein to IVC cortisol ratio is typically >5:1; ✓ aldo and cortisol from 3 sites: right adrenal vein, left adrenal vein, and IVC; then compare adrenal vein cortisol-corrected aldo ratios (PAC/cortisol); ratio >4:1 suggests unilateral aldosterone excess; >10:1 in most APAs; ratio <3:1 suggests bilateral adrenal hyperplasia

Treatment

- Treatment goals: reverse cardiovascular morbidity caused by aldosterone excess, normalize serum potassium, normalize BP
- For unilateral disease (APA or unilateral hyperplasia), Rx is laparoscopic adrenalectomy
- For pts w/ bilateral hyperplasia or in Pts with unilateral disease who are not surgical candidates or unwilling to have surgery, treatment is with MR antagonist
- Unilateral adrenalectomy → marked ↓ in aldosterone secretion and correction of hypokalemia in nearly 100%; HTN improves in nearly 100% and is cured in 35–80%
- Postoperative management: ✓ PAC and PRA to assess biochemical response, d/c potassium supplementation and MR antagonists, and lower other BP medications; risk of ↑ K postop d/t hypoaldosteronism 2/2 chronic contralateral adrenal gland suppression
- Adrenalectomy more likely to cure HTN in Pts with: younger age, shorter duration of HTN, use of ≤2 antihypertensive agents, ↑ ARR, ↑ urine aldosterone, lack of FHx of HTN
- Spironolactone or eplerenone; titrate dose to achieve mid-normal serum K
- K-sparing diuretics (amiloride, triamterene) are an alternative but do not address the CV morbidity caused by persistent hyperaldosteronism and activation of the MR

Rare Entities of MR or ENaC-Induced HTN	
Liddle syndrome	AD; ↑ ENaC function and Na reabsorption in CD; classic triad of HTN, hypokalemia, and metabolic alkalosis at young age; ↓ PRA and ↓ PAC Tx: amiloride or triamterene
Glucocorticoid Remediable Aldosteronism = Familial hyperaldosteronism type 1	AD; ACTH-dependent activation of aldosterone synthase; typical onset of HTN <age 21; ↓ PRA and ↑ PAC Tx: glucocorticoid
Syndrome of apparent mineralocorticoid excess (AME)	AR; deficiency in 11-β-HSD2; ↑ cortisol binding to MR; ↑ urinary free cortisol to cortisone ratio, ↓ PRA, ↓ PAC Tx: amiloride or triamterene or MRA +/– dexamethasone

PHEOCHROMOCYTOMA

Background
- Neuroendocrine tumors derived from chromaffin cells of the adrenal medulla that hypersecrete catecholamines (epinephrine, norepinephrine, and/or dopamine)
- Paragangliomas or "extra-adrenal pheochromocytomas" arise from chromaffin cells of the sympathetic paravertebral ganglia in the thorax, abdomen, or pelvis
- Rare form (<0.2%) of secondary HTN

Presentation
- Classic symptoms: palpitations, headaches, diaphoresis, and paroxysms of hypertension
- Pts do not always present w/ all of these, but paroxysms of BP spikes are common feature
- Pheochromocytoma can occur at any age
- There are no known risk factors except for the presence of certain genetic syndromes including: multiple endocrine neoplasia (MEN) type 2A or 2B, von Hippel–Lindau (VHL) syndrome, and neurofibromatosis type 1 (NF1)
- "10% tumor" because it was commonly thought that ~10% of pheochromocytomas are malignant; ~10% are bilateral; ~10% are pediatric; ~10% are extra-adrenal; and ~10% are familial; but more recent data suggests that up to 25% of pheochromocytomas are inherited

Evaluation
- Indications for testing: classic symptoms, onset of HTN at young age, resistant HTN, FHx of pheochromocytoma, presence of familial synd, or adrenal incidentaloma (>10 HU on CT)
- Testing for plasma-free metanephrine levels has become the most efficient screening test
- A positive screen for plasma-free metanephrines should be followed by more involved 24-hr urine tests for fractionated metanephrines and catecholamines
- After biochemical confirmation: imaging studies w/ CT or MRI to locate the tumor
- If imaging is negative: ^{123}I-Metaiodobenzylguanidine (MIBG) nuclear scan or ^{18}F-fluorodeoxyglucose (18F-FDG) positron emission tomography (PET) scan should be done to search for adrenal tumor too small to appear on CT/MRI
- MIBG also indicated for paragangliomas or large tumors (>10 cm) due to ↑ malignancy risk
- FDG-PET is more sensitive than CT/MRI and MIBG for metastatic disease
- Genetic testing should be considered for Pts w/: paraganglioma, metastatic or bilateral or multifocal dz, + family history, syndromic presentation, onset at young age (<45 yr)

Treatment
- Once a tumor is found, it must NOT be biopsied; can lead to a pheochromocytoma crisis and possibly death
- Definitive therapy is surgical removal of the tumor; adrenalectomy if tumor is in the adrenal gland; specialized approach required for paragangliomas
- Most pheochromocytomas can be removed laparoscopically except for large tumors (>6–8 cm) and those that are clearly malignant
- Perioperatively: combined α- and β-adrenergic blockade to control blood pressure and prevent intraoperative hypertensive crises

Perioperative Medical Management of Pheochromocytoma	
α-adrenergic blockade	Given ~2 wk preoperatively to normalize BP and expand intravascular volume (to prevent severe hypotension after tumor removal)
Nonspecific α-adrenergic blockade	**Phenoxybenzamine:** preferred, conventional drug; long-acting and irreversible; initial dose is 10 mg once or twice daily → increase by 10–20 mg in divided doses every 48–72 hr as needed to control BP → final dose is often between 20 and 100 mg daily; side effects are common and include orthostasis, nasal stuffiness, fatigue, and retrograde ejaculation (men)
Selective α1-adrenergic blockade	Prazosin, terazosin, doxazosin Associated with fewer adverse effects and lower costs
β-adrenergic blockade	Initiated AFTER adequate α-blockade to control tachycardia; usually 2–3 d preoperatively; NEVER first because this can lead to unopposed α-adrenergic receptor stimulation, hypertensive crisis
Calcium channel blockers	Alternative regimen; can also be used as add-on drug; or as intravenous infusion intraoperatively (ie, nicardipine)
Metyrosine	Inhibits catecholamine synthesis; may be used in combination with α-blockade for short period to further stabilize BP

- Followup: Annual biochemical testing to assess for recurrent or metastatic disease

CARDIORENAL SYNDROME (CRS)

Classification of Cardiorenal Syndrome	
Type 1	Acute HF leading to acute kidney injury
Type 2	Chronic HF leading to chronic kidney disease
Type 3	Acute renal failure presenting with fluid overload/HF
Type 4	Chronic renal failure contributes to heart disease (ie, associated with LVH/ diastolic dysfunction, coronary artery disease, arrhythmias)
Type 5	Systemic disorder causes both cardiac and renal dysfunction (ie, sepsis)

Background

- CRS: the interaction between kidney and CV systems where acute or chronic changes in one organ leads to adaptive (or maladaptive) changes in the other organ system
- Risk factors for HF and renal insufficiency overlap. 38–55% of patients had DM (more frequent w/ worsened renal function), 70–80% had a h/o HTN, and advancing age was more common with increasing creatinine (ADHERE J Card Fail 2007;13:422).
- Chronic HF is a/w CKD. Among 80,098 pts w/ HF 63% had any renal dysfunction with 29% being rated as "moderate to severe." Mortality was higher in those with renal dysfunction w/ a stronger effect in those w/ worse renal function (RR 1.48 for any impairment and 1.8 for mild–severe dysfunction) (JACC 2006;47:1987)
- Pts admitted with acute decompensated heart failure (ADHF) may experience worsening renal function (WRF). 27% of 1,004 pts with ADHF experience WRF (JACC 2004;43:61). High R-sided venous pressures correlated best (JACC 2009;53:589)
- WRF may occur in the setting of diuretic use, although some pts may show improvement. In a study of 443 patients ADHF, only 10% worsened w/ diuresis while 27% improved. Larger BP drop was predictor of WRF with cardiac index (CI) and change in RA pressure not being predictive (Eur J Heart Fail 2013;15:433). The frequency of WRF with diuresis varies between studies, ranging from 10–40%.
- In ESRD patients, LVH is very common (>70%) and 40% carry a diagnosis on CHF

Pathogenesis

- <u>Neurohormonal</u>: reduction in cardiac output leads to arterial underfilling → activation of the RAAS, sympathetic nervous system, and endothelin release → arterial vasoconstriction with a reduction in renal blood flow
- <u>Reduced cardiac output</u>: perhaps an overstated contribution to GFR decline, as changes in intraglomerular pressure work to maintain GFR, at least when CI >1.5. In 575 patients with PA catheters in place, there was no association between CI and GFR or WRF (JACC 2016;67:2199), an effect that was confirmed when looking at UNOS registry of patients listed for heart transplantation (JACC 2016;68:874)
- <u>Venous congestion</u>: backward flow from RV dysfunction → venous congestion in an encapsulated kidney → mechanical compression with ↑ in interstitial and intratubular pressure → ↓ GFR. In addition, there is a redistribution of blood flow from the cortical tissue (where glomeruli are) to the medullary compartment. In human studies of HF with renal dysfunction, there is a stronger correlation with RA pressure than CI, an effect that may be modified by systemic arterial pressure. With lower SBP sensitizing patients to a reduction in GFR a/w venous hypertension (Heart Fail Rev 2018;23:291)
- <u>Renal adaptation to HF</u>: in the setting of chronic hypoperfusion, the juxtaglomerular apparatus hypertrophies, glomerulus may undergo ischemic type atrophy with associated progressive interstitial fibrosis or "thyroidization" where tubular atrophy is out of proportion to the degree of fibrosis. These effects are likely worsening by elevated levels of neurohormonal factors (eg, AII) and cytokines (eg, TGF-β)
- <u>Cardiac adaptation to AKI</u>: AKI is a/w fluid retention that results in increased LV end-diastolic pressures. In addition, alteration in Ca^{2+}, K^+, HCO_3^-, all ↓ cardiomyocyte contractility and predispose to arrhythmia. Cytokine release from injury renal tubules have independent effects on mitochondrial oxygen consumption as well as increase pulmonary capillary bed permeability.
- <u>Cardiac adaptation to CKD</u>: chronic fluid overload and HTN lead to progressive LVH. Elevations in RAAS markers, alterations in FGF-23 signaling through the IGF receptor, and oxidative stress all contribute to cardiac fibrosis and impaired relaxation, leading to the rates of CHF >40% in the ESRD population

Treatment

- Loop diuretics: standard of care for ADHF even in renal dysfunction. Torsemide and bumetanide have lower intrapatient and interpatient variability in absorption. Torsemide (c/t furosemide) is a/w ↓ readmission rates 17% vs 32% *(Am J Med 2001;111:513)*
- IV loop diuretics are preferred. In one study, there was no difference in outcomes at 72 hr between continuous vs bolus. However, high-dose group (received ×2.5 their home dose) were ×2 as likely to be able to convert to an oral regimen at 48 hr than low-dose group (continued on their home dose given IV) *(DOSE NEJM 2011;364:797)*
- Add a thiazide diuretic (hydrochlorothiazide, chlorthalidone, or metolazone), spironolactone, or CA inhibitor if refractory edema despite loop diuretics
- ACE inhibition: a mainstay of therapy in HF w/ reduced EF and improves long-term survival. However, its use in these patients has not resulted in reduced risk of renal insufficiency
- Inotropic support: dopamine, dobutamine, or milrinone (requires dose adjustment for CrCl, may ↓ BP with vasodilation) may be considered in persistent CHF despite maximal dose diuretics and/or evidence of low output state

Prognosis of HF With Associated Renal Dysfunction

- Lower eGFR in HF is consistently a/w worse mortality. ↑ RR independent of EF: eGFR 30–59: 1.13; eGFR 15–29: 1.85; and eGFR <15: 2.96 *(Open Heart 2016;3:e000324)*
- WRF during treatment of acute HF is a/w a worse prognosis, with an RR of 1.48 when eGFR declines by 11–15 and 3.2 with a decline >15
- Decongestion (despite WRF) may be a/w improved survival *(Circulation 2010;122:265)*

Prognosis of Renal Failure With Associated Cardiac Disease

- In ESRD pts the presence of HF a/w a doubling of mortality at 2 yr – 16.6% vs 33% *(USRDS 2018 Annual Report)*
- Compared to the general population, patients with CKD are less likely to undergo revascularization and have worse outcomes after cardiac catheterization and CABG. However, revascularized patients do better than those who do not undergo these procedures (reviewed in CAD and CKD)

CORONARY ARTERY DISEASE (CAD)

Background

- Patients with CKD have much higher rates of CAD than the general population: 39.4% of adults >65 yr old have CAD compared to 15.6% in those without CKD
- Even young patients are at risk for CAD. Among patients aged 20–40, 18% on HD carry diagnosis of CAD *(USRDS 2017 Annual Data Report)*, as opposed to only 0.6% of general population *(Circulation 2015;131:e29)*
- Albuminuria on its own is a marker of ↑ risk of CV death. Hazard ratio for CV death (compared to U_{alb} <10 mg/g cr): 11–29 = 1.63, 30–299 = 1.82, >300 = 4.77; an effect that was present throughout all stages of CKD *(CKD Consortium, Lancet 2010;375:2073)*

Pathogenesis

Risk Factors for CKD + CAD		Uremia-specific Factors	
Hypertension	Diabetes	Inflammation	↑ FGF-23
Smoking	Age	↑ Phos, ↑ PTH	Indoxyl sulfate
Hyperlipidemia	Metabolic syndrome	Carbamoylation of LDL	Asymmetric dimethylarginine

- Risk factors for CAD and CKD overlap, but uremia plays a role as well

Treatment of CAD in CKD	
CKD not on HD	**CKD on HD**
Statin Use	
Meta-analysis showed a ↓ cardiac mortality, RR = 0.8 *(Ann IM 2012;157:251)* Simvastatin 20 mg qd + Ezetimibe 10 mg qd: 17% risk ↓ for major atherosclerotic events, driven mainly by ↓ ischemic stroke and revascularizations *(SHARP Lancet 2011;377:2181)*	No clinical benefit in 1255 dialysis pts w/ DM *(4D NEJM 2005;353:238)* Subgroup pts w/ starting LDL >145 had ↓ primary endpoint (HR 0.59), cardiac death (HR 0.48) *(4D CJASN 2011;6:1316)* No difference in primary outcome at 3.8 yr *(AURORA NEJM 2009;360:1395)*

Blood Pressure Control	
↓ CV events w/ similar efficacy as in non-CKD w/ 17% risk ↓ per 5 of ↓ SBP w/o class difference (*BMJ 2013;347:f5680*) Target <130/80 (140/90 if UACR <30 mg/g) (KDIGO CKD 2012), or perhaps 120/80 (*SPRINT NEJM 2015;373:2103; JASN 2017;28:2812*)	No RCT. Observational data suggest a U- or J-shaped curve with ↑ mortality at lower or higher BPs. Pre-HD BP a/w the best outcomes differ between studies and range from SBP 130–159 with DBP 60–99 (*KI 2012;82:570*)
Percutaneous Coronary Intervention (PCI)	
CKD pts w/ NSTEMI are much less likely to undergo PCI (41% stage 4, 20% stage 5), even though CKD pts who undergo PCI are twice as likely to survive to discharge (*JAHA 2018;7:e007920*) In pts w/ eGFR <60, drug eluting stents (DES) vs bare metal stents (BMS), revealed a ↓ all-cause mortality (RR = 0.8), ↓ cardiac death and target vessel revascularization (*J Interv Cardiol 2018;31:319*)	Angiographic success is similar between HD patients and nonuremic controls, but long-term survival is much worse for ESRD patients, with a 3–4 fold ↑ mortality at 1 yr Similar to CKD not HD population, ESRD patients receiving DES have a 18% relative risk reduction in death and a 13% risk reduction in death, MI, and target vessel revascularization (*JACC 2016;67:1459*)
Coronary Artery Bypass Graft Surgery (CABG)	
↑ Mortality, risk of myocardial injury, deep tissue infection, prolonged ICU stay, ventilation (*NDT 2010;25:3654*) ↑ Renal progression at 3 mo (compared to PCI or medical therapy), but no difference at 2 yr. The mortality risk at 24 mo was lower (3.9%) c/w PCI (14.5%) or medical therapy (16.4%) (*Coron Artery Dis 2018;29:8*)	↑ In-hospital mortality (12.2 vs 3.0%), mediastinitis (3.6 vs 1.2%), stroke (4.3 vs 1.7%) (*Circulation 2000;102:2973*) Despite ↑ early mortality, ESRD pts undergoing CABG have lower 1 yr mortality compared to ESRD pts w/ CAD who do not undergo CABG, and lower risk of revascularization compared to patients undergoing PCI

Prognosis
- After ACS (NSTEMI or STEMI), CKD-non HD patients have a higher mortality at 180 d (10.3% vs 3.4%). CAD risk factors are also more common in CKD, after adjustment—each 10 ↓ in CrCl ↑ 180 d mortality with RR = 1.1 (*Circulation 2002;106:974*)
- There is a graded decrement in 2-yr survival patients with CAD, with worse outcomes among patients with worse CKD. 2-yr survival: no CKD: 87.4%, Stage 1–2: 81.1%, Stage 3: 77.6%, Stage 4–5: 67.4% (USRDS 2018 Annual Data Report)

CARDIAC CATHETERIZATION

Background
- More than 1 million cardiac catheterizations performed in the US annually
- Since risk factors for CAD and CKD overlap, many patients requiring catheterization have underlying renal dysfunction. Stage 3A: 17%, 3B: 9.2%, 4–5: 2.9% (*JAHA 2014;3:e001380*)
- Reported rates of AKI after cardiac cath range from 3–20% depending on patient risk factors, procedural factors (eg, contrast dose), and definition of AKI used
- From 2001–2011, number of postcatheterization AKI cases has ↑ 3-fold (*JAHA 2016;5:e002739*)

Pathogenesis of Kidney Injury
- Renal hypoperfusion in ACS, hypotension related to cardiogenic shock
- Cholesterol emboli from procedural manipulation of vasculature
- RBC breakdown products/pigment related to hemolysis from IABP or Impella device

Risk Factors of Kidney Injury	
CKD	Graded increased risk by starting eGFR with values <30 mL/min a/w highest risk of AKI or AKI-D
Diabetes	1.5–2× increased risk compared to non-DM with same eGFR
Age	Each 10 yr increase a/w relative risk 1.1–1.2 for CIN
Hemodynamics	CHF (at presentation or prior), hypotension, and need for intra-aortic balloon pump, all independently increase risk of AKI
Indication	STEMI >> NSTEMI/unstable angina >> elective procedure

Contrast	High osmolar >> Low or iso-osmolar Contrast volume:creatinine clearance ratio: risk of AKI begins to increase at ratios between 2 and 3
Others	Hyperglycemia (w/o diagnosis of DM), anemia, proteinuria (independent of eGFR), NSAIDs, multiple myeloma (possible), complex coronary lesions

Predicting AKI after Catheterization

- Risk of CIN ranges from <1% to >50% in individual patients
- Stratification can identify patients who benefit from additional interventions (see below) to reduce risk of AKI, or identify patients in whom catheterization should be deferred (AHA guideline for PCI JACC 2011;58:24)
- Many prediction equations exist but were generated on data obtained prior to renal sparing interventions, newer contrast agents, and low contrast volume PCI
- Mehran Risk Score includes 11 clinical and procedures factors and has been externally validated (JACC 2004;44:1393)
- National Cardiovascular Data Registry (NCDR) AKI score was developed using >900,000 patients and has been validated in US and overseas, with AKI defined by the Acute Kidney Injury Network criteria, using a modern treatment cohort. 11 clinical characteristics for AKI and 6 clinical characteristics for AKI-Dialysis (JAHA 2014;3:e001380)

Prevention

- Modifiable risk factors with the largest impact are volume status and volume of contrast used. Volume resuscitation avoids hypotension and prevents renal vasoconstriction that could be worsened with contrast administration.
- Frequent examination required as saline administration can be limited by CHF symptoms

Intervention for AKI after PCI	
Fluid	Randomized trial data limited but suggest IV better than unrestricted oral hydration (though oral salt loading may have benefit). Regimens vary ranging from 3 mL/kg for 1 hr to 1 mL/kg for 6 hr prior to cath, continuing postprocedure at 1 mL/kg for 4–6 hr
Type of IVF	NaHCO$_3$ solutions have theoretical benefit of altered urine pH → lower free radical generation → lower AKI. Clinic trials comparing to NS have been mixed with (–) well-designed trials (NEJM 2018;378:603)
LVEDP-guided fluid	Direct measurement of LVEDP during cath detects underfilling as well as avoids giving fluid to patients already at risk for HF. LVEDP-guided fluid administration reduced risk of AKI by 60% (POSEIDON Lancet 2014;383:1814)
Acetylcysteine	Free radical scavenger with mixed results in RCTs. Unlikely to be effective. IV preparation has 3–5% risk of anaphylactoid reaction.
Prophylactic dialysis	Several studies have shown NO benefit of dialysis or hemofiltration prior to contrast or postcatheterization dialysis to remove contrast in hopes of reducing renal toxicity (Am J Med 2012;125:66)
Statins	Mixed results when compared to NS alone, though patients likely to be initiated on statin at time of discharge regardless, may be worth initiating prior to contrast exposure
Diuretics	Diuretics alone do not ↓ risk of AKI and may worsen. Forced diuresis matching IVF to urine output using RenalGuard system may lessen AKI (MYTHOS JACC Cardiovasc Inter 2012;5:90)
Access	Radial access may reduce risk of AKI over femoral access; OR 0.57 (0.35–0.91) (Am J Card 2017;120:2141)

Evaluation

- DDx: prerenal AKI from hypoperfusion/cardiogenic shock, volume depletion in patients who have postprocedural bleeding, cholesterol emboli syndrome
- Unlike other nephrotoxic AKI, urine Na and FE$_{Na}$ is frequently low or unchanged from prior to procedure (NEJM 1989;320:149)
- Cholesterol emboli/renal atheroemboli: presentation is usually subacute over 1–2 wk w/o improvement. Approximately 2/3 will have eosinophilia and 1/3 will have reduced complement levels. Skin findings of livedo reticularis, digital infarcts, and new neurologic deficits are strongly suggestive but not always present.

Prognosis

- In hospital mortality for AKI ~5–10%, with mortality for AKI-D ~20% (JAHA 2016;5:e002739)
- At 1 yr, risk of death remains higher in patients who experienced post-cath AKI, as are rates of reinfarction and target vessel revascularization (Circ Cardiovasc Interv 2015;8:e002475)
- Of all, patients with a 50–99% increase in creatinine between days 3–7, 28% will continue to have elevated creatinine 3 mo later. Those with more severe early AKI, >50% will have sustained loss of function and a more rapid rate of decline in renal function between mo 3 and 24 after exposure (KI 2010;78:803)

ATRIAL FIBRILLATION (AFib)

Background

- The annual incidence of being newly diagnosed with AFib ↑ as renal function declines; 40% of stage 4–5 CKD pts will develop AFib over 2 yr (USRDS 2017 Annual Data Report)
- 18% w/ CKD had AFib (25% >70 y/o), ×2–3 of non-CKD (CRIC AHJ 2010;159:1102)
- AFib is a/w a 67–80% ↑ in rate of ↓ of renal function, including progression to ESRD
- Patients with CKD and AFib are at higher risk for stroke than patients with either condition alone, with those on dialysis having the highest risk. Proteinuria itself is a/w an almost 50% increase in risk (ATRIA Circulation 2009;119:1363)

Pathogenesis

- AFib and CKD share common risk factors. In addition, CKD contributes to HTN (largest population-based risk factor for AFib), volume expansion + LVH → ↑ left atrial volume, electrolytes abnormalities, myocardial fibrosis, and atherosclerosis—all of which may contribute to the ↑ risk.
- Patients with CKD have slower atrial appendage emptying, ↑ frequency of spontaneous atrial appendage echocontrast, ↑ platelet aggregation in response to c-AMP and ET-1, ↑ markers of inflammation and activation of tissue factor pathway, all of which have been a/w an ↑ risk of thrombotic events (JACC 2016;68:1452)

Treatment Considerations

- In addition to having an ↑ risk of thrombotic events, ESRD pts are at higher risk of hemorrhage, w/ ×10 ↑ risk of intracranial bleeds and ×3–4 ↑ risk of GI bleeding
- In non-end-stage CKD pts, balance of risks and benefits favors warfarin use (HR of thrombotic event 0.7 and death 0.65). However, multiple cohort studies in ESRD patients suggests no reduction in stoke (in some studies, higher risk), no reduction in mortality, and a consistent increase in risk of bleeding (Chest 2016;149:951)
- Data regarding Novel Oral Anticoagulants (NOACs) in dialysis patients are limited since most are at least partially eliminated by the kidneys and patients with advanced CKD were excluded from randomized trials. Apixaban at a dose of 2.5 mg BID appears to show similar pharmacokinetics to the 5 mg BID dose in patients with normal renal function (JASN 2017;28:2241) but efficacy studies are not available yet.

SUDDEN CARDIAC DEATH (SCD) AND AICD

Background

- With each stage of CKD, patients experience higher mortality rates (no CKD: 43, stage 1–2: 79, stage 3: 97, stage 4–5: 170 per 1,000 patient-yr). And among those with ESRD, 40% of these deaths are attributed to SCD/Arrhythmia (USRDS 2017 Annual Data Report)
- Common in 1st 2 wk of chronic dialysis (CJASN 2011;6:2642)

Pathogenesis

- Rates of ischemic heart disease approach 40% in dialysis patients. At least part of the elevated risk of SCD related to ischemic events from underlying atherosclerosis, as SCD risk is higher in patients with known CAD and diabetes.
- Electrolyte fluctuations lead to abnormalities in cell membrane stability and polarization. Low K^+ dialysate (<2 mEq/L) was a/w ×2 ↑ risk of SCD (KI 2001;60:350; 2011;79:218)
- Low Ca^{2+} baths have been a/w QTc prolongation and cardiac death (CJASN 2013;8:797)
- Abnormal fluid balance leads to development of CHF, and rapid removal of fluid during dialysis may lead to myocardial hypoperfusion and microvascular ischemia. Increased rates of fluid removal (>13 mL/kg/hr) are a/w ↑ all-cause and CV mortality (KI 2011;79:250)
- The combined impact of additional fluid and electrolyte overload manifests in HD pts as an ↑ risk of mortality during the long (72 hr) interval between dialysis sessions. Compared to other times during the week, the 72-hr interval is a/w a 36% ↑ CV mortality, 23% ↑ in all-cause mortality, and a 90% ↑ risk of dysrhythmia (NEJM 2011;365:1099)

Prevention
- Avoid rapid UF >13 mL/kg/hr and long interdialytic interval (NEJM 2011;365:1099)
- Avoid 0 or 1 K (KI 2001;60:350; 2011;79:218), <2.5 Ca and high bicarbonate (DOPPS AJKD 2013;62:738) dialysate; Avoid digoxin (JASN 2010;21:1550)
- β blockers: in ESRD w/ cardiomyopathy, addition of carvedilol was a/w a 21.5% ↓ in mortality over 2 yr (JACC 2003;41:1438). Among >40,000 pts followed in the Gambro dialysis system, β blocker was a/w an ↑ likelihood of surviving arrest (CJASN 2007;2:491). However, other observational trials have given inconsistent results (AJKD 2018;72:337). Use nondialyzable β blockers (carvedilol) instead of dialyzable β blockers (atenolol, acebutolol, bisoprolol, or metoprolol) (CJASN 2018;13:604; JASN 2015;26:987)
- ACEi/ARBs: fosinopril did not ↓ CV events in ESRD w/ LVH (FOSIDIAL KI 2006;70:1318)

Automated Implantable Cardioverter-Defibrillator (AICD)
- Remains controversial in patients with renal disease
- Patients with renal failure have higher arrhythmia event rates but also higher rates of competing death
- Patients with CKD and eGFR >30 likely benefit. Those with eGFR <30 or advanced age are much less likely to benefit (CJASN 2015;10:1119)
- Ideally, should be placed on side opposite AV access to reduce venous congestion and allow venoplasty or venous stent placement if needed to maintain access patency

PULMONOLOGY

- Interorgan crosstalk between the kidneys and lungs is not limited to "pulmonary–renal" syndromes. AKI/CKD may affect lung function and acute/chronic lung disease may affect kidney function.
- Reduced lung function is a/w several factors that may contribute to the development of CKD: hypoxia (↑ HIF-1α, ↑ RAS activation, ↑ SNS activation); RV dysfunction (↓ perfusion due to ↑ renal venous pressure); chronic inflammation (AJKD 2017;70:675)
- Impaired lung function is common in CKD. In pts w/ ACR ≥30, 15.6/9.8% had obstructive/restrictive lung function. In pts w/ ACR ≥30, OR for obstructive lung function 1.42 and OR for restrictive lung function 1.43 (NHANES AJKD 2016;68:414)
- Reduced baseline lung function (esp. ↓ %-predicted FVC) was a/w ↑ risk of incident ESRD and ↑ risk of CKD progression (ARIC AJKD 2017;70:675)

Acute Lung Injury (ALI)

- AKI is common in patients with ALI: AKIN stage 1: 54.1%, stage 2: 12.3%, stage 3: 15%. AKI defined by change in Cr may be masked in presence of fluid overload. When adjusted for fluid balance, incidence of AKI increased to stage 1: 61.8%, stage 2: 19.3%, stage 3: 17.2%. Patients with AKI that was only diagnosed after adjusting for fluid balance had similar mortality to patients with AKI, and higher mortality than those without AKI (ARDS Network FACTT Crit Care Med 2011;39:2665).
- ALI managed w/ low tidal volume (4–6 mL/kg) ventilator strategy. Low volume → respiratory acidosis → acidemia. Patients in ARDS network study less likely to develop AKI if treated with low tidal volume. Treatment w/ HCO₃ may worsen acidemia in this setting, so earlier initiation of RRT may be needed to prevent complications of acidemia (CJASN 2008;3:578)
- In ALI, conservative fluid strategy (CVP <4, PCWP <8) a/w improved oxygenation index and lung injury vs liberal fluid strategy (CVP 10–14, PCWP 14–18). Baseline Cr good in both groups (Cr 1.24 vs 1.29) and no difference in need for RRT between groups (10 vs 14%). Impact on course of pre-existing AKI or CKD not studied (FACTT NEJM 2006;354:2564)
- Inhaled NO, used in ARDS, a/w ↑ AKI (RR 1.52) in dose-dependent fashion. Risk of AKI not present with low or medium cumulative dose, or when iNO used in absence of ARDS. Possible mechanism: reactive nitrogen species → oxidative injury (Critical Care 2015;15:137)
- Prone positioning may be used in severe ALI → ↑ intra-abdominal pressure, but no effect on renal perfusion or renal function (Anesth Analg 2001;92:1226)

COPD

- The prevalence of CKD is ↑ in COPD, occurring with 2–3× frequency c/w pts w/o COPD. Presence of cachexia and muscle wasting in COPD may mask diagnosis of CKD, as patients may have low GFR with normal creatinine. In pts with COPD exacerbation, more advanced CKD a/w ↑ mortality (Int J COPD 2015;10:2027)

- AKI more common in COPD (1.4 vs 0.6%), esp. among patients with preexisting CKD or CHF. AKI occurring during COPD exacerbations a/w ↑ short-term mortality *(Int J COPD 2015;10:2027; 2013;8:127)*
- ↑ Inflammation → endothelial dysfunction → albuminuria. UACR higher w/ more advanced COPD and albuminuria in COPD a/w ↑ mortality *(Chest 2015;147:56; Eur Respir J 2014;43:1042).*

COPD and Dialysis

- COPD is common (7.5% prevalence) in ESRD on dialysis. Mortality is higher for ESRD w/ COPD (RR 1.20), esp. in active smokers (RR 1.28). COPD pts w/ ESRD are less likely to receive a KT (RR 0.47 for active smokers, 0.54 for nonsmokers) *(AJN 2012;36:287).*
- COPD HD patients are more likely to have prolonged intradialytic hypoxemia, which is associated w/ ↑ risk of hospitalization and ↑ mortality *(CJASN 2016;11:616)*
- With standard HCO_3 dialysate, P_{CO_2} ↑, HCO_3 ↑ and pH ↑ during HD. PO_2 ↓ and A-a gradient ↑ during treatment *(Ann Clin Lab Sci 2011;41:315)*
- Fluid removal >3% of body weight during HD may ↑ FEV_1 and FVC temporarily in COPD *(Hemodial Int 2016;20:68)*
- COPD pts starting on CAPD may have ↓ FVC, ↓ VC, ↓ TLC that reverses within 2 wk, without changes in PO_2, PCO_2, or pH *(Chest 1984;86:874)*

SMOKING AND IDIOPATHIC NODULAR GLOMERULOSCLEROSIS (ING)

- Chronic ischemic/hypoxic conditions can cause ING w/ nodular mesangial sclerosis w/ accentuated glomerular lobularity, mimicking diabetic nephropathy, MPGN, dys-proteinemias, organized glomerular deposition diseases *(JASN 2007;18:2032)*
- ING linked to chronic HTN and cigarette smoking. Patients more likely to be older, white, male; 95.7% with HTN and 91.3% w/ h/o heavy cigarette smoking. Nephrotic-range proteinuria common (70%) but NS uncommon (21%). Mean time from biopsy to ESRD 26 mo. ↑ IF/TA and vascular disease a/w progression to ESRD. Smoking cessation and RAAS blockade a/w better survival *(Human Pathology 2002;33:826)*
- Smoking may cause ING via ↑ AGEs, ↑ oxidative stress, ↑ angiogenesis, ↑ sympathetic activation *(JASN 2007;18:2032)*

PULMONARY HYPERTENSION (PHTN)

- PHTN is common in CKD, and CKD is common in PAH. PHTN (PAP >25 mmHg) occurs in 23% of pt w/ CKD, and severe PHTN (PAP ≥45–50) in 7–29% of HD pts. PD < HD, likely due to differences in comorbidities *(AJKD 2018;72:75; KI 2013;8:682)*
- PHTN in CKD → ↑ mortality (RR 1.4 CKD, 2.3 ESRD, 2.1 after KTx), ↑ CV events (RR CKD 1.7, ESRD 2.3), ↑ CV mortality (RR 2.3) *(AJKD 2018;72:75)*
- CKD occurs in 4–36% of PAH. Prevalence of CKD higher in PAH-associated connective tissue disorder, esp. SSc. CKD in PAH → ↑ risk of death *(Pulm Circ 2017;17:38)*. In pts with PAH and CHF exacerbation, AKI is common (23%), more common if CKD (OR 3.9) and a/w ↑ mortality (OR 5.3) *(J Cardiac Failure 2011;17:533)*
- Mechanisms of CKD: ↑ SNS activity, ↑ RAAS activity → pulmonary/renal vascular remodeling; ↑ RA pressure → ↑ renal vein congestion; endothelial dysfunction in uremia → ↑ pulmonary vasoconstriction; ↑ PCWP *(Pulm Circ 2017;17:38; KI 2013;8:682)*

OBSTRUCTIVE SLEEP APNEA (OSA)

- Common in ESRD (>50%) with similar prevalence in HD and PD. No studies on whether CPAP reduces CV risk and mortality in ESRD patients with OSA, although switching to nocturnal HD a/w improved symptoms *(Semin Dial 2013;26:273)*
- More common in CKD, seen in up to 65%. Nocturnal hypoxemia in OSA is a/w more rapid decline in GFR. Possible mechanisms: endothelial cell dysfunction, ↑ oxidative stress, ↑ RAS activation *(CJASN 2013;8:1502)*
- ↑ Risk of albuminuria independent of the presence of DM or HTN. ↑ UACR may correlate w/ severity of OSA. Treatment of OSA with CPAP is a/w a ↓ in UACR *(Medicine 2016;95:26).*
- Risk factor for developing HTN (risk increased nearly 3-fold in OSA). OSA is a common cause of resistant HTN. OSA patients with resistant HTN treated with CPAP show improvement in BP (↓ 4.78/1.53) *(J Clin Hypertens 2016;18:153)*

CYSTIC FIBROSIS (CF)

- Nephrocalcinosis: 23.2% on u/s, 92% on biopsy *(Turk J Ped 2004;46:22; NEJM 1988;319:263)*
- Nephrolithiasis: 3.0–6.3%. Possible mechanisms: fat malabsorption → ↑ GI oxalate absorption → hyperoxaluria → ↑ CaOx saturation in urine; hypocitraturia

- ↓ *O. formigenes* in GI tract → ↓ breakdown of oxalate in GI tract → ↑ GI oxalate absorption → hyperoxaluria → ↑ CaOx saturation in urine *(AJKD 2003;42:1)*
- Prevalence of CKD (stages 3–5) in CF 2.3%. Disease prevalence doubles with every 10-yr increase in age, reaching 19.2% in patients over 55. Risk of CKD greater in CF-related DM, but not with increasing pulmonary exacerbations of CF *(AJRCCM 2001;184:1147)*
- CF-related DM: microalbuminuria in 14–21%. Patients w/ CF-related DM more likely to have microalbuminuria and less likely to have retinopathy than patients with DM1 *(J Cyst Fibrosis 2008;7:515; Diabetes Care 2007;30:1056)*
- Other causes of intrinsic CKD: AA amyloidosis, IgAN *(CJASN 2009;4:921)*
- AKI in CF most commonly drug-induced from nephrotoxic antibiotics (aminoglycosides, polymyxin B, colistin). NSAIDs used in pediatric patients, may cause AKI if acutely volume depleted *(J Cyst Fibrosis 2008;12:309)*.
- AKI rarely due to acute oxalate nephropathy: fat malabsorption → ↑ GI oxalate absorption → hyperoxaluria → ↑ calcium oxalate deposition in kidney *(AJT 2008;8:1901)*

SARCOIDOSIS *(AJKD 2006;48:856)*

- Granulomas and macrophages make 1-α hydroxylase → ↑ 1,25-(OH)$_2$ vitamin D (calcitriol)
- Hypercalciuria: U$_{Ca}$ >300 mg/d, 50% (m/c renal manifestation); ↑ calcitriol → ↓ PTH → ↓ tubular Ca^{2+} reabsorption
- Hypercalcemia: 10–20%; ↑ calcitriol → ↑ GI Ca^{2+} absorption, ↑ bone reabsorption → ↑ Ca^{2+}
- Prednisone 20–40 mg/d can improve hypercalcemia and hypercalciuria d/t ↓ macrophage 1-α hydroxylase activity
- Noncaseating granulomatous interstitial nephritis: 7–23% on autopsy, most cases clinically silent. Treatment with prednisone 1 mg/kg/d for 6–12 mo improves renal function but most left with CKD. Relapses uncommon (~15%), more likely to occur after prednisone d/c, but also respond to prednisone *(Medicine 2009;88:98)*.
- ESRD rare; KT safe if ESRD develops, but sarcoid GIN can recur in KT *(PLOS One 2014;9:1)*
- Renal tubular dysfunction: common; polyuria from ↑ Ca^{2+}-induced NDI; CDI in neurosarcoidosis; pRTA, dRTA, or Fanconi-like syndrome from tubular damage from ↑ Ca^{2+} or GIN. Tubular abnormalities improve with steroids.

TUBERCULOSIS

- Extrapulmonary TB more common in HIV or organ transplants. 27% of extrapulmonary TB are GU. GU TB occurs in 2–20% of pts with pulmonary TB. GU TB primarily involves the collecting system and less commonly causes parenchymal lesions.
- TB seeding of GU tract can occur with primary infection or reactivation. TB bacilli form granulomas in medulla → rupture into tubular lumen with excretion into collecting system. Descending infection can lead to papillary necrosis, ureteral stricture and obstruction, hydronephrosis, and renal dysfunction. Typically, unilateral; if bilateral can lead to ESRD.
- Urinary symptoms common, systemic symptoms uncommon
- Labs: sterile pyuria and gross or microscopic hematuria
- Renal parenchymal lesions: AA amyloidosis from chronic inflammation; interstitial nephritis; postinfectious GN
- Diagnosis of renal TB: isolation of TB from urine culture or tissue biopsy
- Treatment: anti-TB antibiotics. If obstruction present and renal dysfunction reversible, may require ureteral stenting or nephrostomy. Partial or total nephrectomy may be required in up to 55% *(Am J Trop Med Hyg 2013;88:54)*

INTERSTITIAL LUNG DISEASE (ILD)

- CKD is common in IPF, with 30% of patients having eGFR <60. CKD more common in older patients and patients with HTN. CKD associated with ↓ DLCO and ↓ distance on 6-min walk test. eGFR independent predictor of survival in IPF after adjusting for age and PFTs *(Respiration 2017;94:346)*
- ILD a/w ANCA: usually >65 y/o, MPO (+); pulmonary fibrosis occurs concurrently or predates by several mo to 12 yr; usual interstitial pneumonia is the m/c radiological pattern; ILD has an adverse impact on the prognosis *(Autoimmun Rev 2017;16:722)*

mTOR Inhibitor-Associated Pneumonitis *(Transplantation 2004;77:1215; Ann IM 2006;144:505; Transplant Proc 2018;15:933)*

- In up to 4.3% of txp pts receiving everolimus and up to 11–17% receiving sirolimus
- Not related to drug levels; ~50% of cases occur after >6 mo of drug exposure
- Symptoms: cough, fatigue, fevers, and dyspnea. Pulmonary infiltrates are common and resemble BOOP.

- No formal diagnostic criteria, so r/o infectious etiology. BAL shows lymphocytic alveolitis.
- Treatment: permanent withdrawal of mTOR inhibitor +/– steroids
- Clinical and radiographic recovery typically occur w/i a few weeks of drug d/c

DIFFUSE ALVEOLAR HEMORRHAGE (DAH)

- Caused by disruption of the alveolar-capillary basement membrane; small vessel vasculitis can cause injury to glomerular capillary wall together causing pulmonary renal syndrome
- Life-threatening condition requiring prompt diagnosis and treatment

Conditions Associated With DAH With Renal Impairment (NEJM 2012;367:1540)

- ANCA-associated disease, Anti-GBM disease, SLE +/–, antiphospholipid syndrome
- HSP, mixed cryoglobulinemia, polymyositis, progressive systemic sclerosis, MCTD
- HIV, disseminated cryptococcosis, Legionnaires disease, CMV, strep or staph infection
- Uremic pneumonitis: cardiogenic pulmonary edema d/t HTN and/or volume overload

Clinical Manifestation and Diagnosis

- Hemoptysis may be absent in ~1/3 of cases; should suspect with radiographic opacities (either localized or diffuse) and falling Hb level; PFT: ↑ DLCO
- Confirmed when lavage aliquots are progressively more hemorrhagic
- ✓ ANCA, anti-GBM, ASLO, C3, C4, ANA, RF, cryocrit, APLA, and blood culture
- Biopsy: lung, skin (if rash present), or kidney

Treatment

- Invasive or noninvasive mechanical ventilation, correct coagulopathy, transfusion prn
- Pulse glucocorticoid + PLEX: empirically when autoimmune conditions are suspected

PLEURAL EFFUSION

- Nonmalignant pleural effusion + renal failure 1-yr mortality is 46% (Chest 2017;151:1099)
- 20% of hospitalized HD pts, commonly from hypervolemia (Transplant Proc 2007;39:889)
- Pleuroperitoneal leak in PD: 1.6–10%; pleural fluid/serum glucose >1 (NDT 2012;27:1212)
- Urinothorax: caused by obstructive uropathy (pelvic-ureteral, bladder outlet, pelvic mass), GU procedure, trauma; pleural fluid cr/serum cr >1 (Am J Med Sci 2017;354:44)
- Transudative: hypervolemia, nephrotic syndrome, HF, pleuroperitoneal leak
- Exudative: uremic pleuritic, parapneumonic effusion

EXTRACORPOREAL MEMBRANE OXYGENATION

Background

- Extracorporeal Membrane Oxygenation (ECMO) provides gas exchange for hypoxemia and hypercarbia as well as hemodynamic depending on configuration and indication
- Venovenous (VV): respiratory support
- Venoarterial (VA): respiratory and hemodynamic support
- ECMO use has increased dramatically in recent yr, from 253 in 2006 to 4,297 in 2016 (ECLS registry, 1/2017)

AKI during ECMO

- AKI is common, ranging from 29–86% (pooled estimate 55.6%) with renal replacement therapy (RRT) required in 7–86% (pooled estimate 46%) (Ann Thorac Surg 2014;97:610)
- AKI requiring ECMO is a/w with high mortality (78% vs 20% non-AKI) (NDT 2006;21:2867)

Pathogenesis of ECMO-Associated AKI (Cardiorenal Med 2016;6:50)	
Patient Factors	**ECMO Related**
Hypotension, SIRS, Nephrotoxins, Hypoxia, CKD	Blood flow changes, RAAS dysregulation
	Blood–air interface, Cardiorenal syndrome, Hemo/myoglobinuria, Aortic dissection (VA), Embolism (VA)

- In 50–60%, renal failure precedes the initiation of ECMO (Pediatr Crit Care Med 2016;17:1157)
- In severe ARDS, ECMO use was a/w more days free of RRT and renal failure (EOLIA NEJM 2018;378:1965)

Renal Replacement Therapy (RRT) during ECMO

- RRT frequently initiated earlier for control of volume status
- In one survey, indication for RRT was fluid overload in 43%, prevention of fluid overload in 16%, AKI in 35%, and electrolytes in 4% (ASAIO J 2012;58:407)

- While intermittent HD and PD can be used during ECMO, CRRT or SLED is recommended at least initially until patients are stabilized
- CRRT can be used via a separate double lumen dialysis catheter but central access may be taken by other catheters (cannulate ECMO plus catheters for medication administration) and placement may be risky if on systemic anticoagulation
- Hemofilter may be placed in-line with ECMO circuit distal to ECMO roller pump (providing blood flow) with the venous return line proximal. Effluent needs to be continuously measured with replacement fluid administered to maintain the net filtration balance. In practice, this configuration provides less accurate assessment of fluid balance and more nursing work (CJASN 2012;7:1328)
- CRRT machine can be spliced into the venous limb of ECMO circuit directly. If a centrifugal ECMO pump is used, place the CRRT machine after the pump because of the risk of air entrapment. Return line of CRRT must be prior to oxygenator to trap air or clots (Critical Care 2014;18:675)
- High blood flow used for ECMO can cause high pressure on CRRT circuit. Line pressure adaptor or placement of CRRT access line ± return line before the pump has been tried without air embolism event (ASAIO J 2017;63:48)

Prognosis
- Adult patient survival to discharge in setting of ECMO + AKI ranges from 25–45% with slightly better survival when respiratory failure is the indication (ECLS Registry Report, 1/2017)
- Postcardiotomy AKI requiring ECMO is a/w high mortality ×30.8 in AKIN stage 3, ×12.6 in RIFLE-F (Eur J Cardiothorac Surg 2010;37:334)
- Renal prognosis among adult ECMO patients requiring RRT is poor, with 74% continuing to requiring dialysis in one study (NDT 2013;28:86)
- Among 200 pediatric ECMO + CRRT patients, 68 survived to discharge with 18 requiring continued dialysis (Pediatr Crit Care Med 2011;12:153)
- In pts who survive episode of AKI on ECMO, CKD is common: 12% have proteinuria and 19% have HTN at 8.2 yr, though eGFR >60 (CJASN 2014;9:2070)

GASTROENTEROLOGY

GASTROINTESTINAL SYMPTOMS (Nat Rev Nephrol 2010;6:480)

- Most common symptoms include nausea, vomiting, abdominal pain, constipation, and diarrhea; divided into organic (causal lesion) and functional (no histopathologic) basis and influenced by psychological factors, visceral hypersensitivity and altered GI motility
- Prevalence: 70–79% of pts w/ CKD and ESRD; trend toward increasing Sx w/ duration of renal failure; similar rate of sx in CKD, HD, and PD
- Etiology: uremia/uremic retention molecules, comorbid anxiety, and depression

Constipation
- Prevalence: 63% HD patients and 29% PD patients
- Etiology: ↓ activity, ↓ fiber, ↓ liquid, phosphate binders, and other comorbidities
- Tx: laxatives, stool softeners, enemas; avoid magnesium and phosphate laxatives and enema

Gastroparesis
- Prevalence: up to 36% of patients; ↑ prevalence vs general pop
- Etiology: medications, DM; related to intra-abdominal fluid in PD
- Clinical Sx: nausea, vomiting, abdominal pain, bloating, and weight loss
- Tx: metoclopramide and erythromycin; ↑ dialysis doesn't help

GASTROINTESTINAL BLEEDING (Nat Rev Nephrol 2010;6:480)

Background
- Prevalence: (+) fecal occult ~19%
- Causes: angiodysplasia, GI erosions, ulcers, diverticulosis, and mesenteric ischemia

Upper GI Bleeding
- ↑ Upper GI lesions in renal failure vs general pop
- Duodenal lesions in 61% of ESRD patients w/ (+) fecal occult
- Angiodysplasia and GI erosions most common cause of upper bleeding; angiodysplasia ~20–30% of episodes of upper GI bleeding and cause ½ of recurrent episodes of upper GI bleeding in patients with ESRD (Ann IM 1985;102:588)
- No higher risk of ulceration or H. pylori

- ↑ Acute upper GI bleeding w/ estimated frequency of 21 bleeds per 1,000 patient years; cause 3–7% of ESRD deaths; anticoagulation and antiplatelets are not a risk factor

Lower GI Bleeding

- Angiodysplasia and colonic neoplasms are common causes; angiodysplasia ~20–30% of episodes of lower GI bleeding and are the m/c cause of recurrent lower GI bleeding
- ↑ diverticulosis and diverticulitis in PKD vs general pop

Pancreatitis (*Nat Rev Nephrol* 2010;6:480)

- Prevalence: ↑ pancreatic abnormalities; ↑ risk of acute pancreatitis, PD > HD
- Etiology: similar causes general pop in PD: chronic exposure to icodextrin and high dextrose-containing dialysate are risk factors
- Diagnosis: ↓ clearance of pancreatic enzymes with renal failure → look for amylase >3× ULN, lipase >300 µg/L (>60 IU/L); in PD distinguish from peritonitis; ↑ effluent amylase level >100 U/L; inhibitory effect of icodextrin on serum amylase levels
- Tx: no heparin w/ PD and HD to ↓ risk of pancreatic hemorrhage; stop icodextrin if new

Acute Mesenteric Ischemia (*Nat Rev Nephrol* 2010;6:480)

- Incidence: higher in HD; frequency 0.3–1.9%/pt/yr; 14% of HD pts on autopsy
- Etiology: typically nonocclusive; intradialytic hypotension w/ atherosclerosis
- Common Sx: abdominal pain, fever, guarding, leukocytosis, bloody diarrhea or rectal bleeding; can mimic peritonitis
- Dx: colonoscopy, CT with an opaque enema, surgery; vascular calcification on imaging
- Prevention: avoid excessive UF and normal fluid balance with acute abdominal pain
- Mortality rates from 33–73%

Encapsulating Peritoneal Sclerosis (*Nat Rev Nephrol* 2010;6:480; *KI* 2010;77:904)

- Peritoneal thickening → encapsulation of the bowel and obstructive ileus in PD pts
- Incidence: up to 4% of PD pts; >15% in pts on PD for >15 yr
- Risk factors: PD vintage, prolonged exposure to high glucose dialysate, repeated peritonitis, PD → HD conversion, and no RRF
- Clinical Sx: early satiety, abdominal fullness, obstructive symptoms, UF failure
- Diagnosis: abdominal U/S and CT are not sensitive or specific, gold standard laparotomy/laparoscopy → peritoneal thickening encases intestines
- Tx: tamoxifen; resting peritoneum w/ switch to HD; mortality rates 20–93%, ↑ when on PD for >15 yr

INFLAMMATORY BOWEL DISEASE (IBD) (*J Crohns Colitis* 2016;10:226)

- Kidney Bx findings: IgAN > interstitial nephritis > arterionephrosclerosis > acute tubular injury > proliferative GN > AA amyloidosis (*CJASN* 2014;9:265)

Nephrolithiasis

- Prevalence: 12–28% in IBD; ileocolonic disease > ileal disease (Crohn's > UC); ↑ in Ca Ox and UA stones
- Pathogenesis
  Alkali lost with diarrhea → metabolic acidosis → aciduria → UA stones
  Low urine volume (especially with colon surgery) → CaOx and UA stones
  Bile salt malabsorption → enteric hyperoxaluria (>45 mg/d) (Ca binds to fat and not oxalate) → ↑ oxalate reabsorbed → oxalate stones
  Less *Oxalobacter formigenes* → ↓ intestinal oxalate catabolism → oxalate stones
- Risk factors: bowel surgery, ongoing diarrhea
- Tx: ↑ liquid intake and citrate to alkalinize urine

Glomerulonephritis

- ↑ IgAN in IBD: mucosal inflammation and chronic immune stimulation → dysregulated IgA (*CJASN* 2014;9:265)
- Other GN: IgM nephropathy, membranous, mesangiocapillary, FSGS, Anti-GBM disease
- GN ↑ w/ intestinal disease activity

Tubulointerstitial Nephritis (TIN)

- 5-ASA and sulfasalazine → CIN/chronic interstitial fibrosis > TNF-alpha
- ? Related to underlying disease vs Tx, seen in pediatric population w/o Tx

5-ASA Associated TIN
- Prevalence: CKD in 1–2/1,000; 10% of cases progress to ESRD
- Nonspecific sx, +/– malaise, fever, skin rash, eosinophilia; idiosyncratic often w/ 12 mo of starting
- Tx: d/c; steroids improves function in 40–85% if dx within 10 mo and only 1/3 if dx after 18 mo

AA Amyloidosis
- Incidence: 0.3–10.9% in CD and 0–0.7% in UC; dx 10 yr after IBD diagnosis
- Clinical Signs: m/c AA manifestation renal (90%); Proteinuria, nephrotic syndrome
- Tx: control underlying IBD

SODIUM PHOSPHATE BOWEL PREP (Nat Rev Nephrol 2010;6:480)

Pathophysiology and Risk Factors
- ↑ Serum $[PO_4]$ + volume depletion → ↑ intratubular $[PO_4]$ → precipitation and tissue deposition of CaP salts → luminal obstruction + direct tubular epithelial injury
- Risk factors for AKI: Age, HTN, volume depletion, CKD, ACEi/ARB, NSAIDs, Diuretics

Clinical Manifestation and Diagnosis
- 1–4% w/ oral sodium phosphate prep develop AKI
- U/A often bland sediment, modest proteinuria; Normocalcemic
- Renal Bx: interstitial pattern of CaP deposition +von Kossa stain

Prevention
- Avoid use in patient with CKD
- Use balanced electrolyte solutions containing polyethylene glycol for bowel prep

PROTON PUMP INHIBITORS (KI Rep 2017;2:297)

Pathophysiology and Risk Factors
- AIN → AKI; also linked to CKD and ESRD ? through unresolved AKI
- Duration of exposure up to 720 d (JASN 2016;27;3153)

Clinical Manifestation and Diagnosis
- AIN: idiosyncratic, not dose-dependent, recurrence can occur w/ 2nd exposure
- 2–3× ↑ AKI; 1.2–1.8× ↑ CKD (KI Rep 2017;2:297)
- U/A: +/– sterile pyuria, +/– proteinuria with AIN; Renal Bx: AIN

Prevention
- d/c if possible; consider H-2 receptor blockers (ranitidine or famotidine)

SHORT BOWEL SYNDROME

Pathophysiology and Risk Factors
- Roux-en-Y Gastric Bypass, Jejunoileal bypass → Rapid intestinal transit → fat malabsorption ↓ soluble Ca in the GI tract and insoluble CaOx → 6× ↑ absorption of soluble oxalate and oxaluria
- Bacterial overgrowth, fermentation of unabsorbed carbohydrates → ↑ D-lactate
- Risk factors: CKD and HTN are risk factors for AKI

Clinical Manifestation and Diagnosis
- Intratubular deposition of CaOx crystals with giant-cell reaction and tubular damage + interstitial inflammation and fibrosis; CaOx nephrolithiasis; AKI and CKD
- D-lactic acidosis: ΔMS, slurred speech, seizure, anion gap metabolic acidosis

Prevention
- Consider restrictive procedures if CKD, eg, sleeve gastrectomy

SODIUM POLYSTYRENE (SPS) +/– SORBITOL

- Pathophysiology: cation exchange resin → intestinal necrosis

Clinical Manifestation and Diagnosis
- Ileal and colonic necrosis w/ both oral and rectal SPS–sorbitol reported
- Incidence of bowel necrosis ~0.4% (Clin Nephrol 2016;85:38)

Risk Factors
- Sorbitol containing sodium polystyrene
- CKD, recent surgery, ileus, opiate use, bowel disease and obstruction; use as enema

Prevention
- Use laxatives without sorbitol or alternative potassium binding resins

Electrolyte and Acid/Base Disorder in GI Diseases (CJASN 2008;3:1861)			
(Normal stool: <0.15 L/d Na 20–30 K 55–75 Cl 15–25 HCO₃⁻ 0)			
GI State	**Fluid Composition**	**Electrolyte**	**Acid/Base**
Vomiting/NG suction	0–3 L/d, Hypotonic Na 20–100 K 10–15 Cl 120–160 HCO₃⁻ 0	Hypokalemia: renal loss	Metabolic alkalosis
Inflammatory diarrhea	1–3 L/d, Hypotonic Na 50–100 K 15–20 Cl 50–100 HCO₃⁻ 10	None	+/– Metabolic alkalosis
Secretory diarrhea	1–20 L/d, Hypotonic Na 40–140 K 15–40 Cl 25–105 **HCO₃⁻ 20–75**	Hyponatremia Hypokalemia	Metabolic acidosis
Congenital chloridorrhea	1–5 L/d, Hypotonic Na 30–80 K 15–60 Cl 120–150 HCO₃⁻ <5	Hypokalemia +/– Hyponatremia	Metabolic alkalosis
Villous adenoma	1–3 L/d, Hypotonic Na 70–150 K 15–80 Cl 50–100 HCO₃⁻ Unknown	Hypokalemia	Metabolic alkalosis
Ileostomy drainage (new)	1–1.5 L/d Na 115–140 **K 5–15** Cl 95–125 **HCO₃⁻ 30**	Hyperkalemia w/ acidosis	Metabolic acidosis: HCO₃⁻ loss Metabolic alkalosis: ↑ Cl loss, vol depletion
Ileostomy drainage (adapted)	0.5–1 L/d Na 40–90 **K 5** Cl 20 **HCO₃⁻ 15–30**		

HEPATOLOGY

HEPATORENAL SYNDROME (HRS)

- A variety of causes of AKI/CKD exist in pts w/ cirrhosis/decompensated liver disease
- The approach to differential diagnosis of AKI and CKD can be challenging, as renal biopsy is difficult to perform in cirrhotic pts due to concerns about bleeding/coagulopathy
- Relying on complement testing or FE$_{Na}$ is problematic due to the altered physiology of advanced cirrhosis

Pathogenesis

- Release of vasoactive mediators by failing liver leading to splanchnic vasodilation and renal vasoconstriction: portal hypertension → ↑ nitric oxide production → splanchnic arterial vasodilatation → hypotension → baroreceptor activation → ↑ renin, AII, Aldo, NE, vasopressin → renal vasoconstriction → impaired Na excretion → ascites → impaired H₂O excretion → hyponatremia → ↓ RBF → progressive renal dysfunction
- Precipitants: bacterial infection, GIB, SBP, CKD, acute alcoholic hepatitis, large volume paracentesis with no albumin repletion (NEJM 1999;341:403)

Clinical Manifestation and Diagnosis

Classification of Hepatorenal Syndrome (Hepatology 1996;23:164; 2015;62:986)	
Type (Timing)	**Findings**
Type I (<2 wk)	Rapidly progressive renal failure, Doubling Scr, >2.5 mg/dL UOP <400–500 mL/d, bland urinalysis, <500 mg/g proteinuria No response after 2 consecutive d of diuretic withdrawal and volume expansion with albumin Often precipitant factor(s) Absence of shock, infection, urinary obstruction, nephrotoxins
Type II (Indolent)	Steady and progressive impairment of renal function Related to diuretic resistant ascites Bland urinalysis and <500 mg/g proteinuria Chronic kidney disease

- Diagnosis: mainly established by exclusion, biopsy is high risk

- Volume depletion: large volume paracentesis particularly if done without albumin replacement, bleeding, over diuresis. Responds quickly to holding diuretics and volume expansion
- ATN: prolonged prerenal azotemia, bleeding, shock, nephrotoxins, prolonged renal ischemia in HRS (AJKD 1982;2:363). Expect muddy brown casts. Also bile casts (below)
- Glomerular disease: hepatic IgA nephropathy, hep C associated MPGN, expect an ↑ UPCR, active urine sediment
- Abdominal compartment syndrome: massive ascites, high bladder pressure, bland UA

Prevention

- Use of albumin with large volume paracentesis (8 g/L of ascites removed)
- Primary prophylaxis of SBP with norfloxacin ↓ HRS (Gastroenterology 2007;133:818)
- SBP pts should receive concentrated albumin (1.5 g/kg on d 1, followed by 1 g/kg on d 3). Albumin was a/w lower renal impairment (8.3 vs 30.6%) and mortality (16 vs 35.4%) (Clin Gastroenterol Hepatol 2013;11:123)
- SBP pts should d/c nonselective β blocker (Gastroenterology 2014;146:1680)

Management (J Hepatol 2016;64:717)

- Hold diuretics; volume expansion with crystalloid solutions as initial fluid choice in volume depletion (10–20 mL/kg)
- Albumin 1 g/kg (up to 100 g) on d 1 then 20–40 g/d + vasoconstrictors

Vasoconstrictors for HRS	
Terlipressin	↑ HRS reversal than albumin only (23.7 vs 15.2%) (Gastroenterology 2016;150:1579) ↑ Renal recovery c/w octreotide/midodrine (70.4 vs 28.6%) (Hepatology 2015;62:567)
Norepinephrine w/ MAP goal ↑ 10–15 mmHg	Similar outcome w/ terlipressin (J Hepatol 2012;56:1293)
Octreotide (100–200 μg SQ TID or IV gtt 50 μg/hr) and Midodrine (7.5 mg and ↑ dose at 8-hr intervals up to 15 mg TID)	Octreotide inhibit glucagon, splanchnic vasodilator Up to 3 d, can be attempted prior to norepinephrine

- Other: TIPS, liver transplant, hemodialysis as bridge to transplant (UEG J 2017;8:1100)

Renal Replacement Therapy

- Withhold RRT unless there is reversible component or a plan for liver transplantation (Critical Care 2012;16:R23)
- 30-d and 1-yr mortality 73% and 90% (J Gastroenterol Hepatol 2004;19:1369)
- 6-mo mortality is 84% if not listed for liver txp vs 39% if listed for liver txp (CJASN 2018;136:16)
- Hemodialysis can ↑ ICP worsening hepatic encephalopathy; CRRT preferred

BILE CAST NEPHROPATHY (KI 2015;87:509; WJG 2016;22:27)

- Can occur when bilirubin level >25 mg/dL. Pathology demonstrates pigmented casts occluding tubular lumens, pigmented granular casts seen on urine sediment
- Renal manifestation: direct toxicity to the nephron leading to elevated Scr levels, pigmented bile crystals on urine, natriuresis, and β2 microglobinuria
- Dx: ↑ bilirubin, bland u/a, trace protein and AKI, jaundice, renal biopsy
- Tx: directed at bilirubin reduction which may improve renal function ± hemodialysis

IgA NEPHROPATHY SECONDARY TO LIVER DISEASE (Sem in Nephr 2008;28:27)

- IgAN occurs in association with liver cirrhosis and portal HTN due to poor clearance of IgA by hepatic Kupffer cells that circulate and deposit in the kidney. Most frequently but not exclusive seen with alcoholic liver disease.
- Renal manifestation: proteinuria, microscopic hematuria
- Renal biopsy: mesangial proliferation with IgA deposits
- Tx: treat underlying liver disease

ABDOMINAL COMPARTMENT SYNDROME (J Trauma 2000;48:874; JACC 2013;62:485)

- Definition: sustained intra-abdominal pressure (IAP) >20 mmHg and abdominal perfusion pressure (APP) = MAP – IAP <60 mmHg causing new organ dysfunction
- Epidemiology: occur in liver transplantation, massive ascites, abdominal surgeries, intraperitoneal bleed, pancreatitis

- Renal manifestations: renal vein compression → ↑ venous resistance → impairs venous drainage → progressive reduction in renal blood flow both → ↑ renin, AII, Aldo, NE, vasopressin → ↓ U_{Na} and U_{Cl} → ↑ abdominal pressure → renal dysfunction/ATN
- Dx: ✓ intra-abdominal pressure by bladder pressure; 1 mmHg = 1.36 cmH$_2$O
- Tx: reversible if recognized and decompression is done early (large volume paracentesis, surgical decompression); target APP >60 mmHg

---

ACETAMINOPHEN-INDUCED NEPHROTOXICITY (ACKD 2015;22:376)

- Renal injury in the setting of acetaminophen toxicity
- Epidemiology: acetaminophen remains m/c cause of acute liver failure in the US. ATN can occur in up to 10% of patients.

Renal Manifestations of Acetaminophen Toxicity
ATN: possible mechanisms include direct tubular damage from the toxic metabolite N-acetyl-p-benzoquinoneimine
Anion gap metabolic acidosis: 5-oxoproline (pyroglutamic acid) (CJASN 2014;9:191)

- Dx: clinical, biopsy often not needed
- Tx: supportive management of acetaminophen intoxication

KIDNEY TRANSPLANTATION IN END-STAGE LIVER DISEASE

Indications for Liver and Kidney Dual Organ Transplantation
(CJASN 2017;12:848)
- CKD: GFR ≤60 for >90 consecutive d and eGFR or CrCl ≤30 at or after registration on kidney waiting list or Dialysis (in the setting of ESRD)
- AKI: dialysis for 6 consecutive wk or eGFR or CrCl ≤25 for 6 consecutive wk
- Metabolic disease: aHUS from mutations factor H or factor I, hyperoxaluria, familial nonneuropathic systemic amyloidosis, methylmalonic aciduria may be cured by dual organ transplant
- CKD must be verified by a nephrologist
- Evaluation of MELD-Na score (ACKD 2015;22:391)

ELECTROLYTE AND ACID–BASE DISTURBANCES IN CHRONIC ALCOHOL-USE DISORDER (NEJM 2017;377:1368)

- A variety of electrolyte disturbances occur in patients with chronic alcohol use
- Most severe w/ protein-calorie malnutrition and vitamin deficiency

Hypophosphatemia (<2.5 mg/dL)
- Causes: phosphate deficient diet, deficits in body stores, increased urinary excretion, vitamin D deficiency
- Clinical presentation: skeletal muscle weakness, ± rhabdomyolysis, metabolic acidosis, hemolytic anemia, respiratory failure
- Tx: oral supplements preferred; 42–67 mmol phosphate over 6–9 hr not to exceed 90 mmol/d; IV 10–15 mmol. Check calcium and magnesium levels

Hypomagnesemia (<2.0 mg/dL)
- Causes: intracellular shift from correction of acidosis, administration of glucose-containing fluids leading to insulin release, loop dysfunction and acute pancreatitis
- Clinical presentation: neuromuscular irritability, weakness, anorexia, nausea, tremors, arrhythmias, apathy
- Tx: oral supplements preferred, slow oral replacement 2–8 tablets (5–7 mEq/tablets)/d, parental administration over 8–24 hr, to maintain Mg >1.0 mg/dL in pts with arrhythmias or neuromuscular irritability. Proper replacement of Mg paramount in the effective correction of hypokalemia and hypocalcemia deficiencies

Hypocalcemia (<8.5 mg/dL) (BMJ 2008;336:1298)
- Causes: intracellular shift from correction of acidosis and administration of glucose-containing fluids leading to insulin release
- Clinical presentation: neuromuscular irritability, weakness, tremors, arrhythmias, Trousseau sign, Chvostek sign
- Tx: oral supplements include calcitriol 0.25–0.5 µg twice a day and oral calcium carbonate 1–4 g/d. IV calcium gluconate 1–2 g can be infused over 20 min

Hypokalemia (<3.5 mEq/L) (Drug Alcohol Rev 2002;21:73)
- May occur in nearly 50% of hospitalized pts with alcohol-use disorders

- Causes: inadequate PO intake, GI and urinary losses. Coexisting hypomagnesemia can cause kaliuresis
- Clinical presentation: weakness, paralysis, arrhythmias
- Tx: oral suspension is preferred; if IV KCl is needed give 40–80 mEq/L at rate <20 mEq/hr; administer K before bicarbonate in acidemia disturbance

Sodium Disturbances (ACKD 2015;22:376)

- **Hyponatremia:** Na <135 mEq/L, commonly seen in about 17% in patients with chronic alcohol-use disorders—causes: poor solute intake, hypovolemia, release of vasopressin → ↑ urine osmolality → ↓ free water clearance → hyponatremia
- Clinical presentation: fatigue, nausea, dizziness, vomiting, headaches, confusion, coma
- **Pseudohyponatremia:** alcohol consumption is often associated with hypertriglyceridemia, hence pseudohyponatremia may occur
- **Beer potomania:** vasopressin-independent mechanism of hyponatremia in individuals who drink large quantities of beer without adequate food intake
- **Reset osmostat syndrome:** abnormal osmoreceptor activity due to defective cellular metabolism. Persistent hyponatremia Usom <100 mOsm/kg and natriuresis >40 mmol/L
- **Hyponatremia in Cirrhosis:** d/t hemodynamic changes resulting in an impaired ability to excrete water. Vasodilatation→ activation of endogenous vasoconstrictors → ↑ ADH release → ↓ free water clearance → hyponatremia

Alcoholic Ketoacidosis

- Seen in malnourished pts w/ chronic alcoholism after 1–2 d of drinking cessation
- Present in 25% of pts admitted w/ alcohol-related disorder
- Responds quickly to holding diuretics and volume expansion
- Presentation: abdominal pain, N/V, tachycardia, HTN, ± pancreatitis and volume depletion (Am J Med 1991;91:119)
- Dx: AG metabolic acidosis, due to ketoacids and lact acid, ↑ β-hydroxybutyrate
- Tx: directed at correcting hemodynamic instability and ketogenic process. Volume expansion with 5% dextrose in 0.9% NS. Repletion of coexisting electrolyte abnormalities.

Lactic Acidosis

- Favors the conversion of pyruvate to lactate
- If lactate is >3 mmol/L; consider alternate diagnosis; sepsis or thiamine deficiency
- Tx: volume expansion with 5% dextrose in 0.9% NS

Hyperchloremic Normal-Gap Metabolic Acidosis

- Lowered bicarbonate concentration due to loss of ketoacid salts in urine, which is counterbalanced by an equivalent ↑ plasma chloride

HEPATITIS B VIRUS (HBV)

- HBV infection affects ~2 billion worldwide. HBV-related renal disease is rare in the US and Western Europe d/t the lower prevalence of chronic HBV infection and lower likelihood of childhood infection d/t widespread vaccination. HBV-related glomerular diseases are m/c in endemic areas with high chronic carrier incidence (hepb.org)

HBV-Associated Membranous Nephropathy (MN)

Laboratory and Histology Findings of HBV-Associated MN (Clin Nephrol 2012;78:456)	
HBV-Related MN	**Primary MN**
Younger onset age	Steady and progressive impairment of renal function
High occurrence of microscopic hematuria and renal failure, more nephrotic	Proteinuria ± nephrotic syndrome, ± hematuria, ± anti-PLAR2
Severely low C' (C3 and C4), Neg anti-PLAR2	More severe hyperlipidemia
LM: more segmental glomerular damage, mesangial proliferation, tubulointerstitial damage	**LM:** thickened capillary wall and GBM
IF: polyclonal immunoglobulin and polytypic complement; Granular IgG, C3, and some IgM staining along the GBM	**IF:** granular IgG, C3, and some IgM staining along the GBM
HBeAg in immune deposits (NEJM 1979;300:814)	**EM:** subepithelial immune deposits; extensive podocyte foot processes effacement
EM: extensive podocyte foot processes effacement	

Other Renal Manifestations

- MPGN: microscopic hematuria (dysmorphic RBC and RBC casts), ↓ C4 ± ↓ C3, normal RF, proteinuria ± nephrotic syndrome, ↓ GFR and HTN
- PAN: necrotizing vasculitis of small and med vessels. ↑ ESR, ↑ CRP, neg ANCA. A/w HBe antigenemia and high HBV replication. HBsAg/Ab detected in vessel wall (Am J Pathol 1978;90:619). Can lead to renal infarct, variable degrees of ↓ GFR and HTN.
- Less commonly IgA nephropathy (advanced liver disease) and FSGS

Diagnosis and Workup

- Hepatitis serologies in all patients with CKD
- Kidney biopsy to confirm a glomerular process. For PAN, a different tissue site may be biopsied for diagnosis (skin, nerve, muscle) or renal angiography

Treatment and Immunosuppression

- Acute hepatitis B: supportive treatment
- Antivirals: tenofovir or entecavir. Lamivudine or adefovir monotherapy cause resistance
  - Tacrolimus may have synergistic effect with entecavir (Am J Transl Med 2016;8:1593)
- MN: ~50% children spontaneously remit. IFN ↓ proteinuria (Gastroenterology 1995;109:540) Antivirals therapy ↓ proteinuria, ↑ HBeAg clearance (World J Gastroenterol 2010;16:770) immunosuppression is generally not recommended
- Mild PAN: antiviral therapy plus short course of immunosuppression (prednisone 0.7–1 mg/kg QD, tapered over 4–6 mo) and PLEX (2.5–4 L/session ×6–10, QD or QOD over 2–3 wk) (Arthritis Rheum 2004;51:482)
- Moderate–severe PAN: antiviral therapy and PLEX + prednisone + cyclophosphamide (oral or IV) (Arthritis Rheum 2001;44:666)

ESRD

- About ~1% of dialysis patients are seropositive for HBsAg
- Nosocomial transmission is a risk in HD pts. Machine segregation and proper cleaning and disinfection procedures among HBsAg + pts at HD is essential in the prevention in HBV incidence (Semin Dial 2005;18:52)
- Regular 2–3 mo monitoring of liver enzymes and albumin, liver US annually
- All pts with ESRD should receive HBV vaccination and have HBsAb titers monitored
- HBsAb + after vaccination is a/w ↓ all-cause mortality in dialysis pts (Vaccine 2017;35:814)

Kidney Transplantation and HBV

- All HBV-infected pts should be further evaluated prior to transplantation in order to determine risk of reactivation (HBeAg, serum HBV DNA, and preferably a liver biopsy)
- HBsAg+ a/w ↓ allograft survival, No change in patient survival (Transplant Proc 2015;47:942)
- There are cases of de novo HBV from receipt of kidney from infected donor
- Isolated HBcAb + pts are prophylaxed with lamivudine post-txp to prevent HBV reactivation with IS (Transplant Proc 2007;39:3121; Curr Opin Organ Transplant 2006;11:583)

HEPATITIS C VIRUS (HCV)

- HCV infection affects ~2.8% of the world's population. HCV infection is a risk factor for proteinuria and/or impaired renal function (Contrib Nephrol 2012;176:10)
- HCV infection ↑ incident CKD and prevalent CKD (CJASN 2012;7:549)
- HCV infection doubles the risk of progression to ESRD (Hepatology 2015;61:1495)
- HIV/HCV coinfection: high risk of CKD progression (AJKD 2009;54:43)
- HCV ↑ the risk of morbidity and mortality of dialysis patients (J Viral Hepat 2007;14:697)

Renal Manifestations

- Mixed cryoglobulinemia syndrome (MCS): 30.1% of HCV-infected pts have circulating cryoglobulins (Gastroenterology 2016;150:1599). Symptomatic MCS affects ~2% (J Viral Hepat 2000;7:138)
- Up to 90% of MCS is due to HCV. MCS caused by type II or III cryoglobulins: polyclonal IgG and monoclonal IgM or IgA (type II) or polyclonal IgM/IgA (type III). The IgM has RF activity against Fc portion of the polyclonal IgG. HCV RNA and anti-HCV antibodies have been identified in cryoprecipitates (NEJM 1993;328:465)
- Renal manifestations of HCV MCS: nephritic syndrome, HTN, may also have NS or RPGN
  - Symptoms: palpable purpura, arthralgias, neuropathy, weakness
  - ↓ C3, ↓↓ C4, +RF and +cryocrit
  - Biopsy: MPGN pattern on LM with mesangial and subendothelial proliferation. "Pseudothrombi" are classic. IF positive for IgM, IgG, and C3. EM shows subendo-thelial deposits w/ fingerprint-like substructure
- Mesangioproliferative GN: deposits/proliferation in mesangium. Mild hematuria/proteinuria
- Membranous nephropathy: proteinuria ± nephrotic syndrome, normal C3/C4, normal RF

- PAN: 19% of HCV-associated vasculitis; more severe, variable degrees of ↓ GFR and HTN. Small, medium vessel disease (ANCA neg). ↑ ESR, ↑ CRP *(Arthritis Care Res 2011;63:427)*
- IgA Nephropathy: can be seen in HCV-infected patients with cirrhosis
- Fibrillary and Immunotactoid GN: several cases reported. Hematuria/proteinuria/renal insufficiency with normal C3/C4 and RF *(JSAN 1998;9:2244)*
- FSGS: the m/c lesion seen in patients co-infected w/ HCV and HIV *(Clin Nephrol 2013;79:285)*
- Renal manifestations may be underdiagnosed, autopsy studies and kidney biopsies taken at liver txp show GN in 45–85% *(Intern Med 1998;37:836; Ann IM 2006;144:735)*

Diagnosis and Workup
- All patients evaluated for CKD be screened for HCV
- Evaluate for proteinuria, hematuria, HTN, eGFR, cryoglobulins, complements, RF
- Kidney biopsy recommended if there is hematuria/proteinuria

Treatment of HCV Infection
- √ CrCl, or GFR prior to HCV treatment
- IFN and RBV are renally eliminated. IFN associated with collapsing FSGS and drug-induced lupus. RBV must be dose-reduced for CKD, can cause hemolytic anemia.
- Because of lack of efficacy and because IFN/RBV so poorly tolerated, only 1% of HCV-infected dialysis patients ever received treatment *(Am J Nephrol 2013;38:405)*
- Direct-acting antiviral therapies (DAAs) target the HCV viral proteins with cure rates >95%
- DAAs have many drug–drug interactions *(Clin Pharmacol Drug Dev 2017;6:147)*

DAA Treatment Options for HCV		
Drugs	**Use**	**Comment**
Elbasvir + Grazoprevir (Zepatier®)	Tested in Stage 4–5 CKD/ESRD Genotype: 1a, 1b, 4	Cured 94% of patients with advanced CKD/dialysis s/e: headache, nausea, and fatigue *(C-SURFER Lancet 2015;386:1537)*
Ombitasvir + paritaprevir + ritonavir + dasabuvir (Viekira Pak®)	Tested in Stage 4–5 CKD/ESRD Genotype 1b, add ribavirin for pts w/ 1a	s/e: anemia, nausea, fatigue, diarrhea, headache, peripheral edema *(Gastroenterology 2016;150:1590)*
Sofosbuvir + simeprevir	Genotype 1a and 1b	s/e: insomnia, photosensitivity (simeprevir)
Sofosbuvir–ledipasvir	Genotype 1a, 1b, 4	s/e: headache, fatigue, nausea
Sofosbuvir–daclatasvir	Genotype 1–3	s/e: headache, fatigue, nausea
Sofosbuvir–velpatasvir	Genotype 1–6	s/e: headache, fatigue, nausea
Glecaprevir–pibrentasvir (Mavyret®)	Genotype 1–6	Cured 98% in advanced CKD/dialysis, No treatment-related SAEs *(NEJM 2017;377:1448)*

Treatment of Cryoglobulinemic Glomerulonephritis *(Hepatology 2016;63:408; 2016;64:1473; Clin Gastroenterol Hepatol 2017;15:575)*
- DAAs are safe and effective; curing HCV in >90% patients with MCS
- DAAs alone lead to normalization of complement, and reduction of cryo level in the majority
- DAAs cause complete or partial remission of MCS in ~70% treated with DAAs
- Immunosuppression (Rituximab, steroids +/− PLEX) should be added in patients w severe systemic vasculitis (pulmonary hemorrhage, CNS vasculitis, RPGN) or nephrotic syndrome
- Rituximab does not reduce antiviral efficacy *(Blood 2010;116:343)* and does not lead to hepatitis flares or increase in viremia *(Arthritis Rheum 2012;64:843; 2012;64:835)*

Management of Patients With HCV and Kidney Disease	
Presentation	**Treatment**
Asymptomatic hematuria Normal kidney function Minimal proteinuria	DAA therapy
Suspected GN Subnephrotic proteinuria Stable renal function, eGFR >30	DAA therapy
Suspected GN Subnephrotic proteinuria Stable renal function, eGFR <30	DAAs recommended for eGFR <30 • grazoprevir + elbasvir • glecaprevir + pibrentasvir
Nephrotic syndrome	Biopsy → Rituximab + steroids, DAAs
Rapidly Progressive GN (5%)	Biopsy → PLEX, Rituximab + Steroids, DAAs

Renal Side Effects of DAAs

- Sofosbuvir is not FDA approved for eGFR <30, however analysis of off-label use suggests reasonable safety and efficacy (Liver Int 2017;37:974)
- Sofosbuvir linked to increased rates of AKI events in patients with eGFR <45 compared to those with eGFR >45 (Liver Int 2016;36:807)
- Lupus-like immune complex–mediated GN: sofosbuvir-based therapies (KI Rep 2016;1:135)
- FSGS may occur with/after DAAs (Hepatology 2017;66:658; NEJM 2017;376:2394)

ESRD

- HD is a major risk factor for HCV, HCV prevalence is 10–13% in US dialysis patients
- HCV outbreaks are still reported in dialysis units due to breakdown in infection control techniques (Int J Artif Organs 2015;38:471)
- HCV associated with ↓ survival on dialysis (J Viral Hepat 2007;14:697) and ↑ morbidity (↑ hospitalizations, ↑ transfusions, ↓ QOL) on dialysis (CJASN 2017;12:287)
- Liver-related deaths ↑ in HCV dialysis patients (JASN 2000;11:1896)

Kidney Transplantation and HCV

- HCV is a/w ↑ NODAT, ↑ de novo glomerulopathy, ↑ chronic allograft nephropathy, ↓ allograft survival, ↓ patient survival post-KT (AJT 2005;5:1452; 2001;1:171)
- IFN-based therapies for HCV can provoke acute rejection (Transplantation 1988;45:402)
- No ↑ acute rejection risk with DAAs (KI 2018;93:560)
- Sofosbuvir/ledipasvir: 100% effective in KT recipients with genotype 1/4 (Ann IM 2017;166:109)
- Transplanting HCV positive kidneys (genotype 1 or 4) into HCV negative recipients followed by posttransplant elbasvir/grazoprevir treatment may be safe, and is under active investigation (NEJM 2017;376:2394)

Timing of Kidney Transplantation

- HCV infection dramatically ↓ wait-time for KT (AJT 2010;10:1238)
- Current recommendations are to treat HCV <u>after</u> transplant in patients on dialysis waiting for a deceased donor transplant in centers utilizing HCV+ organs

Timing of Treatment of HCV-Infected KT Candidates on HD (KI 2018;93:560)	
Favors Treating Pre-KT	**Favors Treating Post-KT**
Excellent cure rates for all genotypes	Excellent cure rates for all genotypes
↓ liver disease progression	Does not ↑ risk of rejection
↓ nosocomial transmission in dialysis units	↓ KT waitlist time
↓ post-transplant de novo GN	↑ organ utilization (↓ discard of HCV+ organs)
↓ NODAT risk	↓ cost by shortening time on dialysis

HEMATOLOGY

Possible Hematologic Manifestations of Renal Conditions

- AKI + anemia: hemoglobin ± hemosiderin pigment nephropathy from hemolysis, light chain cast nephropathy with myeloma, TMA, lupus nephritis, undiagnosed CKD
- AKI + thrombocytopenia: TMA including antiphospholipid syndrome, HIT with renal artery ischemia, lupus nephritis, Hantavirus infection, leptospirosis
- AKI + eosinophilia: AIN, renal atheroemboli
- GN + eosinophilia: EGPA
- NS + eosinophilia: parasitic infection, eg, Strongyloides stercoralis (KI Rep 2018;3:14)

Potassium Changes in Hematologic Conditions	
↑ K	Hemolysis, tumor lysis syndrome
	Spurious: leukocytosis d/t cell fragility (Clin Chim Acta 2008;396:95), thrombocytosis (✓plasma) (AJKD 1998;12:116)
↓ K	Hematopoiesis: GM-CSF, folate, vitamin B_{12} treatment
	Spurious: AML (↑ cell uptake)

HEMOGLOBIN AND ERYTHROPOIESIS

- Hb: heme (iron + porphyrin, synthesized in BM and liver) + α-globin + β-globin
- Anemia is defined as Hb <13 (♂) and 12 (♀) (WHO, KDIGO Anemia 2012)

Erythropoiesis: The Production of RBC at Bone Marrow

- Erythropoietin (EPO), a glycoprotein is produced in kidney peritubular interstitial fibroblast-like cells (90%), liver and brain pericytes
- ↓ local oxygen tension → inactive HIF prolyl hydroxylases → ↑ HIF → ↑ EPO → binds to EPO receptors on erythroid precursor cells → ↑ erythropoiesis

- ↑ Local oxygen tension → active HIF prolyl hydroxylases → hydroxylated HIF binds to Von Hippel–Landau (VHL) protein → ubiquitination and degradation of HIF → ↓ erythropoiesis
- Roxadustat: HIF prolyl hydroxylase inhibitor ↑ Hb in CKD ND and CKD 5D (*NEJM* 2019;PMID 31340089; 31340116), Need long term safety data, eg, RCC risk.

ANEMIA OF CKD

- Diagnosis of exclusion: r/o other cause of anemia
- ↑ as GFR declines; 1/3 (♂)–2/3 (♀) at eGFR 15 (NHANES *Arch IM* 2002;162:1401; PAERI *Curr Med Res Opin* 2004;20:1501); ↓ 3% in Hct a/w ↑ 7% death (*JACC* 2001:38:955)

Pathogenesis
- EPO deficiency and resistance: level is not low in CKD, but inappropriate
- Acute and chronic inflammation: ↑ IL-6, IL-1, TNF-α, INF-γ → ↓ erythropoiesis
- **Hepcidin**: ↑ by chronic inflammation, IL-6 and ↓ renal clearance of hepcidin
  - Inhibitor of iron transporter, ferroportin → functional iron deficiency
- Folate, vitamin B_{12} nutritional deficiency ± HD removal → ineffective erythropoiesis and ↓ survival of RBCs
- Blood loss during HD and phlebotomy
- Uremic bleeding: abnormal hemostasis in CKD d/t defects in platelet function
- Aluminum toxicity: BM accumulation → microcytic anemia

Clinical Manifestations
- Dyspnea at rest/on exertion, fatigue, ↓ QOL, LVH (strongly a/w hospitalization, mortality)
- Hb variability is a/w mortality (*NDT* 2010;25:3701; *AJKD* 2011;57:266)

Diagnosis and Monitoring
- ✓ Hb q3mo in CKD3–5 including pts on PD; q1mo in CKD5 pts on HD
- ✓ iron profile: iron, TIBC, and ferritin (reflects storage) periodically
- r/o other causes of anemia: ✓ stool occult blood, reti, MCV, platelet, monoclonal protein; ✓ folate, vitamin B_{12} if ↑ MCV, ✓ reti, LDH, and hapto to r/o hemolytic anemia ✓ PBS if accompanied by thrombocytopenia to r/o TMA
- Homocysteine and methylmalonic acid levels elevated in CKD (*NEJM* 2013;368:149)

IRON DEFICIENCY

Goal and Strategy
- Consider iron initiation if Tsat ≤30% and ferritin ≤500 in CKD (KDIGO Anemia 2012)
- IV iron if ferritin 500–1,200 and Tsat ≤25%: ↑ Hb and Tsat (DRIVE, *JASN* 2007;18:975) and ↓ ESA requirement (DRIVE-II, *JASN* 2008;19:372)
- Iron sucrose high dose (400 mg monthly unless ferritin >700 or Tsat ≥40%): ↓ ESA dose, vs low dose 0–400 mg monthly reactive to ferritin <200 or Tsat <20% (*NEJM* 2019;380:447)

Iron Administration
- In non-CKD, multiple PO iron dose is inefficient d/t ↑ hepcidin. QD or QOD dose is recommended (*Blood* 2015;126:1981). Hepcidin is further ↑ in CKD: consider QD or QOD
- PO iron is generally ineffective in dialysis pts
- Ferric citrate (PO): approved for hyperphosphatemia in dialysis pts and IDA in nondialysis CKD. ↓ IV iron and ESA requirement in dialysis pts (*JASN* 2015;26:493; 2015;26:2578). ↑ Hb and Tsat in CKD (*JASN* 2017;28:1851; *AJKD* 2015;65:728)

IV Iron Agents and Dose	
Iron sucrose (Venofer®)	HD: 100 mg qHD ×10; PD: 300 mg on d 1 and 15, then 400 mg on d 28; Nondialysis pts: 200 mg ×5
Sodium ferric gluconate (Ferrlecit®/Nulecit®)	HD: 125 mg qHD ×8
Ferumoxytol (Feraheme®)	510 mg ×1 then 510 mg in 3–8 d
Iron dextran (INFeD®/ DexFerrum®)	IV or IM; test dose required: 0.5 mL (25 mg), wait for 1 hr then 100 mg; then dose 1,000 mg × 1 or 100 mg × 10
Ferric carboxymaltose (Injectafer®)	750 mg × 2 (at least 7 d apart)
Ferric pyrophosphate citrate (Triferic®)	Added to dialysate; reduced ESA and IV iron dose (*KI* 2015;88:1187)

Side Effects of IV Iron
- Infection: bacteremia ×2.5 in HD pts with Tsat ≥20 and ferritin ≥100 (*Clin Infect Dis* 2004;38:1090); infection is a/w high ferritin (*KI* 2014;86:845)
- No direct evidence of ↑ mortality, CV event, infection, and hospitalization at a systemic review and meta-analysis (*CJASN* 2018;13:457)

- Iron overload: deposition ± injury in liver, heart, pancreas, gonad, and skin; rare with iron administration, but possible (Eur J Haematol 2012;89:87)
- ↓ PO₄ w/ ferric carboxymaltose (BMC Nephrol 2013;14:167); anaphylaxis w/ iron dextran

ERYTHROPOIESIS STIMULATING AGENTS (ESA)

- Benefits: ↓ RBC transfusion, ↓ iron overload, improve QOL, LVH (CJASN 2009;4:755)

ESA Regimen and Dose	
Epoetin α (Epogen®, Procrit®) Epoetin α-epbx (biosimilar, Retacrit®) (CJASN 2018;13:1204)	SC/IV tiw; start with 50–100 units/kg
Darbepoetin α (Aranesp®): ×3 longer half-life than Epoetin α	SC/IV q1–4wk; start with 0.45 µg/kg qwk or 0.75 µg/kg q2wk in dialysis pts and 0.45 µg/kg q4wk in nondialysis pts
Methoxy polyethylene glycol-epoetin β (Mircera®)	SC/IV q2–4wk; start with 0.6 µg/kg q2wk
Peginesatide (Omontys®)	Withdrawn for anaphylaxis and death

Epoetin and Darbepoetin Dose Conversion			
Total Weekly Epoetin α (tiw, units)	Weekly Aranesp (µg)	Total Weekly Epoetin α/Aranesp (µg)	Mircera (µg)
<2,499	6.25	<8,000/<40	120 qmo or 60 q2wk
2,500–4,999	12.5		
5,000–10,999	25	8,000–16,000/40–80	200 qmo or 100 q2wk
11,000–17,999	40		
18,000–33,999	60	>16,000/>80	360 qmo or 180 q2wk
34,000–89,999	100		
≥90,000	200		

Clinical Trials on ESA Use With Hb or Hct Target	
NHCT (U.S.)	HD pts with CHF or CAD. Hct target 42% vs 30%. 28% ↑ death or nonfatal MI (NEJM 1998;339:584; KI 2012;82:235)
CHOIR (U.S.)	CKD (eGFR 15–50); Hb target 13.5 vs 11.3. 34% ↑ death, MI, CHF, CVA (NEJM 2006;355:2085) Post-hoc: inability to reach target Hb and high doses of ESA were each a/w death, MI, CHF, CVA (not the high Hb) (KI 2008;74:791)
CREATE (Europe)	CKD (eGFR 15–35); Hb target 13–15 vs 11–12.5 no difference in CV event; improved QOL; ↑ HTN and headache (NEJM 2006;355:2071)
TREAT (International)	CKD (eGFR 20–60) with T2DM; Hb target 13 vs rescue if <9 no difference in death or CV event and death or ESRD; ↑ nonfatal CVA (NEJM 2009;361:2019)

- ESA dose can be increased to avoid blood transfusion

Recommendations for Target Hb With ESA (KDIGO Anemia 2012)
For nondialysis CKD w/ Hb <10, choice of starting ESA is individualized
For ESRD, use ESA to avoid Hb drop <9
Do not use ESA to keep Hb >11.5, but ok to individualize for QOL if pt aware of risk
Do not use ESA to keep Hb >13

Side Effects

- Hypertension: endothelial cells express EPO receptor → ↑ endothelin → vasoconstriction
- ↑ Mortality and/or tumor progression or recurrence in pts with breast, head/neck, lymphoid, cervical and non–small cell lung cancer (FDA); insufficient evidence on tumor response (Cochrane Database Syst Rev 2012;12:CD003407; Br J Cancer 2012;106:1249)
- High-dose ESA a/w ↑ Incidence of cancer diagnosis (NDT 2016;32:1047)
- AVF/AVG thrombosis (NEJM 1998;339:584)
- Pure red cell aplasia (d/t anti-EPO Ab) with Epoetin α (Eprex®, available in Europe)

ESA Resistance

- Iron deficiency (could be a/w blood loss), infection, inflammation, inadequate dialysis
- Hyperparathyroidism (AJKD 2009;53:823; Clin Nephrol 2011;76:99)

- MDS, multiple myeloma, hemolysis, GI bleeding, Parvo B19
- Possibly a/w deficiency of L-carnitine (CJASN 2012;7:1836), ascorbic acid (AJKD 2006;47:644), and testosterone (NDT 2012;27:709)

INTRAVASCULAR HEMOLYSIS (AJKD 2010;56:780; 2015;65:337)

- TMA: glomerular endothelial injury; MAHA (↓ hapto, ↑ LDH, reti, ⊕ schistocytes) + thrombocytopenia (could be absent making it difficult to diagnose w/o renal biopsy)
- Free Hb from intravascular hemolysis is bound to haptoglobin: glomerulus cannot filter
  - Once haptoglobin is depleted, free Hb is filtered; reabsorbed by megalin–cubilin in PT
  - AKI by direct heme effects (renal vasoconstriction, mitochondrial toxicity, cell damaging enzyme activation) and/or intratubular Hb cast and tubular obstruction
  - Hemosiderin: PT cell deposition (brown on PAS, Prussian blue ⊕) ± AKI

BLOOD TRANSFUSION

Indication
- In CKD, should be determined by symptoms and clinical conditions (acute hemorrhage, unstable myocardial ischemia), not Hb threshold (KDIGO Anemia 2012)
- A restrictive threshold, Hb level 7 is recommended for hemodynamically stable hospitalized adult patients (JAMA 2016;316:2025)

Side Effects
- Volume overload, ↑ K, transfusion-transmitted infection, immunologic sensitization on transplantation candidate, iron overload, transfusion reactions, TRALI
- Acute (<24 hr) and delayed (5–7 d) hemolytic transfusion reaction → AKI
  - Tx: IV fluid ± loop diuretics according to volume status
- Transfusion-associated circulatory overload (Am J Med 2013;126:e29)
  - Risk factors: CKD (×27), HF, hemorrhagic shock; a/w ↑ mortality (×3.2), hospital/ICU stay
- Leukocyte-reduced blood still increases sensitization (Transplantation 2012;93:418)
- Iron overload: chelators are required for conditions requiring chronic transfusion
  - Deferasirox: AKI and Fanconi syndrome are common (Pediatr Nephrol 2012;27:2115; NDT 2010;25:2376; BJH 2014;167:434), reversible w/ d/c w/o long-term kidney injury (BJH 2011;154:387). Dose-dependent hypercalciuria (Bone 2016;85:55), CaOx stone (Ann Hematol 2013;92:263), Avoid in renal dysfunction
  - Deferoxamine: AKI from tubular injury (NDT 2008;23:1061)
  - Deferiprone: no significant renal side effect; preferred in ↓ GFR (NEJM 2018;379:2140)

SICKLE CELL DISEASE (SCD)

Background
- Glu to Val substitution at 6th AA of β-globin chain of HbA → sickled hemoglobin (HbS)
- SCD Genotypes: HbSS, HbSC, HbSβ-thalassemia, HbSD, HbSE, HbSO
- Sickle cell anemia = HbSS (homozygous); most common and severe form of SCD
- Affects millions world-wide. m/c in ancestry from sub-Sahara Africa, Latin America/ Caribbean, Saudi Arabia, India, Italy, Greece, and Turkey
- Renal disease was attributed to cause of death in ~16% (Pediatr Blood Cancer 2013;60:1482)

Pathogenesis (Nat Rev Nephrol 2015;11:161)
- HbS molecule is insoluble upon deoxygenation causing rigid deoxy HbS polymer in RBC
- Leads to hemolytic anemia, inflammation, vaso-occlusion, end-organ damage, and death
- Renal vasculopathy → medulla hypoperfusion + cortex hyperperfusion + vasoconstriction

Clinical Manifestations
- Crisis: vaso-occlusive painful, aplastic, sequestration, and hemolytic
- Acute chest syndrome (ACS), pulmonary HTN, asthma, myocardial ischemia, HF, CVA
- Renal disease develops in 5–40%; CKD → ESRD in 4–12% (Medicine 2005;84:363)
- AKI during vaso-occlusive episode <5%, a/w ACS and pulmonary HTN (NDT 2010;25:2524)
- Glomerular hyperfiltration→ ↑ GFR, albuminuria, proteinuria → glomerulopathy, CKD
- Kidney biopsy: FSGS > MPGN > TMA (Medicine 2010;889:18)
- AKI, NS and red cell aplasia: parvovirus B19/FSGS (Lancet 1995;346:475; BJH 2010;149:289)
- Proximal tubule hyperfunction → ↑ uric acid and Cr secretion: Cr-based equation overestimate GFR (Plos One 2013;8:e69922), ↑ PO_4 reabsorption → hyperphosphatemia

- Distal tubule and collecting duct: metabolic acidosis, ↓ K secretion (incomplete dRTA), enuresis, hyposthenuria 2/2 impaired urinary concentration (Max Uosm after 8 hr H_2O deprivation 400–450 mOsm/kg)
- Interstitium: hematuria (common), papillary necrosis (painless gross hematuria), renal medullary carcinoma, chronic interstitial disease → CKD
- Renal infarction: gross hematuria, pain, vomiting, fever, renin-mediated HTN, ↑ LDH
  - Dx: contrast CT, radio isotope scan, contrast MRI

Treatment
- Fluid for volume depletion; blood transfusions: may ↑ level panel reactive antibody
- Potential ↓ proteinuria with ACE-I (*Cochrane Database Syst Rev* 2015:CD009191)
- Hydroxyurea for 6 mo ↓ albuminuria (*JASN* 2016;27:1847)
- Blood transfusion with Hb goal 10 for stroke, TIA, acute chest syndrome and preop
- Allo-HSCT: curative; sickle nephropathy is an indication (*Haematologica* 2014;99:811)

Prognosis
- ESRD a/w ×2.8 1-yr mortality (*BJH* 2012;159:360)
- HD: high 5-yr mortality (46.3% vs 6.4%) from cardiac arrest and septic shock, low chance to get transplantation (*BJH* 2016;174:148)

Kidney Transplantation
- Better survival than being on dialysis
- 6-yr survival 70%, improved but lower than other disease (*NDT* 2013;28:1039)
- Vascular occlusive crisis on graft (*Human Pathology* 2011;42;1027; *KI* 2008;74:1219) is possible

Sickle Cell Trait (SCT)
- Heterozygous sickle cell mutation on one allele of β-globin chain of HbA, producing HbAS
- ↑ Albuminuria ×1.86, CKD ×1.57 (*JAMA* 2014;312:2115), ESRD ×2.03 (*JASN* 2017;28:2180)
- Microscopic hematuria, papillary necrosis
- HD patients with SCT requires higher-dose ESA (*JASN* 2014;25:819)

Medullary Renal Cell Carcinoma in SCT
- Rare, aggressive form of RCC; almost exclusively in young SCT patient
- Hematuria, flank pain, palpable mass; survival 4–16 mo (*Urology* 2007;70:878)
- Dx: contrast CT or MRI; ultrasound can miss

ERYTHROCYTOSIS

- Polycythemia: ↑ red cell mass
  - Hb >18.5 or packed cell volume >0.52 (♂); Hb >16.5 or packed cell volume >0.48 (♀)

Clinical Manifestations: Hyperviscosity
- Chest/abdominal pain, myalgias, weakness, fatigue, HA, blurry vision, paresthesia

Causes and Pathogenesis (*Am J Nephrol* 2013;37:333)
- **Excess EPO production** (*BMJ* 2013;347:f6667)
  - Tumors: renal cell carcinoma, hepatocellular carcinoma, hemangioblastoma
  - Gastric carcinoma, parathyroid carcinoma, pheochromocytoma, uterine leiomyoma
  - PKD (from epithelial lining of renal cysts), hepatitis (*Am J Med Sci* 1984;287:56)
- **Chronic hypoxia** (via HIF-1): OSA, R→ L cardiac shunt, chronic pulmonary disease, high altitudes, carbon monoxide poisoning, smoking, hemoglobinopathies
- **Polycythemia vera:** acquired *JAK2* V617F mutation in 95%
- **RAAS Activation:** post-transplantation, RAS, chronic severe hypotension
- **Idiopathic:** rare, treated with phlebotomy and close attention to iron levels

Post-Transplantation Erythrocytosis
- Incidence: Hb >17 decreased from 18.7–8.1% (*Clin Transplant* 2009;23:800)
- Risk factors: male, simultaneous pancreas kidney transplantation (*AJT* 2010;10:938), primary disease: PKD and GN
- Pathogenesis: multifactorial; activation of RAAS (angiotensin II type 1 receptor activation stimulates EPO mediated erythroid proliferation), local renal hypoxia, hematopoietic growth factors, eg, IGF-1, serum soluble stem cell factor, endogenous androgens
- Tx: ACE-I or ARB, phlebotomy

Nonvalvular Atrial Fibrillation (NVAF) in ESRD

- Prevalence of AF 10–15% in ESRD (JASN 2011;22:349)
- 1-yr mortality in HD patients with AF is two-fold that of HD pts in sinus rhythm
- AF risk scores have poor predictive value for stroke for the CKD/ESRD population and underestimate stroke risk (CJASN 2016;11:2085)

Anticoagulation for NVAF in CKD and ESRD

- For eCrCl 30–50, noninferior efficacy in prevention of CVA and thromboembolism and likely superior safety of DOAC compared to warfarin (KDIGO Eur Heart J 2018;39:2314)
- Conflicting recommendations on anticoagulation in CKD 4–5. AHA supports for CHA$_2$DS$_2$-VASc score >2, KDIGO does not support

Anticoagulants for NVAF (JACC 2016;68:2272; CJASN 2016;11:2079; 2017;12:1176)			
Drugs (Protein Bound)	**Comments**	**CKD ND**	**ESRD**
Warfarin (99%) Not dialyzable Renal elimination <1% CYP2C9 metabolism to inactive metabolite	Overanticoagulation: ×1.2 in CKD and × 1.5 for ESRD (JASN 2009;20:912) INR variability in ESRD: <45% of time therapeutic (Heart 2017;103:818) CKD: ↓ CVA (CJASN 2016;11:2085) ESRD: 30% ↑ major bleeding w/o ↓ stoke/mortality (Chest 2016;149:951) Stop in calciphylaxis	No adjustment	Avoid for primary prevention (KDIGO KI 2011;80:572)
Dabigatran (35%) ~50–65% dialyzable; Renal elimination ~80% of dose	Major bleeding ↑ 48% in ESRD (Circulation 2015;131:972) HD (BJH 2015;169:603) or idarucizumab (NEJM 2017;377:431) can be used for reversal in bleeding	CrCl 15–30: 75 mg BID CrCl <15: avoid	Avoid
Rivaroxaban (95%) Not dialyzable 35% renal elimination CYP3A4/5 and CYP2J2 metabolize ~50% to inactive metabolite	Noninferior to warfarin in CrCl ≥30 (ROCKET-AF NEJM 2011;365:883) ↑ 38% major bleeding in ESRD; no ↓ w/ 15 mg daily (Circulation 2015;131:972)	CrCl 15–50: 15 mg daily CrCl <15: avoid	15 mg daily; ? 10 mg daily (AJKD 2015;66:91)
Apixaban (87%) 7% dialyzable 30–40% renal clearance CYP3A4/5 metabolism to inactive metabolite	Noninferior to warfarin in CrCl ≥25 (ARISTOTLE NEJM 2011;365:981) ↓ bleeding c/w warfarin (CJASN 2016;11:2079; Circulation 2018;138:1519)	Cr >1.5 and ≥80 y/o or <60 kg; 2.5 mg BID CrCl <15: avoid	5 mg BID; ? 2.5 mg BID (JASN 2017;28:2241)

Prophylactic Anticoagulation in Membranous Nephropathy

- Pts with MN have increased risk of thrombosis (RVT, PE, and DVT)
- No RCT addressed question of prophylactic a/c
- Risk factor: Alb <2.8 a/w RR of 2.5 for thrombosis, ×2 increase for further ↓ albumin of 1. Proteinuria does not correlate with risk (CJASN 2012;7:43)
- Broad spectrum of clinical practice regarding prophylactic anticoagulation in MN
  - A/c if low/intermediate bleeding risk and albumin <3 (KI 2014;85:1412)
- Alb <2.0 w/ prophylactic dose LMWH or low-dose aspirin; 2.0–3.0 w/ low-dose aspirin was successful (CJASN 2014;9:478)

Anticoagulation-Related Nephropathy (Warfarin-Related Nephropathy)

- ↑ Cr by >0.3 w/o other obvious etiology in the setting of INR >3.0 in case of warfarin
- 33% of CKD and 16.5% of no-CKD had ↑ Cr w/i 1 wk after INR >3; a/w 1-yr (31.1 vs 18.9%) and 5-yr mortality (42 vs 27%) and CKD progression (KI 2011;80:181)

- 5/9 did not regain baseline kidney function *(AJKD 2009;54:1121)*
- More common w/i 8 wk of starting warfarin
- Gross or microscopic hematuria after an anticoagulant overdose; minimal proteinuria
- Dx: r/o other causes of AKI (esp RPGN); Bx if Cr does not improve with moderation of anticoagulation; consider risks of bleeding and thromboembolism while off anticoagulation
- Bx: glomerular hemorrhage with RBCs and numerous occlusive RBC casts in tubules
- Dabigatran caused similar pathology in rat *(NDT 2014;29:2228)*
- Rx: d/c or moderation of anticoagulation

MONOCLONAL GAMMOPATHY (MG)

Background

- **Monoclonality**: the abnormally high proportion of one type of light chain (LC) or heavy chain (HC) on serum/urine immunofixation or FLC assays
- M protein: monoclonal protein; BJP: urine M protein
- The type of monoclonal protein determines the type of kidney disease *(NEJM 1991;324:1845)*
- Ig do not cross GBM. LCs are filtered and reabsorbed by PT cubilin–megalin complex
- IgG3: strongest complement activation, highest (+) charge
- sFLC >ULN a/w ↑ mortality (×1.45) and ESRD (×3.25) *(Mayo Clin Proc 2017;92:1671)*
- CD19, CD20 (+) B cells differentiate into CD27, CD38, CD138 (+) plasma cells

HEMATOLOGIC CONDITIONS *(Lancet Oncol 2014;15:e538; NEJM 2006;355:2765)*

Multiple Myeloma (MM)

- Diagnosis: clonal BM plasma cells ≥10% or extramedullary plasmacytoma **AND** any of the myeloma defining events:
  - Evidence of end organ damage that can be attributed to MM: **Ca** > 11 or > 1 higher than the ULN, **Renal** insufficiency (CrCl <40 or Cr >2, LCCN), **Anemia** (Hb <10) **Bone** (osteolytic lesion; MRI or CT more sensitive than plan radiography)
  - Biomarkers: clonal BM plasma cells ≥60%, κ/λ ≥100 or ≤0.01 or >1 focal lesions on MRI
- 17% of newly diagnosed MM had eGFR <30 *(EJH 2013;91:347)*
- Renal biopsy: 3/4 showed MM associated renal disease: LCCN 33%, MIDD 22%, Amyloidosis 21% *(AJKD 2012;59:786)*
- Tx: auto-HSCT if eligible. Proteasome inhibitor (borte-, carfil-, ixazomib), immunomodulatory drugs (lenalidomide, pomalidomide), cytotoxic agents, and CS. Daratumumab and elotuzumab ↓ disease progression or death *(NEJM 2018;378:518; 2015;373:621)*
- Mortality in ESRD: 86.7, 41.4, and 34.4/100 person-yr in the 1st 3 yr *(JASN 2016;27:1487)*

Other Hematologic Conditions Causing MG

- **Smoldering MM (SMM):** serum M protein IgG or IgA ≥3 g/dL or BJP >500 mg/24 hr and/or clonal BM plasma cells 10–60% w/o myeloma defining events or amyloidosis
- **Waldenström Macroglobulinemia (WM):** serum monoclonal **IgM** and ≥10% BM lymphoplasmacytic infiltrate; hyperviscosity syndrome; almost always B cell (CD 20+)
  - Clinical manifestation of IgM subtype of lymphoplasmacytic lymphoma (LPL)
  - Renal biopsy: AL Amyloidosis > IgM deposition/cryoglobulinemia > lymphoma infiltration > LCCN, MIDD *(BJH 2016;175:623; CJASN 2018;13:1037)*
- Chronic lymphocytic leukemia (CLL): MPGN (20%) > interstitial infiltrate (12%) > TMA (12%) > MCD (10%) *(Haematologica 2015;100:1180)*
- Monoclonal B cell lymphocytosis (MBL): B lymphocytes <5,000/μL w/o lymphadenopathy

MG of Undetermined Significance (MGUS)

- **Definition:** serum M protein <3 g/dL, clonal BM plasma cells <10%, no e/o CRAB or amyloid that can be attributed to the plasma cell proliferative disorder
- 1–2% of adults; more common in older age, female, African American
- Progression to MM or lymphoid disorder ~1%/yr (18% at 20 yr, 28% at 30 yr)
  - Risk factors (RF): M protein >1.5 g/dL, abnormal FLC ratio. Progression in IgM/non-IgM MGUS at 20 yr: 55/30% (2 RF), 41/20% (1 RF), 19/7% (no RF) *(NEJM 2018;378:241)*
- f/u pts with IgM MGUS, M protein >1.5 mg/dL or abnormal FLC ratio w/ labs annually
- f/u pts with non-IgM MGUS, M protein <1.5 mg/dL and normal FLC w/ history and P/E

MG of Renal Significance (MGRS) *(IKMG Consensus Report Nat Rev Nephrol 2019;15:45)*

- Any B cell or plasma cell clonal lymphoproliferation with both of the following characteristics:
  - One or more kidney lesions that are related to the produced monoclonal Ig
  - The underlying B cell or plasma cell clone does not cause tumor complications or meet any hematologic criteria for specific therapy; including SMM, smoldering WM, MBL
- Frequently more than 1 type of renal diseases coexist

MG of Clinical Significance (MGCS) (Blood 2018;132:1478)
- MG with related organ damage (kidney, nervous system, or skin) that would otherwise meet criteria for MGUS

DIAGNOSIS AND WORKUP

- ↑ Ca in MM; Igs have Ca-binding site: may ↑ total Ca; ✓ iCa
- ↑ Globulin (total protein − albumin), Low complement in PGNMID, immunotactoid
- AG: ↓ In ↑ IgG (+ charge), ↑ in ↑ IgA (− charge) (CJASN 2011;6:2814)
- **Urine albumin to protein ratio (UAPR)** <25% in LCCN. Sensitivity 0.98, specificity 0.94 vs >25% in amyloidosis and MIDD (CJASN 2012;7:1964)
- **Urine dipstick:** hematuria and proteinuria. Not sensitive to BJP.
- **3% Sulfosalicylic acid precipitation:** detects albumin, BJP, and lysozyme
- **SPEP:** M protein on γ >> β. Low level can be missed. ↓ γ fraction in LC disease is common.

Serum Protein Migration on Electrophoresis	
Region	**Protein**
α1	α1-lipoporteins, α1-antitrypsin, α1-fetoprotein
α2	α2-macroglobulin, haptoglobin, ceruloplasmin, vitamin D binding protein
β1	IgA, ApoB, transferrin
β2	IgM, IgA, C3, C4, fibrinogen, β2 microglobulin
γ	IgG, IgM, IgA, IgD, IgE, LC (κ, λ), CRP, lysozyme

- **SIFE:** more sensitive than SPEP, quantitative
- **FLC:** reference κ/λ ratio varies according to renal function. Non-CKD (0.26–1.65), CKD (0.37–3.1), HD (0.69–2.57), PD (0.32–2.35) (CJASN 2008;3:1684)
- **UPEP/UIFE:** detects BJP
- Cryoglobulin, RF, C3, C4; HCV, SS-A, SS-B (Sjögren's)
- RF: ab against the IgG Fc portion; can be (+) in MG
- **Fat pad biopsy or aspiration:** used for systemic amyloid diagnosis and typing. Fat pad or other organ amyloid + proteinuria >0.5 g/d w/o other explanation (DM or hypertension) is diagnostic for renal amyloidosis (AJH 2005;79:319). Underutilized and can obviate the need for invasive kidney biopsy (Ann Med 2017;49:545).
- **BM biopsy:** evaluate lymphocyte or plasma cell clone. May detect amyloid.
- **Kidney biopsy:** frequently only way to prove MG is responsible for kidney disease Mass spectroscopy types amyloid from formalin-fixed paraffin-embedded specimen Unnecessary if diagnosed as AL amyloid, MM, WM, or CLL and in AKI w/ FLC >150 mg/dL AL amyloidosis a/w factor X deficiency ✓factor X before biopsy (Blood 2001;97:1885)
- Pseudoabnormalities in lab: ↓ Na, Cl, Alb, BUN; ↑ Ca; ↓ or ↑ Cr, CO_2, PO_4 (KI 2012;81:603)

Monoclonal Gammopathy-Associated Kidney Disease	
Type (M Protein)	**Clinical Manifestation**
LC proximal tubulopathy (~100%, κ >> λ)	Fanconi syndrome in 38% (JASN 2016;27:1555) Nonalbumin proteinuria
LC cast nephropathy (~100%, κ = λ)	AKI in nearly all cases; m/c cause of AKI in MM Nonalbumin proteinuria
AL amyloidosis (~100%, κ < λ)	NS, CKD; type 4 RTA, NDI if interstitium, CD is involved (AJM 1960;29:539); MM in 16% (Nat Rev Nephrol 2019;15:45) Nonischemic HF, orthostasis, arthralgia, ecchymoses, macroglossia, hepatosplenomegaly, carpal tunnel
Fibrillary GN (15%; 35% if congophilic) (AJKD 2018;72:325)	Proteinuria, hematuria, NS, CKD (KI 2003;63:1450)
Immunotactoid GN (66%)	
Cryoglobulinemic GN (types I and II; IgM, IgG, IgA; κ > λ in type I)	Type 1: MGUS > MM > LPL (Am J Hematol 2017;92:668) Renal involvement 30% in both types (Blood 2017;129:289) Cold-induced necrotic purpura, ischemic skin
MIDD (90–97%, LC >> LHC, HC; κ > λ)	NS, CKD; MM in 59% (CJASN 2012;7:231) Heart (21%), liver (19%), spleen (8%), PNS (8%) (AJKD 2003;42:1154)
PGNMID (30%, κ > λ)	Proteinuria, hematuria, CKD
Crystalglobulinemia	AKI, proteinuria; Skin, heart, cornea, BM
Lymphoma infiltration	CKD w/o albuminuria

LIGHT CHAIN CAST NEPHROPATHY (LCCN)

- Tamm–Horsfall glycoprotein: synthesized at TAL, binds to LC to form LC cast
- aka myeloma kidney; >95% has MM, rarely CLL and B cell lymphocytosis
- Urine dipstick (sensitive to albumin) protein discrepancy
- Urine albumin/protein ratio: usually <10%, <25% sensitive and specific (CJASN 2012;7:1964)
- Not otherwise unexplained AKI with LC >150 mg/dL is diagnostic for LCCN; consider kidney biopsy if <50 mg/dL (Lancet Oncol 2014;15:e538; Nat Rev Nephrol 2012;8:43)
- Kidney biopsy: eosinophilic distal tubular casts with IF staining of associated Ig chain. Local inflammation with giant cells
- Tx: MM treatment, IV fluid: ↓ LC concentration and correct hypercalcemia
- PLEX: remove LC; didn't improve outcome (Ann IM 2005;143:777)
- High cut-off HD: remove LC (CJASN 2009;4:745); didn't ↓ HD dependence (JAMA 2017;318:2099). Unavailable in the US.
- ↓ FLC is linearly a/w renal recovery; 60% reduction by day 21 a/w 80% renal function recovery. Pt survival is a/w renal recovery (JASN 2011;22:1129).
- Survival on dialysis: 16 mo; 28.9 mo in AL amyloidosis, 18.4 mo in MIDD (CJASN 2016;11:431)

LIGHT CHAIN PROXIMAL TUBULOPATHY (LCPT) (JASN 2016;27:1555)

- aka LC Fanconi syndrome; m/c cause of adult Fanconi; Fanconi in 38%
- MM 25%, smoldering myeloma 15%, MGRS 53%, rarely B cell lymphoma or CLL
- Biopsy: crystalline or noncrystalline inclusions of LC in proximal tubular cells

CRYSTALGLOBULINEMIA (JASN 2015;26:525)

- Monoclonal crystals in vessels or glomeruli; kidney infarction
- Painful purpuric nonblanching rash (occlusive vasculopathy), corneal, BM deposition
- LM: intracapillary crystals; IF: monoclonal Ig; EM: parallel linear array

MONOCLONAL IMMUNOGLOBULIN DEPOSITION DISEASE (MIDD)

- LC >> LHC, HC, κ > λ; M protein 90–97%, MM 34–59% (CJASN 2012;7:231; Blood 2019;133:576)
- NS, CKD; heart, liver involvement; low complement level in HCDD
- LM: nodular mesangial sclerosis, MPGN
- IF: diffuse linear GBM, TBM, and mesangial monoclonal LC or HC
- EM: nonorganized (nonfibrillary), finely granular powdery/punctate EDD
- Tx: bortezomib-based regimen, melphalan-conditioned auto-HSCT (Blood 2015;126:2805)
- Hematologic response a/w good renal outcome
- Txp: no recurrence with sustained remission (Blood 2015;126:2805)
- Prognosis: pt and renal survival MIDD > MIDD + LCCN ≈ LCCN; 33% ESRD, 29% death after ~4 yr (Leuk Lymphoma 2015;56:3357)

PGNMID (JASN 2009;20:2055)

- Proliferative GN w/ monoclonal immunoglobulin deposits: glomerular injury related to monoclonal Ig deposition that cannot be assigned to any other conditions
- IgG3 >> G1 > G2 >> G4, κ > λ; IgA (KI 2017;91:720), IgM (WM) (AJKD 2015;66:756)
- Monoclonal protein in ~30%; BM clone ~30%; hematological malignancy: 5–35%; can develop during f/u; 22% progressed to ESRD
- LM/IF: endocapillary or mesangial proliferative GN, MPGN (IgG3) > MN (IgG1) (CJASN 2011;6:1609). EM: mesangial and subendothelial deposits
- Tx: clone-directed therapy: B cell lymphoma treatment (eg, RTX + prednisone) for B cell clone, MM treatment (eg, CyBorD) for plasma cell clone (KI 2018;94:199)

Transplantation

- Monoclonal protein (+) 4/11 of recurrent MPGN vs 2/15 nonrecurrence (KI 2010;77:721)
- Recur w/ same IgG deposition w/ native PGNMID w/o monoclonal protein (CJASN 2011;6:122)
- Recurrence caused graft failure in 11/25 (44%) during 7-yr f/u (KI 2018;94:159)
- Filgrastim (G-CSF)-induced crescentic RPGN (JASN 2016;27:1911)

RENAL LESIONS WITHOUT MONOCLONAL IMMUNOGLOBULIN DEPOSITION

TMA with MG (KI 2017;91:691)

- Direct or indirect endothelial injury by monoclonal protein
- 13.7% of TMA patients had MG; 21% in ≥ 50 y/o, ×5
- 50% progressed to ESRD vs 33% TMA w/o MG

C3G with MG (Blood 2017;129:1437)
- IgG κ (71%) > IgG λ (22%); MGRS (60%), smoldering MM (30%), symptomatic MM (4%)
- Renal survival was worse in C3G ≥50 y/o w/ MG than w/o MG
- Bortezomib-based regimen induced hematologic response: A/w better renal outcome

GENERAL MANAGEMENT

- **Fluid:** important in ↑ Ca, volume depletion, and LC cast nephropathy
- **BP:** ✓orthostasis in AL amyloidosis. Avoid overdiuresis and α-blockers. Consider midodrine.
- **RAAS blockade:** little evidence supports its use for albuminuria
- Clone-directed therapy may improve renal prognosis. No RCT. Auto-HSCT in eligible pts (Blood 2013;122:3583).

Plasma Cell Directed Treatments	
Cyclophosphamide	Requires adjustment based on renal function s/e: hemorrhagic cystitis (give with MESNA), SIADH
Bortezomib (V)	No renal dosing, require HZV prophylaxis s/e: TMA with AKI (AJH 2016;91:E348), peripheral neuropathy, thrombocytopenia
Lenalidomide (R)	CrCl >50: 25 mg qd 30–50: 10 mg qd <30: 15 mg q48h ESRD: 5 mg qd after HD s/e: birth defects, rash, myelosuppression
Dexamethasone (D)	No renal dosing
Melphalan	High dose: 100–200 mg/m²; standard dose: 10 mg/m² CrCl 10–50: 75% <10: 50%; HD: administer after HD PD: 50% CRRT: 75%

HEMATOPOIETIC STEM CELL TRANSPLANTATION

Background
- Hematopoietic stem cell transplantation (HSCT) is classified into autologous HSCT (auto-HSCT) and allogenic HSCT (allo-HSCT) by donor type
- All auto-HSCT requires myeloablative regimen to replace abnormal replace hematopoietic system. Allo-HSCT can be done with myeloablative (causing pancytopenia), reduced intensity, or nonmyeloablative (lymphopenia w/o significant cytopenia) regimen

AKI
- Mortality of pts with AKI requiring dialysis ~83% (KI 2005;67:1999)
- AKI and mortality decreasing: Cr ×2 50 → 33%, ×3 18 → 10%, dialysis 8 → 5% from reduced intensity of conditioning regimen, reduced hepatic SOS, severe GVHD, infection, amphotericin use (NEJM 2010;363:2091)

CKD
- CKD3–5 after myeloablative allo-HSCT ~17%; ESRD ~4% (NDT 2010;25:278)
- Risk factors: h/o AKI, GVHD, ≥45 y/o, baseline eGFR <90, HTN, high-dose TBI (NEJM 2016;374:2256)
- CKD risk was similar in reduced-intensity and myeloablative allo-HSCT (BBMT 2008;14:658)
- All renal biopsy: MN (36%) > TMA (21%) > MCD (12%) (Adv Anat Pathol 2014;21:330)

Types of HSCT and Associated Complications			
	Autologous Myeloablative	Allogenic Myeloablative	Allogenic Nonmyeloablative
Indications	MM, AL amyloidosis, WM, AML, lymphoma	Leukemia, lymphoma, MDS, aplastic anemia, sickle cell anemia	
AKI	+	+++	++
SOS	++	+++	−
Causes of AKI	Hypotension, volume depletion, sepsis, TLS, TA-TMA, drugs		
Type-specific causes of AKI	Autologous GVHD	CNI toxicity, acute GVHD	
Causes of CKD		Chronic GVHD, MN, CNI toxicity	

Autologous GVHD (One Type of Engraftment Syndrome)
- Within days of neutrophil engraftment in auto-HSCT, usually 8–20 d after HSCT
- Fever, rash, pulmonary edema, weight gain, capillary leak
- Biopsy of involved organ: skin, colon; mononuclear cell infiltrates
- AKI is common; 28% required dialysis, 72% recovered (Am J Hematol 2012;87:51)
- Tx: IV corticosteroid (BBMT 2015;21:2061)

SINUSOIDAL OBSTRUCTION SYNDROME (SOS)/VENO-OCCLUSIVE DISEASE

- Risk factors: myeloablation (busulfan, cyclophosphamide, and TBI), pre-existing liver disease, age, specific treatment (eg, gemtuzumab, ozogamicin) (BBMT 2016;22:400)
- Less common with less intensity conditioning
- Pathophysiology: thrombosis, sinusoidal obstruction, portal HTN, microvascular intrahepatic portosystemic shunting
- Clinical presentation: hepatorenal syndrome ($\uparrow$ bilirubin, AST, ALT, PT, $\downarrow$ urine sodium), hepatomegaly, fluid retention, weight gain
- Doppler U/S: reversal of portal vein flow
- Tx: defibrotide

Transplant-Associated Thrombotic Microangiopathy (TA-TMA) (BMT 2018;53:129)
- 30–35% of allo-HSCT; 45% of all biopsy proven TA-TMA was auto-HSCT (Adv Anat Pathol 2014;21:330). a/w high mortality.
- Risk factors: GVHD, HLA mismatch, high-dose TBI, CNI, genetic (Blood 2016;127:989)
- Clinical manifestation: AKI, proteinuria, edema, HTN
- Arteriolar C4d deposition (Transplantation 2013;96:217)
- Tx: conservative, eculizumab (Transfus Apher Sci 2016;54:181), rituximab

Other Causes of Renal Dysfunction
- Recurrent hematologic disease associated (amyloidosis, MIDD), lymphoma infiltration
- Pigment nephropathy from ABO incompatible HSCT; BKV nephropathy (NDT 2013;28:620)

Nephrotic Syndrome After Allo-HSCT (BBMT 2016;22:975)
- MN (65.5%): PLA2R Ab (+) is rare > MCD (19%) > FSGS (7.7%)
- 87% was a/w acute or chronic GVHD; often a/w immunosuppression reduction
- Tx: reinitiation of immunosuppression, rituximab

Renal Transplantation
- Kidney from HSCT donor or combined txp (NEJM 2008;358:362) may allow IS d/c

ONCOLOGY

TUMOR LYSIS SYNDROME (TLS)

Background and Pathogenesis
- Spontaneous vs induced tumor cell lysis by cytotoxic therapy (chemotherapy; Ab therapy or radiotherapy)$\rightarrow$ Release of intracellular electrolytes (K and Phos) and nucleic acid
- Nucleic acid is metabolized as below by xanthine oxidase (XO) and urate oxidase (UO)

Purine $\rightarrow$ Hypoxanthine $\rightarrow$ Xanthine $\rightarrow$ Uric acid $\rightarrow$ Allantoin
XO XO UO: humans do not have UO

- Water solubility: xanthine < uric acid < allantoin
- UA: precipitation in the distal part of the renal tubules in acidic urine (acute UA nephropathy), renal vasoconstriction
- Hyperphosphatemia: calcium phosphate (CaP) deposition in the renal tubules (a/w hypocalcemia); the deposition starts when $Ca \times P > 60$ mg^2/dL^2
- Xanthinuria: XOI used for TLS prophylaxis can cause accumulation of xanthine $\rightarrow$ Xanthine stone, Xanthine nephropathy (Cancer Res 1981;41:2273)

Cairo-Bishop Definition of TLS (BJH 2004;127:3)
- Laboratory TLS: 2 or more lab changes within 3 d before or 7 d after cytotoxic therapy:
  - UA $\geq$8; K $\geq$6; P $\geq$4.5; Ca $\leq$7 or any change $\geq$25%
- Clinical TLS: laboratory TLS + AKI, cardiac arrhythmia/sudden death or a seizure

Risk Factors of TLS	
Patient-Related	**Tumor-Related**
Pretreatment UA >7.5 CKD Volume depletion Acidic urine	High tumor cell proliferation rate Chemosensitivity of the malignancy **Solid tumors:** rare; mainly when tumor diameter is >10 cm **Hematologic** WBC >50K; Aggressive NHL; ALL; Burkitt lymphoma/leukemia Venetoclax for CLL; Obinutuzumab for diffuse large B-cell lymphoma; Dinaciclib/Alvocidib for ALL or AML

- Spontaneous TLS lacks hyperphosphatemia d/t reutilization of PO_4 in the new tumor cells

TLS Risk Stratification (BJH 2010;149;578)		
	High risk (>5%)	**Intermediate risk (1–5%)**
Prophylaxis	IV fluid + rasburicase	IV fluid + allopurinol
AML	WBC > 100K	WBC 25–100K LDH ≥ 2X ULN
Burkitt lymphoma/leukemia, lymphoblastic lymphoma	Burkitt leukemia Stage III, IV lymphoma LDH ≥ 2X ULN	Early stage lymphoma + LDH <2X ULN
ALL	WBC ≥ 100K LDH ≥ 2X ULN	All others
CLL		Fludarabine, rituximab WBC > 50K
Adult T-cell lymphoma, DLBCL, peripheral T-cell, transformed or mantle cell lymphoma	Adult bulky, LDH > ULN Child stage III/IV, LDH ≥ 2X ULN	Adult non-bulky LDH > ULN Child stage III/IV, LDH < 2X ULN
Others	Intermediate risk + renal dysfunction, ↑ UA, ↑ K or ↑ PO_4	Child anaplastic large cell lymphoma III/IV Lymphoma / leukemia + renal dysfunction Some solid tumors*

*Chemosensitive (eg, neuroblastoma, germ cell, small cell lung) and bulky or advanced stage.

Treatment
- IV fluid to maintain UOP 80 to 100 mL/m²; furosemide only for hypervolemia
- Urinary alkalinization no longer routinely recommended: ↑ CaP deposition. Could consider initially in patients with hyperuricemia w/o hyperphosphatemia (eg, spontaneous TLS)
- Blockers of UA formation through XO inhibition: allopurinol or Febuxostat. Used mainly when UA is still <8. Allopurinol 100 mg/m² q8hr.
- Metabolism of UA to allantoin (water soluble) using exogenous UO: rasburicase 0.2 mg/kg once daily for 5–7 d or 3 mg daily (✓G6PD activity)
  - S/e of rasburicase: anaphylaxis with repeated courses, methemoglobinemia in G6PD def
- RRT if Ca × P ≥70 mg²/dL²; AKI with electrolytes imbalances or hypervolemia

---

CHEMOTHERAPY

Background
- In oncology patients, GFR estimation using BSA-adjusted CKD-EPI is accurate for medication dosage. MDRD tends to underestimate GFR (J Clin Oncol 2017;35:2798)
- Nephrotoxicity is potentiated with: volume depletion, usage of other nephrotoxic agents, obstructive uropathy
- 5-yr incidence of AKI in cancer patients receiving systemic therapy: multiple myeloma (26%), bladder (19%), leukemia (15.4%) (JNCI 2018;PMID 30423160)

Cisplatin
- Mechanisms: organic cation transporter-2 (OCT2) mediated cellular toxicity primarily of the S3 seg of the proximal tubule, vasoconstriction, proinflammatory effect
- Progressive AKI, hypomagnesemia, salt wasting, Fanconi-like syndrome, TMA (when combined with bleomycin or gemcitabine), anemia secondary to epo deficiency
- AKI is dose dependent, nonoliguric
- ↓ Dose: 25% for CrCl 46–60; 50% for CrCl 31–45 (Cancer Treat Rev 1995;21:33)

- Agents to decrease toxicity: (1) amifostine (organic thiophosphate): concerns about possible interference with the antitumor efficacy of cisplatin; (2) sodium thiosulfate for prevention of systemic toxicity of intraperitoneal cisplatin

Ifosfamide
- The metabolite chloroacetaldehyde is directly toxic to the tubular cells
- The metabolite acrolein causes hemorrhagic cystitis (ifosfamide and cyclophosphamide)
- Partial or complete pRTA/Fanconi: hypophosphatemia, glucosuria, bicarbonaturia, aminoaciduria, tubular proteinuria (↑ beta-2-microglobulin excretion), K wasting
- dRTA, nephrogenic DI
- The cumulative dose (>60 g/m²), nephrectomy and concomitant cisplatin ↑ nephrotoxicity

Methotrexate (MTX)
- Precipitate in acidic urine for high doses MTX; transient afferent arteriolar constriction
- Prevention: 50% of dose in CrCl 10–50 and avoid in CrCl <10; avoid drugs inhibiting MTX clearance via OAT1/3: NSAIDs, PCN, salicylates, probenecid, gemfibrozil, TMP-SMZ; IV fluid; Urinary alkalization (target pH ≥7) before starting infusions; leucovorin
- Leucovorin: reduced form of folic acid; competitive inhibitor of MTX

Leucovorin Dose Based on Serial Serum Methotrexate Levels and AKI		
Condition	**MTX Level After Administration**	**Leucovorin Dose**
Normal elimination	~10 μM at 24 hr, 1 μM at 48 hr, and <0.2 μM at 72 hr	PO, IM, IV: 15 mg q6h ×10 beginning 24 hr after the start of infusion
Delayed late elimination	>0.2 μM at 72 hr and >0.05 μM at 96 hr	Continue 15 mg (oral, IM or IV) q6h until <0.05 μM
Delayed early elimination and/ or AKI	≥50 μM at 24 hr, or ≥5 μM at 48 hr, or a doubling of serum creatinine at 24 hr	150 mg IV q3h until <1 μM, then 15 mg q3h until <0.05 μM

- Glucarpidase metabolizes folic acid: used in patients with AKI leading to delayed MTX elimination to decrease systemic toxicity
- HD: limited utility due to the high volume of distribution of MTX leading to rebound

Medication	Pathogenesis and Clinical Presentation	Prevention and Therapy
Platinum		
Carboplatin	Less AKI/ATN than Cisplatin ↓ Mg; salt wasting	Calvert formula* to estimate the dose
Cisplatin	AKI, RTA, ↓ Mg TMA (combination with bleomycin or gemcitabine)	IV fluid, lower dose, amifostine
Oxaliplatin	Rare ATN	No adjustment for GFR >20
Alkylating Agents		
Cyclophosphamide	SIADH with high IV dose Hemorrhagic cystitis	Dose reduction for CKD IV fluid, MESNA
Nitrosoureas (carmustine, lomustine, semustine)	Chronic interstitial nephritis (alkylation of tubular cell proteins → Glomerular sclerosis, interstitial fibrosis)	Delayed toxicity (onset several mo or yr after stopping the medication) Forced diuresis
Streptozocin	Chronic interstitial nephritis Proteinuria (65–75%) Proximal tubular damage	Forced diuresis
Ifosfamide	pRTA, dRTA Nephrogenic DI (polyuria) Hemorrhagic cystitis	IV fluid, N-acetylcysteine, MESNA Toxicity can be delayed
Others		
Mitomycin C	TMA: cumulative dose dependent, delayed clinical onset (few mo)	
Methotrexate (high dose 1–15 g/m²)	Intratubular deposition of crystals SIADH	IV fluid Urine alkalinization (keep urine pH ≥7.0)
Gemcitabine	Cumulative dose dependent TMA	

Cabazitaxel	AKI, hemorrhagic cystitis	
Lenalidomide	AIN	
Interferon	Proteinuria (MCD, FSGS) TMA (mostly with CML), ATN	
All-trans retinoic acid (ATRA), IL-2	Capillary leak w/ edema, weight gain and AKI. Aka "differentiation syndrome" in ATRA	GC or d/c offending drug

*Calvert formula: total carboplatin dose, mg = Target AUC X (estimated CrCl + 25); AUC: 5–7

BIOLOGIC AGENTS

Bevacizumab
- Risk factors for s/e: CKD, renal cell carcinoma
- Usually mild asymptomatic proteinuria; only 2–6% develops nephrotic range proteinuria
- Histology: TMA; local binding of the podocyte-produced VEGF leading to a VEGFR-medicated glomerular endothelial damage (NEJM 2008;359:205)
- HTN w/i days of starting the therapy; the mechanism of HTN seems to be independent from the proteinuria (↑ peripheral resistance; ↓ Na excretion; ↓ NO production; ↑ Endothelin-1)
- Rapidity of the HTN onset depend on the potency of the VEGF inhibitor
- HTN is a surrogate for anticancer efficacy
- TMA rare, reversible in most cases after stopping the drug. Eculizumab is a potential therapy for persistent TMA

Medication	Pathogenesis/Clinical Presentation	Prevention and Therapy
VEGF Pathway Blockers		
Anti-VEGF: bevacizumab, aflibercept	Proteinuria, NS, HTN, TMA, reversible posterior leukoencephalopathy (RPLS) AKI with sunitinib or sorafenib	Proteinuria monitoring Hold for U$_{prot}$ >2 g/d Discontinue for NS
Tyrosine kinase inhibitors: axitinib, pazopanib, sorafenib, sunitinib		
Anti-EGFR		
Cetuximab, panitumumab, necitumumab, matuzumab	Hypomagnesemia d/t wasting, (surrogate of better outcome) → ↓ Ca, ↓ K	Reversible after stopping the therapy
Others		
Rituximab (anti-CD20)	TLS, PRES	
Bosutinib	AKI, CKD	Monitor kidney function
Crizotinib	AKI	Monitor kidney function (first few weeks)
Ibrutinib	AKI	Oral fluid
Vemurafenib and dabrafenib	AKI/CKD (mainly with Vemurafenib)	
Checkpoint inhibitors: PD-1 (pembrolizumab, nivolumab) PD-L1 (atezolizumab, avelumab, durvalumab) Anti-CTLA-4 (ipilimumab,* tremelimumab) Epacadostat	AIN (Immune-related adverse effects)	Prednisone The medication can be resumed after prednisone therapy

*Ipilimumab combined with another checkpoint inhibitors like nivolumab (anti-PD1-Ab) induces AIN with aggressive infiltration of cytotoxic T-cell; therapy requires combination on steroid and/or MMF (KI 2016;90:638).

Hyponatremia	
Pseudohyponatremia	Paraproteinemia
Tumor-induced SIADH	Small cell carcinoma of the lung and other organ, Head and neck cancer
Therapy-induced SIADH	Cyclophosphamide, ifosfamide: occurs and resolves within 24 hr of drug discontinuation
	Melphalan, vinca alkaloids (Vincristine, vinblastine, vinorelbine), Methotrexate
Therapy-induced salt wasting	Cisplatin, carboplatin: salt-wasting through direct tubular damage mainly the loop of Henle

Hypernatremia	
Nephrogenic DI	Ifosfamide

Hypokalemia	
Pseudohypokalemia	Leukocytosis
Tumor-related	ACTH secreting tumor: SCLC, thymus or bronchial carcinoid, thyroid medullary carcinoma, or neuroendocrine tumors
	AML (M4 and M5): lysozyme-mediated tubular injury
	Leukemia blast crisis: cell build up
	Light chain proximal tubulopathy (LCPT) in monoclonal gammopathy
Therapy-related	GM-CSF, Vit B12: cell build-up

Hypomagnesemia	
Therapy-related wasting	Cisplatin
	Anti-EGFR inhibitors (cetuximab and panitumumab): disrupt TRPM6-mediated distal reabsorption of Mg

Hypercalcemia	
Humoral	PTH-rp: squamous cell carcinoma (lung, head and neck), renal cell, ovarian, breast, and esophageal cancers
	$1,25\text{-}(OH)_2$ Vit D: lymphoma, dysgerminoma
	PTH (rare): parathyroid, lung (small, squamous cell), thyroid papillary carcinoma, ovarian cancer
Osteolytic tumor	Osteosarcoma, MM, solid (breast) cancer with osteolytic metastasis

Hypophosphatemia	
Proximal tubulopathy	Ifosfamide, cisplatin, imatinib
Tumor-induced osteomalacia	FGF-23 is release by the tumor (hemangiopericytomas, giant cell tumors, and osteoblastomas) leading to phosphaturia

Metabolic Acidosis	
AGMA	Lactic acidosis: leukemia, lymphoma, Warburg effect
pRTA (NAGMA, glycosuria, aminoaciduria, ↓ K, PO₄)	Ifosfamide: NDI and dRTA can accompany
	Cisplatin
	Light chain proximal tubulopathy (LCPT) in monoclonal gammopathy
dRTA	Ifosfamide

INFECTIOUS DISEASES

Sepsis-Associated AKI

- AKI is common in sepsis, and incidence increases with higher severity of sepsis (>50% in patients with septic shock) (Int J Infect Dis 2009;13:176)
- AKI typically occurs early in clinical course (often w/i first 24 hr of presentation) (JASN 2003;14:1022) and is a/w ↑ mortality, although outcomes are improving over time (AJKD 2015;65:870)
- Although septic AKI is a/w ↑ mortality and ↑ length of hospitalization c/t nonseptic AKI (Crit Care 2008;12:R47), it may carry better renal recovery prognosis in survivors (CJASN 2007;2:431)

Pathogenesis and Workup

- AKI results from both impaired glomerular filtration and tubular dysfunction
- ↓ RBF only if ↓ cardiac output, otherwise ↑ or normal (Crit Care 2005;9:R363)
- Altered intrarenal blood flow and microcirculatory changes can lead to ↓ glomerular capillary pressure independent of RBF → ↓ GFR (KI 2017;91:45)
- Systemic inflammatory response syndrome, tissue hypoxia, ↓ perfusion → tubular cell apoptosis/necrosis
- FE_{Na} >1% and "muddy brown" casts on microscopic sediment

Prevention and Management

- Although maintenance of MAP to preserve renal perfusion pressure is key, no advantage to raising MAP about 65–70, except in subset of patients with chronic HTN (NEJM 2014;370:1583)
- Use of dopamine to increase RBF does not reliably protect against AKI
- Prophylactic fenoldopam results in smaller ↑ SCr, but not ↓ mortality
- Aggressive IVF is a/w inferior outcomes (KI 2009;76:422) and conservative fluid administration strategy after initial resuscitation may be renoprotective (Intensive Care Med 2016;42:1695)
- Balanced crystalloids may provide marginally better renal outcomes compared to NS in critically ill adults (NS has supraphysiologic chloride concentration), although benefit for balanced crystalloids is small (major adverse kidney event [death, new RRT, or persistent renal dysfunction] 14.3% for LR/plasma-lyte vs 15.4% for NS, p = 0.04; no difference in need for new RRT or persistent kidney dysfunction) (SMART NEJM 2018;378:829)
- Artificial colloids (eg, HES) a/w ↑ AKI and ↑ mortality, should be avoided (NEJM 2012;367:124)
- No evidence to support high-volume hemofiltration to clear inflammatory mediators (Intensive Care Med 2013;39:1535)

Renal Replacement Therapy

- Ideal timing of RRT initiation is controversial: early initiation does not appear to provide increased survival or better renal outcomes in septic critically ill patients with AKI
- In patients who require RRT, there is no benefit to high-dose RRT over low-dose RRT, and effluent flow rate of 20–25 mL/kg/hr is considered sufficient (Table)
- Consider higher-dose RRT if refractory acidosis or hyperkalemia

Key Clinical Trials Regarding RRT Management			
Study	**Comparison**	**Primary Outcome**	**Findings**
ATN (NEJM 2008;359:7)	High-intensity RRT (6×/wk HD or CVVHDF with 35 mL/kg/hr effluent) vs low-intensity RRT (HD 3×/wk or CVVHDF with 20 mL/kg/hr effluent)	60-d mortality	No difference in mortality, RRT dependence, organ failure
RENAL (NEJM 2009;361:1627)	CVVHDF with effluent flow 40 vs 25 mL/kg/hr	90-d mortality	No difference in mortality, RRT dependence, length of hospitalization
IVOIRE (Intensive Care Med 2013;39:1535)	High-volume HF vs standard HF in critically ill patients with septic shock and AKI	28-d mortality	No difference in mortality, hemodynamics

ELAIN (JAMA 2016;315:2190)	Early vs late RRT initiation in critically ill patients with stage 2–3 AKI (primarily surgical patients)	90-d mortality	Early RRT→↓ mortality, ↓ RRT duration, ↓ length of hospitalization Extended followup: early RRT ↓ mortality and ↑ renal recovery at 1 yr (JASN 2018;29:1011)
AKIKI (NEJM 2016;375:122)	Early vs late RRT initiation in critically ill patients with stage 3 AKI (80% patients had sepsis)	60-d mortality	No differences in mortality, RRT dependence, length of hospitalization
IDEAL-ICU (NEJM 2018;379:1431)	Early vs late RRT initiation in early septic shock and failure-stage AKI by RIFLE criteria	90-d mortality	Stopped early: no difference in mortality, ICU days, vent d. Delayed → ↓ RRT time

ANTIMICROBIALS

Antibiotic Dosing in AKI
- Patients with AKI display variable alterations in antibiotic pharmacokinetics, so close drug monitoring is required to ensure drug efficacy while avoiding increased drug toxicity (Crit Care Clin 2006;22:255)
- Intravenous route is preferred due to variability in oral drug absorption
- Although some antibiotics will experience ↓ clearance in AKI, third-spacing of fluids, hypervolemia, and ↓ drug-protein binding can ↑ volume of distribution → ↑ dose needed to reach therapeutic drug level (Crit Care Med 2009;37:840)
- Early renal recovery can lead to underdosing d/t ↑ renal drug clearance
- In patients requiring CRRT, antibiotic clearance is highly variable (Crit Care 2015;19:84), and suggested dosing may be inappropriate due to (Nat Rev Nephrol 2011;7:226):
  - Heterogeneity in extraction coefficient: due to variable drug-protein binding
  - Mode of clearance (hemodialysis vs hemofiltration vs hemodiafiltration): convective methods increase clearance of larger solutes
  - Filter adsorption: differs based on filter composition
  - Variability in dialysis dose delivered: dosing recommendations are based on standardized dialysis dose, but there is practice pattern variation in CRRT dosing; in addition, only 68% of patients receive prescribed dose of dialysis
- Consider antibiotic characteristics
  - Concentration-dependent antibiotics (C) require high peak levels: may require increased dose due to factors above, and avoid RRT immediately after dosing
  - Time-dependent antibiotics (T) require prolonged time above MIC: consider prolonged intermittent antibiotic infusions or continuous infusions

Pharmacodynamic Profile and CRRT Monitoring of Antibiotics	
Drug	**CRRT Monitoring/Considerations**
Vancomycin (T)	Daily serum concentration, redose for level <15 mg/L Continuous infusion may be superior in CRRT (J Antimicrob Chemother 2013;68:2859)
Linezolid (T)	No established drug level monitoring parameters, although there is large variability in pharmacokinetics in patients receiving CRRT (J Antimicrob Chemother 2016;71:464)
Daptomycin (C)	Although trough concentrations correlate with peak levels, not routinely checked, as adequate peak levels achieved with 8 mg/kg q48hr (Crit Care Med 2011;39:19) Increase serum CK monitoring frequency (institution-dependent)
Ceftaroline (T)	No data available
Tigecycline (C)	Nonrenal elimination, poorly dialyzed. No adjustments required (J Clin Pharmacol 2012;52:1379)

Piperacillin-tazobactam (T)	No routine drug level monitoring. Higher doses (12 g/d) associated with achieving drug targets, and extended infusion preferred regardless of dose (CJASN 2016;11:1377)
Cefepime (T)	No routine drug level monitoring, although variability in pharmacokinetics in patients on CRRT (Int J Antimicrob Agents 2015;46:413) results in risk of undertreating infection or risk of neurologic side effects
Ceftazidime-Avibactam (T)	Limited data (case report) (Antimicrob Agents Chemother 2017;61:e00464)
Meropenem (T)	No routine drug level monitoring. Consider loading dose prior to dose reduction for CRRT given pharmacokinetic variability (Am J Kidney Dis 2014;63(1):170–1)
Gentamicin (C)	Peak drug level monitoring 30 min after dose delivery (goal 6–8 µg/mL or 8–10 µg/mL depending on severity of sepsis) and redose when level <2 µg/mL (or <1 µg/mL, depending on institution and severity of sepsis) (J Chemother 2012;24:107)
Amikacin (C)	High loading initial dose (≥25 mg/kg) preferred, with peak drug level monitoring (to adjust dose) and extended dosing interval (goal trough <2.5) (Antimicrob Agents Chemother 2016;60:4901)
Polymyxin B (C)	No routine drug level monitoring. No dose adjustment needed for patients on CRRT (J Antimicrob Chemother 2013;68:674)
Colistin (C)	No routine drug level monitoring. Potential role of loading dose (Int J Antimicrob Agents 2016;48:337)
Tobramycin (C)	Peak drug level monitoring 30 min after dose delivery (goal 6–8 µg/mL or 8–10 µg/mL depending on severity of sepsis) and redose when level <1 µg/mL (or <2 µg/mL, depending on institution and severity of sepsis)
Ciprofloxacin (C)	No routine drug level monitoring. Given reliance on achieving desired AUC/MIC ratio for efficacy, consider exceeding recommended dose in severe infection (Clin Infect Dis 2005;41:1159)

Renal Complications of Antimicrobials
- Risk factors of antibiotic-related AKI: CKD, DM, advanced age, other nephrotoxins
- Direct tubular toxicity (ATN) is most common mechanism of injury
- Crystal formation (sulfa, acyclovir) more likely to occur in volume depletion
- Acute interstitial nephritis can complicate therapy with any antibiotic, but commonly with penicillin antibiotics or fluoroquinolones. Classic AIN triad of "rash, fever, and pyuria" occurs only in the minority. Need high index of suspicion or kidney biopsy.
- D-lactic acidosis due to bacterial overgrowth of acid-producing enteric bacteria → anion gap metabolic acidosis

Antibiotic-Associated Renal Toxicity (Nat Rev Nephrol 2009;5:193)	
Drug/Class	**Nephrotoxicity**
Trimethoprim-Sulfamethoxazole	AIN; ENaC inhibition → hyperkalemia, volume depletion induced hyponatremia (AJKD 2013;62:1188) Trimethoprim ↓ tubular Cr secretion → ↑ SCr w/o ΔGFR
Amphotericin B	ATN; ↓ Aquaporin 2 → hypernatremia (nephrogenic DI) ↑ Membrane permeability to cations → hypokalemia, hypomagnesemia, nephrogenic DI, distal RTA
Aminoglycosides	↓ Microsomal protein synthesis, mitochondrial injury (especially in proximal tubule) → ATN, ↓ K, ↓ PO_4, ↓ Mg, Fanconi syndrome (Antimicrob Agents Chemother 1999;43:1003) ↑ CaSR → Bartter-like syndrome (↓ K, metabolic alkalosis)
Linezolid	Mitochondrial toxicity → lactic acidosis (NEJM 2005;353:2305)
Tetracyclines	Proximal tubule ribosome injury → Fanconi syndrome Lactic acidosis
Penicillins	↑ 5-oxoproline, pyroglutamate → anion gap metabolic acidosis AIN: penicillins and other β-lactams can provoke allergy
Fluoroquinolones	AIN: crystal nephropathy (ciprofloxacin)
Vancomycin	Cellular uptake → ATN Vancomycin cast formation → ATN (JASN 2017;28:1723)
Polymyxin B	Tubular cell apoptosis → ATN
Daptomycin	Rhabdomyolysis: possibly via plasma membrane disruption (In Vitro Cell Dev Biol Anim 2010;46:613) → ATN

Antibiotic Toxicity if Inappropriately Dosed for Renal Function	
Drug/Class	Toxicity in Renal Failure
B-lactams	Neurotoxicity: encephalopathy, seizures
Aminoglycosides	Ototoxicity, AKI
Vancomycin	AKI

HUMAN IMMUNODEFICIENCY VIRUS (HIV)

- Prevalence: 38.8 million worldwide and 833,000 in the US (Lancet HIV 2016;3:e361)
- HIV causes primary kidney diseases and is also a risk factor for progression to ESRD
- AKI is common in HIV-infected patients (sepsis, ARV-toxicity) (AIDS 2015;29:1061)
- Glomerular diseases may result from direct infection of podocytes causing HIV-associated nephropathy (HIVAN), immune complex-mediated glomerular disease and endothelial injury causing thrombotic microangiopathy (TMA) (Nat Rev Nephrol 2015;11:150)
- Incidence of HIVAN decreasing with widespread use of ART, although prevalence is increasing as patients live longer (JASN 2005;16:2412). The incidence of FSGS increasing in such patients (NDT 2012;27:2349)
- Increasing survival of HIV-infected patients leading to rise in CKD from other comorbidities (DM and HTN) found in HIV-infected patients and ART nephrotoxicity

Workup and Evaluation

- Recent HIV diagnosis (HIVAN) vs chronic HIV (immune complex-mediated GN)
- Rate of GFR decline: rapid (HIVAN) vs subacute (immune complex-mediated GN)
- Risk factors: HCV co-infection, high viral load
- Workup: HIV activity (CD4 count, viral load), u/a, proteinuria quantification
  - Fanconi syndrome (glycosuria without hyperglycemia, NAGMA, hyperphosphaturia): drug toxicity, especially tenofovir disoproxil fumarate (TDF)
- Kidney biopsy: recommended for suspected TMA, nephrotic proteinuria, or atypical presentations of other renal lesions (typically does not change management)

HIV-ASSOCIATED GLOMERULAR DISEASE

Glomerular Diseases Associated With HIV			
	HIVAN	Immune Complex-Mediated GN	TMA
Risk factors	Advanced HIV, Black race/APOL1 genotype (JASN 2011;22:2129)	Variable stage of HIV (CJASN 2013;8:1524) No racial predilection	Advanced HIV (Scand J Immunol 2008;68:337)
Clinical findings	NS, fast GFR decline, large echogenic kidneys on U/S	GN (proteinuria, hematuria), low complement	↓ plt, MAHA (often nl ADAMTS13)
Biopsy	Collapsing FSGS, microcystic tubular dilation, tubulitis TRIs (IFN footprint)	Immune-complex GN (variable: lupus-like, IgAN, MPGN, IRGN, MN, ITGN, FGN)	Thrombosis, Ischemic glomeruli and tubules, RBC fragments
Treatment	ART, RAASi, GC for rapid progression	ART +/- GC	PLEX and CS if low ADAMTS13, ART
Prognosis	Poor without ARV	Non-IgAN forms have better outcome than IgAN, HIVAN (NDT 2016;31:2099)	Mixed

- The term HIV-associated immune-complex kidney disease (HIVICK) is not recommended for its heterogeneous disease spectrum and potential non-HIV reversible causes (KDIGO KI 2018;93:545)

HIV-Associated Tubulointerstitial Disease

- 11–26% of kidney biopsies from HIV-infected patients show tubulointerstitial disease (*CJASN* 2010;5:798; 2013;8:930). Of these:
  - 70% have a second major diagnosis, ~¾ of AIN attributable to drugs
  - Hematologic (ie, lymphoma) and infectious (TB, MAI) etiologies should be considered

Immune Reconstitution Inflammatory Syndrome (IRIS) (*Semin Nephrol* 2008;28:556)
- Systemic inflammatory response that typically occurs in setting of ART initiation early in course of opportunistic disease (and severe immunocompromised)
- Kidney Bx: granulomatous inflammation
- Tx: steroids

Diffuse Infiltrative Lymphocytosis Syndrome (DILS) (*KI* 2007;72:219)
- Multiorgan lymphocyte infiltration that occurs in setting of uncontrolled HIV infection; commonly affects salivary gland
- Kidney Bx: CD8+ lymphocytic infiltration
- Tx: ART, steroids

Adverse Renal Effects of ART

- Small ↑ Cr w/o true renal dysfunction d/t ↓ tubular cr secretion: dolutegravir (integrase and OCT2 inhibitor) (*Br J Clin Pharmacol* 2013;75:990), cobicistat (CYP3A4 and MATE inhibitor) (*JAIDS* 2012;61:32). ↑ Cr >0.4 should be evaluated for its cause (NIH https://aidsinfo.nih.gov/).
- Nucleoside/tide reverse transcriptase inhibitors (NRTIs) stavudine and didanosine may cause lactic acidosis and rhabdomyolysis. Rarely used in developed world.

Proximal Tubulopathy
- Tenofovir disoproxil fumarate (TDF) and Adefovir inhibit mitochondrial DNA γ-polymerase and cause renal tubular mitochondrial toxicity and Fanconi syndrome. TDF is most common cause of Fanconi syndrome.
- Secreted by OAT1 (basolateral) and MRP4 (apical) in the PT (*Lab Invest* 2011;91:852)
- Lab: ↓ PO₄, glucosuria, aminoaciduria, nonalbumin proteinuria (*AIDS* 2015;29:941)
- Kidney Bx: tubular damage; EM w/ change in mitochondrial shape, enlargement, or depletion
- TDF causes osteopenia d/t hypophosphatemia, ↓ 1-α-hydroxylase activity, and loss of vitamin D binding protein in urine
- Early detection and d/c may prevent further decline of renal function (*JID* 2013;207:1359)
- Tenofovir alafenamide (TAF): newer formulation w/ safer renal and bone s/e profile due to 90% lower serum tenofovir levels. Less renal adverse events and proteinuria with TAF than TDF (*JAIDS* 2016;71:530)

Crystalluria
- Protease inhibitors (Indinavir and Atazanavir) can cause nephrolithiasis and intratubular crystal formation. Indinavir caused renal colic in 8%, Atazanavir (case reports) Radiolucent stones comprised of the medicine (*Ann IM* 1997;127:119)

HIV Drug-Associated Nephrotoxicity (*Nat Rev Nephrol* 2015;11:150)		
Drug	**Class**	**Comments**
Tenofovir	NRTI	ATN from mitochondrial toxicity Proximal tubulopathy (TDF>>TAF) w/ tubular proteinuria: failure to reabsorb low MW proteins Fanconi syndrome: phosphaturia, glucosuria, acidosis (insufficient ATP to power sodium-glucose cotransporter and perform ammoniagenesis) Renal osteodystrophy: PO₄ wasting, loss of Vitamin D binding protein, low 1-α-hydroxylase production Biopsy: ATN and characteristic mitochondrial enlargement/distortion Treatment: drug discontinuation → good prognosis
Didanosine	NRTI	Fanconi syndrome, Lactic acidosis, Rhabdomyolysis
Lamivudine, Stavudine	NRTI	RTA
Efavirenz	NNRTI	Nephrolithiasis (*Am J Med Sci* 2016;351:213)
Indinavir, Atazanavir	PI	Crystals, stones, AKI

KIDNEY TRANSPLANTATION

- Transplantation improves survival compared to HD in HIV+ patients with ESRD
- HIV viral load should be undetectable prior to transplantation
- No increase in HIV progression after transplant (*NEJM* 2010;363:2004)
- Safety and efficacy of HIV+ to HIV+ transplantation established (*NEJM* 2015;372:613)

Drug Interactions
- Generally continue with same pretransplant ART regimen
- CYP450-3A inhibited by CNI and PI; expect to use ~20% of typical CNI dose via extended dosing interval (*Transplantation* 1999;68:307)
- Avoid MMF + zidovudine or stavudine: myelosuppression, ↓ zidovudine efficacy (*AJT* 2009;9 Suppl 4:S263)

Outcomes
- Pt & graft survival worse than non-HIV, but similar to other high-risk (*NEJM* 2010;363:2004)
- Increased rates of rejection compared to HIV-negative recipients
- Worst outcomes if HCV co-infected (*JASN* 2015;26:2222)

DIABETES MELLITUS

DIABETIC KIDNEY DISEASE (DKD)

Background
- Most common cause of CKD and ESRD in the US (USRDS)
- About ¼ of diabetic patients develop DN
- Albuminuria with strong predictive value for CKD progression
  - Microalbuminuria on spot morning void: HR 4.4 for progression (*NEJM* 2001;345:861)
  - A/w all-cause mortality, CV events at all GFR's (*JAMA* 2010;303:423)
- Moderately increased albuminuria (microalbuminuria): 30–300 mg/g or mg/d
- Severely increased albuminuria (macroalbuminuria): >300 mg/g or mg/d
- Of diabetes with eGFR <60, 16% have microalbuminuria, 61% macroalbuminuria
- Of those with microalbuminuria, 20% progress in 8 yr, 50% stable, 30% improve
- Possible to progress directly to ESRD without evidencing overt proteinuria

Pathogenesis and Risk Factors
- Hyperglycemia and advanced glycation end products drive diabetic complications: glomerular hyperfiltration (*JASN* 2017;28:1023)
  - ↓ Afferent arteriole resistance from tubuloglomerular feedback (TGF) inhibition, ↑ NO bioavailability, hyperinsulinemia
  - ↑ Efferent arteriole resistance from ↑ AII, endothelin 1, ROS
    Inflammation/fibrosis from cytokines and growth factors (eg, TNF-α, VEGF, TGF-β)
    Direct podocyte effects, eg, ↓ nephrin expression, podocyte-specific insulin signaling
- Older age, African ancestry, smoking, and obesity increase risk for DKD
- No single gene has been identified, familial clustering is common

Screening
- Annually from DM2 diagnosis, annually 5 yr after DM1 diagnosis
- ✓ Cr, eGFR calculation, urine microalbumin to creatinine ratio (UACR) (ADA, KDIGO)

Workup and Diagnosis
- Urinalysis: bland sediment, although hematuria can be seen, especially in severe DN
- Urine protein measurement
  - Dipstick: affected by urine concentration, usually "+" indicates >300 mg/d
  - 24-hr collection: gold standard
  - Spot UPCR and UACR: acceptable and easier for patients, accuracy affected by creatinine generation (large muscle mass, cachexia)
  - Urine microalbumin sensitive for low levels of albuminuria
  - Protein electrophoresis: distinguishes albumin and nonalbumin proteins (light chains)
- Biopsy (*CJASN* 2013;8:1718)
  - Of biopsied diabetic patients, 1/3 with DN, 1/3 with nondiabetic renal disease (NDRD), and 1/3 with both DKD and NDRD
  - m/c NDRD: ATN, FSGS, IgA nephropathy, HTN glomerulosclerosis

Kidney Biopsy Decision in Patients With DM	
Pursue Biopsy	**Defer Biopsy**
CKD of short duration	Stable proteinuria
Rapid worsening of GFR	Inactive sediment
Vasculitic symptoms	Known retinopathy
New onset nephritis/nephrosis	
Low C3/C4	
Monoclonal gammopathy	

Pathologic Classification of Diabetic Nephropathy (JASN 2010;21:556)	
I: GBM thickening	II: mesangial expansion
III: nodular (Kimmelstiel–Wilson lesion) sclerosis (<50% global glomerulosclerosis)	IV: advanced sclerosis (>50% global glomerulosclerosis)

- Interstitial fibrosis and small vessel disease frequently coexist (JASN 2010;21:556)

Treatment
- Nephrology referral: GFR <30, UACR >300 mg/g, 25% drop in GFR (KDIGO)
- Lifestyle changes: exercise, BMI <25; no clear benefit to protein restriction
- BP goal: <140/90 (ADA, KDIGO, JNC), <130/80 if proteinuria (KDIGO), <130/80 (2017 ACC/AHA)
  - Every 10 mmHg drop in SBP ↓ mortality (×0.87), albuminuria (×0.83), CV events (×0.89), stroke (×0.73), retinopathy (×0.87) (JAMA 2015;313:603)
  - Diuretics usually necessary to achieve BP control, loop preferred in advanced CKD (eGFR <30, or heavy proteinuria)
- RAS inhibition: first line for BP and proteinuria control; ↓ intraglomerular pressure
- ACEi or ARB: renoprotective (IDNT NEJM 2001;345:851; RENAAL NEJM 2001;345:861)
  - ↑ >30% cr: acceptable, ✓BMP, risk of AKI ↑ w/ diuretics, NSAIDs or volume depletion
  - ↑ >30% cr: consider workup for renal artery stenosis
  - Continue in advanced CKD unless ↑ K (try ↓ dose + diuretic) or sudden ↓ eGFR
  - Not recommended for primary prevention in normotensive, UACR <30 mg/g
- ACEi + ARB a/w worse outcomes and no benefit (ONTARGET, NEJM 2013;369:1892)
- MRA + ACEi or ARB for further antiproteinuric and anti-HTN; can initiate K ≤4.5 and eGFR ≥30; ↑ K frequent: low-K diet, loop diuretic, no NSAID, close BMP monitoring
- Glycemic control: strict control prevents onset of microalbuminuria (NEJM 1993;329:977)
  - A1c ⦸ appropriate in CKD to avoid complications of hypoglycemia (ADA, KDIGO)
  - A1c correlates with Hgb and pH, can be confounded in CKD due to anemia, acidosis
  - Fasting and postprandial fingersticks generally more reliable than A1c
- Proteinuria control: ↓ 50% albuminuria, ↓ 18% CV event (RENAAL KI 2004;65:2309)
  - CCB: non-DHP more antiproteinuric than DHP (KI 2004;65:1991)
  - Pentoxifylline ↓ eGFR decrease, albuminuria (JASN 2015;26:220)
- CV comorbidities: statin with LDL goal <100, smoking cessation, aspirin 81

Antihyperglycemic Agents for Impaired eGFR (JASN 2017;28:2263)	
Medication	**Comments and Doses for CKD**
Biguanides (Metformin)	eGFR 30–60: hold before iodinated contrast; restart in 48 hr eGFR 30–45: can continue; eGFR <30: d/c do not initiate
Sulfonylureas	
Glipizide	No adjustment
Glyburide	eGFR <60: d/c
Glimepiride	Caution in CKD, use reduced 1 mg dose; ESRD: d/c
Thiazolidinediones (pio-, rosiglitazone)	No adjustment; Advanced CKD watch for ↑ BP, fluid retention from ENaC activation
SGLT–2 inhibitors	Recommended for CKD (ADA Diabetes Care 2019;42:S124) ↓ Wt, BP; ↓ glom HTN by TGF s/e: AKI w/ concurrent NSAID, UTI, Fournier gangrene (Ann IM 2019;PMID 31060053), lower limb amputation, euglycemic ketoacidosis (BMJ 2018;363:k4365)
Canagliflozin	eGFR 45–59: 100 mg daily, eGFR <30: d/c ↓ CKD progression (JASN 2017;28:368), ↓ albuminuria (NEJM 2017;377:644) ↓ ESRD (CREDENCE NEJM 2019;380:2295)
Dapagliflozin	eGFR <30: d/c In CKD 3b-4, ↓ albuminuria (NDT 2018;33:2005)
Empagliflozin	eGFR <45: d/c; ↓ 39% CKD (NEJM 2016;375:323)

DPP4 inhibitors	N/V/D can cause AKI (Diabetes Care 2009;32:e22)
Linagliptin	No adjustment; ↓ albuminuria (Diabetes Care 2013;36:3460)
Semaglutide	↓ albuminuria (NEJM 2016;375:1834)
Sitagliptin	eGFR 30–50: ½ dose; eGFR<30: ¼ dose
Saxagliptin	eGFR <50: ½ dose
GLP-1 receptor agonists	Recommended for CKD (ADA Diabetes Care 2019;42:S124)
Exenatide	eGFR 30–50 caution; eGFR <30: d/c
Dulaglutide	No adjustment; ↓ albuminuria, eGFR decline (Lancet 2019;PMID 31189509)
Liraglutide	No adjustment; ↓ albuminuria (NEJM 2017;377:839)
Lixisenatide	eGFR <60: monitor; eGFR <15: d/c
Semaglutide	No adjustment; ↓ nephropathy (NEJM 2016;375:1834)
α-glucosidase inhibitors	eGFR <30: d/c

GLUCOSE DISARRAY IN PATIENTS ON DIALYSIS

- Susceptible to hyperglycemic episodes
  No urinary glucose excretion postprandially, adsorption of insulin by dialyzer
  Hypoglycemic episodes → counterregulatory hormones that are poorly cleared
- Susceptible to hypoglycemic episodes
  No renal gluconeogenesis, no renal clearance of insulin → prolonged half-life
- Recommended target for Hgb A1c: 6–8% (Nat Rev Nephrology 2015;11:302)
- Treatment: no glucose-free dialysate
  Aim for pt's glucose to be wnl before HD to prevent shifts during treatment
  Titrate insulin to nutritional status as malnutrition/inflammation → ↑insulin resistance
  Increased pt self-monitoring on dialysis days to catch post-HD hyperglycemia

DIABETIC KETOACIDOSIS (NEJM 2015;372:546)

Pathophysiology

- Insulin deficiency/resistance → impaired peripheral tissue glucose metabolism, ↑ fatty acid oxidation and lipolysis, ↑ glycogenolysis and gluconeogenesis
- Fatty acids overwhelm Krebs cycle and excess Acetyl CoA → Acetoacetic acid
- Loss of ketones in urine → ECF contraction → AG acidosis when ketoacids retained in severe volume depletion

Clinical Manifestations and Workup

- N/V, abd pain, ∆MS; ✓ Insulin use, ischemic symptoms, ingestions, infection
- Exam: volume depletion (orthostasis, flat neck veins, dry axillae), hyperventilation
- Labs: +urine/serum ketones, AG acidosis, sGlu usually ~400–800 although can have euglycemic DKA especially in setting of SGLT2 inhibitors

Treatment

- Monitoring: hourly glc, q2hr BMP, cardiac monitor
- Volume resuscitation: bolus 1–2 L NS via large-bore access; continue fluids 250–500 cc/hr
- Potassium repletion
  - If K <3.5, hold insulin until repleted >3.5
  - If K <5.0, 40 mEq KCl with each L of NS
  - If K >5.0, monitor q2hr
- Phosphate repletion: avoid, unless phosphate <1.0 mg/dL, then 20 mEq Na-phos
- If pH<6.9, 100 mEq NaHCO3 in 500 cc w/ 20 mEq KCl and repeat until pH >7.0
- Insulin: 0.1 u/kg regular insulin IV bolus, then 0.1 u/kg/hr continuous infusion
  - Repeat bolus if sGlu does not drop >50 mg/dL in first hr
  - Once sGlu <200 mg/dL, change IVF to D5 ½ NS at 250 cc/hr
  - When AG acidosis resolves, start subq rapid acting 0.1 u/kg q2hr
  - Overlap 2 hr of insulin GTT with subq p/t stopping GTT
- Treat potential underlying disorder: infection, ACS, intoxication

METFORMIN ASSOCIATED LACTIC ACIDOSIS

Pathophysiology

- ↑ conversion of glucose to lactate in GI tract and inhibiting mitochondrial respiratory chain complex 1 → ↓ lactate use in hepatic gluconeogenesis

Diagnosis

- History: N/V, abd pain, ∆MS, dyspnea; documented metformin use when eGFR <30
- Exam: tachycardia and hypotension in setting of severe acidosis
- Labs: AG acidosis, negative w/u for infection or other causes of severe lactic acidosis

Treatment *(Crit Care Med 2015;43:1716)*

- Volume resuscitation with isotonic IVF if hypotensive; avoid bicarbonate administration
- 1 g/kg IV dextrose if hypoglycemic
- Dialysis if: lactate >20, pH <7.0, shock despite fluid resuscitation, ongoing ∆MS >2 hr

---

HYPORENINEMIC HYPOALDOSTERONISM (TYPE IV RTA) IN DM

Pathophysiology

- Chronic interstitial inflammation and effect of hyperinsulinemia on WNK4 signaling lead to low renin levels and hypoaldosteronism *(NEJM 2015;373:548)*. Volume expansion from CKD can elevate atrial natriuretic peptide which directly inhibits renin and hyperkalemia-induced aldosterone secretion.
- Hypoaldosteronism → ↓ Na absorption → ↓ lumen electronegativity → ↓ K^+/H^+ excretion
- Hyperkalemia → impaired excretion of ammonium → H^+ retention

Diagnosis

- r/o alt causes of hypoaldosteronism:
  Primary adrenal insufficiency; chronic interstitial nephritis: HIV, Tb, sarcoid, EBV/CMV
  Drug-related: NSAIDs, CNIs, heparin, ACEI/ARB, K-sparing diuretics, trimethoprim
- Labs: non-AG acidosis, hyperkalemia, +UAG, urine pH <5.5, low plasma renin, aldosterone

Treatment

- If p/w HTN or edema, low K diet with thiazide or loop diuretic
- If not, then patiromer (potassium binding resin)

ELECTROLYTE DISORDERS IN DIABETES *(NEJM 2015;373:548)*

- Dysnatremia: intra → extracellular fluid shifts and osmotic diuresis from hyperglycemia
- Hyperkalemia: potassium shifts due to insulinopenia and acidosis, Type IV RTA
- Hypomagnesemia: renal Mg wasting due to osmotic diuresis
- Hypophosphatemia: renal Phos wasting due to osmotic diuresis
- Hypermagnesemia/Hyperphosphatemia: in DKA due to acidosis and insulinopenia

HYPERLIPIDEMIA

- CVD is a/w death in ESRD (50% of deaths, 20% of which is related to CAD)
- Dyslipidemia is a/w incidence and progression of kidney disease
- Risk stratification: 10-yr risk for atherosclerotic cardiovascular disease (ASCVD) *(Circulation 2014;129:S1)*; available AHA/ACC website, app (ASCVD Plus, QxMD®)

HMG CoA Reductase Inhibitors (Statin)

Intensity of Statins (mg) *(ACC/AHA Circulation 2019;139:e1046)*			
	Low	**Moderate**	**High**
↓ LDL goal	<30%	30–49%	≥50%
Statin dose		Atorva: 10–**20**	Atorva: 40–80
		Rosuva: 5–**10**	Rosuva: 20–40
	Simva: 10	Simva: 20–**40**	
	Prava: 10–20	Prava: **40**–80	
	Lova: 20	Lova: 40	
	Fluva: 20–40	Fluva: 40 BID or XL **80**	
		Pitava: 1, **2**, 4	

Bold: Recommended dose for CKD 3–5, including CKD 5D or w/ KT *(KDIGO Lipid 2013)*

2° (18 y/o) and 1° (40–75 y/o) Prevention of ASCVD *(ACC/AHA Circulation 2019;139:e1046)*	
Conditions	**Treatment**
Multiple major ASCVD or 1 major ASCVD + multiple high-risk conditions*	Maximal tolerated statin; if LDL ≥70 add ezetimibe then PCSK9-I
History of ASCVD event	High or moderate statin
LDL ≥190	Maximal tolerated statin; if LDL ≥100 add ezetimibe then PCSK9-I

LDL 70–189 and DM	Moderate statin; if multiple ASCVD risk (50–75 y/o) high statin
LDL 70–189 and 10 yr ASCVD ≥20%	High statin
LDL 70–189 and 10 yr ASCVD ≥7.5 to <20%	Moderate statin; consider risk enhancers# and coronary artery Ca score
LDL 70–189 and 10 yr ASCVD ≥5–<7.5%	Selective moderate statin; risk discussion considering risk enhancer#
LDL 70–189 and 10 yr ASCVD <5%	Lifestyle and risk discussion
LDL <70	Assess lifetime risk

CKD3–4 (eGFR 15–59) is one of high-risk conditions* and risk enhancing factors#

Statin Myopathy
- Dose-dependent; lowest with prava- and fluvastatin
- Prava-, fluva-, pitava-, and rosuvastatin are less affected by CYP3A4 inhibitors
- Drugs causing myopathy with statin: cyclosporine, gemfibrozil, protease inhibitors

Statin and AKI
- No ↓ kidney failure but ↓ proteinuria and rate of eGFR decline (AJKD 2016;67:881)
- Preoperative use is not a/w ↓ postoperative AKI (Sci Rep 2017;7:10091)
- Statin should not be recommended solely for renal protection and proteinuria

Hyperlipidemia in CKD
- Cholesterol level is predictor of mortality in HD pts: lowest in 200–219 (KI 2002;61:1887)
- Pravastatin 40 mg 28% ↓ CV death or recurrent nonfatal MI in CrCl <75 w/ previous MI (CARE Ann IM 2003;138:98); 23% ↓ new MI, CV death, or cardiac intervention in eGFR 30–60 (mean 55) (PPP Circulation 2004;110:1557)
- Simvastatin 20 mg + ezetimibe 10 mg 22% ↓ 1st major atherosclerotic event in non-dialysis Cr >1.7 ♂ >1.5 ♀; no effect in dialysis population (SHARP Lancet 2011;377:2181)
- Simvastatin + ezetimibe: better than simvastatin alone (JASN 2017;28:3034)
- Atorvastatin 20 mg did not lower CV death, nonfatal MI, and stroke in HD pts with T2DM. There was 18% ↓ cardiac events (4D NEJM 2005;353:238). If LDL >145, 31% ↓ cardiac death, nonfatal myocardial infarction, or stroke (CJASN 2011;6:1316)
- Rosuvastatin 10 mg did not lower CV death, nonfatal MI, or nonfatal stroke and all-case mortality in HD pts (AURORA NEJM 2009;360:1395). In post hoc analysis of DM pts, 32% reduction in cardiac events (AURORA JASN 2011;22:1335)

Pharmacologic Treatment of CKD (KDIGO Lipid 2013)	
18–49 y/o, CKD	Statin if CAD, DM, prior ischemic stroke or 10-yr risk >10%
≥50 y/o, eGFR ≥60	Statin
≥50 y/o, eGFR <60	Statin or statin/ezetimibe
ESRD	If pt is already on a statin, continue it. Do not routinely initiate it

OBESITY

Background and Definition
- By BMI (kg/m^2): overweight 25–29.9; class I 30–34.9; class II 35–39.9; class III ≥40
- Prevalence: increasing; 33.7 (2007–2008) → 39.6% (2015–2016) (JAMA 2018;319:1723)
- Waist circumference is a/w mortality in CKD (AJKD 2011;58:177)
- a/w low GFR and albuminuria (KI 2017;91:1224), inflammation (AJKD 2017;70:817)
- Risk factor of ESRD: overweight ×1.87, class I ×3.57, class II ×6.12 (Ann IM 2006;144:21)

Medical Causes of Obesity
- Cushing (including iatrogenic), hypothyroidism, PCOS, hypothalamus injury
- Atenolol, metoprolol, propranolol, MAO inhibitors, TCA, paroxetine, lithium, escitalopram, clozapine, olanzapine, risperidone, valproate, divalproex, mirtazapine, progestins, insulin, sulfonylureas, thiazolidinediones, meglitinides (Circulation 2012;125:1695)

Nonsurgical Treatment
- Behavioral intervention: dietary changes (energy deficit ≥500 kcal/d), physical activity, self-monitoring and in-person counseling (USPSTF Ann IM 2012;157:373; JAMA 2014;63:2985)
- Orlistat: lipase inhibitor; AKI (Arch IM 2011;171:703), oxalate nephropathy (AJKD 2007;49:153)
- Phentermine: used with topiramate; sympathomimetic; ↑ BP, HR; avoid in glaucoma
- Topiramate: cause hypokalemia, distal RTA → nephrolithiasis
- Liraglutide: ↓ new albuminuria (NEJM 2017;377:839)

- Lorcaserin: serotonin agonist; no significant CV side effect (*NEJM* 2018;379:1107); improved renal function and albuminuria (*Circulation* 2019;139:366)

OBESITY-RELATED GLOMERULOPATHY (*Nat Rev Nephrol* 2016;12:453)

- Glomerular hyperfiltration → glomerular hypertrophy > podocyte hypertrophy (*JASN* 2012;23:1351) → podocyte detachment → FSGS
- Bx: glomerulomegaly, FSGS (perihilar common), segmental foot process effacement
- Proteinuria: subnephrotic (52–90%), normal albumin, NS is uncommon (<6%)
- Tx: wt loss, RAASi induce proteinuria reduction >nonobese (*JASN* 2011;22:1122)
- Prognosis: 10–33% progressive renal failure and ESRD

GASTRIC BYPASS SURGERY

Indications (AACE Guidelines *Obesity* 2013;21:S1)
- BMI ≥40 w/o excessive risk of bariatric surgery
- BMI ≥35 with ≥1 severe obesity related comorbidities:T2DM, HTN, HLD, OSA, obesity-hypoventilation, NAFLD, NASH, pseudotumor cerebri, GERD, asthma, venous stasis, severe urinary incontinence, debilitating arthritis, considerably impaired QoL
- BMI 30–34.9 with diabetes or metabolic syndrome may be offered

Types of Surgery
- Malabsorptive: biliopancreatic diversion with or without duodenal switch
- Restrictive: adjustable gastric banding and sleeve gastrectomy
- Malabsorptive + restrictive hybrid: roux-en-Y gastric bypass (RYGB)

General Effects of Bariatric Surgery
- Lower mortality (1.3%) in 4.3 yr than matched cohort (2.3%) (*JAMA* 2018;319:279)
- ↑ Remission of HTN, DM, HLD (*JAMA* 2018;319:291)
- Deficiencies of iron, vitamin B_{12}, D, and thiamine. Gallstone, sagging skin
- ↑ Additional GI op (×2.0), op for obstruction (×10.5), peptic ulcer (×3.4) (*JAMA* 2018;319:291)

Renal Effects of Bariatric Surgery
- Postoperative AKI 8.5% (↑ 50% cr or dialysis requirement). Risk factors are higher BMI, HLD, intraop hypotension and preoperative use of ACEi/ARB (*CJASN* 2007;2:426)
- Renal function predicts postop complication: 4.6 (CKD1) – 9.9% (CKD5) (*JASN* 2012;23:885)
- ↓ Proteinuria, albuminuria (*Pediatr Nephrol* 2009;24:851; *Clin Nephrol* 2008;70:194)
- 27 kg weight reductions with RYGB: ↓ absolute mGFR (↓ glomerular hyperfiltration), unchanged mGFR adjusted for BSA. ↑ creatinine-based eGFR (overestimation d/t ↓ muscle mass), unchanged cystatin C-based eGFR (*BMC Nephrol* 2017;18:52)
- Improvement in KDIGO CKD risk categories (*JASN* 2018;29:1289)
- At median f/u of 4 yr, 58% ↓ eGFR decline ≥30%, 57% ↓ ESRD or cr doubling (*KI* 2016;90:164)

Calcium Oxalate Nephropathy
- Saponification of calcium/insoluble calcium oxalate complexes formation → excessive reabsorption of oxalate by the gut
- Malabsorptive procedure ↑ urine oxalate excretion, oxalate nephropathy (*KI* 2007;72:100; *CJASN* 2008;3:1676) kidney stone and CKD (×1.96) (*KI* 2015;87:839)

CKD-MINERAL AND BONE DISORDER

Definition (*KI Suppl* 2010;78:S10)
- Systemic disorder of mineral metabolism, bone, and vascular calcifications
- Abnormalities of Ca, PO_4, PTH, vitamin D metabolism
- Renal osteodystrophy refers to the bone component of CKD-Mineral and Bone Disorder (CKD-MBD) and is a spectrum of disorders in bone <u>turnover</u>, <u>mineralization</u>, and <u>volume</u> in CKD

Background
- Linked to vascular calcification: the leading cause of mortality in dialysis patients
- Clinical outcomes in CKD-MBD are increased risk of CV events and fractures
- Risk of CKD-MBD and (–) clinical outcomes ↑ with severity of CKD (usually eGFR <40)
- CKD: ↑ risk of falls 2/2 frailty and sarcopenia, ↑ fragility fracture and related mortality (2.5× 1-yr mortality rate after hip fracture) compared to general pop (*AJKD* 2000;36:1115)
- Renal osteodystrophy is a form of osteoporosis: osteoporosis is defined as a disorder of bone that increases risk of fracture

Pathogenesis

- Phosphorus retention with ↓ ionized Ca and vitamin D → 2° hyperparathyroidism
- In early CKD, ↑ fibroblast growth factor 23 (FGF-23) peptide → suppression of 1-α-hydroxylase → ↓ calcitriol production → ↑ PTH → phosphaturia with further GFR decline → hyperphosphatemia → osteoblastic transformation of vascular smooth muscle → vascular calcification
- Vascular calcification: media >intima → vascular stiffness and LVH. FGF-23 linked to LVH and CV events (atherosclerotic and death) in CKD (*JASN* 2014;25:349)

Adynamic Bone Disease

- Very low rate of bone formation (1 SD below normal mean, <20 μg^3/μm^2/yr bone formation) secondary to PTH suppression by inflammatory cytokines → low osteoblast activity and bone formation rates
- 55% of HD patients (*JBMR* 2011;26:1368)
- Increased incidence when PTH <100 pg/mL (PPV >90%)
- ↑ Serum calcium secondary to reduced bone uptake; ↓ alkaline phosphatase
- Some evidence that it is associated with increased risk of arterial calcification

Osteomalacia

- Low bone turnover with abnormal mineralization
- Previously from deposition of aluminum containing binders; now ↓ incidence (3%) (*JBMR* 2011;26:1368)

Hyperparathyroidism (34%)

- "High bone turnover disease" ↑ rates formation and resorption PTH >600 pg/mL
- Secondary to calcitriol deficiency, hyperphosphatemia, hypocalcemia, and excessive FGF-23 in early CKD

Relatively Low PTH

- Associated with ↑ mortality (U-shaped mortality curve with ↑ PTH) secondary to calcium-based binders, dialysate bath, assay differences, excessive active Vit D repletion

Vitamin D Deficiency

- ↓ 1,25(OH)$_2$D$_3$ active metabolite secondary to worsening CKD. Supplementation associated with improved survival in CKD and HD patients
- ↓ 25(OH)D (<30 ng/mL) associated with ↑ mortality in HD patients, supplementation with nutritional/inactive D2 (ergocalciferol) or D3 (cholecalciferol) results in reductions in PTH that are more appreciable in patients with less severe CKD

Hyperphosphatemia and Hypophosphatemia

- Phosphorus <3 and >6–7 associated with ↑ mortality

Hypercalcemia and Hypocalcemia

- Both associated with increased CV mortality
- Hypocalcemia (↑ PO$_4$ retention, ↓ calcitriol, PTH resistance) → ↑ PTH → abnl bone remodeling
- Hypercalcemia → extraskeletal calcification

Increased Alkaline Phosphatase (Hyperphosphatasemia)

- Linear a/w all-cause and CV mortality (pyrophosphate hydrolysis → vascular calcification) and hip fracture risk in HD pts (*NDT* 2014;29:1532). ↓ w/ vitamin D and calcimimetics

OSTEOPOROSIS

Definition

- Disease of low bone mass, disrupted bone architecture, and skeletal fragility
- Osteoporosis: dual energy x-ray absorptiometry (DXA) T-score ≥2.5 SD below young adult mean OR fragility fracture
- Low bone mass (previously osteopenia): T-score ≥1–2.5 below young adult mean
- Normal: within 1 SD of young adult mean

Background

- US prevalence 9.9 million, 2 million fractures annually (*Osteoporos Int* 2014;25:2359)
- CKD: lower bone mineral density (BMD) and 2× the fracture risk of age matched controls
- ESRD: up to 40% prevalence of fragility fractures

Screening

- All postmenopausal women and men >50 should be evaluated for fracture risk
- DXA recommended for all women ≥65 or <65 with equal or greater fracture risk on Fracture Risk Assessment Tool (FRAX): 10-yr risk ≥9.3% (USPSTF *Ann IM* 2011;154:356)
  - FRAX is available at www.sheffield.ac.uk/FRAX

Clinical Risk Factors for Fracture

- Advanced age, previous fracture, family hx of fracture, low body weight

Risk Factors for Osteoporosis-Related Fracture (Office of the Surgeon General US 2004)	
Lifestyle	Alcohol abuse, immobilization, low calcium intake, vitamin D deficiency, smoking, hypervitaminosis A
Genetic	CF, osteogenesis imperfecta, porphyria, Marfan syndrome, Ehlers–Danlos syndrome, hemochromatosis, homocystinuria, Gaucher disease, glycogen storage disease
Hypogonadal states	Anorexia nervosa, panhypopituitarism, premature menopause (<40 yr), hyperprolactinemia, androgen insensitivity, Turner syndrome, Klinefelter syndrome
Endocrine	Cushing syndrome, DM, hyperparathyroidism, thyrotoxicosis, central obesity
GI disorders	Celiac disease, IBD, malabsorption, PBC, gastric bypass, pancreatic disease
Hematologic	Hemophilia, leukemia/lymphoma, multiple myeloma, sickle cell disease, thalassemia
Rheumatologic	RA, SLE, ankylosing spondylitis
Neurologic and musculoskeletal	Epilepsy, MS, muscular dystrophy, Parkinson disease, spinal cord injury, stroke
Medications	Aluminum, anticoagulants, anticonvulsants, aromatase inhibitors, barbiturates, chemotherapeutic drugs, depomedroxyprogesterone, glucocorticoids (>2.5 mg/day prednisone for >3 mo), GnRH agonists, methotrexate, PPIs, SSRIs, TZDs, thyroid hormones, parental nutrition
Miscellaneous	HIV/AIDS, amyloidosis, COPD, CHF, ESRD, sarcoidosis, post-transplant bone disease

Glucocorticoid-Induced Osteoporosis (ACR *Arthritis Rheumatol* 2017;69:1521)

- Monitoring and prevention for patients taking >2.5 mg/d prednisone for >3 mo
- Osteoprotegerin inhibition & ↑ RANKL synthesis → osteoclast proliferation
- Inhibited gonadotropin secretion→ ↓ androgens and estrogens → ↓ bone resorption
- ↑ Osteoblast apoptosis → ↓ bone formation
- High fracture risk during early rapid bone loss phase (first 3–6 mo) and subsequently correlates to dose and duration of glucocorticoid treatment

Clinical Manifestations

- None until there is a fracture (often no preceding trauma)
- Vertebral fracture most common (~2/3 asymptomatic, usually incidentally found on other imaging, signs: height loss and kyphosis)

Workup and Fracture Risk Assessment (*Osteoporosis Int* 2014;25:2359)

- DXA for BMD of hip and spine: spine BMD has limited use in CKD to predict fracture risk 2/2 extraosseous calcification and focal osteosclerosis
- Vertebral imaging (lateral T and L-spine X-ray or lateral assessment on DXA) in setting of low bone density/risk factors to assess for vertebral fracture (indication for treatment)
- FRAX: calculator to estimate 10-yr probability of major osteoporotic or hip fracture for untreated patients age 40–90. Can be used with or without BMD at the femoral neck
- Bone turnover markers: not routinely used, possible role in monitoring response to tx
- Evaluation for secondary etiologies if recent/multiple fractures or very low BMD

TREATMENT (*Nat Rec Nephrol* 2013;9:681; *CJASN* 2018;13:962)

- Conventional osteoporosis meds effective in mild CKD when CKD-MBD excluded (normal PTH, Ca, and PO$_4$)
- Insufficient evidence for fracture reduction in stage 4–5 CKD
- Initiate treatment if eGFR <30 with fragility fracture or osteoporosis (KDIGO MBD 2017)

- Exclude adynamic bone disease prior to bisphosphonates (theoretical ↓ in bone formation)
- Exclude hyperparathyroid bone disease in patients with CKD prior to anabolic treatment

Nonpharmacologic Treatment
- Diet (1,200 mg/d calcium, 800–1,000 IU/d Vit D), lifestyle (exercise and fall prevention)
- In CKD patients, limit calcium intake to 500–800 mg daily, replete 25-OH vit D to 30 and manage metabolic disturbances a/w CKD-MBD (hyperparathyroidism, hypocalcemia, hyperphosphatemia, vitamin D deficiency) prior to starting treatment for osteoporosis

Estrogen
- ↓ Fractures, initiate within 10 yr of menopause given CV risk. Dose-reduce in CKD.
- Avoid estrogen–progestin combo d/t VTE, CVA, CAD, and breast CA risk

Selective Estrogen Receptor Modulators (SERMs)
- Raloxifene ↓ vertebral fractures in eGFR <45, ↑ L-spine BMD in stage 4–5 CKD
- ↑ VTE risk and 1.4× higher serum levels in CKD (KI 2003;63:2269)

Bisphosphonates
- ↓ Fracture rate by 50% in postmenopausal osteoporosis (AJM 2009;122:S14), effectiveness correlates with degree of bone-turnover
- Fracture reduction comparable in mild CKD, but data lacking in stage 4–5 CKD (small ↓ BMD in ibandronate-treated HD patients) (Am J Nephrol 2012;36:238)
- Prevents resorption by binding mineralized bone surface—half bound with remaining half excreted unchanged by the kidney. Cleared by HD.

Teriparatide: Recombinant Human PTH$_{1-34}$ Peptide
- Anabolic effect with daily SQ injections
- ↑ BMD and ↓ fractures in mild CKD, ↑ BMD in adynamic bone disease (Kidney Blood Press Res 2010;33:221). No evidence to support use in CKD-MBD.

Denosumab
- Monoclonal ab against RANKL (osteoclast-differentiation cytokine)
- Antiresorptive, nonrenally excreted, no restriction with CrCl <35
- ↓ Vertebral fracture in mild CKD (JBMR 2011;26:1829)
- Risk of severe symptomatic hypocalcemia in late stage CKD (JBMR 2012;27:1471). No evidence to support use in CKD-MBD.

Strontium Ranelate: Incorporated into Bone in the Place of Calcium
- Used outside the US for postmenopausal osteoporosis
- Renally cleared, no safety data to recommend use in CKD-MBD

Osteoporosis Pharmacotherapy in CKD (Nat Rev Nephrol 2013;9:681; KI 2012;82:833)		
Drug	Comments	FDA Label
Alendronate	Not recommended for CrCl <35	2013
Risedronate	Not recommended for CrCl <35	2013
Ibandronate	Not recommended for CrCl <30	2013
Zoledronic acid	Not recommended for CrCl <35	2013
Teriparatide	Caution in recent urolithiasis Benefit in CKD, low PTH and low BMD	2009
Denosumab	Risk of hypocalcemia in CrCl <30 May be useful to treat hypercalcemia	2013
Calcitonin	No renal adjustment Probably safe, weak effects, no data in CKD	2012
Raloxifene	No renal adjustment Pilot data with beneficial effects in HD patients	2007
Estrogen	Limited data in CKD 4–5; appropriate in premenopausal women with CKD and amenorrhea	2011

PROGNOSIS AND MONITORING

- 8–35% excess mortality within 1 yr of hip fracture (Osteoporos Int 2009;20:1633)

Monitoring
- eGFR >30: BMD testing 1–2 yr after initiation of therapy, q2yr thereafter
- eGFR <30:
  - q4mo serum calcium, phos, 25(OH)D; calcium 10 d after starting denosumab
  - Annual Cr monitoring on bisphosphonates
  - Repeat DXA may be useful for response to tx (not for assessing fracture risk)
  - Markers of bone turnover not recommended

PRIMARY HYPERPARATHYROIDISM

Definition and Pathogenesis
- 1° Hyperparathyroidism (PHPT): one or more parathyroid gland(s) secretes excessive PTH with elevated or high-normal serum calcium and replete vitamin D
  - Adenoma (80–85%), hyperplasia (10–15%), carcinoma (<1%)
- 2° HPT: renal failure (impaired calcitriol production and hyperphosphatemia), vitamin D deficiency (may be present in PHPT and lower serum calcium to normal range), meds (lithium, thiazides), calcium malabsorption, renal calcium loss, inhibited of bone resorption
- 3° HPT: after longstanding 2° (glands remain hyperfunctioning despite correction of 2°)
- Normocalcemic PHPT: variant with normal total and ionized calcium, elevated PTH, and no 2° causes. Progression to hypercalcemia (19%), renal stones, fracture, decline in BMD, and hypercalciuria (40%) over 3 yr (JCEM 2007;35:123)
- Familial hypocalciuric hypercalcemia (FHH): benign mild Ca elevation 2/2 AD inactivating mutation in the parathyroid and kidney calcium-sensing receptor (CaSR)
- PTH inhibits NHE3 and bicarbonate reabsorption in PT. Clinical pRTA is uncommon (KI 1985;28:187)

Clinical Manifestations
- Most commonly asymptomatic hypercalcemia; asymptomatic nephrocalcinosis
- Renal stones in 55%, osteoporosis in 63%, vertebral fractures in 35% (JCEM 2015;100:1309)
- Nonspecific sx related to hypercalcemia: weakness, anorexia, fatigue, polyuria/polydipsia, cognitive/neuromuscular dysfunction
- Parathyroid bone disease: osteitis fibrosa cystica (<5%) excessive osteoclast activity → subperiosteal bone resorption in middle phalanges, tapering of distal clavicles, bone cysts, brown tumors (fibrous tissue and poorly mineralized bone) → bone pain. Reduced cortical BMD and increased risk of fracture
- CV: HTN, LVH, diastolic dysfunction, coronary atherosclerosis
- Atypical: parathyroid crisis (1–2%) symptomatic severe hypercalcemia (mean 17.5 mg/dL)

Workup
- Serum calcium: repeat to confirm. Most <1.0 mg/dL above ULN
- PTH: elevated in 80–90%, wnl 10–20%. No performance differences between 2nd gen "intact" and 3rd gen "whole molecule" 1–84 assays (JCEM 2014;99:3570)
- Creatinine: for calculation of CrCl; 60 is the threshold of parathyroidectomy
- 24-hr urinary calcium: elevated (>200–300 mg/d) in 40%, correlates with risk of renal complications. FE$_{Ca}$ < 0.01 sens/spec of 85%/88%, PPV 85% (Clin Endocrinol 2008;69:713)
- 25-Hydroxyvitamin D (25-OH vit D): <20 may lead to a false-positive dx of PHPT. Repletion increases urinary calcium excretion

Differential Diagnosis for PHPT				
	PTH	Ca	Vitamin D	Urinary Ca
PHPT	↑ or high nl	↑	Nl, low-nl, or ↓	↑ or high nl
FHH	Nl, ↑ (15–20%)	↑	Nl	↓
PHPT w/ Vit D deficiency	↑	nl	↓	Low nl or ↓
2° HPT d/t Vit D deficiency	↑	nl or ↓	↓	↓
Normocalcemic PHPT	↑	nl	nl	nl

- Genetic testing (CaSR, AP2S1, GNA11) for FHH. Indications: positive family hx, young age, multigland involvement, concern for multiple endocrine neoplasia (MEN 1)
- Renal imaging: u/s, CT, or plain film for stone and nephrocalcinosis detection
- Bone mineral density (BMD): decreased particularly at cortical sites (forearm and hip), not required for dx. Imaging for vertebral fracture recommended if DXA negative for osteoporosis d/t increased risk
- Neck imaging (ultrasound, technetium-99m sestamibi scan, dynamic CT, MRI) not indicated for dx, used for surgical localization

Surgical Treatment: Parathyroidectomy
- Symptomatic hypercalcemia or nephrolithiasis

Indications for Parathyroidectomy in Asymptomatic PHPT	(JCEM 2014;99:3561)
Age	<50
Renal	CrCl <60, 24-hr urine calcium >400 mg/d with increased stone risk, nephrolithiasis or nephrocalcinosis on imaging study
Bone	DXA T score <-2.5 at lumbar spine, total hip, femoral neck, or distal 1/3 radius OR Vertebral fracture by x-ray, CT, MRI, or vertebral fracture assessment on DXA
Serum Ca	>1 mg/dL above the upper limit of normal

Medical Treatment

- For nonsurgical candidates or failure of cure after surgery
- Dietary Ca 1,000–1,200 mg/d: dietary Ca & vit D def ↑ PTH: should not be restricted
- Vit D repletion (goal >30 ng/mL) ↓ PTH (17%) and ↑ L-spine BMD (2.5%) (JCEM 2014;99:1072)
- Thiazide: ↓ PTH, urinary Ca (JCEM 2017;102:1270). Monitor serum Ca level.
- Calcimimetics: serum Ca >1 above ULN. Cinacalcet normalizes Ca in 75%, no change in BMD, preferred in patients with nl BMD (Eur J Endocrinol 2015;172:527)
- Bisphosphonates: osteoporosis and/or fracture risk. Improves BMD without change in serum calcium. Combo therapy with cinacalcet can be used to reduce serum Ca levels but has not been studied in RCTs.
- Estrogen–progestin: significant increases in BMD in postmenopausal PHPT. Not recommended 1st-line tx d/t breast cancer, stroke, and CHD risk.

Prognosis

- Surgery as the only definitive therapy
- Significant increases in BMD and reduced risk of renal stones (NEJM 1999;341:1249)
  - Comparable BMD improvements with bisphosphonates alone (JCEM 2010;95:1653); Reduced fracture risk observed but not demonstrated in RCTs
- No change in postop renal function (JCEM 2014;99:2646)
- Excess mortality (RR 1.7 male, 1.8 female) 2/2 cardiovascular disease persists after surgery, unclear relationship to severity of underlying disease (Eur J Clin Invest 1998;28:271)
- Small nonspecific differences in postop neuropsychiatric sx that favor surgery

URIC ACID (UA)

Background

- UA ↔ Urate⁻ + H⁺, pKa 5.75; potential to crystallize in acidic milieu (pH <5.5)
- UA is the result of metabolism of purine in the liver; diet can provide ~40% of urate
- UA excretion via the GI tract (1/3) and the kidney (2/3)
- <5% protein bound; most UA is filtered at the glomerulus

PCT Handling of UA	
Process (Proportion of UA, PCT Segment)	Transporter
Reabsorption (~99%, S1), postsecretory reabsorption (~40%, S3)	URAT1, OAT4 (apical) GLUT9 (basolateral)
Secretion (~50%, S2)	OAT1, OAT3 (basolateral) MRP4, ABCG2, NPT1, NPT4 (apical)

URAT, urate anion exchanger; OAT, organic anion transporter; GLUT, glucose transporter; MRP, multidrug resistance-associated protein; ABCG, ATP binding cassette subfamily G member; NPT, sodium-dependent phosphate transporter

- FE_{UA} ~10%; >20% in ATN
- Females have lower levels by 1–1.5 (estrogen-mediated renal urate excretion) (Hum Reprod 2013;28:1853). After menopause level ≈ male's level (Arthritis Res Ther 2008;10:R116)

Pathogenesis of Clinical Conditions Associated With Uric Acid

- Hyperuricemia: 85–90% underexcretion; 10–15% overproduction (Arthritis Rheum 2002;47:610)
- Hyperuricemia is risk factor for renal and cardiovascular diseases (potential mechanism: activation of the RAAS, ↓ NO, ↓ glutathione formation an antioxidant and dysfunction of intrahepatic fructose metabolism)
- CKD progression: ↑ oxidative stress, endothelial dysfunction → systemic and glomerular HTN; alteration of RAAS→ ↑ renal vascular resistance, ↓ renal blood flow (NDT 2013;28:2221)

- Autosomal dominant tubulointerstitial kidney disease (ADTKD), aka medullary cystic kidney disease can be cause by mutations of *UMOD*, *REN*, and *MUC1* gene: familial CKD/ESRD, chronic tubulointerstitial nephritis, CKD, and hyperuricemia/gout
- Hypouricemia associated with uricosuria may be associated with recurrent exercise-induced AKI resulting from mutations in URAT or GLUT9 transporters

Factors Affecting Uric Acid Level		
	Hyperuricemia	Hypouricemia
Diet	Alcohol, red meat, seafood, high fructose diet	Low-fat dairy products, coffee, plants proteins
Medication	Thiazide, loop diuretics, niacin, low-dose ASA, CNI, pyrazinamide, ethambutol, pancreatic extract (for CF)	Allopurinol, febuxostat Losartan, fenofibrate
Pathologic conditions	Volume depletion, Vit B_{12} def, pre-eclampsia	Mutation of URAT1, GLUT9, pRTA, SIADH, cerebral salt wasting

HYPERURICEMIA

Clinical Manifestations and Management of Hyperuricemia		
Diagnosis/Labs	Pathogenesis	Prevention/Therapy
Acute Uric Acid Nephropathy		
AKI + UA >15 Urine UA/creat >1	UA overproduction: TLS, seizure Lesch–Nyhan Sd	IV fluid (HCO₃ controversial) XOI, rasburicase
Chronic Urate Nephropathy		
CKD + UA >9 for Cr ≤1.5 UA >10 for Cr 1.5–2 UA >12 for Cr >2	Deposition of sodium urate crystals in the medullary interstitium → chronic interstitial fibrosis DDx: lead nephropathy	CKD management UA lowering agents
Uric Acid Nephrolithiasis		
CT, stone analysis	Low urine pH, high urine UA	Urine alkalinization ↑ UOP >2 L/d XOI in hyperuricosuria (no RCT)
Gout		
UA can be nl within 2 wk of an acute attack Urate crystals on polarized light microscopy	Deposition of urate crystal: acute gouty arthritis (starts mostly at night d/t low body temp) Chronic gouty arthropathy Tophaceous gout (connective tissue deposits)	Acute attack treated w/ colchicine, steroid (intra-articular/po) or NSAIDs UA <6 (<5 +tophi) w/ XOI
Asymptomatic High Uric Acid		
2/3 of ↑ UA is asymptomatic UA >8	The degree of ↑ UA is a/w ↑ risk of gout and nephrolithiasis Uncertain role of UA in CKD progression	Consider tx of male w/ UA >13, female w/ UA >10 (*JAMA IM* 2018;178:1526; *AJKD* 2015;66:945)

General Management
- Goal: lower UA levels by ≤1–2/mo
- Weight loss, purine restricted diet
- Diet modifications: ↓ total calories, refined carbohydrates, saturated fat, meat and fish, ↑ low-fat dairy products, plant proteins
- Cherries reduces recurrence of gout; Vit C (500 mg/d) reduce UA levels by 0.5

Xanthine Oxidase Inhibitors (XOI)
- Initiate w/ anti-inflammatory drugs to prevent acute flare-up
- Do not use w/ 6-mercaptopurine and azathioprine; metabolism is inhibited by XOI
- Allopurinol: a/w lower incident renal disease than febuxostat (*Ann Rheum Dis* 2017;76:1669) Start w/ 50 mg qd in CKD4–5; 100 mg qd otherwise; uptitrate dose monitoring toxicity (can exceed 300 mg/d) (ACR Guidelines *Arthritis Care Res* 2012;64:143)

Allopurinol hypersensitivity (dose-dependent): high risk if +HLA-B*5801; ✓ in Han Chinese, Thai, Korean, African American (Semin Arthritis Rheum 2017;46:594); AKI, fever, rash, eosinophilia, ↑ LFTs

Other s/e: vasculitis, AIN, xanthine or oxypurinol crystalluria and urolithiasis
- Febuxostat: start w/ 40 mg qd; No cross-reactivity w/ allopurinol
  s/e: ↑ all cause and CV morality c/t allopurinol in pts with coexisting CV conditions (NEJM 2018;378:1200); ↑ LFTs, myopathy and rhabdomyolysis in CKD (CJASN 2017;12:744)

Anti-Inflammatory Drugs
- Treatment of acute gout and initiation of XOI
- Colchicine, corticosteroid ≈ NSAIDs (J Rheumatol 2018;45:128)

Uricosuric Agents
- When urine UA excretion is <800 mg/24 hr
- Avoid in CaOx nephrolithiasis; use w/ XOI
- Probenecid, losartan (inhibit URAT1), fenofibrate
- Lesinurad: inhibit URAT1, OAT4; use w/ XOI, otherwise a/w AKI (Rheumatology 2017;56:2170)

HYPOURICEMIA

Background
- Low serum UA <2 mg/dL
- Hypouricemia is pathological in conditions a/w renal urate reabsorption defects (ie, hypouricemia due to hyperuricosuria)

Etiologies
- Decreased UA production:
  - XOI therapy, liver disease
  - Hereditary xanthinuria (deficiency in XO): xanthine stones treated with hydration and urine alkalinization, myopathy
  - Purine nucleoside phosphorylase (PNP) deficiency: recurrent infections
- UA oxidation: rasburicase
- Decreased UA tubular reabsorption
  - Fanconi syndrome, volume expansion, SIADH, salt wasting
  - Familial renal hypouricemia: non-Ashkenazi Jews and Japanese, mutation in URAT1 or GLUT9 leading to decrease urate reabsorption, GLTU9 more severe symptomatology than URAT1, recurrent nephrolithiasis and exercise-induced AKI

Exercise-Induced AKI in Familial Renal Hypouricemia
- UA is an antioxidant and AKI is due to an oxidative stress induced by exercise; other potential etiology could be due to the increase of uric acid excretion that is exacerbated by exercise leading to intratubular UA precipitation
- Some patients were successfully treated with allopurinol
- Prognosis is good with recovery of renal function

RHEUMATOLOGY

- Many autoimmune disease (AID) present with renal manifestations, eg, SLE; conversely lupus nephritis may develop w/o systemic manifestation of SLE

Rheumatologic Conditions and Kidney	
Systemic diseases/conditions associated with kidney involvement	SLE, systemic sclerosis, IgA vasculitis (HSP), Cryoglobulinemia, ankylosing spondylitis (IgAN) Allergic interstitial nephritis: Sjögren syndrome Medication-associated AID: immune checkpoint inhibitor (NEJM 2018;378:158)
AID causing AA amyloidosis	AID a/w 60% of AA amyloidosis. RA (33%) is m/c (NEJM 2007;356:2361)
Treatment of rheumatologic conditions a/w kidney involvement	NSAIDs: vasoconstriction, interstitial nephritis, papillary necrosis Allopurinol: interstitial nephritis, DRESS Sulfasalazine: interstitial nephritis Anti-TNF agents: lupus nephritis, pauci-immune crescentic, IC-mediated (NDT 2005;20:1400)
Renal disease affecting course of rheumatologic conditions	Exacerbation of gout by diuretics/CKD

ANA Staining Pattern, Possible Antigens, and Conditions
- Homogeneous (histone, DNA, and DNA–histone complexes): SLE, RA, SS, MCTD
- Speckled (U1 RNP, Scl-70, Sm, and La): dcSSc, SLE, MCTD
- Centromere: lcSSc, dcSSc
- Nucleolar (fibrillarin, RNA polymerase I and III, Th, PM-Scl, and RNA helicase): SLE, dcSSc

SYSTEMIC SCLEROSIS (SSc)

- An autoimmune disorder causing vasculopathy and **fibrosis** of skin and multiple organs
- Skin: edema and redness → thickening/sclerodactyly, fingertip pitting pitting ulcer

Classification of SSc Based on Skin Involvement	
Limited cutaneous SSc (lcSSc)	Diffuse Cutaneous SSc (dcSSc)
Skin involvement on extremities distal to elbows and knees >face	Skin involvement on trunk, distal, and proximal extremities and face
CREST syndrome: calcinosis cutis (soft tissue calcification), Raynaud phenomenon, Esophageal dysmotility, Sclerodactyly, and Telangiectasia PAH >pulmonary fibrosis	Scleroderma renal crisis: more common Restrictive cardiomyopathy
Anticentromere Ab	Antitopoisomerase-1 (Scl-70) Ab Anti-RNA polymerase III Ab

- Vascular involvement: Raynaud phenomenon, telangiectasia
- Albuminuria (25%), intermediate MW proteinuria (31.3%) a/w GI involvement and dcSSc (Clin Nephrol 2008;70:110); MPO-ANCA crescentic GN (Clin Nephrol 2007;68:165)
- Penicillamine: used as antifibrotic; a/w MN, MPO-ANCA GN (J Rheumatol 2006;33:1886)
- Myeloablative auto-HSCT improved event-free and overall survival (NEJM 2018;378:35)

Scleroderma Renal Crisis (SRC)
- Prevalence: 5–10% of systemic sclerosis (Rheumatology 2009;48:iii32)
- Risk factors: diffuse SSc, CS ≥15 mg/d prednisone (Arthritis Rheum 1998;41:1613), anti-RNA polymerase III Ab (25% risk vs 2% if –) (Rheumatology 2009;48:1570), fine speckled ANA
- Less common w/ anticentromere Ab (QJM 2007;100:485)
- AKI not explained by other causes, malignant HTN: abrupt onset or worsening of HTN, ↑ PRA, retinal hemorrhage and exudates
- TMA: MAHA (schistocytes, ↑ retics, ↓ hapto, ↑ LDH, ↑ indirect bili) + ↓ plt
- Urinalysis: normal or mild proteinuria with few cells or casts
- Kidney Bx: TMA, onion skin hypertrophy from intimal proliferation and thickening; vascular thrombosis, glomerular ischemic collapse, and peritubular C4d deposits a/w poor renal outcome (Hum Pathol 2009;40:332)
- Treatment: indefinite ACEi (↑ patient and renal survival) (Ann IM 1990;113:352; 2000;133:600). ARB unproven; avoid glucocorticoids; ? PLEX (NDT 2012;27:4398)
- Prognosis: ESRD (54%), death (41%) despite ACEi on 45.8 mo f/u (Rheumatology 2012;51:460); Kidney may recover in up to 18 mo of dialysis on ACEi (Ann IM 2000;133:600)
- Transplantation: wait for 6–18 mo for recovery; patient survival is better than on dialysis 90.1% (vs 81.1%), 79.5% (vs 54.6%) at 1 and 3 yr (AJT 2004;4:2027); avoid CNI (Br J Rheumatol 1994;33:90) and high-dose CS

RHEUMATOID ARTHRITIS (RA) (Rheum Dis Clin North Am 2018;44:571)

Background
- eGFR <60 more common (25–34%) than general population (AJKD 2014;63:206; Clin Rheumatol 2017;36:2673); chronic inflammation mediated CVD and metabolic changes
- Hydroxychloroquine use is a/w ↓ CKD (CJASN 2018;13:702)
- Rheumatoid Factor: IgM antibody against IgG Fc portion; elevated in various conditions:
  - Rheumatologic: RA, type II & III cryoglobulinemia
  - Aging, infection (endocarditis, HBV, HCV, TB) sarcoidosis, silicosis, asbestosis, PBC

Methotrexate (MTX)
- MTX is excreted by glomerular filtration and tubular secretion
- Rheumatologic dose of MTX does not cause crystal nephropathy as in oncologic high dose
- MTX cause bone marrow suppression in CKD (Renal Fail 2006;28:95)
- CrCl 31–50: reduce dose by 50%; CrCl ≤30: contraindicated (ACR Arthritis Rheum 2008;59:762)

Glomerular Disease

Renal Biopsy Findings in RA (Arthritis Rheum 1995;38:242; Clin Exp Nephrol 2017;21:1024)			
Region	Mesangial GN	Amyloidosis	MN
Finland (n = 110)	36%	30%	17%
Japan (n = 52)	4%	21%	63%

- AA amyloidosis (17.2 yr) and mesangial GN (12.9 yr) are a/w longer disease duration than MN (3.8 yr) (Arthritis Rheum 1995;38:242); **Fat pad aspiration** can diagnose AA amyloidosis
- Drugs a/w MN, bucillamine, penicillamine, gold, and auranofin are now rarely used

---

SJÖGREN SYNDROME (SS)

Background and Extrarenal Manifestations

- Lymphocytic infiltration around epithelial ducts of exocrine glands (salivary, lacrimal) gland
- Sicca syndrome: keratoconjunctivitis sicca (dry eyes), xerostomia (dry mouth)
- Secondary form (a/w RA, SLE, scleroderma) has extraglandular findings: ILD, cutaneous vasculitis, peripheral neuropathy
- ↑ Lymphoma (NHL) ×6.5, in primary and secondary form (Blood 2008;111:4029)
- (+) Anti-Ro/SS-A, Anti-La/SS-B
- Kidney biopsy: TIN (71%) >> MPGN (8%), cryoglobulinemic GN, FSGS (CJASN 2009;4:1423)

Tubulointerstitial Nephritis (TIN) in Sjögren Syndrome

- CD4+ T lymphocyte dominant; Granulomatous TIN is rare (CJASN 2009;4:1423)
- Tx: prednisone, AZA, rituximab, MMF (BMC Musculoskelet Disord 2016;17:2)

Other Renal Manifestations

- No CKD4 progression to ESRD (CJASN 2009;4:1423). The other study showed 11% ESRD (Arthritis Rheum 2013;65:2945)
- GN: a/w ↑ death, CKD, lymphoma (Arthritis Rheum 2013;65:2945)
- Cryoglobulinemic GN: 32.5% (m/c noninfectious cause); 22.5% Sjögren's only; 10% Sjögren's + hematologic malignancy (JASN 2016;27;1213)
  - Sjögren's w/ cryoglobulinemia has ↑ mortality (×4.36) than w/o (Rheumatology 2016;55:1443)
- dRTA >> pRTA: absence of H⁺-ATPase in CCT (JASN 1992;3:264); Ab against CA-II (Am J Med 2005;118:181); severe hypocitraturia → CaP nephrocalcinosis; stone 4/24 (CJASN 2009;4:1423)
- Hypokalemia: dRTA, sodium wasting (QJM 1993;86:513); rarely Gitelman syndrome-like metabolic alkalosis with anti-NCC Ab (AJKD 2008;52:1163)
- Nephrogenic DI: polydipsia can be attributed to xerostomia

VASCULITIS

Large Vessel Vasculitis

- Takayasu arteritis: renovascular HTN >50%
- Giant cell arteritis: rare renal involvement; ANCA GN may present (Rheumatology 2014;53:882)

Medium Vessel Vasculitis

- Polyarteritis nodosa: a/w HBV frequently; renal artery microaneurysm → rupture, peri-renal hematoma, renal infarctions; mild proteinuria, CKD, HTN (d/t RAS activation)
- Skin: retiform (angulated) purpura ± palpable purpura

Small Vessel Vasculitis

- IgA vasculitis (HSP), staph-associated IgA dominant IRGN, ANCA-associated GN, cryoglobulinemia
- Renal manifestation: GN with hematuria and proteinuria
- Skin: palpable purpura, telangiectasia, ulcer, urticaria
- Skin biopsy: leukocytoclastic vasculitis; direct IF should be performed
  IgA deposition in IgAV, IgM deposition in cryoglobulinemia, pauci-immune in ANCA

PAIN MEDICINE

ANALGESIC NEPHROPATHY

- CKD due to years of consuming at least 2 analgesics, usually containing codeine or caffeine (AJKD 1996;27:162); can also occur with single agents
- Most cases were due to phenacetin, much less common since banned in 1983 by FDA
- Phenacetin also linked to urothelial malignancies
- Chronic acetaminophen: possible (NEJM 2001;345:1801); aspirin: unlikely (JAMA 2001;286:315)
- NSAIDs cause AKI and worsening of preexisting CKD, but unclear if causes incident CKD (Arch IM 2004;164:1519; Am J Med 2007;120:280)

Pathogenesis (AJKD 1996;28:S39)

- Phenacetin metabolized to acetaminophen and other metabolites, which concentrate in renal papilla, causing damage by lipid peroxidation; most damage in renal medulla
- Aspirin potentiates effect of acetaminophen by further depleting glutathione, which normally detoxifies acetaminophen

Clinical Manifestations, Workup, and Treatment

- Renal papillary necrosis, chronic interstitial nephritis, ↓ urinary concentrating capacity (KI 2007;72:517)
- Often clinical diagnosis based on history, bland urine, minimal proteinuria
- Noncontrast CT: indented kidneys and papillary calcifications but low sensitivity, especially in absence of phenacetin (5–26%) (JASN 2006;17:1472)
- Sensitivity of ultrasound likely even lower sensitivity, but frequently first-line imaging
- Urinalysis with spot proteinuria (usually <1.5 g) (KI 2007;72:517)
- Tx: no specific treatment other than stopping offending analgesics

Prognosis

- If analgesics are stopped, eGFR can stabilize if there is not heavy proteinuria or CKD is not advanced; heavy proteinuria can develop due to nephron loss
- Monitor patients with a history of phenacetin use for transitional cell malignancy

---

NEPHROTOXICITY OF NSAIDs

- Mostly associated with AKI but can worsen preexisting CKD and may cause incident CKD; no established safe dose/duration in setting of CKD, risk higher with lower GFR
- Topical NSAIDs with far less systemic absorption than oral, fewer side effects (Semin Arthritis Rheum 2016;45:S18); case reports of renal failure after topical use; not well studied in CKD, cannot routinely recommend currently
- COX-2 inhibitors: risk of AKI may be lower with celecoxib than naproxen or other nonselective NSAIDs (RR 1.5 vs 2.4 and 2.3, respectively) (Am J Epidemiol 2006;164:881)

Pathophysiology and Risk Factors

- Inhibit renal prostaglandin (PG) synthesis; PG → renal afferent arteriolar vasodilation and natriuresis; in normal circumstances, not very important
  - In setting of hypoperfusion, renal PG needed to counteract excessive renal vaso-constrictive effects of AII and SNS to preserve renal blood flow and GFR
  - NSAIDs block PGs, leading to vasoconstriction, renal ischemia, ↓ GFR, and fluid retention
- **AKI risk factors:** CHF, cirrhosis, nephrotic syndrome, hypercalcemia, volume depletion (all conditions that lead to decreased effective arterial volume); also CKD, elderly
  - Concurrent ACEI/ARB + diuretic + NSAIDs combo increase risk (BMJ 2013;346:e8525)

Clinical Manifestation

- Hemodynamically mediated AKI, ATN, AIN, MN, MCD, chronic tubulointerstitial nephritis, hypertension (NEJM 1984;310:563)
- Usually minimal proteinuria (<0.5–1 g), with acellular urine; heavier proteinuria suggests MN or MCD, or from preexisting CKD; sterile pyuria suggests AIN

Electrolyte Derangements

- Hyperkalemia: NSAID-mediated decrease in aldosterone release, hyporenin state from decrease in PGs, and any concurrent renal failure
- Hyponatremia: increased ADH activity from decrease in PGs, and concurrent renal failure which limits free water clearance

Treatment

* Supportive, volume repletion, hold NSAIDs/ACEI/ARB; may need biopsy if no improvement in few days, or if atypical labs such as >1 g proteinuria or cellular urine that would suggest a lesion other than ATN (eg, membranous, AIN)

PAIN CONTROL IN CKD AND ESRD (Semin Dial 2014;27:188)

* Most data in HD, prevalence 21–81%, similar in PD and nondialysis stage 5 CKD; nearly 73% in one study of CKD 1–5 patients (Clin Nephrol 2010;73:294)
* Adjunctive nonpharmacologic therapies (eg, exercise, behavioral therapy) should be tried
* Pharmacokinetics of analgesics are different in CKD vs non-CKD

General Approach to Chronic Pain

Modified WHO Analgesic Ladder (JASN 2006;17:3198)	
Step 1	Acetaminophen
Step 2	Hydrocodone, oxycodone, tramadol
Step 3	Hydromorphone, methadone, fentanyl, oxycodone

* Avoid NSAIDs, meperidine (causes seizures)
* If ineffective add tramadol, or switch to low-dose opioids with slow titration if needed

Neuropathic Pain

* Common in CKD given high prevalence of DM
* Tx: start w/ SNRI or gabapentin/pregabalin; cautiously use TCA; often need combo therapy
  - Lidocaine patches if localized; add-on acetaminophen +/− opioids/tramadol if needed

Carpal Tunnel Syndrome

* 9–63% incidence in ESRD, increases with duration of time on dialysis; due to deposition of β2-microglobulin amyloid, extracellular calcification, and ischemia related to AV access
* Tx: usually splinting, CS injection, or surgical decompression for severe/refractory cases

ADPKD

* Pain due to enlarging cysts, stones, cyst hemorrhage/infection, polycystic liver disease
* Tx: consider surgery if medications/conservative therapy fail, cyst aspiration, sclerotherapy

Dialysis Removal and Renal Dosing of Analgesics (Semin Dial 2014;27:188)		
Medication	**Removal**	**Comments and Maximum Dosing**
Acetaminophen	HD: yes; PD: no	No dose changes, first-line analgesic
Codeine	HD: no; PD: unlikely	**Not recommended.** Metabolized to morphine derivatives; can cause CNS/respiratory depression, hypotension
Tramadol	HD: yes; PD: ?	eGFR 10–30: 50–100 mg BID; eGFR <10 or HD: 50 mg BID; dose after HD
Morphine	HD: yes (parent/active metabolites); PD: no	**Not recommended.** Metabolites accumulate in CKD causing sedation, confusion, respiratory depression, myoclonus
Hydromorphone	HD: yes (active metabolite); PD: ?	Better tolerated than morphine, fewer toxic metabolites
Fentanyl	HD/PD: no	Inactive metabolites, safe to use if monitored
Buprenorphine	HD/PD: yes	Generally safe to use
Oxycodone	HD: yes; PD: ?	Generally safe to use, case reports of toxicity
Methadone	HD/PD: no	Similar plasma levels as non-CKD, may help with neuropathic pain, generally safe
Gabapentin	HD: yes; PD: ?	s/e: CNS depression, myoclonus if overdosed CrCl <15: dose after HD; 300 mg QD; start 100 mg after HD or 100 mg QOD if not ESRD; CrCl 15–29: 300 mg BID; CrCl 30–49: 300 mg TID; CrCl 50–79: 600 mg TID
Pregabalin	HD/PD: yes	eGFR <15: dose after HD; 75 mg QD; start 25 mg after HD or 25 mg QOD if not ESRD; eGFR 15–30: 150 mg QD; eGFR >30: 150 mg BID

Duloxetine	HD/PD: no	30–60 mg daily; eGFR <30: do not use
TCA (amitriptyline, nortriptyline)	HD/PD: no	Use cautiously esp. in cardiac patients, can cause QT prolongation and arrhythmias, start low (ie, 10 mg QD); nortriptyline may be better tolerated with less sedation
Topical capsaicin	HD/PD: ?	Useful for local pain (eg, knee osteoarthritis)

PSYCHIATRY, SLEEP MEDICINE, AND NEUROLOGY

CHRONIC LITHIUM TOXICITY

- Lithium (Li) commonly used to treat bipolar disorder, mania, and depression

Pathogenesis
- Li freely filtered at glomerulus; reabsorbed at various points in nephron (JASN 2016;27:1587)
- In proximal tubule, small amount of transcellular and paracellular reabsorption
- In thick ascending limb, paracellular movement due to favorable luminal gradient created by potassium efflux into tubule via ROMK channel
- In distal tubule/collecting duct, reabsorbed by principal cells through ENaC, causes nephrogenic DI (NDI) by downregulating aquaporin-2; DI also caused by increased prostaglandins, which inhibit aquaporin-2 expression
- Hypercalcemia due to hyperparathyroidism, raising threshold for calcium sensing receptor in parathyroid gland (Lancet 2012;379:721; JCEM 1984;59:354)

Clinical Manifestations
- Nephrogenic DI: polyuria/polydipsia, hypernatremia, dilute urine, nocturia
- CKD: chronic tubulointerstitial disease, renal microcysts, can progress to ESRD (1.5% in Li users, 6–8× higher than general population) (JASN 2016;27:1587)
  - Typically subnephrotic proteinuria (<1 g/d usually), but can develop FSGS and increased proteinuria; also rarely nephrotic range proteinuria with MCD
- Hyperparathyroidism with hypercalcemia—up to 25% (KI 2003;64:585)

Workup
- ✓ BMP, U/A with spot proteinuria and osmolality, PTH, U/S: microcysts
- Renal bx: proximal tubular atrophy and chronic interstitial fibrosis, FSGS, microcysts originating from distal tubule/collecting duct, distal tubular dilatation (KI 2003;64:585)

Nephrogenic DI (NDI)
- First option always d/c Li if possible
- NDI can improve if treatment begins prior to onset of severe concentrating defect
- Preferred: if continuing Li, start amiloride 5–10 mg daily, competes with Li for ENaC, blocking entry into principal cells and ↑ urine osmolality, if concentrating defect not severe (NEJM 1985;312:408); monitor Li level as can ↑ due to amiloride-induced volume depletion and increased proximal tubular reabsorption
- Other options similar for any cause of NDI: (1) NSAIDs which ↓ prostaglandins and concentrate urine, but contraindicated with CKD; (2) low salt diet/thiazides → hypovolemia, causes ↑ proximal urinary reabsorption, and ↓ urine output, monitor Li levels closely; (3) Acetazolamide (experimental) (NEJM 2016;375:2008)

CKD
- Stopping Li can stabilize or modestly improve renal function if CKD not advanced, otherwise can still progress; may be a "point of no return" around eGFR <40 where renal function continues to decline even if Li is stopped (KI 2003;64:585)
- 7/9 patients with Cr >2.5 progressed to ESRD despite stopping Li (JASN 2000;11:1439)
- Greater proteinuria a/w poorer prognosis and higher rates of ESRD, possibly due to superimposed FSGS (JASN 2000;11:1439)

Other Treatments
- **Hypercalcemia treatment:** if severe consider cinacalcet (AJKD 2006;48:832)
- Cautious use of ACEI/ARB and thiazides which ↑ Li levels; monitor levels closely, usually need empiric Li dose reduction

ANXIETY IN CKD (Semin Dialysis 2015;28:417)

- SSRIs can be used for generalized anxiety disorder
- Benzodiazepines can be used, most hepatically metabolized and no dose adjustment needed; Chlordiazepoxide has active metabolites → 50% dose reduction; other benzodiazepines would start lower than usual dose

PSYCHOSIS IN CKD (Semin Dialysis 2015;28:417)

- Aripiprazole and quetiapine have similar pharmacokinetics in CKD and non-CKD
- Risperidone should be dose reduced with CKD due to active metabolite
- Haloperidol not well studied but unlikely to need dose adjustment
- Monitor for side effects including prolonged QTc

DEPRESSION IN CKD

- Prevalence ~22% in both dialysis and nondialysis CKD, and is associated with increased mortality (KI 2013;84:179; AJKD 2013;62:493)
- Adverse outcomes in CKD patients with depression may be due to increased inflammation, nonadherence, autonomic/endocrine imbalances
- Likely underdiagnosed; routine screening controversial, unclear if treatment improves outcomes; depression scales should be adjusted with higher thresholds in ESRD (eg, Beck Depression Inventory threshold ↑ from >9 to 14–16) (KI 2006;69:1662)

Treatment

- RCT data lacking, ideally should be combination meds/behavioral changes
  - Undertreated (<50% on meds) in ESRD (KI 2006;69:1662)
  - Nonpharmacologic treatment: limited data show benefit for CBT and exercise
  - Meds: SSRI generally first line; in general, any medication should be started at low dose with slow titration

Antidepressants in CKD (KI 2012;81:247; AJKD 2009;54:741; Aust N Z J Psychiatry 2014;48:530)	
Medication	Dose and Comments
SSRI	
Citalopram	Citalopram: start 10 mg/d; active metabolites, cautious use if eGFR <20 although probably safe based on small studies (Ren Fail 2007;29:817)
Fluoxetine	Fluoxetine: start 20 mg/d; no renal dose adjustment, use cautiously because long half-life, small studies showed safety in ESRD (Int J Psychiatry Med 1997;27:71)
Sertraline	Sertraline: start 50 mg/d; active metabolite but no renal dosing
Paroxetine	Paroxetine (immediate release): accumulates with eGFR <30, start at 10 mg/d, increase slowly to max 40 mg/d Class s/e: nausea, hyponatremia, sexual, HA, ? bleeding Relative good safety record with cardiovascular disease
SNRI	
Venlafaxine	Venlafaxine: toxic metabolites, avoid if eGFR <10, ↓ dose by 50% for eGFR 10–50; start ER 37.5 mg/d; side effects: HTN, sexual
Duloxetine	Duloxetine: start 30 mg/d; do not use if eGFR <30; side effects: nausea, dry mouth, fatigue
Trazodone	No dose adjustment but start low (150 mg immediate release) in divided doses; can be used for insomnia (start 25–50 mg QHS); side effects: sedation, priapism, dry mouth
Bupropion	Toxic metabolites, can cause cardiac dysrhythmia Not recommended for CKD
Mirtazapine	Antidepressant/anxiolytic effects; sedating properties; accumulates in ESRD, use with caution (Hum Psychopharmacol 1998;13:357)
TCA	
Amitriptyline	Can have cardiac side effects including QTc prolongation and arrhythmias, and anticholinergic effects; use with caution
Nortriptyline	Start with low dose (10 mg/d) and increase slowly
Desipramine	Can be useful for neuropathic pain

SLEEP DISORDERS IN CKD

Insomnia and Poor Sleep Quality (Semin Nephrol 2015;35:359)

- Prevalence ~20–40% and increases even in early CKD; a/w co-morbid conditions including fatigue, depression, and anxiety; may increase risk of mortality in ESRD (NDT 2008;23:998)
- Contributors: comorbid conditions (eg, CHF, depression), medications, pruritus, pain, dialysis schedules, physical inactivity, nocturia, substance abuse
- History: if heavy snoring, restless legs, parasomnias, refer to sleep specialist to rule out more serious sleep conditions (eg, OSA)

- Nonpharmacologic treatment: preferred over medications
- Start with trial of sleep hygiene, treat comorbidities, modify any culprit meds
- Cognitive behavioral therapy has efficacy in ESRD (KI 2011;80:415)
- Pharmacologic treatment: limited data in CKD, always start at low doses
  - No dose adjustment for nonbenzodiazepine benzodiazepine receptor agonists such as zolpidem, zaleplon, eszopiclone (hepatically metabolized)
  - Melatonin receptor agonist ramelteon not well studied in CKD, no dose adjustment
  - Benzodiazepines and trazodone can be used as well (see above sections)

Restless Leg Syndrome (RLS)

- Definition: an urge to move legs during periods of rest, usually worse at night, accompanied by discomfort, and relieved by movement
- Distinguish from periodic limb movement disorder, characterized by increased limb movements in sleep
- Prevalence: much higher in ESRD than general population (30%), significantly lowers quality of life (KI 2013;85:1275); nondialysis CKD similar to general population
- Risk factors in ESRD: low iron/hemoglobin and diabetes (Sleep Med 2014;15:1532)
- Treatment (KI 2013;85:1275)
  - Improves with transplantation (Mov Disord 2002;17:1072)
  - Fix iron stores/anemia, remove SSRI/TCA (may exacerbate RLS), dopamine agonists (first-line medications), gabapentin/benzodiazepines (second-line)

Sleep Apnea Syndrome (KI 2006;70:1687)

- Definition: disturbed sleep from periods of apnea → oxygen desaturation and arousal
- Prevalence: >50% in ESRD vs 2–4% in general population; ↑ risk of CVD
- Different phenotype: in general population, usually obstructive, in ESRD even distribution between central/obstructive/mixed; possibly due to uremic toxins, volume overload, altered chemoreceptor sensitivity affecting respiratory control
- Treatment: CPAP, nocturnal hemodialysis (NEJM 2001;344:102), transplantation Hanging style

---

STROKE AND CEREBROVASCULAR DISEASE

- CKD is an independent risk factor for stroke; ↑ risk 41% with eGFR <60 (BMJ 2010;341:c4249)
- Dialysis patients have 10× ↑ risk of CVA and carotid endarterectomy vs general population, ischemic stroke most common, embolic most common subtype; high mortality and worse neurologic outcomes (AJKD 2009;54:468; Neurology 2012;78:1909)
- Perfusion abnormalities, subclinical white matter disease, brain atrophy, and silent infarcts more common in CKD, especially dialysis (Semin Nephrol 2015;35:311)
- Besides traditional stroke risk factors, nontraditional risk factors more common in CKD (anemia, inflammation, oxidative stress, uremic toxins, sleep dysregulation)

Stroke Prevention in Setting of Atrial Fibrillation (Afib)

- Afib common in CKD, exact management unclear
- Warfarin use appears to reduce stroke risk, but may increase bleeding risk in CKD, particularly in dialysis patients, and anticoagulation risk needs to be individualized (BMJ 2015;350:h246; JAMA 2014;311:919)
- Warfarin may have other adverse effects in CKD; associated with ↑ vascular calcification in animal models, by interfering with matrix gla protein, which is a potent inhibitor of vascular calcification; also ↑ risk for calciphylaxis (Semin Dial 2014;27:37)
- Novel anticoagulants require dose adjustment in CKD, none well studied in ESRD where warfarin is still drug of choice; in retrospective cohort study apixaban 5 mg BID reduced risk of stroke, bleeding, death vs warfarin while apixaban 2.5 mg BID reduced risk of bleeding but not death/stroke vs warfarin (Circulation 2018;138:1519)

Stroke Treatment

- Therapies less likely to be utilized in CKD (Semin Nephrol 2015;35:311)
- No dose adjustment for tPA, but outcomes less favorable in CKD (Neurology 2013;81:1780)

COGNITIVE DECLINE AND DEMENTIA

- **Epidemiology:** even mild-to-moderate CKD is a risk factor for cognitive decline
  - Cognitive impairment in 30–60% of HD patients (JASN 2013;24:353)
- Manifests as a vascular-type dementia with impairment in memory and executive function (Nat Rev Neurol 2009;5:542); may also raise risk of nonvascular dementia

- **Pathophysiology:**
  - Traditional and nontraditional (anemia, inflammation, oxidative stress, uremic toxins, sleep dysregulation, endothelial dysfunction) risk factors clustered in CKD
  - ↓ cerebral blood flow, ↑ subclinical cerebrovascular disease on MRI
- Potential improvement after transplantation (NDT 2006;21:3275)

NEUROPATHIES (Nat Rev Neurol 2009;5:542)

Uremic Neuropathy
- Only in ESRD; prevalence 60–90%, chronic process
- **Clinical Manifestations:** symmetric length-dependent polyneuropathy, starting with sensory deficits, paresthesia, loss of ankle reflexes; can eventually involve motor nerves → muscle atrophy and weakness
- **Differential:** diabetes, paraprotein disease, vasculitis, inflammatory demyelinating neuropathies (associated with FSGS and membranous, usually much more acute)
- **Diagnosis:** nerve conduction studies
- **Treatment:** ensure achieving adequate clearance on dialysis; transplantation may reverse symptoms; pain management

Carpal Tunnel Syndrome (Semin Dial 2014;27:188)
- Common in ESRD: 9–63% prevalence, increases with duration of time on dialysis
- **Clinical manifestations:** sensory symptoms initially (numbness, paresthesia) which can progress to muscle atrophy in medial nerve territory; can worsen on dialysis
- **Pathophysiology:** multifactorial; deposition of β2-microglobulin amyloid, extracellular calcification, ischemia related to AV access
- **Treatment:** usually splinting, corticosteroid injection, or surgical decompression for severe/refractory cases

Autonomic Neuropathy
- ~60% of patients with CKD
- **Clinical manifestations:** has been detected even in early CKD
  - Intradialytic hypotension, orthostasis, erectile dysfunction, cardiac arrhythmias
  - Higher resting HR, lower HR variability predict ESRD and hospitalization (JASN 2010;21:1560)
- **Treatment:** may improve with transplantation (Proc Eur Dial Transplant Assoc 1979;16:261)
  - Midodrine for intradialytic hypotension
  - Sildenafil for erectile dysfunction, has most data for CKD; consider holding on dialysis days if intradialytic hypotension

ACUTE UREMIC ENCEPHALOPATHY

- Due to buildup of uremic toxins; results in irritability, confusion, headache, nausea, tremor, asterixis, myoclonus, coma (in severe cases); treatment is dialysis
- Treatment is dialysis, overly aggressive dialysis on initial treatment with high BUN can precipitate dialysis disequilibrium syndrome

DIALYSIS DISEQUILIBRIUM SYNDROME (Semin Dial 2008;20:493)

- Clinical manifestations: headache, nausea, fatigue, seizures/coma (severe cases)
- Risk factors: old age, very high BUN, initial treatment, neurologic disease
- Pathophysiology: cerebral edema due to osmotic shifts; rapid decline in plasma BUN causes water to shift intracellularly, also possibly from paradoxical CSF acidosis induced by rapid correction of serum bicarbonate levels with dialysis
- Prevention: slow, gentle dialysis aiming for no more than 40% urea reduction during first session; eg, 2 hr, blood flow 200 mL/min, with small filter; IV mannitol/hypertonic saline for prevention, but data limited; increases dialysate sodium 143–146 mEq/L may be helpful if high-risk
- Treatment: supportive, reduce dialysis blood flow; terminate dialysis if significant symptoms; IV mannitol or hypertonic saline may be useful; key is prevention

UREMIC MYOPATHY

- Up to 50% of dialysis patients; proximal muscle weakness/wasting, especially legs
- Pathophysiology unclear; ? role for hyperparathyroidism, vitamin D deficiency, uremic toxins, malnutrition; muscle biopsy nonspecific
- Treatment: correct metabolic disarray, nutritional status, anemia

DRUG-INDUCED ENCEPHALOPATHY IN CKD

- Numerous common medications implicated, especially when incorrectly dosed
- H-2 antagonists: infrequently causes altered mental status and delirium, improves with withdrawal (Am J Med Sci 2005;330:8)
- Baclofen: presents w/ altered mental status, respiratory depression, somnolence; avoid with eGFR <60, no safe dosing guidelines in CKD; treatment is daily dialysis (Semin Dial 2015;28: 525)
- Gabapentin: entirely renally cleared; useful in CKD for neuropathic pain, uremic pruritus, restless legs; improper dosing can lead to accumulation causing myoclonus, altered mental status, coma (Pain Med 2009;10:190)
- Acyclovir (AJKD 1992;20:647) and valacyclovir in PD; cefepime

CEREBRAL EDEMA AND RENAL REPLACEMENT THERAPY (Semin Dial 2009;22:165)

- Cerebral edema and elevated intracranial pressure can be seen with trauma, hemorrhage, stroke, liver failure, tumor, infection
- Pathophysiology: intermittent HD (iHD) can worsen cerebral edema by removing solutes from plasma, causing an osmotic gradient favoring movement of water intracellularly; also rapid correction of plasma bicarbonate, which cannot readily cross blood–brain barrier, can combine with hydrogen ions → CO_2 formation → diffuses into CSF → intracellular acidosis → generation of intracellular osmoles and water movement intracellularly
- CRRT preferred over iHD, due to less osmotic shifts and greater cardiovascular and intracranial pressure stability; aim for lower clearance than usual
- If iHD must be used: start low blood flow (50 mL/min increasing to maximum 250 mL/min), short sessions (2 hr), daily treatments, cool dialysate (35°C), higher dialysate sodium (up to 10 mEq/L higher than plasma), lower bicarbonate dialysate
- Hypertonic saline boluses can be used during iHD or CRRT to maintain sodium 145–155

SODIUM DISORDERS

- Hyponatremia occurs with stroke, infection, trauma, hemorrhage

Neuropsychiatric Drugs Causing SIADH (NDT 2014;29 suppl2:i1; AJKD 2008;52:144)

- Antidepressants: TCA (amitriptyline, protriptyline, desipramine), SSRI (escitalopram, fluoxetine, paroxetine, sertraline), SNRI (venlafaxine), MAOI
- Antipsychotics: phenothiazines (thioridazine, trifluoperazine), haloperidol
- Antiepileptics: carbamazepine, oxcarbazepine, sodium valproate, lamotrigine

Subarachnoid Hemorrhage

- 57% in one series, with 20% developing sodium <130; more commonly due to SIADH than cerebral salt wasting (69% vs 7.5%) (Clin Endocrinol 2006;64:250); although true incidence unknown given diagnostic challenges
- Cerebral salt wasting usually within 10 d, resolves by 3–4 wk (NDT 2000;15:262)

Comparison of SIADH and Cerebral Salt Wasting		
	SIADH	**Cerebral Salt Wasting**
Urine sodium	Elevated; >40	Elevated; >40
Urine osmolality	Elevated; >100, often higher	Elevated; >100, often higher
Serum uric acid	Usually low	Usually low
Volume status	Euvolemic/slightly hypervolemic	Hypovolemic
Physical exam/ Other Lab	Typically normal	↓ Skin turgor, hemoconcentration, ↑ BUN/Cr ratio, orthostasis, relative hypotension
Pathophysiology	Inappropriate ADH secretion	Unknown; ? ↓ sympathetic reducing PT Na absorption, possible unidentified natriuretic factor (NDT 2000;15:262)
Response to IV normal saline challenge	Does not improve; may even worsen if U_{osm} >300 as infused sodium is excreted but some water is retained; U_{osm} does not change significantly	Should improve hyponatremia as restoring volume turns off ADH, causing excretion of dilute urine; of note, this is not always the case as there may be co-existing SIADH

Treatment	Fluid restriction or vasopressin antagonist; however if SAH, cannot fluid restrict d/t risk of vasospasm, give hypertonic saline to ensure volume and sodium correct (≤6 ↑ /24 hr)	Volume expansion with IV normal saline; +/− fludrocortisone; given diagnostic difficulty with SIADH, start hypertonic saline if sodium not improving

Transsphenoidal Pituitary Surgery (*J Neurosurg* 2007;106:66; *Pituitary* 2006;9:93)
- Both SIADH and DI can occur postoperatively, though DI more common
- Associated with classic triphasic pattern, although incidence of this pattern is low
  1. Polyuria and **hypernatremia** from CDI (19% incidence; usually first 48 hr)
  2. **Hyponatremia** from release of stored ADH (9% incidence; 4–7 d postop)
  3. **Hypernatremia** from CDI when stored ADH depleted
- Tx: depends on phase; DDAVP during DI, fluid restriction or hypertonic saline during SIADH
- Monitor sodium 1 wk following surgery as outpatient to check for SIADH
- 80% of DI resolved at 3 mo at one center

OBSTETRICS

PREGNANCY AND KIDNEY

- Weight gain: 1–1.5 kg during 1st trimester (~12 wk), 0.45 kg/wk during 2nd (13–27 wk), and 3rd trimester (28–40 wk) (*NDT* 1998;13:3266). Overweight/obese mothers gain more weight; underweight gain less weight (*Obstet Gynecol* 2015;125:773)
- ↓ SVR, ↑ CO, ↓ MAP (nadir at 18–24 wk); glomerular hyperfiltration, ↑ GFR by 37–40%; ↑ Kidney size by 1 cm, dilatation of the collecting duct R > L (*CJASN* 2012;7:2073)
- Adverse pregnancy outcome is lower with eGFR 120–150 (*CJASN* 2017;12:1048)

Effects of ↑ Progesterone (LH Surge ~4 wk before Delivery) and its Binding to Mineralocorticoid Receptor (MR)	
Normal	Antagonistic; Potassium retention
1° Aldosteronism	Antagonistic; Resolution of HTN and hypokalemia
Geller syndrome	GOF mutation of MR; progesterone and spironolactone become agonist; HTN and hypokalemia (*Science* 2000;289:119)

- ↓ PT reabsorption: glycosuria, amino aciduria, tubular proteinuria w/o true pathology
- Hypokalemia and metabolic alkalosis: d/t vomiting; ↓ serum albumin
- Gestational DI: vasopressinase produced by placenta; polyuria throughout pregnancy, recurs w/ each pregnancy, responds to both DDAVP and AVP
- Other DI: a/w HELLP, acute fatty liver: 3rd trimester; decreased metabolism of vasopressinase; responds only to DDAVP
- Preterm and early term birth is a/w later CKD likely d/t ↓ nephron (*BMJ* 2019;365:l1346)

MEDICATIONS IN PREGNANCY

Medicines to Avoid in Pregnancy and Alternatives (FDA Category) (*KJ* 2016;89:995)		
Indication	Medicines to Avoid	Possible Alternatives
HTN, Proteinuria	ACEi (D): CNS and CVS malformation in 1st trimester (*NEJM* 2006;354:2443); urogenital and renal malformation in 2nd trimester Aliskiren (D), ARB (D), Spironolactone (D) β blockers (*Ann IM* 2018;169:665)	Labetalol (C), hydralazine (C), methyldopa (B), nifedipine (C), HCTZ (B) Amlodipine (C: limited data) ? Amiloride (B) (*Obstet Gynecol* 2011;117:512)
Immunosuppression	CYC, MTX, MMF, sirolimus, leflunomide, Rituximab (C: spontaneous abortion, hematologic abnormalities in fetus)	Glucocorticoids (B): adrenal insufficiency, cataract and infection w/ large dose AZA (D), CNI (C), HCQ (C), Eculizumab (C) Belatacept (C, limited data)

| Hyperlipidemia | Statins (X) | Bile acid sequestrants: cholestyramine (C), colestipol, colesevelam (B) Fibrates: fenofibrate (C) |
| Anticoagulation | Warfarin | LMWH, UFH |

- Dose requirement is increased d/t ↑ volume of distribution, hepatic metabolism, GFR, and ↓ albumin and drug protein binding

Medication during Breastfeeding
- For a list of medication use in breastfeeding, please refer to the LactMed Database: https://toxnet.nlm.nih.gov/newtoxnet/lactmed.htm
- Enala-, capto-, and quinapril do not pass into breast milk; warfarin is safe for breastfeeding
- Most antihypertensives are present at breast milk; labetalol and nifedipine acceptable; avoid atenolol

HYPERTENSIVE DISORDERS OF PREGNANCY (HDP)

Gestational Hypertension
- New onset of HTN (SBP ≥140 and/or DBP ≥90) at ≥20 wk of gestation in the absence of proteinuria or new signs of end-organ dysfunction
  - HTN at <20 wk is chronic HTN, not gestational HTN
- a/w sustained HTN and CV disease later in life (J Hypertens 2010;28:826)

Treatment
- BP control may prevent maternal end-organ damage
- BP control may ↓ placental perfusion; a/w ↓ birth weight (J Obstet Gynaecol Can 2002;24:941)
- Tight control (DBP goal 85) not a/w ↓ pregnancy loss, high-level neonatal care, maternal complication including preeclampsia (NEJM 2015;372:407)
- Salt restriction close to delivery is not recommended to avoid volume depletion
- Ca (>1 g/d): 35% ↓ HTN and 55% ↓ preeclampsia (Cochrane Database Syst Rev 2010;CD001059)
- Weight loss during pregnancy: not recommended; gain goal (kg): 11.2–15.9 in BMI <25; 6.8–11.2 in BMI 25–29.9; <6.8 kg in BMI ≥30 (Rev Obstet Gynecol 2008;1:170)
- Weight loss after delivery: recommended (BMJ 2017;358;j3024)
- BP control in mild–moderate HTN: unclear benefit (Cochrane Database Syst Rev 2014;CD002252)
- Severe HTN: >150/95 (ESG Eur Hear J 2011;32:3147) ~160/105 (ACOG Obstet Gynecol 2013;122:1122) should be treated w/ antihypertensive
- Avoid NSAIDs: frequently used for peripartum analgesia
- Follow up no later than 7–10 d postpartum; if severe w/i 72 hr (Obstet Gynecol 2018;131:e140)

Prognosis
- HTN development w/i 10 yr is 14% (vs, 4% in non-HDP) (BMJ 2017;358;j307)
- Half of postpartum stroke occurs w/i 10 d of discharge (Obstet Gynecol 2018;1:70)
- Chronic HTN (×2.8), T2DM (×1.7), hypercholesterolemia (×1.4) (Ann IM 2018;169:224)

PREECLAMPSIA

Pathogenesis
- Placental hypoperfusion inducing soluble fms–like tyrosine kinase 1 (sFlt-1, soluble VEGF receptor 1, sVEGFr1): circulating antagonist to VEGF and placental growth factor (PlGF); ↑ sFLT-1/PlGF (NEJM 2016;374:13)
- Deficiency of Apela/ELABELA, placental angiogenesis mediator (Science 2017;357:707)
- Endothelial dysfunction (↓ NO, ↑ endothelin); injury of multiple organs

Definition (ACOG Guideline Obstet Gynecol 2013;122:1122)
- BP >140/90 after 20 wk of gestation, previously normal BP AND one of following:
  - Proteinuria >300 mg/24 hr or spot urine prot/creat 0.3 g/g
  - Platelet <100K; Cr >1.1 or doubling in the absence of other renal disease
  - Liver transaminases >×2 the normal; pulmonary edema; cerebral or visual symptoms

Severe Features: Any of Following (ACOG Guideline Obstet Gynecol 2013;122:1122)
- BP >160/110 ×2 >4 hr apart on bed rest
- Platelet <100K; Cr >1.1 or doubling in the absence of other renal disease
- Liver transaminases >×2 the normal or RUQ or epigastric pain not explained otherwise
- Pulmonary edema, new-onset cerebral or visual symptoms

Clinical Manifestations

- AKI: TMA (endothelial injury)
- Seizure (eclampsia), cerebral hemorrhage, hepatic rupture, pulmonary edema, bleeding related to thrombocytopenia, abruptio placenta, or fetal growth restriction
- 10–20% HELLP (hemolysis, elevated liver enzymes and low platelet) syndrome
- m/c cause of prematurity
- Diagnosis in ESRD is challenging: proteinuria and renal function cannot be evaluated
- Uterine and umbilical artery Doppler U/S: ↑ pulsatility index + fetal growth restriction

Risk Factors and Prevention

- Risk assessment is available: https://fetalmedicine.org/research/assess/preeclampsia
- Recovered AKI (×4.7) (*JASN* 2017;28:1566), fetal APOL1 risk allele (*AJHG* 2018;103:367)

Aspirin Prophylaxis for Preeclampsia (USPSTF *Ann IM* 2014;161:819)	
High risk factors	Renal disease, h/o preeclampsia, esp. accompanied by an adverse outcome, multifetal gestation, chronic HTN, Type 1 or 2 DM, SLE, APS
Moderate risk factors	Nulliparity, BMI >30 kg/m^2, mother or sister's h/o pre-eclampsia, African American race, low socioeconomic status, ≥35 y/o, low birth weight or small for gestational age, previous adverse pregnancy outcome, >10-yr pregnancy interval

Aspirin 81 mg qd if ≥1 high risk factors or several moderate risk factors from 12 wk to 5–10 d before expected delivery

- Aspirin ↓ delivery w/ preeclampsia before 37 wk in high risk group (*NEJM* 2017;377:613)
- Ca supplementation (>1 g/d): 55% ↓ preeclampsia (*Cochrane Database Syst Rev* 2010;CD001059)
- Weight loss (*Obstet Gynecol* 2010;116:667); bariatric surgery (*JAMA* 2008;300:2286)

Monitoring and Diagnosis

- U/S to screen for fetal growth restriction; if present umbilical artery Doppler velocimetry
- Kidney biopsy not always necessary

Treatment

- CS for lung maturity if <34 wk with severe features
- MgSO$_4$ pre- and postpartum for severe features to prevent seizure; ✓ DTR, ✓ Mg in mother and baby; half dose for ESRD mother
- BP control: antihypertensives for severe HTN >150/95 ~ 160/105
- Delivery (placental removal): only definitive treatment; consider regardless of gestation age if uncontrollable severe HTN, eclampsia, pulmonary edema, abruption placentae, DIC, nonreassuring fetal status (ACOG Guideline *Obstet Gynecol* 2013;122:1122)

Prognosis

- ↑ CKD esp w/i 5 y: ×3.9 (delivery < 34w) ×2.8 (delivery 34–36w) (*BMJ* 2019;365:l1516)
- ↑ ESRD ×5; ×9.2 if preterm; ×7.1 if preeclampsia in 2 pregnancies (*PLoS Med* 2019;e1002875)
- 41.5% had HTN 1 yr after severe preeclampsia (*Hypertension* 2018;71:491)
- a/w dementia, esp. vascular type (*BMJ* 2018;363:k4109)
- Regarded as risk-enhancing factor of ASCVD (ACC/AHA *Circulation* 2019;139:e1046)

AKI IN PREGNANCY

- Absence of ↓ Cr during pregnancy is sign of renal dysfunction
- AKI requiring dialysis: 1/10,000; 4.3 vs 0.01% died; ↑ preterm birth, low birth weight, small for gestational age. 69% experienced complications (preeclampsia, TMA, HF, sepsis, or postpartum hemorrhage) (*JASN* 2015;26:3085).

Possible Causes of AKI in Pregnancy (*KI Rep* 2018;3:247)	
1st	Septic abortion, hyperemesis gravidarum
2nd–3rd	Pre-eclampsia/HELLP (after 20 wk), TTP, complement-mediated HUS (aHUS), acute fatty liver of pregnancy
Anytime	LN, APS

- Acute fatty liver of pregnancy: ↓ antithrombin activity; AKI 14–90%, HTN/preeclampsia 26–70% (*J Obstet Gynaecol Res* 2014;40:641)

GLOMERULAR DISEASES AND PREGNANCY

Background
- Proteinuria, ↑ BP and CKD are a/w adverse outcome
- Pregnancy can potentially worsen proteinuria, HTN, edema in NS
- In IgAN w/ Cr ≤1.2, pregnancy was not a/w difference in kidney function (AJKD 2010;56:506)

Infant Survival Rates (%) (CJASN 2017;12:1862)			
IgAN	70–100	FSGS	55–94
MN	67–76	MCD	71–76

NS during Pregnancy (KI 2017;91:1464)
- Causes: FSGS > IgAN, MN > Fibrillary, MPGN, C3G, MCD
- ↑ preterm, preeclampsia (27 vs 3.4%), C-section

Kidney Biopsy during Pregnancy
- ↑ complication than postpartum (7 vs 1%); major bleeding at 23–26 wk (BJOG 2013;120:412)
- Bx after 32 wk gestation is not recommended (BJOG 1987;94:932)

ATYPICAL HUS (aHUS) AND PREGNANCY

- Alternative complement activation. Pregnancy is frequent triggering event.
- Not all patients have genetic mutations
- Risk factors: h/o HUS, aHUS (26%) (JASN 2018;29:1020)
- Common between 36 wk to postpartum; similar severity w/ nonpregnancy aHUS; rare death; 27–57% ESRD (CJASN 2017;12:1237; KI 2018;93:450; JASN 2018;29:1020)
- Overlapping features with pre-eclampsia including biopsy finding (TMA)
  - aHUS does not resolve with delivery vs preeclampsia resolve with delivery
- Eculizumab: used in pregnancy safely; no ESRD out of the 22 cases (KI 2018;93:450)

SLE AND SJÖGREN SYNDROME AND PREGNANCY

Background
- Risk factors of active nephritis during pregnancy: active disease w/i 6 mo before conception, h/o multiple flares, d/c of hydroxychloroquine (Rheum Dis Clin North Am 2007;33:237), past kidney disease, low C4; low C3 or dsDNA Ab alone are NOT (CJASN 2017;12:940)
- Risk factors of adverse pregnancy outcome: (+) lupus anticoagulant, antihypertensive use, thrombocytopenia, maternal severe flare, disease activity, high BMI (Ann IM 2015;163:153)

Clinical Manifestation/Prognosis

Fetal and Maternal Pregnancy Outcome in SLE (%): ↑ premature Births and Maternal HTN With LN and APLA (+) (CJASN 2010;5:2060)			
Spontaneous abortion	16.0	SLE flare	25.6
IUGR	12.7	HTN	16.3
Stillbirth	3.6	Nephritis	16.1
Neonatal death	2.5	Preeclampsia	7.6
Premature births of all live births	39.4	Eclampsia	0.8

- Neonatal lupus: heart block and rash caused by SS-A and/or SS-B Ab transfer from mother; all mother w/ SLE, Sjögren syndrome should be screened for fetal heart block
- All mother of fetus with congenital heart block should be screened for SS-A, SS-B; asymptomatic mother can progress to SLE and/or Sjögren (Ann Rheum Dis 2009;68:828)

Prevention and Treatment
- Recommend against conception within 6 mo of active class III and IV LN
- ✓antiphospholipid Abs in pregnant women with suggestive APS history
- HCQ in SLE: ↓ flare (Ann Rheum Dis 2018;77:855)
- HCQ in refractory APS: a/w ↑ live births in refractory APS (Autoimmun Rev 2015;14:498)
- Active LN class III or IV: treat with CS ± azathioprine

CKD AND PREGNANCY

Pregnancy Outcome in CKD

- Preterm and early term birth is a/w later CKD likely d/t ↓ nephron (BMJ 2019;365:I1346)
- Infertility and sexual dysfunction are common in advanced CKD and ESRD
- In CKD adverse maternal events happened in 11.5% (2% in non-CKD control). Premature birth 13% (vs 6% in non-CKD) (CJASN 2011;6:2587)
- CKD a/w preeclampsia (×10.36), premature delivery (×5.72), small for gestational age/low birth weight, C-sec, and failure of pregnancy (CJASN 2015;10:1964)
- CKD stage shift or RRT start was: 7.6% (CKD1), 12.6% (CKD2), 16.2% (CKD3), 20% (CKD4-5). Adverse outcome is a/w HTN and proteinuria (JASN 2015;26:2011).
- ↑ proteinuria in DN during pregnancy. Insulin is recommended during pregnancy.
- In CKD w/ Cr >1.4 pregnancy ↓ GFR 6 mo postpartum in 31%; progression was highest in Cr >2.0 and uncontrolled HTN (NEJM 1996;335:226)

Laboratory Changes in CKD

- HCG: 36.7 kDa, degraded and excreted by kidney; can be elevated in CKD w/o pregnancy. Ultrasound should be used to diagnose pregnancy.
  - Elevated HCG level may lead to misdiagnosis of molar pregnancy (Contraception 2015;92:84)
- AFP: ↓ level is used to screen fetal Down syndrome; can be falsely elevated in CKD

General Management

- Delay conception until txp if <35 y/o. Risk discussion if >35 y/o (J Nephrol 2012;25:450).

ESRD AND PREGNANCY

Pregnancy Outcome in ESRD

- Live birth/1,000 person-yr: dialysis (1.26) < Transplanted (16) < General population (60.27); PD (1.06) < HD (2.54); among pregnancies on dialysis 79% achieve live birth; 53.4% preterm, 65% low birth weight (Nephrology 2013;18:276)
- HD has lower incidence of small for gestational age than PD (NDT 2016;31:1915)
- High BUN (KI 2009;75:1217) and shorter dialysis (NDT 2016;31:1915) is a/w adverse outcome

General Management

- Iron, Epoetin alfa (C), and darbepoetin (C) can be used; ESA requirement goes up
- Cholecalciferol 4,000 IU is safe (JCEM 2013;98:2337). May need PO Ca for hypocalcemia
- PO$_4$ binder is usually unnecessary d/t high intensity dialysis; use Ca-based binder
- Noncalcium binder and active vitamin D are not well studied

Hemodialysis

- Intensive HD with goal predialysis BUN <50 (18 mmol/L); weekly Kt/V 6–8; requires daily HD ~36 hr/wk
- May need Mg and PO$_4$ supplement and 3 K, 3 Ca bath for low level d/t intensive HD
- Assess DW weekly and ↑ based on expected weight gain (1–1.5 kg during 1st trimester and by 0.5 kg/wk in 2nd and 3rd trimesters) and physical examination
- Avoid hypotension to keep uterine blood flow
- Heparin can be used

Peritoneal Dialysis

- May need to ↓ fill volume and ↑ frequency; may need HD conversion for clearance

---

KIDNEY TRANSPLANTATION RECIPIENTS AND PREGNANCY

- Delay conception to 1 yr after KT, stable graft function, minimal proteinuria
- Higher risk of preeclampsia (27.0 vs 3.8%), gestational diabetes (8.0 vs 3.9%), C-section (56.9 vs 31.9%), and preterm delivery (45.6 vs 12.5%) (AJT 2011;11:2388)
- Pregnancy does not affect graft or patient survival (Transplantation 2006;81:660)
- CNI: relatively safe; need to ↑ dose, 20–40% for ↑ hepatic metabolism
  - Tacrolimus ↑ gestational DM
- MMF/MFA: switch to AZA

CONTRAST-INDUCED NEPHROPATHY (CIN)

- CIN: ≥0.5 rise in serum Cr or a 25% ↑ in serum Cr occurring within the first 24 hr after contrast exposure and peaking up to 5 d after (NEJM 2018;378:603)
- 2–5% in patients with no risk factors; 10–30% among those at risk (Semin Nephrol 2011;31:300)

Risk Factors

- **Patient factors:** CKD, DM, CHF, hypovolemia, concomitant nephrotoxic medication usage and multiple myeloma
- **Procedure-related factors:** higher dose of contrast, multiple contrast studies performed within short period, ionic contrast, hyperosmolar contrast
- IV contrast may have no or low risk (Ann Emerg Med 2018;71:44; Radiology 2017;285:414)
- Risk prediction tools for CIN from coronary angiography (JACC 2004;44:1393; Am Heart J 2008;155:260) are available at QxMD® app

Pathogenesis

- Renal vasoconstriction → medullary hypoxia → ATN (mediated by effects of viscosity and by alterations in nitric oxide, endothelin, and/or adenosine)
- Direct cytotoxic effects of contrast agents on tubular epithelial cell → ATN (mediated by reactive oxygen species partly) (JACC 2008;51:1419)
- Cellular events occurs within first 60 min after administration of the contrast agent with greatest risk in the first 10 min (AJKD 1998;32:64; AJR 2004;183:1673)

Clinical Manifestations

- Rise in creatinine, generally within 24–48 hr after contrast exposure
- The creatinine usually peaks and then starts to decline within 3–7 d
- Severity range from nonoliguric transient fall in GFR to severe renal failure requiring dialysis in generally 1% (Am J Cardiol 2002;90:1068)
- Urine sediment → muddy brown granular/renal tubular epithelial cell cast
- Absent or mild proteinuria (contrast agents may induce false positive proteinuria)
- FE_{Na} often <1% (as opposed to ischemic/toxin-induced ATN)
- A persistent nephrogram on intravenous pyelogram or contrast-enhanced CT scan may be suggestive of CIN (Br J Radiol 1997;70:897)

Prevention

- Avoid volume depletion and NSAIDs
- No proven benefit of holding ACE inhibitors/ARBs (AJKD 2012;60:576)
- Avoid repeated studies that are closely spaced (within 48–72 hr)
- Contrast: lowest effective dose (<30 mL if diagnostic, <100 mL if diagnostic + intervention); low or iso-osmolar (Iodixanol is nonionic and iso-osmolal) (KDIGO AKI 2012)
- Volume expansion with isotonic NaCl in pt at risk (KDIGO AKI 2012)
  - Outpatient: 3 mL/kg starting 1 hr preprocedure and 1–1.5 mL/kg/hr during and for 4–6 hr postprocedure
  - Inpatient: 1 mL/kg/hr for 6–12 hr pre-, intraprocedure, and for 6–12 hr postprocedure

Preventive Interventions	
Intervention	Results
LVEDP-guided vs standard IVF	LVEDP guidance ↓ CI-AKI and benefit sustained through 6 mo (POSEIDON Lancet 2014;383:1814)
0.9% NaCl vs 1.26% NaHCO₃	Similar rate of AKI, dialysis at 90 d or persistent kidney impairment and death (PRESERVE NEJM 2018;378:603)
N-acetylcysteine	Conflicting or no benefit (AJKD 2004;43:1; Am Hear J 2006;151:140; PRESERVE NEJM 2018;378:603)
Statins	Support use of statins in statin-naïve patients Higher dose superior to lower dose (JACC 2014;114:1295; Ann IM 2016;164:406)
RRT	No benefit (Am J Med 2012;125:66)

NEPHROGENIC SYSTEMIC FIBROSIS (NSF)

- Most gadolinium containing agents are excreted by kidneys. Low renal function prolongs half-life of gadolinium.

- NSF is a fibrosing disorder seen exclusively in patients with CKD or ESRD due to exposure to gadolinium containing contrast agents (NDT 2009;24:856)
- Characterized by marked expansion and fibrosis of dermis leading to thickening and hardening of skin overlying trunk and extremities
- Incidence of NSF in patients with renal dysfunction may vary from 0.19–4% (JASN 2006;17:2359; Curr Opin Rheumatol 2003;15:785)

ACR Classification of Gadolinium-based Agents Relative to NSF		
Group I	The greatest number of NSF cases	Gadodiamide (Omniscan®) Gadopentetate dimeglumine (Magnevist®) Gadoversetamide (OptiMARK®)
Group II	Few, if any, unfounded cases of NSF	Gadobenate dimeglumine (MultiHance®) Gadobutrol (Gadavist®) Gadoterate acid (Dotarem®) Gadoteridol (ProHance®)
Group III	Limited data, but for which few, if any unconfounded cases of NSF reported	Gadoxetate disodium (Eovist®)

Pathogenesis
- Inciting event is tissue deposition of gadolinium → direct stimulation of bone marrow to produce CD34+ fibrocytes → aberrant activation of circulating fibrocytes → accumulation of fibrocytes in the tissues and production of collagen → local tissue fibrosis
- Activation of TGF-beta-1 pathway
- Associations: use of ESA, placement of dialysis catheters, chronic liver disease, hepatorenal syndrome, peritransplant period after liver transplant

Clinical Manifestations
- Skin manifestations: fibrotic, indurated papules, plaques, or subcutaneous nodules. Lesions are symmetrical, bilateral, and centrifugal in distribution. May give "cobblestone" "woody" or peau d'orange appearance (Am J Dermatopathol 2001;23:383)
- Systemic manifestations: muscle induration, joint contracture, involvement of lungs, diaphragm, myocardium, pericardium, pleura, sclera, and dura mater
- A fulminant form w/ flexion contractures and immobility in 5% (Curr Opin Rheumatol 2003;15:785)
- Course: death (28%), no improvement (28%), modest improvement (20%) (Semin Arthritis Rheum 2006;35:238)

Workup
- Elevation in serum CRP, serum ferritin, ESR, and reduction in serum albumin
- Skin lesions can be visualized by [^{18}F]-FDG whole-body PET
- Skin biopsy: proliferation of dermal fibrocytes in early lesions, marked thickening of the dermis, with a florid proliferation of fibrocytes and long dendritic processes in fully developed cases
- Immunohistochemistry: CD34 and procollagen-I⊕ spindle cell infiltration

Prevention
- US FDA recommends avoidance of gadolinium in patients with eGFR <30, receiving dialysis, or with AKI (U.S. Food and Drug Administration. September 2007)
- If study has to be performed in at-risk patients, avoid Group 1 agents
- Lowest dose of gadolinium that is needed should be used in at-risk patients
- Elimination of gadolinium with PD is much lower than with HD (Acad Radiol 1998;5:491)
- Gadolinium is effectively cleared by HD (Acta Radiol 2001;42:339; Radiat Med 2006;24:445)
- HD soon after the procedure and a repeat HD w/i 24 hr can be considered among pts on HD but no proven benefit (ACR Committee on Drugs and Contrast Media 2017)

Treatment
- No proven therapy
- Imatinib, oral and topical steroids, plasmapheresis, extracorporeal photopheresis, UVA phototherapy have been studied with inconsistent results
- Intensive physical therapy to reverse disability from joint contractures
- Restoration of renal function with kidney transplant can slow or stop disease progression Renal transplantation may offer benefit in patients who are candidates for transplantation (AJKD 2005;46:763; NDT 2011;26:1099; Clin Transplant 2008;22:803)

- NSF has a chronic and unremitting course in most patients
- More severe and rapid progression of the skin disease is a/w a poor prognosis

DERMATOLOGY

CALCIFIC UREMIC ARTERIOLOPATHY (CUA, CALCIPHYLAXIS)

- Microvascular occlusion of arterioles in subcutaneous adipose tissue and dermis by medial calcification, subintimal fibrosis, and thrombosis
- 5th decade of life, M < F (1:2), whites (AJKD 2015;66:133)
- a/w obesity, liver disease, CS use, CaxP >70, Aluminum >25 ng/mL (JAAD 2007;56:569)
- a/w DM, high BMI, Ca, P and PTH; nutritional vitamin D, cinacalcet, warfarin, multiple insulin dose (JASN 2016;27:3421); thrombophilia (Mayo Clin Proc 2016;91:1395)
- 50% used vitamin K antagonists (VKA) (NDT 2017;32:126)
- Possible in pts w/ eGFR >60; VKA and obesity are risk factors (Mayo Clin Proc 2018;93:1202)

Pathogenesis
- Oxidative stress, inflammation, recurrent skin trauma
- ↓ Arteriolar blood flow, endothelial injury; PTH-induced ischemic skin necrosis
- Inhibitor of vascular calcification: fetuin-A (reduced in CUA pts) (NDT 2017;32:126)
- Impaired Vit K dependent carboxylation of Matrix Gla Protein, inhibitor of vascular calcification → dermal arteriolar calcification (JASN 2017;28:1717)

Clinical Manifestations
- Dysesthesia only in early stage; pruritic surrounding area
- Painful violaceous, plaque-like subcutaneous nodules; sometimes livedo reticularis pattern
- Ischemic, necrotic ulcers with eschars; can be infected
- Site: frequently abdomen, buttock, and thigh; possibly acral and penile
- 1 yr survival ~50% (JAAD 2007;56:569). Mortality >80% w/ ulcer (KI 2002;61:2210).

Diagnosis
- Skin biopsy: arteriolar medial calcification (von Kossa stain), thrombosis of dermal vessels, ischemic necrosis w/o vasculitis; biopsy may complicate w/ ulceration, infection, bleeding
- X-ray using mammography technique (AJKD 2006;48:659), bone scan

Treatment
- d/c VKA; DOAC safe alternative (Int J Dermatol 2017;56:1065)
- Low Ca bath (2.25–2.5 mEq/L) d/c calcium containing binder, vitamin D analogues
- Lower phos with noncalcium containing binder to keep phos <5.5 and CaxP <55
- Cinacalcet PO to ↓ PTH <300; ↓ CUA ×0.31 (EVOLVE CJASN 2015;10:800), etelcalcetide IV
- Sodium thiosulfate IV: antioxidant; 25 g (diluted in 100 mL of NS), infused over 30–60 min during the last hr of each HD session; effective in 70% (Nephrology 2018;23:669)
  - s/e: AG metabolic acidosis, N/V, bad taste w/ periorbital tingling
- Intralesional sodium thiosulfate (JAMA Dermatol 2013;149:946)
- Hyperbaric oxygen (Nephrology 2015;20:444), bisphosphonates (Nefrologia 2012;32:329)
- Surgical debridement, parathyroidectomy a/w ↓ mortality (Mayo Clin Proc 2016;91:1384)
- Vitamin K 10 mg TIW clinical trial ongoing (NEJM 2018;378:1704)

UREMIC PRURITUS

- 42% of prevalent HD pts a/w 17% higher mortality (DOPPS NDT 2006;21:3495)
- 18% are very much or extremely bothered by itching (DOPPS CJASN 2017;12:2000)
- ↑ With inadequate dialysis, anemia, ↑ BUN, PTH, CaxP, Mg, CRP, IL-2, ↓ albumin
- Polyarylethersulfone > polysulfone membrane dialyzer (BMC Nephrol 2015;16:184)
- a/w xerosis: dry skin from sweat gland atrophy
- Affects quality of life and sleep; fatigue, agitation, depression
- Pathogenesis: systemic inflammation, calcification, opioid receptor imbalance

Treatment
- Adequate dialysis, control CaxP, PTH; topical capsaicin, topical tacrolimus
- If occurs during HD only, consider changing heparin formulation, dialyzer
- Glycerol/paraffin emulsion esp. in xerosis (dry skin) (CJASN 2011;6:748)
- Gabapentin (AJKD 2017;70:638), pregabalin is better than doxepin (Hemodial Int 2017;21:63)
- Nalfurafine (κ opioid agonist, unavailable in USA)

ACQUIRED PERFORATING DERMATOSIS (Br J Dermatol 1996;135:671)

- Similar to the primary perforating dermatosis, Kyrle disease
- Common in CKD, DM, and African American; 11% of dialysis pts
- Skin biopsy: ulcer craters showing perforation of both collagen and elastic fibers
- Pruritic dome-shaped papules w/ central crusts on the trunk & extensor limb surfaces
- Treatment: topical steroid, retinoid

DRUG REACTIONS WITH EOSINOPHILIA AND SYSTEMIC SYMPTOMS (DRESS)

Drugs Causing DRESS

- Xanthine oxidase inhibitors: allopurinol >> febuxostat (AJM 2017;130:e67)
- Antiepileptics: phenytoin, carbamazepine, oxcarbazepine, lamotrigine
- Sulfonamides, sulfasalazine; vancomycin, dapsone, minocycline, lenalidomide

Clinical Manifestation

- 2–8 wk after use of the culprit drug; symptoms may persist after stopping offending drug
- Renal involvement: **interstitial nephritis**; 40%; higher (68%) renal involvement with allopurinol cases; baseline CKD (×24) is risk factor (Arch Dermatol 2010;146:1373)
- Maculopapular rash, purpura, exfoliative dermatitis, lymphadenopathy
- Fever, facial edema, hepatitis, pneumonitis, myocarditis, hemophagocytosis, shock, death
- Eosinophilia, atypical lymphocytosis, elevated aminotransferase (ALT)

Differential Diagnosis: Stevens-Johnson Syndrome/Toxic Epidermal Necrolysis

- Similar offending drugs: allopurinol, antiepileptics, sulfonamides
- AKI from **volume depletion**/hemodynamic change; extensive mucosal involvement
- 4–28 d after use of the culprit drug; leucopenia instead of eosinophilia

Treatment

- d/c offending drug; systemic corticosteroids for interstitial nephritis

OTHER SKIN CHANGES IN CKD

- Xerosis: dry skin from sweat gland atrophy
- Uremic frost: crystallized urea from sweat evaporation (NEJM 2018;379:669)
- Lindsay's nails (half-and-half nails): distal pink nail bed and proximal white band; found in CKD (NEJM 2015;372:1748)

Skin Changes and Associated Renal Pathology	
Skin Manifestation	**Renal Pathology**
Purpura: nonblanchable red–purple, 3–10 mm (<3 mm petechiae; >10 mm ecchymoses); RBC leakage; leukocytoclastic vasculitis (LCV)* on skin biopsy; Skin ulcer	Small vessel vasculitis: IgAV, staph-associated IgA dominant IRGN (Clin Nephrol 2013;79:302), ANCA GN, cryoglobulinemia (immune thrombi in small blood vessel)
Livedo reticularis: mottled, reticulated; congested venules	TMA: APS, TTP; Crystalglobulinemia
	Medium vessel vasculopathy: APS, SLE, PAN, cholesterol emboli a/w Raynaud phenomenon
Pyoderma gangrenosum	ANCA GN (Autoimmun Rev 2017;16:1138)
Maculopapular rash	Acute Interstitial nephritis

*LCV: small vessel vasculitis with neutrophil infiltrate; 44% has renal involvement; IgAV/HSP (30%), ANCA (10%), cryoglobulinemic (4%) (Mayo Clin Proc 2014;89:1515)

Genetic Conditions Affecting Skin and Kidney		
Conditions	**Skin Manifestations**	**Renal Manifestations**
Tuberous sclerosis	Hypopigmented spots, malar angiofibromas, periungual fibromas, connective tissue naevi, cafe-au-lait spots	Angiomyolipomas: hematuria, RP bleeding; 59% CKD3–5 (AJKD 2015;66:638); Benign cysts, lymphangiomas, RCC
VHL disease	Capillary malformations, hemangioma	Clear cell RCC

Fabry disease	Telangiectasias and angiokeratomas at groin and hip; Hypo- or anhidrosis	Proteinuria w/ lamellated lysosome membrane structures: myeloid (zebra) bodies
Nail–patella syndrome	Hypoplastic nails, webbing, absence of distal dorsal phalangeal skin creases	Proteinuria, CKD with type III collagen deposition in lamina densa and/or FSGS

Renal Manifestation of Dermatologic Diseases	
Psoriasis	IgAN ×4.75 in mod–severe disease (BJD 2017;176:1366) Mesangioproliferative GN (Int Urol Nephrol 2012;44:509)
Hidradenitis suppurativa	AA amyloidosis. Can progress to ESRD. Tx: Infliximab (Eur J Intern Med 2008;19:e32)

OPHTHALMOLOGY

Age-related Macular Degeneration (AMD)
- m/c cause of blindness in the developed world; ×3.2 in eGFR <60 (JASN 2008;19:806)
- Drusen: extracellular deposits between Bruch membrane and the retinal pigment epithelium (RPE). Early sign of AMD.
- CFH, alternative complement pathway regulator variation, Y402H is a/w AMD
- VEGF produced by RPE → ↑ CFH → regulate alternative pathway (JCI 2017;127:199)
- Dry AMD: geographic atrophy of the retinal pigment epithelium; degeneration of light-sensitive cells and supporting tissue + vision loss
- Wet AMD: choroidal neovascularization; rapid and severe visual loss and retinal edema
- Clinical manifestations: loss of vision, visual distortion
- Intravitreal anti-VEGF for wet AMD: rarely may be associated with TMA (HTN, proteinuria, AKI) in native (AJKD 2011;57:756) and txp kidney (Transplantation 2015;99:2382)

Diabetic Retinopathy (DR)
- m/c cause of visual loss worldwide; ×2.0 in renal dysfunction (JASN 2004;15:2469)
- T1DM (+) DN almost always have microvascular disease, such as DR and neuropathy
- T2DM (–) DR is a predictor of nondiabetic renal disease. (+) DR is a predictor of ESRD (Diabetes Res Clin Pract 2011;92:198); (+) DR does not necessarily predict DN
- Nonproliferative DR: cotton wool spots, intraretinal hemorrhages, microaneurysms
- Proliferative DR: neovascularization
- Clinically significant macular edema: retinal thickening and macula edema
- Treatment: photocoagulation for proliferative DR, severe nonproliferative DR; intra-vitreal anti-VEGF for proliferative DR and clinically significant macular edema

Hypertensive Retinopathy
- Grade 1: generalized arteriolar narrowing; 2: Focal narrowing and AV nicking/nipping; 3: 2 + exudates, hemorrhages, and cotton wool spots; 4: 3 + optic disc swelling
- Grades 3 and 4: a/w malignant HTN, requiring urgent tx to prevent irreversible damage
- Retinopathy, microaneurysms, retinal hemorrhages, soft exudates, and AV nicking were a/w renal dysfunction (JASN 2004;15:2469)

Uveitis With Tubulointerstitial Nephritis
- Causes: sarcoidosis, Sjögren syndrome, TINU, ANCA vasculitis
- Anterior uveitis: pain, photophobia, ciliary flush; more systemic involvement
- Posterior uveitis: floaters, reduced visual acuity

Tubulointerstitial Nephritis and Uveitis (TINU)
- 1–5% of IN, common in adolescent (median 15 y/o), ♀; typically bilateral and anterior uveitis; 58% developed uveitis after TIN dx: easily misdiagnosed (CJASN 2014;9:21)
- Modified CRP: target Ag (CJASN 2011;6:93); predict late onset uveitis (CJASN 2014;9:21)
- Eosinophilia, pyuria, pRTA/Fanconi; ↑ Urine β2-microglobulin (JAMA Ophthalmol 2015;133:140)
- Prednisone 1 mg/kg; topical corticosteroids/cycloplegics for uveitis
- May spontaneously resolve. CKD in many cases despite steroids (NDT Plus 2008;1:112).

Ocular Effects of Hydroxychloroquine (HCQ)
- Corneal deposits: reversible w/ d/c of HCQ
- Retinopathy: Bull's eye maculopathy with a central patchy depigmentation surrounded by a concentric pigmentation
Risk factors: HCQ dose >400 mg/d, cumulative dose >1,000 g, >5 yr use, renal or liver dysfunction, concomitant tamoxifen, retinal disease, obesity (HCQ is lipophobic)
- Pretreatment and annual fundus examination: d/c HCQ if there is retinal damage

Ocular Manifestation of Renal Conditions	
SLE	Keratoconjunctivitis sicca (2° Sjögren), retinal vasculopathy w/ cotton wool spot, optic neuropathy, scleritis, anterior uveitis
C3G	Drusen, retinal pigment epithelium detachment, choroidal neovascularization
GPA	Conjunctivitis, corneal ulceration, episcleritis/scleritis, optic neuropathy, retinal vasculitis, and uveitis
Alport syndrome	Anterior lenticonus (20–30% of X-linked) Subcapsular cataracts, perimacular granulations
Fabry disease	Corneal opacity (cornea verticillata), subcapsular cataracts
Cystinosis	Corneal cystine crystals/photophobia
Nephronophthisis	Retinitis pigmentosa (tapetoretinal degeneration)/blindness
CKD	Narrowed retinal microvasculature (CJASN 2011;6:1872)
Corticosteroid	Glaucoma, cataract, central serous chorioretinopathy
Hemodialysis	↑ Intraocular pressure; Tx: hypertonic sodium, mannitol (NEJM 1980;18:702), glucose (AJKD 2014;63:500)

GERIATRICS

Background
- Adjusted ESRD incidence rate highest in population >75 yo, though declining since 2010 (USRDS.org)
- For age >65 yo risk of ESRD exceeds risk of death only once eGFR <15 (JASN 2007;18:2758)
- In the elderly, frail population dialysis may not provide survival advantage c/t optimal medical management and is a/w a functional decline (CJASN 2012;7:185; NEJM 2009;361:1539; 2009;361:1612)

Kidney Changes in Ageing (JASN 2017;28:407; 2017;28:2838)
- Structural changes in healthy aging: cortical volume loss, increase in simple renal cysts, ↑ glomerulosclerosis (upper limit vary with age; NDT 2015;30:2034, available at QxMD®), ↑ interstitial fibrosis, ↑ tubular atrophy, ↑ arteriosclerosis, decrease in nephron number
- Normal GFR decline with aging is 0.75 mL/min/yr
- Tubular dysfunction: ↓ sodium reabsorption and potassium excretion, and ↓ urine concentrating ability
- Increasing susceptibility to AKI particularly ischemic and toxic ATN

LIFE EXPECTANCY AND PROGNOSIS

Prognosis by Modality	
Modality	**Prognostic Information**
HD	• Remaining life in yr age 75–79: ESRD 3.2 (male) and 3.5 (female) vs Gen Population 9.8 (male) and 11.4 (female) usrds.org • Quartiles of life expectancy in yr: Age 75–79: 0.5 yr (lowest), 3.7 yr (highest) Age 80–84: 0.4 yr (lowest), 3 yr (highest) (KI 2012;82:261) • Median survival >65 yo in yr – Vent + dialysis (HD): 0.9; post CPR + HD: 0.8; feeding tube + HD: 0.4 (JASN 2014;25:143) • Nursing home population, cumulative mortality: 24% (3 mo), 41% (6 mo), 58% (12 mo) (NEJM 2009;361:1539)
PD	• 5.7% of prevalent ESRD patients age 75 and older are on PD (usrds.org) • Retrospective study of French PD registry and patients >76 yo showed median survival of 27 mo (NDT 2010;25:255) • Mortality benefit of PD over HD modified by age, HD may be favored after 90 d in age >65 yo (JASN 2010;21:499) • No difference in 12-mo survival and hospitalization rate and QOL at 6 and 12 mo between HD and PD patients age 70+ (Perit Dial Int 2002;22:463)

Medical management	• Median unadj survival 37.8 mo RRT and 13.9 mo medical management (CJASN 2009;4:1611)
	• Low comorbidity: median survival 36.8 mo RRT and 29.4 mo medical management; High comorbidity: no survival benefit RRT vs medical management (NDT 2011;26:1608)
	• Renal supportive care clinic: mean survival 20 mo, median survival 16 mo. RRT patients: mean survival 36 mo, median survival 46 mo (CJASN 2016;10:260)
Transplantation	• Age 70+: adjusted relative risk of death 41% lower in transplant vs wait-listed patients. Risk of death among transplant recipients higher than wait listed until 125 d after surgery. Transplant recipient survival worse than waitlisted until 1.8 yr after transplant. At 4 yr, adjusted survival of transplant recipients 66% compared with 51% for waiting list candidates. Subgroup analyses showed a significant transplant survival benefit for ages 70 to 74 yr, ages 75 and older, DM and HTN, ECD kidneys (Transplantation 2007;83:1069)

- Gait speed & timed get up and go test predictive of mortality in CKD (JASN 2013;24:822)
- Other prognostic risk factors for mortality (see palliative care chapter)

FRAILTY

- A physiologic state of increased vulnerability to stressors that results from decreased physiologic reserves. High vulnerability for adverse health outcomes including disability, dependency, falls, and mortality.
- Characterized by slowness/weakness, poor endurance/exhaustion, physical inactivity, unintentional weight loss
- Starts early in CKD and increases as eGFR declines. High prevalence in CKD. Independent RF for death, hospitalization, and need for dialysis (CJASN 2013;8:2091; AJKD 2012;60:912)

HEMODIALYSIS VASCULAR ACCESS

- Fistula first may not be appropriate in the elderly with a limited life expectancy. Patient-centered approach that considers risk to develop ESRD, overall survival, risk of primary access failure, patient preferences, and quality of life should be considered.

AVF

- Older age is risk factor for 1° failure (AJKD 2003;42:1001; JASN 2006;17:3204; CJASN 2008;3:437)
- Higher prevalence of CAD and PAD; both risk factors for 1° failure (JASN 2006;17:3204; KI 2005;67:2462)
- Lower cumulative survival of AVF (J Vasc Surg 2007;45:420; J Vasc Access 2009;10:199)
- a/w with repeat vascular access placement compared to AVG (CJASN 2015;10:1791)
- a/w HD initiation with a catheter compared to AVG (JASN 2015;26:448)
- Patient factors affecting AVF placement, even among pts w/ AVF + catheter, may explain ≥ 2/3 of the mortality benefit observed in pts w/ AVF (JASN 2017;28:645)
- Timing: placing an AVF >6–9 mo predialysis is not a/w greater success and is associated with increased number of vascular procedures (JASN 2015;26:448)

AVG

- AVG use has declined with a concomitant increase in AVF and catheters in this population (CJASN 2007;2:1043; AJKD 2003;42:1013; Hemodial Int 2012;16:233)
- AVG survival superior to AVF survival, in the first 18 mo after access placement, when primary failure rates included (CJASN 2010;5:2438)
- Some studies show no mortality benefit of AVF over AVG (JASN 2013;24:1297; Semin Dial 2007;20:606), others have shown some small benefit to AVF (CJASN 2015;10:1791)

Hemodialysis Catheter

- Higher mortality than AVF and AVG (JASN 2013;24:1297)
- Majority of patients start with a catheter (JASN 2013;24:1297; JASN 2017;28:645)

MEDICAL MANAGEMENT/CONSERVATIVE CARE

- Defined as planned holistic patient-centered care that includes intervention to delay the progression of CKD and minimize risk of adverse events and complications, as well as shared decision making, advanced care planning, active symptom management, and psychological and social support. Does not include dialysis in the treatment plan (KDIGO KI 2015;88:447; CJASN 2016;11:1909)
- Guidelines recommend informing all patients of this treatment option in addition to RRT; include toolkit (RPA/ASN Revised Guideline. Shared Decision Making; CJASN 2010;5:2380)
- Palliative care can run concurrently with curative treatment

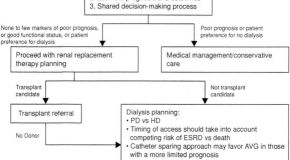

FLOW SHEET FOR MANAGING ELDERLY PATIENTS WITH ADVANCED CKD

1. Assess goals of treatment, including patient preferences
2. Estimate prognosis and outcomes
3. Shared decision-making process

None to few markers of poor prognosis, or good functional status, or patient preference for dialysis

Proceed with renal replacement therapy planning

Poor prognosis or patient preference for no dialysis

Medical management/conservative care

Transplant candidate

Transplant referral

No Donor

Not transplant candidate

Dialysis planning:
• PD vs HD
• Timing of access should take into account competing risk of ESRD vs death
• Catheter sparing approach may favor AVG in those with a more limited prognosis

PALLIATIVE CARE

Background
- High health care utilization and low hospice use compared to other end organ failure (Arch IM 2012;172:661)
- High symptom burden, high prevalence of uncontrolled pain, and low health-related quality of life (NEJM 1985;312:553; JASN 2005;16:2487; ACKD 2007;14:82)

Definition
- Palliative care is an approach to care focused on improving quality of life of patients and their families facing a life-threatening illness through prevention and relief of suffering by means of impeccable assessment and treatment of pain and other problems, physical, psychosocial, and spiritual (http://www.who.int/cancer/palliative/definition/)
- Can run concurrent with curative treatment
- Guidelines recommend palliative care services and advanced care planning to all AKI, CKD, and ESRD patients who suffer from their disease burden (CJASN 2010;5:2380)

Identifying Patients Most Likely to Benefit (CJASN 2010;5:2380; JASN 2000;11:1340)	
Identifying Factor	**Measurement**
High mortality risk	Age ≥75 yr
	Dementia
	High comorbidity score: charlson comorbidity index ≥8 (CJASN 2010;5:2380)
	Marked functional impairment: Karnofsky performance score <40, nonambulatory (AJKD 1994;23:463)
	Serum albumin <2.5
	Frailty
	Surprise question—No: provider would not be surprised if patient died in 1 yr
	Cohen score (CJASN 2010;5:72; available at QxMD®)
	Berger score (CJASN 2012;7:1039)
High symptom burden	Dialysis symptom index
	Edmonton symptom assessment scale
	Palliative care outcome Scale—Renal (Qual Health Care 1999;8:219)
	Pain assessment
Difficulty with determining goals of care	Advanced care planning

Nephrology Palliative Approach

- **Advanced Care Planning** (JASN 2000;11;1340; CJASN 2010;5:2380)
- Purpose: help the patient understand their condition, identify GOC, and prepare for future decisions needed as the condition progresses over time
- Specific goals: written advanced directives including health care proxy or power of attorney, DNR or POLST form when appropriate
- When: when considering RRT, with sentinel events, when question raised by patient or families, no to the surprise questions, routine care plan
- **Treatment of Symptoms:** pain assessment scale and distinguish nociceptive vs neuropathic pain

WHO Ladder for Analgesic Therapy (JASN 2006;17:3198)			
Pain Score (#)	Mild (1–4)	Moderate (5–6)	Severe (7–10)
Treatment	Acetaminophen ±[a]Adjuvant for neuropathic pain	Hydromorphone or Tramadol ±[a]Adjuvant for neuro pain	Hydromorphone[b] ±[a]Adjuvant for neuro pain
Dose	Acetaminophen: max daily dose 3.2 g/d	Hydromorph: 0.5 mg q4h prn Tramadol: 25 mg/d to 75 mg BID	0.5 mg q4h standing
Administration route	Oral	Oral to start and IV PRN	PO standing, IV PRN

[a]Adjuvants include gabapentin, pregabalin, desipramine, some antiepileptics and tricyclics.
[b]Can be converted to fentanyl or methadone.

- Morphine should not be used in CKD and ESRD
- A bowel regimen should be prescribed with opiates
- Pruritus: gabapentin effective in CKD and ESRD, dose adjust for GFR
- Reference: www.kidneysupportivecare.org; www.who.int/cancer/palliative/painladder

ULTRAFILTRATION (UF)

Hemodialysis (HD)/Hemofiltration (HF)
- Driving force: **hydrostatic pressure gradient** across the membrane, transmembrane pressure (TMP, mmHg)
- UF coefficient (K_{uf}, mL/hr/mmHg): water permeability of dialyzer
- HD pump applies TMP = desired UF (mL/hr)/K_{uf} (mL/hr/mmHg)
  - High flux dialyzer (K_{uf} >20) requires lower TMP to achieve desired UF

Peritoneal Dialysis (PD)
- Driving force: **osmotic gradient** between dialysate and blood, created by glucose (1.5%, 2.5%, or 4.25% glucose), or a poorly absorbed carbohydrate polymer, icodextrin in dialysate
- UF rate is maximum at the beginning of dwell and decreases as glucose is absorbed

CLEARANCE

Types of Clearance		
	Diffusion	**Convection**
Concept	Movement of solutes across a semipermeable membrane along a **concentration gradient** between the blood and dialysate compartment	Movement of solutes across a semipermeable membrane resulting from **"solvent drag"** during UF of plasma solutes across a semipermeable membrane
Removal	Small solute	Middle and some large solutes
Modality	HD (predominant), PD	HF, PD; hemodiafiltration (HDF)

Types of Solutes (MW)
- Small solutes (<500 D): urea (60), Cr (113), Na^+, K^+, H^+, glc, HCO_3^-, lactate
- Middle solutes (500–5,000 D): inulin, Vit B_{12} (1355), aluminum/deferoxamine complex (700), vancomycin, aminoglycosides
- Large solutes (>5 kD): PTH (9 kD), β2 microglobulin (11.8 kD), myoglobin (17.8 kD), κ LC (22.5 kD), α1 microglobulin (33 kD), λ LC (45 kD), albumin (68 kD)
- Protein bound solutes: indoxyl sulfate, p-cresyl sulfate, p-cresol glucuronide (proinflammatory *JASN* 2013;24:1981); homocysteine, indoles; only small portion of nonbound form can be cleared by HD

Determinants of Convective Clearance
- UF: replacement fluid (RF) is infused to allow for increased total UF to achieve convective clearance, yet maintain desired net fluid balance
- Sieving coefficient: the ratio of the concentration of the solute in the ultrafiltrate over the plasma; important factor in middle MW solutes; 1 in small MW solutes

Determinants of Diffusive Clearance
- Flux (J): the rate of solute movement is based on Fick principle

$$\text{Flux (J)} = \text{Diffusivity} \times \text{Area} \times \text{Concentration Gradient}$$

- Diffusivity (D, permeability): dependent on membrane composition (pore size, pore density, membrane thickness, membrane charge, solute, and solvent)
- Area (A): effective membrane surface area (typically 1.7–2.0 m^2)
- The mass transfer coefficient (K_oA) = permeability (K_o) × surface area (A)
  K_o: membrane- and solute-specific constant
  K_oA determines maximal clearance at infinite blood flow (Qb) and dialysate flow (Qd)
  Actual diffusivity is affected by stagnant fluid layer, Qb and Qd
- Concentration gradient: dependent on dialysate solute concentration, Qb, Qd, stagnant fluid films, geometry of flow (parallel vs antiparallel)
- Flow: **small** solutes clearance is dependent on **Qb** and **Qd**; higher flows help to maintain the concentration gradient across which diffusion occurs, up to optimal flows which, in turn, is determined by the **K_oA** of the dialyzer
- Time: **large** solutes clearance is dependent on **length** of treatment (ie, contact time across the dialysis membrane) d/t slow diffusion and to a lesser extent by the K_oA of the dialyzer

High Flux Membrane

- High rate of water transfer, the ultrafiltration coefficient (K_{uf}) >20 mL/hr/mmHg
- Removes ~10–15 kD (middle and some large) solute; does not remove albumin
- Back-filtration of bacterial endotoxin from dialysate into blood is possible
- No Δ in mortality and hospitalization rate (HEMO *NEJM* 2002;347:2010)
- Survival benefits in DM or patients w/ albumin ≤4 (MPO *JASN* 2009;20:645)
- High flux membranes use is a/w ↓ CV mortality ×0.83 (*Cochrane Database Syst Rev* 2012;CD005016) and low CV event in pts with AVF and DM (EGE *JASN* 2013;24:1014)

Other Terms Used for Types of Membrane

- **High permeability:** higher clearance of the middle solute (eg, β2-microglobulin)
  - β2-microglobulin clearance >20 mL/min; ≈high flux membrane
- **High efficiency:** high urea clearance >210 mL/min and urea K_oA >600 mL/min
- **High cut-off (HCO):** remove ~100 kD solutes, eg, Ig LC (*CJASN* 2009;4:745); myoglobin; Cons: albumin loss
- **Medium cut-off (MCO):** remove 15–45 kD solutes; less loss of albumin than HCO
  - Greater clearance of large solutes (eg, λ LC) than high flux (*NDT* 2017;32:165)

SUBSTITUTION FLUID

Dialysate

- Electrolytes and buffer containing fluid used to generate concentration gradient
- Produced by adding acid and base concentrate to treated water
- Separated by dialyzer from blood

Replacement Fluid (RF)

- Electrolytes and buffer-containing sterile fluid that is given to replace fluid removal
- Administered into systemic circulation before or after hemofiltration
- Prefilter RF: less extracorporeal circuit (filter) clot; prefilter RF flow rate is added to plasma water flow rate, lowering filtration fraction
- Postfilter RF: more efficient clearance

FORMS OF RRT

Forms of RRT			
Column Title	Fluid	Clearance	Comment
Hemodialysis (HD)	Dialysate	Diffusive >> Convective	Convective clearance proportional to UF amount
Hemofiltration (HF)	RF	Convective	Small solute clearance correlate w/ UF rate
Hemodiafiltration (HDF)	Dialysate and RF	Diffusive and Convective	Not used for maintenance of RRT

- HDF: online ultrapure substitution fluid (dialysate and RF) production ↓ the cost
  - No ↓ mortality, CV events (vs low flux HD). High volume HDF ↓ mortality, CV event (CONTRAST *JASN* 2012;23:1087)
  - No ↓ mortality, CV events (vs high flux HD). High volume HDF ↓ overall and CV mortality (*NDT* 2012;28:192)
  - ↓ Mortality, hypotension, hospitalization (vs 92% high flux HD) when convective volume 23–24 L/session (ESHOL *JASN* 2013;24:487)
- Peritoneal dialysis (PD): utilizes the peritoneal membrane to facilitate fluid and solute transfer between dialysate in the peritoneal cavity and the bloodstream

Modalities Available in Hospital Setting Only

- Continuous venovenous HD (CVVHD): slow form of HD
- Continuous venovenous hemofiltration (CVVH): slow form of HF
- Continuous venovenous hemodiafiltration (CVVHDF): combined CVVHD + CVVH
- Slow continuous ultrafiltration (SCUF): UF only. No dialysate/RF.
  - Minimal convective clearance
  - In decompensated HF, ↑ Cr, adverse events in SCUF group, c/w diuretic group (*NEJM* 2012;367:2296)

RRT INITIATION

RRT Initiation in CKD

The IDEAL Study (NEJM 2010;363:609)
- 828 pts in Australia and New Zealand (mostly white patients) were randomized based on BSA-corrected CrCl by Cockcroft–Gault equation to early (10–14) vs late (5–7) initiation of dialysis. Clinicians were allowed to initiate dialysis based upon the presence of uremic symptoms and volume overload in addition to CrCl. The mean CrCl was 12 in the early start group vs 9.8 in the late start group.
- The median time to the initiation of dialysis was 1.8 and 7.4 mo after randomization in the early and late start groups, respectively
- At a median followup of 3.6 yr, there was **no difference** in survival between groups or in cardiovascular events, infections, or dialysis complications

NKF-KDOQI and KDIGO (AJKD 2015;66:884; KDIGO CKD 2012)
- Based primarily based on assessment of s/s a/w uremia, progressive deterioration in clinical status refractory to dietary intervention, inability to control blood pressure, volume overload, or metabolic abnormalities with medical therapy
- Not based on a specific level of kidney function in the absence of symptoms

Canadian Society of Nephrology (CMAJ 2014;186:112)
- Intent-to-defer dialysis until a clinical indication is present or eGFR has declined to 6 mL/min or less (even in the absence of symptoms), whichever occurs first

European Renal Best Practice Advisory Board (NDT 2011;26:2082)
- In patients with an eGFR <15 mL/min when a clinical indication arises
- When close supervision is not feasible and in patients whose uremic symptoms may be difficult to detect, a planned start of dialysis while still asymptomatic may be preferred

General Indications of RRT Initiation in CKD
- The optimal time of dialysis initiation in CKD is controversial
- Most patients will develop uremic symptoms with eGFR 5–10 mL/min. Younger pts and those without multiple comorbidities may remain asymptomatic at lower levels of eGFR.
- Uremic pericarditis or pleuritis, uremic encephalopathy
- Declining nutritional status (anorexia, weight loss, evidenced by decrease in dry weight and serum albumin level)
- Persistent or difficult-to-treat volume overload, refractory HTN or recurrent admissions for HF
- Metabolic acidosis, hyperkalemia, and hyperphosphatemia refractory to medical therapy
- Cognitive impairment (consider time-limited trial of dialysis to see if ΔMS improves)
- Other uremic symptoms: nausea, vomiting, pruritus, fatigue, pain, muscle cramps, sleep disturbance, altered taste, sexual dysfunction

RRT Initiation in AKI

- The initiation of RRT in patients with AKI prevents uremia and immediate death from the adverse complications of renal failure
- Emergent indications: K ≥6.5, metabolic acidosis w/ pH <7.1, fluid overload especially with increasing oxygen requirements in patients who are oliguric or anuric; uremic pericarditis or uremic encephalopathy; certain intoxications (eg, methanol, ethylene glycol, lithium, metformin)
- Elective indications: K >6.0 or metabolic acidosis w/ pH <7.2 despite optimal medical therapy, repeated positive fluid balance despite aggressive attempts at diuresis
- RCTs have compared strategies of early vs delayed initiation of RRT (in the absence of emergent indications) in critically ill patients with AKI with the majority of them not showing a difference in mortality at 60 or 90 d, the risk of dialysis dependence, length of ICU or hospital stay, or recovery of renal function (AKIKI NEJM 2016;375:122; AJRCCM 2018;198:58; BMC Nephrology 2017;18:78)
- However, in the delayed initiation groups (48–72 hr) a significant amount of patients did not receive RRT, the majority of them because they recovered renal function, but a few but died before RRT was initiated (low likelihood that this would have been prevented with dialysis) (NEJM 2018;379:1431; NEJM 2016;375:122)
- In hemodynamic instability, ACS, acute brain injury, or fulminant hepatic failure CRRT may be a better option compared to intermittent hemodialysis

- Kidney transplant when feasible is the best option for ESRD. However, if a decision to start dialysis is made, adequate patient education and shared-decision making are key factors in determining what is most suitable for the patient.
- Patient should be informed about pros and cons of in-center HD and home dialysis modalities (peritoneal dialysis, conventional, short-daily, or nocturnal home hemodialysis)

Comparison of In-Center Hemodialysis vs Peritoneal Dialysis		
	Hemodialysis (HD)	Peritoneal Dialysis (PD)
Frequency	3–4 hr on machine in a dialysis unit ×3 times/wk	CAPD: 4 manual exchanges/d CCPD: cycling machine at night
Benefits (ACKD 2011;18:428)	Less patient responsibility Opportunity for socialization More frequent monitoring Preferred in bed-bound patients, those with multiple comorbidities	Lower cost, patient autonomy, adapted to lifestyle Higher satisfaction and quality of life Preferred in young, high functioning people with residual renal function Maintenance of residual renal function
Risks (ACKD 2011;18:428)	Access complications Central venous catheters (CVC): infection (bacteremia), thrombosis, venous stenosis Fistula: body image problem	Infection (peritonitis) Loss of UF (membrane failure) Patient and caregiver burnout Body image problem with PD catheter Higher dropout rate mostly due to peritonitis or inadequate dialysis
Access and dialysis initiation	Allow 2–3 mo for fistula to mature before use; usually around 2 wk for graft before use CVC can be used immediately	Routine PD: start 2–4 wk after catheter insertion to allow for abdominal wall to heal before use Urgent PD: start within 2 wk
Training time	No training needed	Usually 1–2 wk
CV complications	Angina, MI, and stroke can be precipitated by low BP Marked K changes can lead to cardiac arrhythmias	Safer for pts with low BP and CV disease More gentle fluid removal
Other complications	Access malfunction Disequilibrium syndrome Muscle cramps	Access malfunction Hyperglycemia and weight gain Encapsulating peritoneal sclerosis with long-term PD (>5 yr)
Absolute Contraindications (Int J Nephrol 2011;2011:739794)	Lack of vascular access Intolerance to HD procedure	Absence of a functional peritoneal membrane (eg, extensive abdominal adhesions, pleuroperitoneal communication) Active abdominal wall infection (cellulitis, abscess, peritonitis) Severe intestinal disease (eg, IBD, ischemia) Severe mental impairment Lack of suitable home environment AKI in pregnancy
Relative Contraindications (Int J Nephrol 2011;2011:739794)	Severe heart failure Severe ischemic heart disease Thrombosed central veins Needle phobia Long-distance to closer dialysis unit	Ostomy, abdominal hernias, multiple abdominal surgeries Frailty or physical impairment Poor personal hygiene Severe malnutrition Morbid obesity Medication nonadherence GERD or ileus

CONTINUOUS RENAL REPLACEMENT THERAPY

Introduction

- A renal replacement therapy (RRT) modality for acutely ill or hemodynamically unstable patients unable to tolerate intermittent hemodialysis (iHD)
- Continuous renal replacement therapy (CRRT) offers the advantage of gradual correction of fluid electrolyte abnormalities in renal failure due to slow flow rates, smaller dialysis dialyzer surface areas, and extended duration of therapy used in this form of RRT. As a result, this is the preferred modality in unstable patients particularly in the ICU

Indications (Chest 2019;155:626)

- Acute indications are the same as those for initiating any form of RRT
  - Severe acidosis (pH <7.15), diuretic resistant fluid overload, uremia and certain drug intoxications, and poisoning cases
- The role of early initiation of CRRT in AKI is not established. There is currently no strong evidence to support the early introduction of CRRT, the choice of one modality over another, or a specific clearance dose
- CRRT has been used for the removal of toxins with large volumes of distribution effectively with rebound: metformin (Eur J Drug Metab Pharmacokinet 2012;37:249), lithium, methotrexate, dabigatran

TYPES OF CRRT

Slow Continuous Ultrafiltration (SCUF)

- Primarily designed for volume removal with slow UF rates. SCUF does not provide meaningful clearance of solutes and is used in volume overload states, eg, refractory CHF

Continuous Venovenous Hemofiltration (CVVH)

- A **convective** method of CRRT where hydraulic pressure across the dialyzer membrane ultrafilters plasma water. The clearance delivered is directly proportional to ultrafiltration volume.
- Replacement fluid (RF) can be added to the circuit either before the blood enters the dialyzer (predialyzer) or after it leaves the dialyzer (postdialyzer)
  - Predialyzer RF dilutes the blood entering the circuit somewhat decreasing the concentration and thus the clearance of solutes. Predilution is the primary circuit setting used in the United States.
  - Postdialyzer dilution maintains concentration and thus efficiency but the higher hematocrit at the end of the dialyzer resulting in decreased plasma volume increases risk of dialyzer clotting

Continuous Venovenous Hemodialysis (CVVHD)

- Employs **diffusive** clearance where dialysate is circulated in a countercurrent fashion to facilitate maximal diffusion from the blood side. The diffusive clearance delivered is proportional to the dialysate flow rate. Diffusive clearance is less effective at removal of larger molecules including so called "middle molecules."

Continuous Venovenous Hemodiafiltration (CVVHDF)

- Uses both dialysis and RF which allows for both **diffusion** and **convection** clearance. This modality limits the loss of clearance by limiting the volume of RF used by adding dialysate fluid used to dilute the blood entering the dialyzer. Newer circuits allow for the use of both pre- and postdialyzer addition of RF allowing for considerable customization of the circuit.

PRESCRIPTION

- CRRT differs from intermittent RRT in several respects as below
  - **Blood flow rates:** much slower, 100~300 mL/min
  - **Dialysate flow rates:** when dialysate is used, the flow rates are much lower at 20~25 mL/kg/hr (eg, for a 70-kg person, 1.5~2.0 L/hr with CRRT vs >24.0 L/hr with iHD).
  - Since fluid is continuously removed at a low rate with CRRT, there is less chance of hemodynamic instability
  - **RF flow rate:** when prescribed, this is done at a rate similar to dialysate and expressed as mL/kg/hr
  - **Net ultrafiltration rate:** rate of goal net fluid removal from the patient expressed as mL/hr. Net ultrafiltration rate is determined by patient's volume status. CRRT prescriptions are written either to maintain net even balance or negative balance.

- **Total UF volume** is the sum of the RF (including the volume of fluid used for anticoagulation) and the net UF volume removed from the patient
- **Effluent** volume is the sum total of the total ultrafiltrate and the dialysate fluid (if used) that is discarded
• Given the relatively low flow rates and assumed sieving coefficient of 1 (ie, that the equal concentration of solutes in the blood is equal to the effluent) for low MW substances, small molecular clearance is:
  - $U \times V/P$, U: effluent concentration, V: effluent volume, P: blood concentration
  - It is equal the total effluent volume (V) in mL/kg/hr as $U/P = 1$
• However, predialyzer RF decrease the U/P ratio by ↓ the solute concentration entering the dialyzer compared to the solute concentration in the patient. ↑ RF rates and ↓ blood flow rates lower the clearance delivered (*Int J Artif Organs* 2012;35:413).

DOSE

• Currently delivered dose of CRRT recommended is 20–25 mL/kg/hr (KDIGO AKI 2012)
• When prescribing RRT as supportive therapy for AKI, a weekly Kt/V of >3.6 is reasonable and translates to an approximate goal of 20–25 mL/kg/hr
• The prescribed dose may need to be increased to ensure that the target dose is actually delivered. Dose reductions may be required in the presence of severe metabolic alkalosis (given the high concentration of bicarbonate in the dialysate solutions), or if the primary indication was volume management in the absence of metabolic derangements.
• Time off CRRT usually lowers delivered dose by 20–30% per day
• Effluent volume underestimates the total dose especially when sieving coefficient is <1 and in prefilter CVVH and CVVHDF
  - In these cases, the % decrease in clearance is = $1 - [Q_b/(Q_b + Q_{RF})]$ where Q_b is blood flow rate and the Q_{RF} is the replacement flow rate
  - Delivered dose is effluent volume $\times [Q_b/(Q_b + Q_{RF})]$
• CVVH is the preferred modality to remove large MW substances including myoglobin in cases of severe rhabdomyolysis (*NEJM* 2009;361:1627; *Cochrane Database Syst Rev* 2014;CD008566)

ANTICOAGULATION

• Anticoagulation of the CRRT circuit is necessary to ensure viability of the circuit and avoid blood loss that result when the circuit clots
• Unfractionated heparin: low dose, 300 units/hr; traditional circuit anticoagulation
• Regional citrate anticoagulation: pts at high risk of bleeding or in postoperative setting
  - The administration of citrate predialyzer to chelate all the calcium and repletion of calcium before returning the blood to the patient
  - Citrate is metabolized to bicarbonate and can contribute to metabolic alkalosis
  - Failure to metabolize citrate in liver failure or shock can result in metabolic acidosis
  - Hypocalcemia may occur when there is an imperfect balance between the amounts of citrate administration and calcium repletion
  - Citrate anticoagulation is now the preferred method (*Crit Care Med* 2015;43:1622)

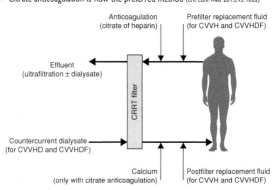

Anticoagulation (citrate of heparin)

Prefilter replacement fluid (for CVVH and CVVHDF)

Effluent (ultrafiltration ± dialysate)

CRRT filter

Countercurrent dialysate (for CVVHD and CVVHDF)

Calcium (only with citrate anticoagulation)

Postfilter replacement fluid (for CVVH and CVVHDF)

PRACTICAL CONSIDERATIONS

- Good vascular access with a double lumen catheter placed in a large blood vessel is necessary to ensure adequate flow. Lower blood flow rates make recirculation an infrequent concern. Patients with ESRD and a working fistula need a catheter as well as long term cannulation of the fistula is considered unsafe (Contrib Nephrol 2007;156:275)
- Given the slow rate of removal, iHD is the preferred treatment modality for the management of acute hyperkalemia (Crit Care 2015;19:s9)
- Large variance between the prescribed and delivered dose of dialysis is common for ICU patients due to the device being turned off for a variety of reasons. This should be taken into consideration by checking the total effluent volume for the preceding 24 hr and taken into prescribing subsequent flow rates. Alternatively, increase the prescribed dose by 20–25% (Crit Care 2015;19:s9)

COMPLICATIONS

Electrolyte/Acid–Base Complications
- Hypophosphatemia is common especially when feeds are held. Unlike iHD, the gradual rate of removal allows phosphate to move from the intracellular compartment. Can potentially delay ventilator weaning. Either PO and slow IV repletion of phosphate is often necessary (Semin Dial 2018;31:213)
- Metabolic alkalosis results commonly from diffusion of bicarbonate from the dialysate solution or from direct mixing of the bicarbonate in the RF. Bicarbonate concentration in most fluids is 32–35 mEq/L and this may impact the prescribed flow rates.
- Hypocalcemia and hypomagnesemia are uncommon occurrences given the presence of calcium and magnesium in fluid solutions. Hypocalcemia when using citrate anticoagulation requires an increase in the calcium supplementation rate.
- Sodium concentrations in most dialysate and replacement fluid is 140 mEq/L. This is of concern when initiating a patient with either hyponatremia or hypernatremia on CRRT which may result in a rapid change in concentration of serum sodium which should be avoided (KI Rep 2019;4:59; Nephron Clin Pract 2014;128:394)

Inadequate Drug Dosing
- When possible, drug dosing should be titrated either using clinical response or therapeutic drug monitoring. Most drugs require at least some dose adjustments for patients on CRRT and subtherapeutic drug concentrations are common (Semin Dial 2014;27:441)
- Drugs with a small volume of distribution, low protein binding, low molecular weight are impacted to a greater extent but the amount of drug removed depends on the delivered dose of clearance and whether the clearance was convective (greater drug removal) or diffusive. Dialyzer size and membrane may also impact this (Crit Care Med 2012;40:1523)

Circuit Clotting: A Frequent Complication and Can Result From
- Inadequate anticoagulation
- Inadequate vascular access → frequent alarms → cessation of flow in the circuit
- High filtration fraction: the goal filtration fraction is <20%
  - Filtration fraction = ultrafiltration volume/plasma water flow rate
  - Plasma water flow rate = blood flow rate (1 − Hct) + predialyzer RF rate
  - This can be lowered by decreasing the rate of ultrafiltration or increasing the plasma water flow rate (by adding predialyzer RF or increasing the blood flow rate)

Other Complications
- Catheter-related complications include catheter infections, bleeding, and clotting
- Anticoagulation of the circuit can ↑ the risk of bleeding especially in susceptible patients
- Given the ability of glucose to diffuse from the blood to the effluent, rare instance of normoglycemic ketoacidosis have been reported
- Hypothermia resulting from the use of fluids in large volumes at room temperature is primarily a concern in pediatric and small adult patients. Fluid warmers should be considered in these situations (AJKD 1998;32:1023)
- Thrombocytopenia has been reported; usually responds to cessation of therapy or the use of a dialyzer with a different membrane type (Ann Pharmacother 2018;52:1204)

DISCONTINUATION

- The most important predictor of successful cessation of CRRT is urine volume at the time of cessation particularly achieved without diuretics (Crit Care Med 2009;37:2576)
- Standardized protocols for initiation and discontinuation of CRRT have been associated with lower mortality (CJASN 2017;12:228)

HEMODIALYSIS INITIATION

Indications

- AKI, CKD: for control and correction of fluid and electrolyte imbalance that cannot or no longer be managed conservatively by diet and medications, for control and correction of acid–base abnormalities, and for the uremic syndrome
  - Early (eGFR 10–14) vs late (eGFR 5–7) HD start did not result in improved outcomes at 1 yr of followup (IDEAL NEJM 2010;363:609)
- Intoxication: lithium, ethylene glycol, methanol, aspirin, phenytoin, barbiturates, theophylline

First Three Hemodialysis Sessions

- Low intensity to prevent dialysis disequilibrium; avoid UF >2 L for 1st session

Examples of First Three Sessions of HD Initiation				
	Time (hr)	Qb (mL/min)	Qd (mL/min)	Needle, Dialyzer
1st	1.5–2	150–200	400	17 G, Low K_oA dialyzer
2nd	2.5–3	250–300	500	16 G
3rd	3–4	300–350	600	15 G, High K_oA dialyzer

DIALYZER

- Dialyzer K_oA = permeability × surface area: determines maximal clearance
- Currently available dialyzers are hollow-fiber (capillary)

Dialyzer Type by Membrane Material			
Type	Biocompatibility	Example	Comment
Cellulose	Low	Cuprophane	Low-flux
Substituted (modified) cellulose	Intermediate	Cellulose acetate Cellulose diacetate Cellulose triacetate (Exeltra®)	High-flux
Synthetic	High	Polysulfone (F, FX, Optiflux®) Polyethersulfonem Polyarylethersulfone (Revaclear®) Polymethyl methacrylate (PMMA)	High-flux Protein adsorption esp. PMMA Reflect dialysate impurities

- Polyacrylonitrile membrane: chest pain and dyspnea in pts on ACEi. Unavailable.
- Sterilized by gamma irradiation, ethylene oxide, or electron beam

FLUID REMOVAL AND ULTRAFILTRATION (UF)

Estimated Dry Weight (EDW): Various definitions

- EDW is the optimal weight patients should reach after HD
- The weight at which the pt is asymptomatic w/o signs of volume depletion or overload
- The weight at which patient is normotensive without antihypertensive medications
- Failure to achieve EDW is a/w ED visit and hospitalization (JASN 2018;29:2178)

Methods to Assess EDW

- Empiric ("trial-and-error"/traditional method): lowest post-HD weight tolerated without intradialytic hypotension (IDH) or symptoms (cramps, N/V, dizziness, near syncope)
- Blood volume monitoring (BVM): monitoring of relative contraction of intravascular volume due to hemoconcentration from UF of the blood to help determine the maximal rate of UF-tolerated and the lowest post-HD weight achievable without the development of IDH
- Bioimpedance measurement: measure of total body water (TBW); not in routine clinical use
- DW assessment protocol ↓ mortality; orthostatic BP may help (CJASN 2019;14:385)

UF Amount and UF Rate (= UF amount/dialysis treatment time)

- UF rate >10–13 mL/kg/hr (AJKD 2016;68:911; KI 2011;79:250) and IDWG >4 kg (Circulation 2009;119:671) are a/w mortality

Strategies to Lower UF Rate
Increase treatment time (duration of each session or frequency)
Decrease interdialytic weight gain (IDWG)
Restrict fluid intake (including IV fluid for inpatient) to <1 L/d
Restrict sodium intake
Loop diuretics: ↓ intradialytic hypotension, hospitalization (CJASN 2019;14:95)
Lower dialysate sodium gradually to 135 as tolerated

HEMODIALYSIS PRESCRIPTION

Prescription of Maintenance Hemodialysis	
Blood flow (Qb)	400–450 mL/min 200 mL/min: initial, restart; hypotension, cerebral edema (CRRT preferred)
Dialysate flow (Qd)	600–800 mL/min for high flux dialyzer Should be 1.5–2 × Qb for optimal clearance
Length	Initially <50 kg: 3 hr, 50–90 kg: 3.5 hr, >90 kg: 4 hr Adjust based on adequacy, UF requirement, lab (K, PO$_4$)
Frequency	≥3×/wk for minimal residual renal function Incremental HD based on RRF is an option (AJKD 2014;64:181)
Needle	Max Qb: 300 (17 G), 400 (16 G), 450 (15 G)
Ultrafiltration (UF)	
UF amount	Commensurate with EDW
UF modeling	Higher UF rate (when the patient is at a higher volume and capillary refill is presumably more rapid) → Lower UF rate Various profiles available: stepwise, linear, or exponential decline Rarely lower → higher UF rate for intradialytic HTN worse in late part
Dialysate	
Temperature	36.5°C; Low temperature (35–35.5°C) promote peripheral vasoconstriction and aid in hemodynamic stability during HD; s/e: cramps, chilling
Sodium (132–155 mEq/L)	Low Na: ↓ BP, IDWG (Ren Fail 2007;29:143); may cause cramps, N/V High Na: may stimulate thirst and ↑ IDWG Rapid Na reduction may cause cerebral edema Rapid Na rise may cause osmotic demyelination; safe correction limit is unclear: 15–20 (Semin Dial 2011;24:407) In severe hyponatremia CRRT with customized substitution fluid or postfilter hypotonic fluid may be considered (CJASN 2018;13:787)
Sodium profiling (modeling)	Higher dialysate Na (to allow for higher UF rate) → Lower dialysate Na Various profiles available: stepwise, linear, or exponential decline Stepwise profiling is effective (Hemodial Int 2017;21:312) s/e: potential Na loading → ↑ thirst and fluid intake with higher IDWG; a/w ↑ all-cause & CV mortality (CJASN 2019;14:385)
Potassium (0–4 mEq/L)	4: rarely used in advanced CKD 3: pre-HD K <4; 2: pre-HD K 4–6 0–1: pre-HD K >6; a/w cardiac arrest (KI 2011;79:218; CJASN 2012;7:765)
Potassium profiling	Higher K initially → lower K later in treatment allows for gradual fall in serum K (JASN 2017;28:3441) with less K gradient (NDT 2018;33:1207)
Calcium (2–3.5 mEq/L)	2.5: typical 3.0–3.5: hypocalcemia in hungry bone syndrome after parathyroidectomy 2.0: hypercalcemia; a/w low BP, sudden cardiac death (CJASN 2013;8:797)
Bicarbonate (30–40 mEq/L)	35: typical; adjust to have pre-HD HCO$_3$ level 21–22 (AJKD 2004;44:661) High dialysate bicarbonate ↓ BP (NDT 2009;24:973), ↑ death (AJKD 2013;62:738)

Heparin Anticoagulation
• Prevents clotting within the dialysis circuit
• AVF/AVG: 25–50 u/kg; 60% bolus at initiation then 40% as infusion over duration of HD; held last 60 min of therapy for hemostasis (eg, 1,000 u bolus + 500 u/hr)
• TDC: 50–75 u/kg heparin; 60% initial bolus: 40% as maintenance infusion – held last 30 min before completion of HD (eg, 2,000 u bolus + 1,000 u/hr)
• Alternatively, the entire dose given as a bolus at the start of HD

Heparin-Free Dialysis
• Indication: active or recent GI bleed, hemorrhagic or ischemic stroke, surgery w/i the past 24 hr or a known/suspected allergy to heparin, HIT

- Options:
  1. Periodic flushing of the dialyzer with 50–100 cc NS every 15–20 min
  2. Citrate infusion into the arterial side of the dialyzer (to bind Ca and inhibit pro-coagulant factors) w/ Ca-free dialysate and repletion of calcium on the venous side
  3. Citrate containing dialysate; ✓ ionized calcium (iCa) after HD in (2) and (3)

Dialysis Catheter Thrombosis
- Prevention: 4% sodium citrate or tPA lock
- Tx: tPA (alteplase, tenecteplase) to each port for 30–45 min; if it does not dissolve thrombosis, catheter exchange

MBD AND HEMOGLOBIN IN DIALYSIS PATIENTS

Considerations in MBD and Hb Management in Dialysis Patients	
Conditions	**Considerations**
High PO$_4$ (>5.5)	Dietary restriction: 750–1,000 mg/d ↑ PO$_4$ binder dose; ✓ compliance and timing: right before or w/ meals Readdress the need for active and inactive vitamin D R/o rhabdomyolysis, hemolysis, tumor lysis syndrome Pseudohyperphosphatemia: high Ig, bili, or lipid
Low PO$_4$ (<3.5)	Lower or stop PO$_4$ binder If PTH is high, start or increase active vitamin D If PTH is within goal, consider low-dose active vitamin D (but maintain PTH within goal)
High PTH (>600–770)	Control PO$_4$ If Ca × P >70, avoid active vitamin D and consider PO cinacalcet or IV etelcalcetide if Ca is not low; consider parathyroidectomy If Ca × P 55–70, start low dose or titrate up active vitamin D If Ca × P < 55, start or titrate up active vitamin D
Low PTH (<150–170)	Lower active vitamin D dose and d/c inactive vitamin D If s/p parathyroidectomy, do not d/c active vitamin D for low PTH—titrate active vitamin D to maintain serum Ca ≥8.4 If Alk phos is low, possible adynamic bone; stop active vitamin D and convert Ca containing PO$_4$ binder to non-Ca containing one; consider low Ca bath
High Ca	Convert Ca containing PO$_4$ binder to non-Ca containing binder Readdress the need for vitamin D R/o: malignancy, granulomas, hypothyroidism, immobility If PTH is above goal, consider cinacalcet or etelcalcetide
Low Ca	Use albumin corrected Ca level; Control high PO$_4$ Stop calcimimetics (PO cinacalcet or IV etelcalcetide) if it is given If PO$_4$ is controlled, consider active ± nutrient vitamin D
High Hb	Lower (Hb 11–12) or stop (Hb >12) ESA dose R/o malignancy (RCC, HCC, hemangioblastoma), polycythemia vera
Low Hb (<10)	Start of increase ESA dose to avoid transfusion Initial ESA dose: epoetin 100 u/kg TIW or darbepoetin 0.45 µg/kg/wk ESA resistance: requiring >75 u/kg epoetin 3×/wk (225 u/kg/wk) or equivalent dose r/o other causes of anemia including iron deficiency (could be a/w blood loss), inflammation, malignancy, folate or vitamin B$_{12}$ deficiency, TMA, inadequate solute clearance, hyperparathyroidism (AJKD 2009;53:823) Proactive iron sucrose high dose (400 mg monthly unless ferritin >700 or Tsat ≥40%) ↓ ESA dose c/t reactive low dose 0–400 mg monthly reactive to ferritin <200 or Tsat <20% (NEJM 2019;380:447)

Initial Active Vitamin D Dose (TIW for IV) Based on PTH			
PTH	**300–600**	**600–900**	**>900**
Paricalcitol (IV)	0.04 µg/kg	0.07 µg/kg	0.1 µg/kg
Doxercalciferol (IV)	0.025 µg/kg	0.04 µg/kg	0.055 µg/kg
Calcitriol (IV)	0.015 µg/kg	0.025 µg/kg	0.035 µg/kg
Calcitriol (PO)	total weekly IV dose and divide into a daily PO dose		

Examples of Dose Adjustment Based on Serial monthly PTH			
Change in PTH	PTH <150	PTH 300–600	PTH >600
Fall >60%	↓ 25%	↓ 25%	↓ 25%
Fall 40–60%	↓ 25%	Maintain	Maintain
Fall <40%	↓ 25%	Maintain	↑ 25%

Examples of ESA Dose Adjustment			
↑ Hb >0.5/wk	↓ −25%	Hb 11–11.5	↓ −25%
↑ Hb <0.5 over 2 wk	↑ −25%	Hb 11.5–12	↓ −50%
Hb >12	hold until <11.5 and then resume at a ↓ dose (−25%)		

HD ADEQUACY

Adequate HD
- Solute clearance, BP, and volume status are considered

SOLUTE CLEARANCE

Urea Reduction Rate (URR, %)

$$URR = \frac{(pre\ HD\ BUN - post\ HD\ BUN)}{pre\ HD\ BUN} \times 100$$

- Limitations: does not consider urea volume change and generation; inability to incorporate the patient's residual kidney function; cannot compare treatments with different frequency
- Should be ≥65% (68% if no UF during HD); KDOQI not recommending the use

Normalized Urea Clearance, Kt/V
- Dimensionless, urea clearance normalized to distribution volume of urea
- K = Urea clearance; t = Dialysis time; V = Volume of distribution of urea

Single Pool Urea Clearance, spKt/V
- Per treatment normalized urea clearance based on the single pool variable volume urea kinetic model estimated by the Daugirdas II equation (*JASN* 1993;4:1205, available at QxMD®):

$$\frac{spKt}{V} = -Ln(R - 0.008 \times t) + (4 - 3.5 \times R) \times \frac{UF\ volume\ (L)}{post\text{-}HD\ weight\ (kg)}$$

$R = \dfrac{post\text{-}HD\ BUN}{pre\text{-}HD\ BUN}$ t = dialysis time (in hr)

- spKt/V should be >1.2 with target 1.4 (KDOQI *AJKD* 2015;66:884)

Equilibrated Urea Clearance, eKt/V
- Similar to spKt/V except uses a post-HD BUN drawn 30 min after the completion of HD to allow for the initial rapid rebound and transcellular re-equilibration of urea
- eKt/V should be >1.05: approximately ≈ spKt/V 1.25
- Computed from the spKt/V and session length (t) using, for example, the Tattersall equation (*KI* 1996;50:2094):

$$\frac{eKt}{V} = \frac{spKt}{V} \times \frac{t}{t + C}$$

t = session duration (min)
C = time constant, specific for type of access and type solute being removed. For urea, C should be 35 min for arterial access (AVF/AVG) and 22 min for TDC

Standard Normalized Urea Clearance, stdKt/V
- An estimation of <u>weekly</u> urea clearance on continuous or intermittent therapy
- On intermittent therapy, use the Leypoldt formula to calculate stdKt/V (*Semin Dial* 2004;17:142, calculator is available at www.hdcn.com)
- Typically used for treatment prescriptions other than 3×/wk dialysis sessions
- stdKt/V should be ≥2.0 if residual renal function is not measured or negligible
- A spKt/V of 1.2 delivered 3×/wk yields a stdKt/V of 2.0

Normalized Urea Clearance from Residual Renal Function, Kt/V$_{renal}$

- K: urea clearance from 24-hr urine prior to the first HD of the wk and the predialysis BUN (can put urine volume in dL and multiply by 0.07 = 100/1,440)

$$K \text{ (mL/min)} = \frac{\text{Urine urea (mg/dL)} \times \text{Urine volume (dL/day)}}{\text{predialysis BUN (mg/dL)}} \times \frac{100 \text{ mL}}{dL} \times \frac{day}{1440 \text{ min}}$$

- t: 1 wk = $60 \times 24 \times 7$ = 10,080 min
- V: the urea space, or total body water (TBW) as: (a) dry weight TBW 0.6 (in men) or 0.5 (in women) (b) alternatively, use the Watson V formula
- Kt/V$_{renal}$ >2.0 indicates sufficient residual renal function to not require dialysis
- No residual renal function (RRF) is a/w mortality RR 17.66 compared to Kt/V$_{renal}$ >0.84 (c/w C$_{urea}$ 3.5 mL/min in 70 kg man) (JASN 2004;15:1061)

Total Weekly Kt/V

- stdKt/V + Kt/V$_{renal}$ should be >2.0; for PD total Kt/V >1.7 is considered sufficient
- Example: 50-yr-old man male produces 10 dL of urine/24 hr with a urea nitrogen of 405.7 mg/dL. His EDW is 71 kg. Treatments are 3.5 hr with 2-kg interdialytic weight gain and pre-BUN is 75 mg/dL and a post-BUN is 25 mg/dL.
  - Estimated TBW or urea space is 0.6×71 kg = 42.6 L = 42,600 mL
  - Residual urea clearance = $(405.7 \times 10/75) \times 0.07$ = 3.79 mL/min
  - Kt/V$_{renal}$ = (3.79 mL/min $\times$ 10,080 min/wk)/42,600 mL = 0.90

Calculation of Total Kt/V			
	Method	×3/wk	×2/wk
spKt/V	Daugirdas II formula*	1.27	1.27
stdKt/V	Leypoldt formula*	2.07	1.37
Total	Kt/V$_{renal}$ + stdKt/V	2.97	2.27

*Use online calculator

Conclusion: this patient could treat ×2/wk at this point

Normalized Protein Catabolic Rate (nPCR, g/kg/d)

- Estimate of dietary protein intake based on the assumption of a steady state equilibrium between dietary protein intake and protein catabolism
- Can be estimated based on interdialytic (ID) BUN and interval (Blood Purif 1997;15:157)

$$nPCR = 0.22 + \frac{0.036 \times \text{ID rise in BUN} \times 24}{\text{ID interval (hrs)}} + \frac{\text{Urine urea nitrogen (g)} \times 150}{\text{ID interval (hrs)} \times \text{weight (kg)}}$$

- Can be estimated based on pre-HD BUN and spKt/V if there is no significant renal urea nitrogen excretion, C$_{urea}$ <2 mL/min (JASN 1996;7:780)

nPCR = preHD BUN/[a + (b × spKt/V) + (c/spKt/V)] + 0.168					
	×3/wk HD			×2/wk HD	
	1st	2nd	3rd	1st	2nd
a	36.3	25.8	16.3	48.0	33.0
b	5.48	1.15	4.30	5.14	3.60
c	53.5	56.4	56.6	79.0	83.2

- nPCR at least 1.0–1.2 g/kg/d; optimal nPCR is 1.2–1.4 g/kg/d
- Inadequate dialysis is associated with poor oral intake and decreased nPCR
- Renal urea clearance corrected nPCR and its changes are a/w high albumin and low mortality (CJASN 2017;12:1109)

Clinical Implication of Solute Clearance

- Weekly time-averaged BUN (TAC$_{urea}$) 50 (vs 100) was a/w less hospitalization in nondiabetic ESRD w/o residual renal function. TAC$_{urea}$ is an imperfect measure of urea clearance alone as confounded by and not separated from urea generation rate (nPCR) (NCDS NEJM 1981;305:1176)
- spKt/V >0.8–0.9 was a/w less hospitalization (NCDS KI 1985;28:526)
- spKt/V goal of 1.65 (vs 1.25) and high flux dialyzer did not improve mortality and hospitalization rate (HEMO NEJM 2002;347:2010)
- High flux dialyzers (K$_{uf}$ >20 mL/hr/mmHg) did not improve overall mortality. It produced survival benefits in DM or patients w/ albumin ≤4, presumably related to better middle molecule clearance (MPO JASN 2009;20:645).
- High flux dialysis a/w low CV event in pts with AVF and DM (EGE JASN 2013;24:1014)

- ×6 vs ×3/wk HD for 12 mo (stdKt/V 3.54 vs 2.49) resulted in ↓ death or ↓ LV mass progression (HR 0.61), ↑ access intervention (×1.71) (FHN NEJM 2010;363:2287). 3.6-yr followup showed ↓ mortality (×0.56) (FHN JASN 2016;27:1830)

Solute Clearance Goal (KDOQI AJKD 2015;66:884)			
	spKt/V (×3/wk)	stdKt/V (if not ×3/wk)	URR (approximate)
Minimum	1.2	2.1	65%
Target	1.4	2.3	70%

CAUSES OF INADEQUATE DIALYSIS

Causes of Inadequate Solute Clearance
- Lower Qb than prescribed: inappropriate needle position; small diameter needle
- Inadequate treatment time: late arrival, early termination
- Dialysis noncompliance
- Access recirculation: inflow and outflow stenosis

Causes of Inadequate Fluid Removal
- Overestimated DW: volume overload; large interdialytic volume gain
- Inadequate treatment time
- Dialysis noncompliance, excessive dietary sodium, and fluid intake
- Dialysis associated symptoms: cramping, hypotension

HD WATER TREATMENT

- Water for HD is pretreated through a series of purification steps before it is used to dilute the dialysate concentrate to generate the final dialysate solution
- Chlorine dioxide, chloramine: added in municipal water supply to prevent bacterial (eg, Legionella) growth
- Conventional HD requires 600–800 mL/min (100–200 L/session) of dialysate flow
- The process consists of having water pass through a series of membranes and filters

Components of Water Treatment	
Heating	Warmed to 25°C (77°F) for optimal RO membrane performance
Multimedia filters	Remove large particulate matters; aka sediment filter aka sediment filter
Water softener	Remove Ca^{2+}, Mg^{2+}, iron, and manganese Ion exchange resin: exchange with Na Prevents Ca^{2+} scaling on RO membrane
Carbon filter (activated carbon)	Remove chorine, chloramine, organic contaminants Usually 2 in series, the 1st "worker" tank and the 2nd "polisher" tank Empty bed contact time (EBCT) should be ≥10 min High pH of water to ↓ copper, lead and chlorine cause ↓ efficiency of carbon filter ✓ Chlorine, chloramine between 1st and 2nd carbon tank at each shift
Reverse osmosis (RO) membranes	Remove inorganic (aluminum, zinc, fluoride, copper), organic contaminants, bacteria, viruses, endotoxins Uses high pressure, rapid filtration of the water across a 300-Da pore membrane to generate the deionized water Chlorine can damage RO membranes ✓ Conductivity of product water continuously
Deionizers (optional; used with RO membrane)	Remove ionized contaminants; do **not** remove bacteria, endotoxins Exchange cations for H^+ and anions for OH^- Either 2 tanks (cation and anion exchanger) or combined in 1 tank ✓ Resistivity continuously
Ultramicron filter	Remove any remaining bacteria and bacterial products (endotoxins) Cartridges filters with pore size <1 μm in diameter

Bacteria and Endotoxins
- Pyrogenic reaction is esp. a/w dialyzer reuse and high flux dialyzers
- The presence of low levels of bacteria and endotoxin are a/w chronic inflammation and potential ↑ risk for accelerated atherosclerosis and CV morbidity/mortality

- Cytokine-inducing substances: endotoxin, peptidoglycans, bacterial DNA and its fragments lead to chronic inflammation: ↑ ESR, hsCRP, IL-6 which may contribute to accelerated atherosclerosis, CV disease, ESA resistance
- Ultrapure water is required for high flux HD or HDF to reduce risk of backfiltration of bacterial products

Bacteria and Endotoxin Limits in Water Used for HD			
	CMS (AAMI 2004)	Europe, AAMI 2014	Ultrapure
Bacteria (CFU/mL)	<200	<100	<0.1
Endotoxin (EU/mL)	<2	<0.25	<0.03

Potential Water Contaminants

Water Contaminant		
Contaminant	Manifestation	Potential Cause
Chloramines	Hemolysis, methemoglobinemia, ESA-resistant anemia Damage RO membrane	Short EBCT Chlorine contamination → carbon filter failure
Aluminum	Dementia, myoclonus, seizures, delirium, ESA-resistant anemia, osteomalacia	Acid concentrate pumped via low pH incompatible tubing
Fluoride	Pruritus, headache, nausea, hypotension, Vfib	Saturated deionizer
H_2O_2	Methemoglobinemia	Incomplete rinsing
Copper, Zinc	Hemolysis	Metal pipes
Lead	Abdominal pain, myopathy	Pipes
Cyanotoxin	Neurotoxicity, hepatotoxicity	Contaminated water

HD COMPLICATION

DIALYSIS DISEQUILIBRIUM SYNDROME

Epidemiology
- Risk Factors: high BUN, low bicarbonate, CKD (>AKI), brain injury (stroke, seizure, trauma), cerebral edema (hyponatremia, hepatic encephalopathy, malignant hypertension)
- Rarely w/ CRRT with high intensity (effluent flow 40 mL/kg/hr) (NEJM 2009;361:1627) or significant osmolality drop (CKJ 2013;6:526)

Pathogenesis
- Intracellular osmotic equilibration in ESRD or AKI of relatively long duration
  → Rapid osmolytes and fluid shifts at the initiation of dialytic therapy
  → Osmotic disequilibrium across cellular membranes and fluid shifts into cells
  → Acute cell swelling and, in the brain, cerebral edema

Clinical Manifestations
- Range from mild (headache, nausea) to severe (confusion, restlessness, altered sensorium, blurred vision, seizures, coma, brainstem herniation, and death)
- MRI: demyelinating white matter injury

Prevention
- Initial HD URR <30% with low Qb (150–200 mL/min) and short treatment times (1.5–2 hr) based on body weight (and estimated total body water or urea space), UF <1 L
- Followed by gradual uptitration of dialysis time (usually 30 min increments) and blood flow (50–100 mL/min) until HD adequacy is achieved
- +/− mannitol 75 g IV during first 1–3 HD session

Treatment
- Mild: ↓ Qb; consider d/c of HD according to indication
- Severe: d/c HD, IV fluid, consider mannitol 10–75 g, 23% hypertonic saline 5 mL
- Seizure: airway protection, lorazepam 4 mg IV or diazepam 5 mg IV

TYPE A DIALYSIS MEMBRANE REACTION

Pathogenesis
- IgE-mediated type 1 hypersensitivity reaction (anaphylaxis) to ethylene oxide
- Non-IgE mediated anaphylactoid reaction to acrylonitrile membrane + ACEi use

Clinical Manifestation

- Typically, within the first few min of initiation of dialysis
- Burning at the access site, chest pain, dyspnea, bronchospasm, urticaria, hypotension

Treatment

- Stop dialysis immediately; do not return the blood in the extracorporeal circuit
- Epinephrine, IV steroids, and H1-blockers; proper sterilization for prevention

---

TYPE B DIALYSIS MEMBRANE REACTION

Pathogenesis

- Alternate pathway complement activation; PMN sequestration in the pulmonary vascular bed and degranulation with release of inflammatory cytokines

Clinical Manifestation

- Typically, within the first 30–45 min of initiation of dialysis; Chest and back pain
- More common with the modified cellulosic membranes than synthetic membranes
- Neutropenia during the event and have a postdialysis rebound neutrophilia (common occurrence: not clinically significant in the absence of systemic symptoms)

Treatment

- Symptomatic, supportive

CRAMPS

- Frequent cause of HD early termination and inability to achieve dry weight
- Causes: below DW, high interdialytic weight gain (dietary noncompliance), high UF rate, hypotension, hyponatremia, hypovolemia, carnitine deficiency

Treatment and Prevention

- NS, 25% mannitol 50–100 mL, 50% dextrose 25–50 mL
- Readdress DW, dietary counseling to educate on weight gain <1 kg/d
- Higher sodium dialysate or Na modeling
- If fluid removal is needed, ↑ treatment time and/or frequency to ↓ UF rate
- Vitamin E 400 IU HS (Am J Ther 2010;17:455), Carnitine 300 mg PO bid (AJKD 2008;52:962)
- Quinine: may cause severe allergic reaction and TMA; not recommended

---

INTRADIALYTIC HYPOTENSION (IDH)

Background and Clinical Implication

- Minimum SBP <90 a/w mortality (JASN 2015;26:724)
- IDH in >10% of HD ↑ CV mortality 22% (CJASN 2014;9:2124)
- a/w residual renal function loss (KI 2002;62:1046), cerebral ischemia (KI 2015;87:1109), access thrombosis (JASN 2011;22:1526)
- Myocardial stunning: recurrent myocardial ischemia, regional wall motion abnormalities (CJASN 2008;3:19) → fibrosis → dysfunction (CJASN 2009;4:914; KI 2013;84:641)
- HD early termination, ↑ EDW → chronic hypervolemia → LVH, HF (Semin Dial 2016;29:425)

Causes

- Contraction of the intravascular volume which occurs when the rate of UF exceeds the rate of capillary refill from the interstitial space reaching a critical point where the patient's CV system can no longer compensate to maintain systemic BP
- UF rates >13 mL/kg/hr (Hemodial Int 2018;22:270); volume depletion: below DW
- High predialysis osmolality (AJKD 2015;66:499)
- Paradoxical withdrawal of reflex vasoconstriction (JCI 1992;90:1657)
- Dialysate: acetate, low Na, low Ca, high HCO₃ vasodilation (NDT 2009;24:973)
- Bleeding, distributive (sepsis, adrenal insufficiency), cardiogenic, obstructive shock

Clinical Manifestation

- Asymptomatic, lightheadedness, N/V, cramps, hoarseness (thinning of vocal cords), vagal symptoms (yawning, sighing) (CJASN 2014;9:798)
- Stroke, myocardial and bowel ischemia, shock

Treatment

- Stop UF, head-down (Trendelenburg) position, ↓ Qb if solute clearance is not an issue
- Administer NS, hypertonic saline, albumin or mannitol; address causes

Strategies to Prevent IDH	
Ultrafiltration (UF)	↓ UF rate <13 mL/kg/hr: ↑ dialysis time, additional HD session ↓ IDWG: restrict fluid (<1 L/d) and Na intake; lower dialysate Na may ↓ thirst; loop diuretics if UOP >200 mL/d (CJASN 2019;14:95) UF profiling/modeling: greater UF earlier when the patient is more volume overloaded and a lower UF rate late in HD as the patient approaches the EDW and is more prone to IDH Reassess volume status and EDW: may need to ↑ EDW
Osmolality change	Na profiling/modeling: high Na dialysate to prevent fluid shift into cells; stepwise profiling is effective (Hemodial Int 2017;21:312) s/e: may cause (+) Na balance and ↑ thirst leading to ↑ IDWG; routine use is a/w ↑ mortality (CJASN 2019;14:385) Sequential UF: UF w/o dialysis for 1–2 hr while BUN concentration remains high; followed by HD with no or less fluid removal Low Qb (CJASN 2018;13:1297)
Vasoconstriction	d/c antihypertensive or dose after HD ↓ dialysate temperature (35–35.5°C): promote vasoconstriction to maintain BP; ↓ IDH (NDT 2006;21:1883; CJASN 2016;11:442), ↓ regional wall motion abnormalities (CJASN 2006;1:1216) High dialysate Ca (NDT 2009;24:973); may cause (+) Ca balance Low dialysate bicarbonate (NDT 2009;24:973) Midodrine: α1 agonist; 2.5–10 mg 15–30 min before HD; removed by HD; additional small dose can be given during HD; ↑ SBP of 12.4 (NDT 2004;19:2553); no additional effect to cool dialysate (AJKD 1999;33:920). s/e: urinary retention, supine HTN Droxidopa: NE prodrug; no benefit w/ ↑ s/e (Postgrad Med 2015;127:133)
Others	Avoid food intake during HD; manage anemia Blood Volume Monitor (BVM): helps determine the maximum rate of UF that a patient can tolerate before developing IDH; monitor for the relative contraction of intravascular volume (goal <8%/hr or 16%/session). No clear benefit (CJASN 2017;12:1831; 2019;14:385). Switch to PD High predialysis BP does not prevent IDH (Nephron Clin Prac 2006;103:c137)

INTRADIALYTIC HYPERTENSION

Background and Clinical Implication
- Common: 21.3/100 HD session (Int J Artif Organs 2012;35:1031)
- a/w ↑ ambulatory BP (CJASN 2011;6:1684)
- ↑ Short-term mortality, hospitalization (Am J Hypertens 2018;31:329)
- ↑ Long-term adverse CV events and death (AJKD 2009;54:881, KI 2013;84:795)

Pathogenesis and Causes
- Volume overload: inadequate dialysis (NDT 2010;25:3355)
- Activation of the RAAS ± SNS, removal of antihypertensives, high sodium dialysate
- ESA ↑ endothelin-1 (ET-1, vasoconstrictor); endothelial dysfunction (CJASN 2011;6:2016)
- Low SaO_2 → sympathetic activity, ET-1 (NDT 2018;33:1040)
- Dietary salt and high [Na] (KI 2012;81:407). Serum to dialysate sodium gradient (Am J Nephrol 2013;38:413)

Treatment
- DW reduction: ↓ 1 kg ↓ SBP by 6.6, DBP by 3.3 (DRIP Hypertension 2009;53:500)

Management of Interdialytic Hypertension	
Early	**Late**
↓ Target EDW ↓ Dialysate Na ↑ Antihypertensives	↓ Dialysate Na: 5 mEq/L below serum level (AJKD 2015;65:464) If being used, d/c Na profiling/modeling Add or ↑ nondialyzable RAAS inhibitor (ARB or fosinopril) SNS blockade (α- and β-adrenergic blockade) Carvedilol 50 mg bid: ↓ ET-1 release (CJASN 2012;7:1300)

- Consider addition of RAAS blockade (ACEi/ARB) and/or SNS blockade (carvedilol)

PERICARDIAL DISEASE

Causes
- Inadequate dialysis solute clearance > volume overload

Clinical Manifestations
- Dyspnea, pleuritic chest pain, fever, pericardial rubs
- Tachycardia (in tamponade; can be absent in uremia), cardiac tamponade, death

Workup
- r/o other causes: infection (Tb, fungal, viral—Coxsackie, enteroviruses, adenovirus, echoviruses, CMV), MI, hypothyroidism, malignancy, autoimmune (SLE, MCTD)
- EKG: diffuse ST elevations, PR segment depression, low-voltage QRS complexes
- Echocardiography: pericardial effusion
  - Tamponade physiology respiratory variation in transvalvular velocities

Treatment
- Pericardiocentesis: tamponade, large effusions (usually resistant to intensive dialysis) (J Nephrol 2015;28:97)
- Intensive dialysis: w/o tamponade, daily heparin free HD or PD
  - Failure is a/w admission temp >102°F, rales, admission SBP <100, JVD, PD only because of hemodynamic instability, WBC >15K, large effusion (Am J Med 1984;76:38)

PULMONARY HYPERTENSION

- Cause: chronic volume overload or ↑ venous return to the RV from a high flow AVF or AVF, typically in >2 L/min
- Echocardiogram to evaluate for elevated RV pressures

Treatment
- Attempt to reduce DW; banding of AVF to reduce flow through the access

---

AIR EMBOLISM

Cause
- Air leak within the extracorporeal circuit

Symptoms
- Chest pain, dyspnea/wheezing, tachycardia, hypotension (can progress to overt shock)

Treatment
- Terminate dialysis
- Place patient in the left lateral decubitus position and in Trendelenburg (to trap air in RA/RV)
- Monitor oxygen saturation; supplemental high flow oxygen
- Echocardiogram and/or Chest CT angiogram (if needed) to confirm air embolism
- Vasopressors for shock; mechanical ventilation for respiratory therapy

---

HYPERKALEMIA

Background
- Hyperkalemia is more common in pts on HD (K > 6 –5%) (KI 2003;64:254) than PD
- High pre-HD K a/w mortality (CJASN 2007;2:999; AJKD 2017;69:266)
- Low (<2) K dialysate use is a/w cardiac arrest (KI 2011;79:218; CJASN 2012;7:765)
- HD diffusive clearance is decided by serum-dialysis K gradient: reduced after 2 hr of HD and after using hyperkalemia treatment for intracellular shift
- HD pts have ×2–3 colonic K secretion mediated by AII/aldosterone (Semin Dial 2014;27:571); –35% of daily intake is removed by colonic secretion (CJASN 2018;13:155)
- Each HD session removes 50–100 mEq K according to dialysate K, time, Qb

Causes of Hyperkalemia in HD Patients (Semin Dial 2014;27:571; CJASN 2018;13:155)	
↑ Intake	Dietary indiscretion, transfusion, IV or PO supplementation
↑ Transcellular shift	Metabolic acidosis Cell lysis: hemolysis, rhabdomyolysis, trauma, tumor lysis Prolonged fasting: D/t ↓ insulin secretion High Na dialysate (JASN 2000;11:2337)
Inadequate HD	Recirculation; Missed, shortened, or low dose (Qb, Qd) HD
↓ Renal K excretion	In pts with significant residual renal function: RAAS inhibitors, loss of residual function
↓ Colonic K secretion	Constipation: ↓ wet stool weight, RAAS inhibitors

Prevention
- Prolonged fasting: D10W 50 mL/min + regular insulin 10 U/L if diabetic
- Dietary K restriction: 2–3 g (51–77 mmol) diet; d/c RAAS inhibitors
- Potassium exchange agents: sodium polystyrene sulfate, patiromer (NEJM 2015;372:211), sodium zirconium cyclosilicate (NEJM 2015;372:222)

Treatment
- Prior to HD: dextrose + insulin; NaHCO₃ only is not effective in HD pts; albuterol 10–20 mg neb; Ca gluconate 1 g IV if EKG changes
- HD: low K bath according to pre-HD potassium; long session
- K profiling: from moderate (2 mEq/L) to low K (1 mEq/L) less arrhythmogenic (NDT 2008;23:1415; JASN 2017;28:3441)

HEMOLYSIS

Causes
- Contamination: chlorine/chloramine (inadequate removal by carbon membranes), copper, nitrate, bleach, formaldehyde, peroxide
- Mechanical trauma to RBCs due to a malfunction of the blood pump, kinked tube
- High flow through narrow needle
- Hypotonic dialysis from erroneous electrolytes mixing, overheated dialysate
- All other causes of hemolysis: medication induced, TMA, autoimmune hemolysis

Clinical Manifestation
- Chest pain, dyspnea, back pain, bradycardia due to severe hyperkalemia
- Port wine appearance of blood in venous line, pink plasma in centrifuged specimen
- Acute anemia

Treatment
- If severe, d/c HD; do not return hemolyzed blood to patient; ✓ K, Hb, LDH, retic count

THROMBOCYTOPENIA

Causes
- Heparin induced: rinsing of the circuit (Hemodial Int 2017;21:E30), catheter lock
- Electron beam sterilization of membrane (JAMA 2011;306:1679)

Treatment of Heparin-Induced Thrombocytopenia
- d/c heparin; ✓ heparin-PF4 Ab by ELISA and confirm with serotonin release assay
- Consider nonheparin anticoagulation for ≥3–6 mo if (+) thrombosis
- HD anticoagulation: heparin free HD, argatroban (KI 2004;66:2446)
- Apixaban approved for Afib/ESRD (Circulation 2018;138:1519) can be considered
- Bivalirudin can be removed by HD

HD VASCULAR ACCESS

Background

- Vascular access patency is crucial for patients with ESRD. A significant amount of hospitalizations in ESRD patients is related to vascular access problems. Also, dialysis catheter infections are associated with higher morbidity and mortality.
- In 2016, 80% of patients of ESRD in the US were using a catheter at hemodialysis (HD) initiation. After 90 d, 69% of patients were still using catheters. The percentage of patients with a functional or maturing AV fistula at time of HD initiation was increased from 28.9% in 2005 to 33% in 2015 (USRDS 2018 Annual Data Report)
- The US has higher rate of grafts and dialysis catheters compared to Japan and many European countries within 5 d of first dialysis treatment (KI 2003;63:323)
- Optimal vascular access planning should begin when eGFR <20 mL/min
- Without early planning patients often end up requiring placement of temporary dialysis catheters with increased risk of infections and higher mortality

Types of Access

Types of HD Vascular Access	
Access	**Time to Use**
Arteriovenous fistula (**AVF**): connection between native artery and vein, typically constructed with end-to-side vein to artery anastomosis	Although some AVF may be ready for cannulation at 30 d, a longer time (up to 6 mo) may be needed before they provide reliable HD access (KI 2005;67:2399)
Arteriovenous graft (**AVG**): a connection between an artery and a vein using a prosthetic graft	Can usually be cannulated within 2–3 wk Immediate use AVG (within 24–72 hr of placement) is an option (J Vasc Access 2011;12:248)
Dialysis central venous catheter (**CVC**)	Can be used immediately, but require verification of proper positioning prior to use

Selection of the Appropriate Dialysis Access

- The choice of optimal access for an individual patient depends on multiple factors: timing of referral, personal preference, life expectancy, comorbidities, frailty, patient anatomy, institutional resources, and surgeon experience

Factors that can Influence Vascular Access Selection	
Repeated venipuncture, peripheral IV catheters, CVC, PICC lines (Ann IM 2019;PMID 31158846); previous dialysis access; history of neck/thoracic surgery or CABG	May lead to phlebitis, venous sclerosis, stenosis and thrombosis which may interfere with future AVF placement In CKD 3-5, avoid PICC (JASN 2012;7:1664; CJASN 2016;11:1434) Dorsal veins of the hand are the preferred location for phlebotomy or peripheral access Internal jugular vein is the preferred location for central access (J Vasc Interv Radiol 2000;11:1309)
Cardiac devices (AICD, pacemakers, CRT)	May lead to central vein stenosis Create AVF in contralateral upper limb Avoid central venous catheters If possible, avoid transvenous leads Consider leadless pacemakers, subcutaneous ICDs, or epicardial leads (J Vasc Access 2018;19:521)
Potential for early kidney transplant	Preemptive transplantation is always preferred if feasible Adverse effects of posttransplant outcomes on dialysis therapy are duration dependent No mortality difference between HD or PD prior to transplant (Transplant Proc 2009;41:117)
Estimated life expectancy	For elderly patients with frailty, functional and cognitive impairment or severe comorbidities always discuss palliative care If a trial of dialysis is desired, may benefit from a CVC, AVG or assisted-PD (KI 2019;95:38)

Background
- An AVF is a direct surgical anastomosis between an artery and a vein
- Advantages of AVF: lowest morbidity and mortality, lowest need for intervention, and it has the best long-term patency (AJKD 2006;48:S1; KI 2005;67:2399; CJASN 2010;5:1787). In most patients it should be the initial hemodialysis (HD) access (AJKD 2006;48 Suppl 1: S176).
- Disadvantages of AVF: longer maturation time, potential for vascular steal syndrome, aneurysm formation
- AVF are more likely to experience primary failure (access never usable or failed within 3 mo of use) than AVG
- In order to be usable, several characteristics must be present in an AVF. These include adequate blood flow, adequate maturation, reliable repeated cannulation, and accessibility in sitting position.
- In order to determine the best location to create an AVF, evaluation should start distally in the forearm of the nondominant arm and then move proximally. A radiocephalic AVF (1st choice, Figure 1) should be done if feasible. Alternative vessels may be used if needed (Figures 2 and 3)
- AVG or prosthetic bridge grafts are surgically created artificial conduits that connect an artery to a vein and are superficially tunneled under the skin to allow easy cannulation
- The conduit can be looped (Figure 4) or straight (Figure 5). Forearm looped grafts are preferred (J Vasc Surg 2015;62:1258).
- In older patients or those with poor vascular anatomy an AVG may be preferred. There is no clear AVF patency advantage in pts >65 yo compared to AVG (Semin Dial 2007;20:606). AVF may be more difficult to cannulate than AVG, particularly during initial use.

Timing of AVF Creation and Time to Use
- Evaluation for vascular access includes clinical exam and vascular mapping by Doppler US
- A number of events take place before a successful AVF is created: referral to surgery, surgical evaluation, scheduling for surgery, a period of maturation, and the possibility of a need for salvage procedure to achieve usability which may be followed by another waiting period before the AVF is finally declared suitable for use
- Although a minimum time for AVF maturation may be 1 mo, we generally try to place AVF 6–12 mo prior to anticipated dialysis
- When created at least 4 mo prior to starting HD there may be a lower risk of sepsis and mortality (JASN 2004;15:1936)
- Minimum time for maturation in older pts should be longer (>3 mo) (JASN 2015;26:448)
- Polytetrafluoroethylene (PTFE) AVG can typically be cannulated in 2–3 wk. Polyurethane AVG can be cannulated in as little as 24–48 hr if needed (J Vasc Access 2011;12:248).

Concepts of AVF Maturation
- Once an AVF is created, the blood vessels involved are subjected to marked changes in hemodynamic forces and increases in wall shear stress that trigger vascular remodeling, resulting in an increase in vessel diameter and wall thickness which are needed for a successful cannulation (J Vasc Access 2014;15:291)
- Blood flow through the AVF will increase providing adequate delivery to the dialysis machine. In addition, appropriate AVF depth, length, and location, which contribute to successful cannulation, are critically important.

Evaluation of AVF Maturation
- A thorough evaluation of a new AVF 4–6 wk after creation should be considered mandatory to assess for AVF maturation and to detect problems as soon as possible
- Physical exam by an experienced practitioner has >80% accuracy for predicting AVF maturation (Radiology 2002;225:59)

Rule of 6's: More Likely to Be Useable if AVF Meets Following Criteria at 6 wk After Creation (KDOQI AJKD 2006;48:S176)	
Depth	<0.6 cm below skin surface
External diameter	>0.6 cm
Blood flow	>600 mL/min

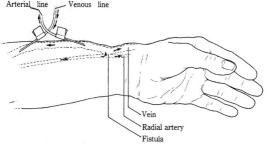

Figure 1. The radiocephalic AVF with the usual position of the access needles. (From Daugirdas JT, ed., *Handbook of Dialysis*, 4th ed. 2007)

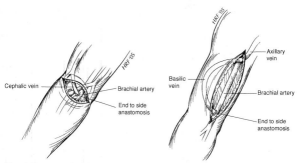

Figure 2. Brachiocephalic AVF. (From Zelenock GB, ed., *Mastery of vascular and endovascular surgery*, 1st ed. 2006)

Figure 3. Brachiobasilic AVF. (From Zelenock GB, ed., *Mastery of vascular and endovascular surgery*, 1st ed. 2006)

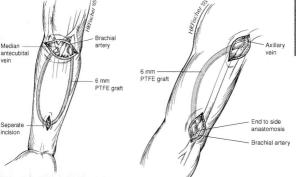

Figure 4. Brachial-antecubital forearm loop AVG. PTFE, polytetrafluoroethylene. (From Zelenock GB, ed., *Mastery of vascular and endovascular surgery*, 1st ed. 2006)

Figure 5. Brachioaxillary straight AVG. (From Zelenock GB, ed., *Mastery of vascular and endovascular surgery*, 1st ed. 2006)

Physical Exam of HD Vascular Access (*J Vasc Access* 2019;20:7)		
History	Difficulty placing needles, low Kt/V, low blood flow	Inflow stenosis
	Prolonged bleeding after removal of needles, high venous pressure during HD, large aneurysms	Outflow stenosis
Inspection	Ipsilateral arm swelling	Subclavian vein stenosis
	Ipsilateral arm and face swelling	Brachiocephalic vein stenosis
	Bilateral arm and face swelling	Superior vena cava stenosis
	Enlarged veins on chest	Central vein stenosis
	Long scar in forearm or arm	Transposed or superficialized AVF
	No collapse of AVF with arm raise	Outflow stenosis
	Aneurysm with pain, enlargement, skin erosion	Impending rupture
	Cold and painful hand, gangrene of fingertips	Steal syndrome
Palpation	Compression of loop AVF	Pulsation felt in arterial portion
	Hyperpulsatile access	Outflow stenosis
	Compression of access with palpation between arterial anastomosis and occluding finger (Augmentation test)	Poor augmentation suggests inflow stenosis
Auscultation	High-pitched predominantly systolic bruit	Stenosis

- If there are abnormalities in the routine exam of the new AVF that has failed to mature, this should be further evaluated as soon as possible, usually using duplex US and/or contrast angiography. Some parameters such as AVF internal diameter and volume flow are typically assessed by U/S (*CJASN* 2016;11:1817)

Surgical Procedures for AVF Maturation
- Superficialization: used often in obese patients and those with deep veins
- Transposition: used mainly in AVF using the basilic vein, since this vein is more medial it requires lateralization
- Translocation: with a vein translocation AVF, a vein is removed from its normal anatomic location to another location and thus requires the creation of a VV anastomosis and a VA anastomosis. The construction of a vein translocation AVF is similar to the placement of an AVG. The only difference is that a native vein is used instead of prosthetic material.

Cannulation Technique
- AVF: rotating site (**rope-ladder**) technique with sharp needle or constant site (**buttonhole**) with blunt needle. Constant site cannulation offers some advantages: less hematomas, less need for interventions. However, it may be associated with higher infection rate and more difficult cannulation compared to rotating site technique (*NDT* 2010;25:225; *CJASN* 2012;7:1632)
- AVG: must use rotating site technique with sharp needle

AVF FAILURE

Primary Failure
- AVF that has never been usable for dialysis or that fails within the first 3 mo of use. It is essentially a failure of maturation (*CJASN* 2006;1:332).
- The primary failure rate for the brachial-basilic transposed AVF has been reported to be the lowest, followed by the brachial-cephalic, and then the radial-cephalic with the highest rate (*CJASN* 2009;4:86)
- Failure in the first mo is often due to technical errors in fistula construction or vessel selection (*JASN* 1992;3:1)

Late Failure
- Mature AVF that fails after at least 3 mo of normal usage. Usually caused by stenosis (venous or arterial), flow stasis (excessive fistula compression after HD or due to sleeping position), hypotension or hypovolemia, hypercoagulability, endothelial injury (*JASN* 1992;3:1)

Evaluation of AVF
- The best validated and most widely recommended method for access surveillance for detecting hemodynamically significant stenosis is monthly access flow (Qb) measurement
- In one study, access with >35% decrease in Qb had a 14-fold increased risk of thrombosis compared to those without change (*KI* 1998;54:1714)

- Several techniques are available for Qb measurement: ultrasound dilution, conductivity dialysance, duplex U/S. Measurement of static and dynamic pressures is less effective for access monitoring.
- The m/c indications for AVF intervention are inadequate blood flow during dialysis, thrombosis, and failure to mature. Specific endovascular interventions include angiography, thrombectomy, angioplasty, and stenting all of which are performed with fluoroscopy in a dedicated facility by adequately trained staff. Surgical interventions are now rarely needed.
- Signs and symptoms suggestive of access dysfunction are edema, decreased delivered dialysis dose, excessive negative pressures, prolonged bleeding time after needle withdrawal

Percutaneous Balloon Angioplasty

- Angioplasty is indicated if the stenosis is >50% and is associated with clinical or physiologic abnormalities (KDOQI AJKD 2006;48:S176)
- In AVF the m/c stenosed site is the "swing point" or "juxta-anastomotic area," the portion of native vein mobilized during creation of the AV anastomosis (Clin Nephrol 2003;60:35)
- Treatment of stenosis increases access blood flow and longevity, reduces access thrombosis and reduces vascular-access related hospitalizations (AJKD 2008;51:93)
- Successful angioplasty is defined as no more than 30% residual stenosis and resolution of physical indicators of stenosis (KDOQI AJKD 2006;48:S176)

Stents

- There is no clear access patency benefit of primary stent use versus angioplasty alone within a stenotic access or central vein (CJASN 2008;3:699)
- Stents should be considered in the setting of failed balloon angioplasty (an elastic lesion), when there are few remaining access sites, if the patient is not a surgical candidate for a new access, or when an outflow vein ruptures after balloon angioplasty (Radiology 1997;204:343)

COMPLICATIONS OF AVF AND AVG

Local Complication

- Easy bruising: hematomas may also result from improper cannulation technique
- Skin rashes: allergic reactions to iodine, Betadine, antibiotic cream are not uncommon
- Prolonged access bleeding should raise suspicion for elevated intra-access pressure and outflow stenosis

Infections

- Bacteremia frequently occurs during cannulation without actual AV access infection
- Dialysis pts with uncomplicated catheter-related bacteremia are treated with systemic antibiotics for 3 wk. Those with metastatic infection (eg, endocarditis or osteomyelitis) should receive 6 wk of antibiotic therapy (AJKD 2009;54:13)

Venous Hypertension

- Usually occurs in pts with central venous stenosis or valvular incompetence
- May present as edema, skin discoloration, dilated collateral veins, or access dysfunction. Although mild extremity swelling is common following access surgery, it usually subsides. If the problem persists beyond 2 wk an underlying problem should be suspected

Aneurysm and Pseudoaneurysm

- True aneurysms: abnormally dilated focal regions of a blood vessel that contain all the layers of the vessel wall
- Pseudoaneurysm: a focal disruption of the vessel with a collection of blood outside the vessel that is contained by fibrous tissue
- Complications: rupture, infection, bleeding, erosion of the underlying skin, difficulty with cannulation

Hand Ischemia (Vascular Steal Syndrome)

- Placement of AVF can reduce perfusion of the more distal extremity as a result of shunting of arterial blood flow into the AVF (J Vasc Access 2011;12:113)
- More common after creation of a high flow upper arm AVF than a more distal AVF (Eur J Vasc Endovasc Surg 2004;27:1)
- It can cause paresthesias, sense of coolness, loss of sensation, weakness. Symptoms often worsen during HD.
- Tx: if symptoms are severe and persistent pts may require MILLER banding, distal revascularization, and AVF ligation

High Output Heart Failure and Pulmonary Hypertension
- In addition to dyspnea on exertion and fluid retention, pts may have a hyperkinetic precordium and wide pulse pressure in the high output state. Access should be hypertrophied, located in the upper arm, with high (>2 L/min) access flow rates.
- The Nicoladoni–Branham sign can be elicited by brief manual compression of the AVF. The response to this diagnostic maneuver is an immediate ↓ in pulse rate and an ↑ in BP, which occur as a result of the sudden restoration of normal blood flow to the systemic circulation coincident with occlusion of the AVF
- Definite diagnosis of high output state requires right heart catheterization. High cardiac output, low-normal systemic vascular resistance and pulmonary HTN are characteristic (Hemodial Int 2011;15;104)
- Evaluation of other etiologies of high output heart failure should be done
- Tx: ↓ AVF inflow by banding techniques or surgical ligation of the access

Coronary Steal
- Symptomatic steal from an internal mammary artery CABG from an Ipsilateral upper extremity AVF can cause myocardial ischemia (AJKD 2002;40:852)

Thrombosis Infections and Seromas
- Occur more frequently with AVG than AVF

USE OF HD CVC

Advantage
- Can be used immediately. Does not require cannulation.
- Option if an AVF or AVG is contraindicated (eg, severe heart failure), or if the expected duration of dialysis is less than 1 yr
- Used temporarily with a failing AVG or AVF until these are repaired

Disadvantage
- ↑ infection, sepsis, and mortality, and the development of central venous stenosis or thrombosis, which comprises further access in the upper limbs (KI 2002;61:305)
- The annual Medicare expenditures for pts with a CVC average approximately $20,000 more than for pts with an AVF (USRDS 2006 Annual Data Report)

Location of Catheter
- The right internal jugular vein is the preferred vein for HD access because the vein takes a straight path directly into the SVC (J Vasc Interv Radiol 2013;24:1295)
- In cases of occlusion of all central veins, alternative sites for catheter insertion are the IVC which can be accessed via a percutaneous translumbar approach (J Vasc Interv Radiol 2013;24:997) or the hepatic vein (Ann Vasc Surg 2013;27:332)

Types of Catheter
- Tunneled dialysis catheter (TDC) or nontunneled dialysis catheter (NTDC)
- TDC: dual lumen, composed of silicone, polyethylene, PU, PTFE and contain a subcutaneous cuff for tissue ingrowth to immobilize the catheter below the skin surface
- NTDC are preferred for pts who require emergent HD
- TDC are associated with lower rates of infectious complications and greater blood flow rates compared with NTDC. Tissue ingrowth into the cuff seals off the catheter tunnel and reduces risk of infection (NDT 2008;23:977)
- Real-time U/S guidance is recommended for venous access during the placement of CVC. Once inserted, positioning of the tip of the catheter often needs to be verified by imaging.

Duration of Catheter
- Due to the increased risk of infection over time, the duration of use of NTDC is limited. Usually <2 wk for IJV catheters and <3 d for femoral catheters.
- If there is a longer anticipated duration of dialysis a cuffed TDC should be used
- The overall survival of TDC is variable when used as a permanent access. One study showed 74% 1-yr and 43% 2-yr catheter survival (NDT 1992;7:1111)

Care and Maintenance of Catheter
- Before and after each use dialysis CVC should be disinfected with chlorhexidine, flushed with saline to evacuate residual blood and locked with antithrombotic prophylaxis to prevent catheter malfunction
- Common solutions to lock TDC are normal saline, heparin, 4% sodium citrate, tPA
- The available data do not support use of routine systemic antithrombotic prophylaxis for HD catheters to prevent catheter dysfunction (J Vasc Access 2016;17:S42)
- Antibiotic coating appears to be effective in preventing intravascular catheter infections in the short term, but no data is available in the long term (Crit Care Med 2009;37:702)

COMPLICATIONS OF HD CVC

Complications of Catheter Placement
- Bleeding, usually due to arterial puncture or venous laceration
- Pneumothorax, air embolism, cardiac dysrhythmias, atrial perforation, pericardial tamponade

Catheter Infection
- Exit site infections: localized cellulitis confined to 1–2 cm where the catheter exits the skin
- Tunnel track infections: involves space surrounding the catheter >2 cm from the exit site
- Risk factors for catheter-related bacteremia: poor personal hygiene, use of occlusive transparent dressing, accumulation of moisture, nasal and skin colonization with Staph aureus and bacterial colonization of HD catheters
- m/c organisms of dialysis catheter-related bacteremias are coagulase negative Staphylococcus, S. aureus, Enterococci and gram-negative rods (AJKD 2004;44:779)
- Patients often present with fever or chills. Patients with severe sepsis can develop hemodynamic instability, altered mental status or acidosis.
- The diagnosis of dialysis catheter-related bacteremia requires one of the following:
  - Concurrent positive blood cultures of the same organism from catheter and peripheral vein
  - Culture of the same organism from both the catheter tip and at least one percutaneous blood culture
  - Cultures of the same organism from two peripherally drawn blood cultures and an absence of an alternate focus of infection
- Broad spectrum antibiotic coverage should consist of vancomycin plus either tobramycin or cefepime. Antibiotic regimen should be modified based on sensitivity.

Catheter Removal in Infection
- NTDC removal: in all bacteremia
- TDC removal: in severe sepsis, hemodynamic instability, metastatic infection (eg, endocarditis or vertebral osteomyelitis), exit-site or tunnel infection, persistent fever or bacteremia >72 hr after initiation of antibiotics, bacteremia caused by S. aureus, Pseudomonas, fungi or mycobacteria, or multidrug resistant organisms (IDSA Guideline Clin Infect Dis 2009;49:1)
  - In this setting, a temporary NTDC is placed for short-term dialysis access until the bacteremia resolves. Then, a new TDC can be inserted.
- If there are absolutely no alternative sites for catheter insertion catheter exchange over a guidewire can be performed (KI 1998;53:1792)
- In pts without indications for immediate removal of TDC the principal options are guidewire catheter exchange or instillation of antibiotic lock solution as adjunctive therapy to systemic antimicrobial treatment (AJKD 2007;50:289)

Central Venous Stenosis
- Stenosis of superior vena cava (SVC) or brachiocephalic/subclavian vein
- Risk factors: subclavian catheter (ASAIO J 2005;51:77), duration and number of prior catheter, pacemaker, younger age at dialysis initiation (CJASN 2019;PMID 30765534)
- Often these are initially asymptomatic, but the stenosis may manifest after the creation of a peripheral AVF in the ipsilateral extremity
- It may present as edema or elevated venous pressures on dialysis (KI 1988;33:1156)
- Severe extremity edema may lead to patient discomfort, skin ulceration, and infection
- SVC syndrome: SVC stenosis or obstruction or bilateral brachiocephalic vein occlusion
  - Presents with edema of both upper extremities, face, neck along with multiple dilated collateral veins over chest and neck
- Prevention: avoid catheterization especially subclavian including PICC (CJASN 2016;11:1434)

Catheter Malfunction
- Adequate catheter function is the ability to sustain a Qb >300 mL/min
- It is often suspected when blood cannot be withdrawn from the catheter or saline cannot be infused into it; also when during dialysis there are high pressures and low flow rates
- The mechanism of the obstruction may be mechanical (kinking or improper positioning of the catheter tip) or thrombotic (catheter-associated thrombus or a fibrin sheath)

Exposed TDC Cuff
- A TDC with an exposed cuff can be easily pulled out
- The exposed cuff also suggests that the catheter tip is no longer at the proper location and delivery of blood through the catheter may be inadequate

PD CONCEPTS

PERITONEAL TRANSPORT

Peritoneal Membrane Anatomy
- The peritoneal membrane is semipermeable
  - Mesothelial cells with microvilli cover the peritoneal cavity
  - Microvilli increase the surface of exchange
  - In females, the fallopian tubes and ovaries are connected to the peritoneal cavity (during menses PD fluid may turn red given the appearance of hemoperitoneum)
- In PD, the peritoneal membrane serves as the dialysis membrane; surface area of 1–2 m^2
- The peritoneal cavity serves as the dialysate compartment
- The lymphatic system drains the peritoneal cavity

The Three Pore Model (KI 2014;85:750)		
Pores	**Size**	**Comments**
Large	100–250 Å	<10% of solute removal
Small	40–50 Å	>90% of solute removal + 60% of water transport
Ultra-small	2.5 Å	Aquaporin-1, transport water only

Large pores < Aquaporins << Small pores in number

- Nearest capillary hypothesis (Perit Dial Int 1996;16:121)
  - Capillaries closer to the mesothelial cells have a greater contribution to transport across the peritoneal membrane
  - Transport is dependent on surface area, distance from mesothelial cell layer and the extent of perfusion of capillaries (increased capillary perfusion in peritonitis)

WATER TRANSPORT

Osmosis
- Osmotic gradient is created by the additives to the PD solution, glucose, or icodextrin
- 40% of water moves through aquaporin-1 channels
- 60% of water moves through paracellular transport between cells, ie, via small pores

Hydrostatic Pressure
- Hydrostatic pressure gradient is the difference between intraperitoneal pressure and peritoneal capillary pressure
- Higher when patient is supine compared to standing

SOLUTE TRANSPORT

Diffusion
- Based on Fick law: transfer rate of a solute is determined by
  - The diffusive permeability of the membrane to a solute
  - The surface area available for transport, ie, the surface area of the peritoneal membrane and capillaries
  - The concentration gradient: solute moves from high to low concentration
- The concentration gradient: highest at the beginning of a dwell → fastest removal
- In PD, creatinine, urea, K^+, H^+, and phosphate are mainly moved by diffusion

Convection
- Occurs with ultrafiltration and is determined by:
  - The mean concentration of the solute, ie, the dialysate fluid concentration. The higher the dialysate concentration → the higher the gradient between the dialysate and blood → faster movement of water across pores.
  - Of note, dextrose from the dialysate fluid is absorbed during dialysis and therefore the concentration gradient is reduced as dwell time is prolonged
  - **Water flux:** depends on the number of small pores and aquaporins which varies among patients
  - The specific solute **reflection coefficient** of the membrane: ranges from 0 to 1. Reflection coefficients closer to 0 indicate faster transport
  - Dwell time ie, short and frequent dwell times are the most effective because longer dwell times allow for equilibration of solutes between blood and dialysate

Barriers to Effective PD
- Effective surface area of peritoneal membrane available, ie, number of capillaries and area in contact with dialysate
- Intrinsic permeability of the peritoneal membrane that allows solutes to be transported ie, number of pores
- Peritoneal fluid is absorbed at a rate of 1–2 mL/min (Physiology of Peritoneal Dialysis. In *Handbook of Dialysis*, 3rd ed. 2001:281)

PD PRESCRIPTION

Peritoneal Dialysis (PD) Solutions

PD Solutions					
Solution (Color)	**Na (mEq/L)**	**Lactate (mEq/L)**	**Bicarbonate**	**Glucose (mg/dL)**	**Osmotic Agent**
1.5% (Yellow)	132	40	0	1,360	Dextrose
2.5% (Green)	132	40	0	2,270	Dextrose
4.25% (Red)	132	40	0	3,860	Dextrose
7.5% (Purple)	132	40	0	0	Icodextrin

Advantages of Icodextrin over Dextrose-based Solutions
- 1/3 of icodextrin is absorbed through lymphatics over 12 hr → can be used for longer dwells because oncotic pressure is maintained for ultrafiltration
- Greater UF in high transporters (*AJKD* 2002;39:862)
- Improved glycemic control (*JASN* 2013;24:1889)

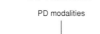

PD MODALITIES

PD modalities

Continuous or Intermittent

Manual or Automated

Continuous Ambulatory Peritoneal Dialysis (CAPD)
- Multiple exchanges during the day followed by a night dwell

Automated Peritoneal Dialysis (APD) Combined with Day Dwell

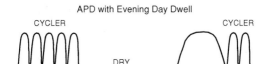

APD with Morning Day Dwell

CYCLER   CYCLER

DRY

10 pm   7 am   12 noon   10 pm

APD with Evening Day Dwell

CYCLER   CYCLER

DRY

10 pm   7 am   5 pm   10 pm

(From Daugirdas JT, ed., *Handbook of Dialysis*, 5th ed. 2015)

Continuous Cyclic Peritoneal Dialysis (CCPD)
• A cycler performs multiple night dwells followed by a day dwell

APD with Long Day Dwell (CCPD)

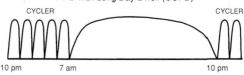

(From Daugirdas JT, ed., Handbook of Dialysis, 5th ed. 2015)

Nocturnal Intermittent Peritoneal Dialysis (NIPD)
• A cycler performs multiple night dwells; No day dwell is used

"Day Dry" APD (NIPD)

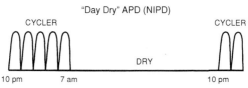

(From Daugirdas JT, ed., Handbook of Dialysis, 5th ed. 2015)

PD PRESCRIPTION

Patients Choose the Modality that Fits Their Lifestyle
• CAPD needs less training than APD
• APD offers more flexibility for maintaining a good lifestyle

Calculate the Required Total Dialysate Volume
• Daily Kt/V$_{urea}$
  - Kt = 24-hr dialysate volume × D$_{urea}$/P$_{urea}$
  - D: the urea concentration in 24 hr effluent dialysate collection
  - P: the serum concentration of urea
  - V$_{urea}$: the volume of distribution of urea ≈ total body water = ideal body weight × 0.6 in male; × 0.5 in young female
• The target is weekly Kt/V$_{urea}$ ≥1.7 = daily Kt/V$_{urea}$ ≥0.24 in anuric patient
• The initial prescription usually assumes that the patient has average membrane transport and that the plasma and dialysate urea are in full equilibrium; D$_{urea}$ ≈ P$_{urea}$
  - Daily Kt = 24-hr dialysate volume
• eg, in a man with ideal body weight 70 kg V$_{urea}$ is 42 L
• Required Kt is 0.24 × 42 L = 10 L of urea clearance per day. 10 L is the amount of dialysate that should be drained per day to achieve the goal weekly Kt/V 1.7.
• In a patient who has residual kidney function, residual renal Kt/V should be calculated. This is then subtracted from 1.7. The resultant number will be the target Kt/V used to calculate the dialysate amount.

Determine the Fill Volume per Exchanges and the Number of Exchanges
• The initial fill volume is usually 30–35 mL of dialysate per kg per exchange, or 1,500 mL/m^2 of BSA per exchange, or 2.5 L/1.73 m^2 of BSA per exchange
• The initial fill volumes should not increase intraperitoneal pressure >18 cm H$_2$O
• In patients with residual renal function, it is possible to avoid a daytime dwell

Determine Ultrafiltration Needs
• The initial dialysate composition depends on the volume status of the patient and their residual kidney function
• Euvolemic patients with residual kidney function can start with 1.5% dialysate
• In hypervolemic patients, 2.5% dialysate can be initially used
• UF can be increased by using dialysate with higher dextrose concentration, by decreasing dwell time, increasing dwell volume, and increasing the number of exchanges

Adjust Prescription Based on:
- The total UF (dialysate and urine), changes in body weight, volume status
- Uremic symptoms and dialysis adequacy
- 4 wk following prescription, ✓ peritoneal transport rate

PERITONEAL TRANSPORT RATE MONITORING

Peritoneal Membrane Variability
- Variability in peritoneal membrane transport between different individuals
- Changes in efficiency of peritoneal membrane over time
- Therefore, PD prescriptions should be individualized

Tests to Evaluate PD Transport Rate
- Multiple tests have been advocated:
  - Peritoneal equilibration test (PET)
  - Standard permeability analysis (SPA)
  - Peritoneal dialysis capacity (PDC) measurement
  - Dialysis adequacy and transport test (DATT)

Peritoneal Equilibration Test (PET)
- PET is the most commonly used test
- The PET is a 4-hr standardized test with several steps
- It should be done no earlier than 1 mo after initiating PD. PET can also be performed after bouts of peritonitis as well as with UF failure.
- A dwell of 2 L (200 mL/min for 10 min) of 2.5% dextrose dialysate is used
- Drain 200 cc at 0, 0.5, 1, 2, and 4 hr. 10 cc is sampled and the rest is reinfused
- The dwell is drained at 4 hr, and total volume of dialysate is calculated. Ultrafiltrate is then inferred.

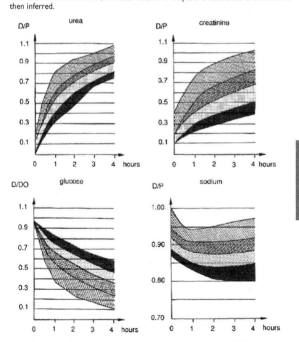

Peritoneal membrane transport types are based on 4-hr equilibration ratios for urea, creatinine, glucose, and sodium. (From Daugirdas JT, ed., Handbook of Dialysis, 5th ed. 2015)

- 4 hr after the dwell, sodium, potassium, urea, creatinine, glucose, and total protein are measured in both the serum and the dialysate
- High transporters remove waste products fast but are not effective at UF
  - Tx: short dwells and frequent exchanges, ie, CCPD
- Low transporters remove waste products slowly but are effective at UF
  - Tx: longer dwells and less frequent exchanges, ie, CAPD

Peritoneal Membrane Failure

- The peritoneal membrane properties change over time. This is related to the exposure to dialysate and to inflammation in the membrane. Peritonitis increases the risk of membrane failure.
- Peritoneal membrane failure is defined as a UF <400 mL after a dwell time of 4 hr using 4.25% dextrose solution in the absence of any catheter malfunction or fluid leaks
- Type I membrane failure is characterized by high solute transport
  - Tx: shortening dwell time and doing more frequent exchanges
- Type II membrane failure is characterized by decrease solute transport and water transport
  - Tx: d/c of PD and switching to HD
- Type III membrane failure is due to lymphatic absorption
  - Tx: shorter dwell time and using 4.25% dextrose or icodextrin solution

PD ADEQUACY

Adequate Dialysis

- Effective dose that maintains fluid balance and prevents metabolic complications

Measurement of Adequate Dialysis

Urea Clearance (K) in PD Patients	
Peritoneal Daily Kt	**24-hr dialysate volume × D_{urea}/P_{urea}** D_{urea}: dialysate urea concentration, P_{urea}: plasma urea concentration
Renal Daily Kt	**24-hr urine volume × U_{urea}/P_{urea}** U_{urea}: urine urea concentration, P_{urea}: plasma concentration of urea ✓ residual renal function at least once every 4 mo using 24-hr urine collections if urine volume is >100 mL/d (AJKD 2006;48 Suppl 1:S98)
Weekly Kt/V	(Peritoneal daily Kt/V + Renal daily Kt/V) × 7 × (1.73/BSA) V: urea volume of distribution; BSA: body surface area (m²) Should be measured in the 1st mo and at least once every 4 mo Goal is ≥1.7 (Ademex JASN 2002;13:1307; KI 2003;64:649)

Factors Affecting PD Adequacy

- Residual Renal Function (RRF)
  - PD prescription should be adjusted as residual renal function decreases over time
  - Higher RRF is associated with decreased odds ratio for death (AJKD 1999;33:523; CANUSA JASN 2001;12:2158)
  - ACEi (Ann IM 2003;139:105) and ARB (AJKD 2004;43:1056) may help to preserve RRF
- Higher solution osmolality increases UF and can increase solute clearance by convection
- Higher fill volume can increase solute clearance
- Higher frequency of exchanges can ↑ the concentration gradient between dialysate and blood which leads to better solute clearance
- Peritoneal transport type (described below)
- Patient position: the supine position ↑ the peritoneal surface area available for exchange
- Catheter malfunction

Fill and Exchange Volume

- Can be estimated using the following formula: $V_{max} = V + \{(18-IAP)/2\} × 1,000$ mL
  - V_{max}: the maximum dwell volume tolerated by the patient
  - IAP: the intraperitoneal hydrostatic pressure which should be <18 cmH₂O in the supine position. IAP is lowest in the supine position, highest in the sitting position and intermediate in the standing position.
  - V: the intraperitoneal volume
- Daily dwell volume = [kt/v × V]/t × D/P_{urea} (V = volume distribution of urea, t = time in d)

Peritoneal Transport Type

- Fast Transporter: require short dwells, ie, PD regimens that include frequent exchanges
- Slow Transporter: require long dwells and high fill volumes, ie, CAPD or APD

PD COMPLICATION

PERITONITIS

Background and Pathogenesis

- Presentation: abdominal pain, cloudy effluent fluid
- Bacterial peritonitis: effluent WBC >100 cell/μL with >50% neutrophils
  - Majority Gram-positive organisms: *S. epidermidis* > *S. aureus* > *Enterococcus*
- Fungal or mycobacterial peritonitis: lymphocytic predominance of the effluent WBC
  - *Candida albicans* is the most common organism in fungal peritonitis
  - Recent antibiotic use is a risk factor
- Mycobacterial peritonitis: lymphocytic predominance of the effluent WBC
  - PCR is more sensitive and can yield faster results than acid-fast smears
- Eosinophilic peritonitis: >10% eosinophils in effluent fluid
  - Related to allergic reaction, drug exposure, fungal and viral infections
- Icodextrin-associated sterile peritonitis: (−) peritoneal cultures
  - Can occur any time after exposure to icodextrin
  - Cloudy effluent with macrophage and eosinophil predominance

Workup

- PD fluid total cell count and differential, Gram stain and cultures
- If the suspicion for peritonitis is high and cell counts are low, resend cell count and culture after a dwell time of at least 2 hr
- Swab of the catheter exit site if there is purulence

Treatment

	Stepwise Treatments of Bacterial Peritonitis
1	Empiric antibiotics while awaiting cultures: • Vancomycin (15–30 mg/kg every 7 d) or 1st-generation cephalosporin (ie, cefazolin 15–20 mg/kg daily) for gram-positive organisms • Aminoglycoside (ie, gentamicin 0.6 mg/kg daily) or 3rd-generation cephalosporin (ie, cefotaxime 500–1,000 mg/d) for gram-negative organisms
2	Followup daily effluent counts
3	If clinical manifestations of peritonitis persist beyond 48–72 hr or if effluent cell counts remain positive for >5 d → treatment failure and need for catheter removal
4	Antibiotics are narrowed when culture sensitivities are back

- Antibiotic course: usually 2 wk; *Staph aureus* and *Pseudomonas* are treated for 3 wk
- IP administration of antibiotics is superior to IV administration in treating peritonitis. No specific antibiotic appears to have superior efficacy for preventing treatment failure or relapse of peritonitis (*Cochrane Database Syst Rev 2014;CD005284*).
- Oral antifungal prophylaxis (fluconazole or nystatin) with each antibiotic course may reduce the risk of fungal peritonitis (*Cochrane Database Syst Rev 2017:CD004679*)
- Relapsing peritonitis: 2 peritonitis episodes caused by the same organism or 2 sterile peritonitis episodes within 4 wk of each other
- Refractory peritonitis: peritonitis that persists for >5 d
- Indications of PD catheter removal: relapsing or persistent peritonitis (*Cochrane Database Syst Rev 2014;CD005284*), pseudomonal peritonitis, and fungal peritonitis (high risk of death)
- Mycobacterial peritonitis: 6–9 mo of isoniazid, pyrazinamide, ofloxacin, and IP rifampin followed by a maintenance antimycobacterial regimen

EXIT-SITE AND TUNNEL INFECTION (ISPD Guidelines *Perit Dial Int* 2017;37:141)

- Exit-site infections: purulent discharge at the catheter–epidermal interface
- Tunnel Infection: the presence of inflammation (erythema, edema, tenderness, or induration) or collections along the tunnel
- Exit-site infections or tunnel infections can occur at the same time
- Investigation includes sending any drainage from the site for gram stain and culture
- Catheter care should be continued during treatment of an exit-site infection. Please refer to catheter care in the "PD Catheter" chapter
- Empiric antibiotic therapy of exit-site and tunnel infections includes oral antibiotics that cover *S. aureus*. Patients who have a history of MRSA or *P. aeruginosa* should receive oral antibiotics that cover those organisms.

- Consider nystatin for prophylaxis against fungal peritonitis
- If the cultures grow *P. aeruginosa*, then patients should be given two antibiotics for coverage, one of which being an oral fluoroquinolone. Of note, quinolones should not be given at the same time as phosphorus binders.
- Duration of therapy for exit-site and tunnel infections is typically 2 wk, except in cases of *P. aeruginosa* where the duration of therapy is 3 wk
- Exit sites should be observed closely to evaluate response to therapy
- ✓ U/S of the tunnel to document clearance of any fluid collections
- Remove the catheter if fail to respond to antibiotics after 3 wk of therapy and in patients whose exit-site or tunnel infection progresses to peritonitis
- A new catheter can be replaced immediately after removal of an infected catheter in patients with exit-site and tunnel infections only. In those with concomitant peritonitis, a new catheter should be placed no sooner than 2 wk after catheter removal.

MECHANICAL COMPLICATIONS

Hernias
- Can develop secondary to increased intra-abdominal pressure

Encapsulating Peritoneal Sclerosis
- Sclerosis of the peritoneal membrane → bowel encapsulation and intestinal obstruction
- The causes are not well understood but longer duration on PD is a risk factor. Many patients present after stopping PD.
- Clinical manifestations: partial or complete bowel obstruction, hemoperitoneum, abdominal masses, abdominal pain, poor ultrafiltration among others
- CT is the imaging modality of choice; peritoneal thickening and calcifications, bowel thickening, tethering, dilatation, obstruction, and loculated ascites
- Tx: discontinuation of PD, supportive care in case of bowel obstruction, nutritional support. Enterolysis can be considered for recurrent or severe symptoms.

PD Catheter-related Mechanical Complications	
Impaired dialysate flow	Can be seen during inflow or drainage Can be related to constipation → laxative regimen Can be related to catheter tip migration → Abdominal X-rays can detect migration Entrapment of the catheter by the omentum Fibrin → add heparin to the dialysate
Pain	From abdominal irritation of the catheter tip From the dialysate flow against the bowel
Leakage of dialysate	Can be related to high dialysate volume → ↓ dialysate volume Can be related to weak abdominal muscles → supine exchanges
Hydrothorax	PD catheter migrates into the pleural space → a communication between the pleural space and the abdomen Presents with respiratory distress and lung collapse. High glucose in the pleural effusion is a clue to the diagnosis Tx: temporary discontinuation of PD or diaphragm patching

Hemoperitoneum
- PD catheters may erode into mesenteric vessels or internal organs
- Other causes of hemoperitoneum include: menstruation, ovarian cyst rupture, renal cyst rupture, carcinoma in the abdomen, abdominal organ infections, splenic rupture, and sclerosing peritonitis
- ✓ effluent counts, culture, amylase and CBC. Hct >2% is suggestive of intraperitoneal bleeding and requires further workup of intra-abdominal bleeding.
- Oral contraceptives can stop bleeding related to menstruation
- Tx: rapid exchanges (2–3 hr) with 500 units of heparin per liter of dialysate. This prevents clot formation that can result in catheter malfunction

Metabolic Derangements With PD and Causes	
Hyperglycemia	Absorption of glucose from the PD solutions
Hyperlipidemia	Not completely understood, possibly due to hypoalbuminemia and hyperglycemia
Hyponatremia	Fluid overload and low dialysate sodium
Hypokalemia	Low dialysate potassium concentration/continuous dialysis/use of diuretics
Hypercalcemia	High dialysate calcium concentration
Hypermagnesemia	High dialysate magnesium concentration
Hypoalbuminemia	1–2 g losses/L of drained dialysate

PD CATHETER

Relative Contraindications to PD Catheter Placement
• Previous abdominal surgeries; abdominal wall hernias

Types of Catheters
• Tenckhoff (most widely used), Missouri swan neck, Toronto western catheter

PD Catheter Segments	
Intraperitoneal	The section inside the peritoneal cavity with side holes to drain the dialysate No difference in function between straight intraperitoneal segments compared to coiled
Double Cuff	Superficial cuff is in the subcutaneous portion of the abdominal wall Deep cuff is in the rectus abdominis muscle
Extraperitoneal	The section within the abdominal wall and outside the body

Preplacement Recommendations
• Laxatives to avoid postoperative constipation
• Antibiotics prior to PD catheter insertion: cephalosporins (ISPD *Perit Dial Int* 2017;37:141)
• Pre/perioperative intravenous vancomycin may reduce the risk of early peritonitis in the first few wk (<1 mo) following PD catheter insertion but has an uncertain effect on the risk of exit-site/tunnel infection (*Cochrane Database Syst Rev* 2017;CD004679)

Periplacement Care (but before use)
• PD catheters are flushed with dialysate followed by immediate drainage to maintain patency
• Heparin is flushed to avoid clots
• Catheter is covered. Trauma and change of dressing should be avoided for at least 1 wk
• PD is started at least 10–14 d after catheter insertion
• Showers should be avoided until the exit site is healed
• Urgent start PD is started 24–72 hr after PD catheter insertion. This is done in patients who need dialysis urgently but want to avoid hemodialysis.
• Early start PD is started 72–14 d after PD catheter insertion
• Both urgent start and early start PD should be done by trained staff, using low volume exchanges in the supine position

PD Catheter Maintenance
• Wash PD exit site daily with antiseptic, either chlorhexidine or povidone iodine
• Topical antimicrobial agent should be applied daily: Mupirocin, Gentamicin
• Non-occlusive dressing should be used to cover the site
• Catheter should be immobilized with tape to prevent injury to the site
• If patients report trauma to their catheter site → 3 d of cephalosporins
• Patients should avoid baths and swimming
• Pets should not be in the room when exchanges are being done, windows and doors should be closed
• Mechanical and infectious PD catheter malfunction causes 50–70% of patients to switch to hemodialysis.

Background
- Kidney Txp ↓ death and ↑ survival compared to remaining on dialysis *(NEJM 1999;341:1725)*
- Pre-emptive txp: the optimal treatment for ESRD. Waiting time on dialysis is one of the strongest independent modifiable risk factor for txp outcomes *(Transplantation 2002;74:1377)*

Transplantation Evaluation Referral
- Early referral is important to avoid the development of comorbidities associated with dialysis and to increase chance for pre-emptive transplantation *(Transplantation 2002;74:1377)*
- Refer all medically appropriate pts w/ CKD stage 4,5 (eGFR <30) *(AJKD 2007;50:890)*
- Patients can begin to accrue wait time on the waitlist once eGFR or CrCl ≤20 or when they are receiving chronic dialysis therapy (http://optn.transplant.hrsa.gov)

Goal of Evaluation
- To assess patient's medical, surgical, social, and psychological suitability for transplant
- To educate the patient about the risk vs benefit of transplant
- To discuss donor options: living vs deceased donor, Kidney Donor Profile Index (KDPI) >85%, Public Health Service Increased Risk (PHS IR)
- <u>KDPI</u> combines a variety of donor factors (age, height, weight, ethnicity, HTN, DM, cause of death, Cr, HCV status, donation after circulatory death status) into a single number that summarizes the likelihood of graft failure after DDKT (eg, a kidney with a KDPI of 85% is expected to have shorter longevity than 85% of recovered kidneys)
- <u>PHS IR</u> identifies donors at increased risk of transmitting HBV, HCV, and HIV

Contraindications of Transplantation *(AJKD 2007;50:890)*
- Chronic illness that shortens life expectancy significantly; Poor functional status
- Reversible renal failure. Chronic or active infection (needs treatment prior transplant).
- Active malignancy: needs treatment prior transplant and must be in remission
- Uncontrolled psychosis; active substance abuse; ongoing noncompliance

Cardiac Disease
- Cardiovascular disease is the leading cause of death after kidney transplantation
- Se, Sp of noninvasive cardiac tests in CKD/ESRD pts are very low *(Hypertension 2003;42:263)*
- Immunosuppressive agents can worsen HTN, hyperglycemia, and dyslipidemia, and thereby accelerate CAD (calcineurin inhibitors, sirolimus, steroid)
- Asymptomatic for CAD: ≥3 risk factors (age >60, DM, HTN, dyslipidemia, obesity, h/o angina pectoris, LVH, previous cardiac events, smoking history, (+) family history, HD duration ≥2 yr), or ≥1 CAD risk equivalent (DM, atherosclerosis in other vascular beds, history of stroke) → noninvasive cardiac stress test *(Semin Dial 2010;23:595)*
- Symptomatic for CAD, type 1 DM complicated with ESRD, cardiomyopathy with reduced EF, (+) noninvasive cardiac stress test → coronary angiogram
- (+) Coronary angiogram → If amenable, revascularization before txp *(AJKD 2007;50:890)*
- Pretransplant LVH and elevated LA volume are associated with reduced survival after kidney transplantation *(Transplant Res 2014;3:20)* → Echocardiogram should be obtained in those with suspected valvular disease or CHF → Patients with severe irreversible cardiac dysfunction should not be listed for kidney transplantation alone (may be candidates for combined heart-kidney transplantation) *(CMAJ 2005;173:S1)*

Infectious Disease
- ✓ HIV, HBV, HCV, tuberculosis, CMV (risk stratification), EBV, toxoplasmosis
- ✓ If from endemic areas for: coccidomycosis, histoplasmosis, strongyloidiasis

HIV
- Not an absolute contraindication. Needs HIV-specialist consultation.
- Should be on stable antiretroviral regimen, should have no detectable viral load, and should have CD4 count >200 cells/mm^3
- Protease inhibitor can increase serum concentration of calcineurin inhibitors
- Short-term outcomes comparable to general kidney txp patients. Higher acute rejection rate. No increase in HIV-associated complications *(NEJM 2010;363:2004)*.
- For HIV-infected ESRD patients, kidney transplantation is associated with a significant survival benefit compared with remaining on dialysis. Adjusted RR of mortality at 5 yr is 79% lower after kidney transplantation compared with dialysis *(Ann Surg 2017;265:604)*.

Liver Cirrhosis
- HBV-, HCV-positive patients should undergo liver biopsy and hepatic venous pressure gradient measurement (>10 mmHg: clinically significant portal HTN)
- Pts w/ cirrhosis and portal hypertension needs evaluation for combined liver–kidney txp *(AJKD 2007;50:890)*. A contraindication for KT alone due to increased mortality

HCV (Nat Rev Nephrol 2015;11:172): needs hepatology referral
- HCV-infected patients have a lower mortality following KT c/w mortality on dialysis
- HCV-infected renal transplant recipients have worse patient and allograft survival after transplantation compared with noninfected recipients
- An HCV-positive organ may reduce waiting time substantially → Consider postponing antiviral treatment until after transplantation to maintain eligibility for an HCV-positive organ as long as disease severity does not warrant earlier treatment

HBV (World J Hepatol 2017;9:1054): needs hepatology referral
- Immunosuppression ↑ HBV reactivation → HBsAg-positive-recipients are at high risk
- Both, patients with chronic HBV (HBsAg-positive) as well as resolved HBV (HBsAg-negative, anti-HBc-positive) should be initiated on antiviral therapy around the time of transplantation (Gastroenterology 2015;148:215)
- The use of antiviral therapy to prevent reactivation has improved long-term patient and graft outcomes → Similar 5-yr patient and graft survival when compared to HBV-negative recipients (CJASN 2011;6:1481)

Malignancy
- Immunocompromised patients are at increased risk for recurrent and de novo malignancy
- All patients need age-appropriate screening. If malignancy is diagnosed, the cancer should be treated and cured before transplantation.

Minimum Tumor-Free Waiting Period (CMAJ 2005;173:S1; AJKD 2007;50:890)			
Cancer	**Minimal Wait Time**	**Cancer**	**Minimal Wait Time**
Bladder	In situ: none Invasive: 2 yr	Breast	Early in situ: 2 yr Other: 5 yr
Cervix	In situ: <2 yr Invasive: 2–5 yr	Prostate	At least 2 yr
Colorectal	Duke's A or B1: 2–5 yr Other: 5 yr	Renal	Small, incidental tumors: none Other: 2–5 yr
Lymphoma	2–5 yr	Basal cell	None
Lung	At least 2 yr	Melanoma	5 yr

Hematologic Disease (AJKD 2007;50:890)
- ~15–20% of ESRD pts have hypercoagulable state (eg, activated protein C resistance, factor V Leiden gene mutation, prothrombin gene mutation, and APLA)
- History of thrombosis (DVT, PE, recurrent dialysis access clotting), and/or recurrent spontaneous abortion/preeclampsia → ✓ hypercoagulability workup
- Plan pre-, peri-, and postoperative anticoagulation: hematology referral for bleeding risk

Glomerular Disease
- Transplant should be delayed until disease is quiescent. Not absolute contraindication.

Risk of Primary Kidney Disease Recurrence (CJASN 2008;3:800)			
Disease	**Rate**	**Disease**	**Rate**
Primary FSGS	20–30%	MPGN	Type 1: 20–30% Type 2 (DDD): 50–100%
MN	10–30%	ANCA GN	17%
IgAN	20–60%	Anti-GBM disease	15%
SLE	2–10%	HUS/TTP	Noninfectious: 60%

Neurologic Disease
- History of convulsion: avoid anticonvulsants which can interfere with CNI metabolism (carbamazepine, fosphenytoin, phenobarbital, and phenytoin may decrease serum concentrations of calcineurin inhibitors) → neurology referral
- History of CVA: needs neurology evaluation. Modifiable risk factors should be addressed.

Pulmonary Disease
- Smoking cessation. CXR & PPD/IGRA (Quanitferon-TB Gold®) → isoniazid if indicated
- History of extensive smoking and/or any signs of obstructive or restrictive lung disease → PFT/CT chest → pulmonary referral

Psychiatry
- Mild cognitive impairment is not an absolute contraindication, esp w/ good social support
- Stable and controlled mental illness is not a contraindication
- Compliance should be documented prior transplantation
- Substance abuse should be eliminated prior transplantation
- Needs psychosocial evaluation in conjunction with a transplant social worker to assess support network, determine suitability, and develop a plan to avoid adverse post-transplantation psychosocial outcomes

LIVING DONOR EVALUATION

- Living donation: 25% of transplants performed in the US in 2016. The rate remains stable, compared to rising deceased donation since 2011 (AJT 2018;18 Suppl 1:18)
- Racial disparities in donation—donors: 12.3% black (36.4% waitlist pts) vs 65.1% white (33.2% waitlist pts) (AJT 2018;18 Suppl 1:18)
- Commercial donation, a common practice in some countries, comprises 10% of transplants. It had fallen after the Declaration of Istanbul on Organ Trafficking and Transplant Tourism (Lancet 2008;372:5; KI 2019;95:757).
- Superior outcomes compared to deceased donor transplant: 10-yr graft failure 34.2% vs 51.6% and 10-yr death-censored graft failure 18% vs 26.2% (AJT 2018;18 Suppl 1:18)

MEDICAL EVALUATION

- Informed consent mandated by UNOS: evaluation process; surgical procedure; alternative treatment for recipient; medical and psychological risk; financial and insurance factors; voluntarism and the right to opt out of donation at any time
- ✓ The operative cardiac, pulmonary, bleeding risks and anesthesia-related complications
- H&P: includes focus on kidney disease history and risk factors: AKI/ CKD, DM, HTN, gestational DM/gestational HTN, hematuria, proteinuria, kidney stones, UTI, congenital genitourinary anomalies, medications review including NSAIDs, PPI, herbal supplements, genetic or familial kidney disease, family history of HTN/DM
- Social history including adequate support, psychiatric disease history and behaviors meeting Public Health Service (PHS) high-risk criteria
- Compatibility testing: ABO typing (×2) including group A subtype; HLA typing for MHC Class I (A, B, C), Class II (DP, DQ, DR). Donor specific Anti-HLA antibodies in recipients.
- ID screening: HIV, HCV, HBV, CMV, EBV, Syphilis, TB testing w/in 28 d of surgery
- Age-appropriate cancer screening

Evaluation of Renal Function and Albuminuria and Selection Recommendation (KDIGO Transplantation 2017;101 8S Suppl 1:S1)

	GFR	Albuminuria
Screening	CKD-EPI eGFR by creatinine	Random UACR
Confirmation	(1) mGFR using an exogenous filtration marker* (2) mCrCl using 24-hr urine* (3) CKD-EPI eGFRcreat-cys (4) CKD-EPI eGFRcr	24-hr urine albumin, repeat random UACR if collection cannot be done
Donation	≥90	<30 mg/d
Individualization	60–89	30–100 mg/d
No donation	<60	>100 mg/d (KDIGO) >300 mg/d (ERBP, CARI)
Comments	Most centers exclude eGFR <80	ERBP NDT 2013;28:ii1 CARI Nephrology 2010;15:S106

*UNOS requires mGFR or mCrCl

- Hematuria (KDIGO Transplantation 2017;101 8S Suppl 1:S1)
  Persistent ×2–3 of 2–5 RBC/hpf. r/o infection (UA), malignancy (cystoscopy), nephrolithiasis (stone panel), glomerular disease: TBMN, IgAN (kidney biopsy).
  TBMN does not preclude donation (in absence of proteinuria and with normal BP)
- HTN (Transplantation 2017;101 8S Suppl 1:S1)
  ✓ Office BP ×2. If indeterminate, confirm w/ ABPM. Not an absolute contraindication if controlled on 1–2 antihypertensives w/o end-organ damage (LVH, albuminuria)
- Imaging: MRI or CTA. In case of functional and anatomical disparities, the kidney with smaller size and/or lower function kidney is to be procured
- Additional considerations: dependent on each transplant center preference and based on the individual's lifetime ESRD risk.
  - Obesity: BMI >40: absolute contraindication. In the general population, BMI >30 a/w CKD (JASN 2006;17:1695; JAMA 2004;291:844; AJKD 2005;46:587), 3.57 fold ↑ in ESRD (Ann IM 2006;144:21) and 1.16 (NEJM 2016;374:411) in otherwise healthy potential donors, albuminuria, and glomerulopathy
  - Smoking: relative contraindication at most centers despite association with renal injury. Advised to quit before donation (Transplantation 2017;101 8S Suppl 1:S1)
  - DM is an absolute contraindication. Screening with 2-hr GTT or A1C.

- Role of APOL1 testing is unclear. Testing is advisable among young donors of African ancestry with ESRD family history although precise risk is not quantified. APOL1 high-risk genotype donors have lower eGFR pre and post donation compared to low-risk black donors w/ 0–1 high-risk variant (57 vs 61.7, 12 yr) *(JASN 2018;29:1309)*.
- Surgical Technique: hand-assisted laparoscopic donor nephrectomy (LDN) widely used compared to open nephrectomy (ON). LDN is 51 min longer but has less blood loss, shorter hospital stay, and time to return to work compared to ON *(Transplant Proc 2013;45:65)*

OUTCOMES

Short-term Outcomes
- 90-d mortality is 0.03% *(JAMA 2010;303:959)*
- Perioperative complications encountered in 6.8% of donors: 4.4% GI, 3% bleeding, 2.5% respiratory, 2.4% surgical/anesthesia-related injuries, 6.6% other *(AJT 2016;16:1848)*. Similar rates compared to patients undergoing cholecystectomies or appendectomies but lower than nephrectomies for cancer *(CJASN 2013;8:1773)*.

Long-term Outcomes
- Physiologic changes post donation:
  - 50% immediate reduction in GFR with subsequent compensatory hyperfiltration by increased RBF and thus SNGFR ultimately leading to 30% GFR decrease
  - Physiologic adaptation: at 36 mo post donation, 1.47 mL/min/yr increase in GFR in donors vs 0.36 mL/min/yr decrease in healthy controls *(AJKD 2015;66:114)*. And 0.20 mL/min/1.73 m^2/yr at 12.2 ± 9.2 yr *(NEJM 2009;360:459)*.
- No accelerated loss of kidney function *(Transplantation 2001;72:444)*
- At 12.2 ± 9.2 yr after donation, among 255 donors: 85.5% GFR ≥60 *(NEJM 2009;360:459)*
- Proteinuria: same estimate across studies: 12% (N = 4,793, 7 yr) *(KI 2006;70:1801)*; 12.7% (1.2% >300 mg/d, N = 255, 12.2 ± 9.2 yr) *(NEJM 2009;360:459)*; 13% (3% with >1 g/d, N = 331, 18 mo–16 yr) *(AJKD 2015;66:114)*. It correlates to longer time since donation *(NEJM 2009;360:459)* and HTN *(AJKD 2015;66:114)*.
- HTN: developed in 32.1% *(NEJM 2009;360:459–469)* to 38% *(Transplantation 2001;72:444)* of normotensive donors. Risk similar to age matched nondonors in men but lower in women *(Transplantation 2001;72:444)*. 85% of white HTN donors had BP <140/90 at 6 and 12 mo after donation but readings are higher than normotensive donors. Cr, UACR were similar *(Transplantation 2004;78:276)*.
- CV events: no difference in death/CVD events between donors and nondonors at 6.2 yr after donation *(Transplantation 2008;86:399)*. In Norway, the risk increases among donors by ×1.4 at 15.1 yr *(KI 2014;86:162)*.
- Older donors: in the US, 5,717 donors with age >55 from 1996–2006. Compared to age-matched donors (mean age 59) with median followup 7.8 yr, no difference in mortality or combined outcome death/CVD *(AJT 2014;14:1853)*.
- Pregnancy: gestational HTN/pre-eclampsia are more common among living kidney donors (11%) than among nondonors (5%, OR 2.4); Preterm birth (8% vs 7%) and low birth weight rates (6% vs 4%) are similar *(NEJM 2015;372:124)*
- Quality of life: donors physical-health summary score and mental-health summary score are above the US population norms *(NEJM 2009;360:459)*. In Canada, Scotland, and Australia both scores are comparable *(AJT 2011;11:463)*.
- ESRD rate
  - 1.8/10,000/yr vs 2.68/10,000/yr in the general population (f/u 22.5 yr) in white dominant donors *(NEJM 2009;360:459)*
  - In another study, ESRD rates in donors 30.8/10,000 vs 3.9/10,000 in matched nondonors. Although higher than in the general population, the risk remains low *(JAMA 2014;311:579)*
  - The 15-yr risk in donors is ×3.5–5.3 higher than the estimated projected risk of nondonors. Long-term ESRD risk varies by age at donation and race *(NEJM 2016;374:411)*.
- Obesity: BMI >30 86% ↑ risk of ESRD compared to nonobese donors *(KI 2017;91:699)*
- Life expectancy similar to nondonors *(Transplantation 1997;64:976; NEJM 2009;360:459)*

Other Considerations
- Kidney paired donation: incompatible donor/recipient swap for matched kidneys. Chains often initiated by nondirected donors. The National Kidney Registry facilitated 1,748 transplants, through 344 chains, 78 loops from 2008–2015/2016 *(AJT 2017;17:2451)*
- Financial impact from eval to 3 mo after donation: median out-of-pocket expenses Can $1254 (531-2589) and the median for lost donor productivity costs: can $0 (0-1908) (12 centers in Canada 2009–2014) *(JASN 2018;29:2847)*
- Potential donors are more willing to take potential health risk compared to potential recipients and health care professionals *(KI 2008;73:1159)*
- Kidney donors on the waitlist: 56 donors were listed as of 2/2002 *(Transplantation 2002;74:1349)*. From 1993–2005, 102/8,889 donors were on the waitlist. Black donors 14.3% of donors but 44% of donors reaching the waitlist *(Transplantation 2007;84:647)*

Background
- ABO blood type antigens and the human leukocyte antigen (HLA) system provide the major immunologic barriers to renal transplantation
- Transplant across ABO barriers is generally contraindicated (can be done in experienced centers, but at increased cost and risk of rejection)

HLA Antigens		
Class	Expressed by:	Control the Action of
Class I (**A**, **B**, C)	All nucleated cells	CD8+ cytotoxic T lymphocytes
Class II (DP, DQ, **DR**)	Antigen-presenting cells B cells	CD4+ "helper" T lymphocytes

- HLA-**A**, -**B**, and, -**DR** are the primary antigens considered for HLA matching between recipient and donor; 2 alleles at each locus = 6 antigens total: A recipient will therefore have 0–6 HLA "mismatches" with a particular donor

Significance of HLA Matching	
Deceased-donor KTR	↑ #s of HLA mismatches are associated in a stepwise fashion with decreased long-term graft survival (*Transplantation* 2016;100:1094)
Living-donor KTR	Aside from zero-mismatch donor-recipient pairs (who have the best long-term graft survival), the number of mismatches has little effect on graft survival

The Sensitized Patient
- Patients may have preformed antibodies to HLA antigens as a result of prior transplants, pregnancies, blood transfusions, and (rarely) viral/bacterial infections
- Such patients are referred to as "sensitized," and comprise approx. 1/3 of patients awaiting renal transplant in the US
- Preformed donor-specific antibodies (DSA) is associated with ↑ incidence of AMR and ↓ allograft survival compared to DSA-negative pts (*AJT* 2008;8:324)
- Crossmatch (XM): tests reactivity of recipient serum against allogeneic cells or HLA molecules (see table); can be performed against a specific donor or against "panels" of cells/antigens representative of the general population

Antibody Detection Methods (*NEJM* 2016;374:940)			
Assay	Components	Readout	Sensitivity
Complement-dependent cytotoxic (CDC) XM	Donor lymphocytes, recipient serum, and complement	% killing of donor cells	Low (requires high Ab levels for positive result)
Flow-cytometric XM	Donor lymphocytes, recipient serum, and fluorescein-labeled antibodies against human IgG	Binding of antibodies to donor lymphocytes (quantified as mean fluorescence intensity or "MFI")	Intermediate
"Virtual" XM (via solid-phase assays, eg, Luminex®)	Recipient serum, beads coated with purified HLA molecules tagged with unique, identifying immunofluorescence	Binding of antibodies to beads (quantified as MFI); allows precise definition of DSA specificity	High (can detect low Ab levels)

Immunologic Testing Prior to Deceased Donor Transplantation
1. HLA typing of recipient
2. Use solid-phase assay to detect and define anti-HLA antibodies present in recipient serum
3. List "unacceptable" HLA antigens based on center-specific MFI threshold. Recipients will not receive offers for donors who possess unacceptable antigens.

4. Calculate the calculated panel-reactive antigen (CPRA): CPRA reflects the probability of a CDC XM+ based on the listed unacceptable antigens and their frequency in the general population (pts with CPRA >80% are considered "highly sensitized" and given higher priority for HLA-matched kidneys)
5. Final crossmatch: CDC crossmatch performed just prior to transplant using fresh serum from recipient

Immunologic Testing for Living Donor Transplantation

1. HLA Typing of recipient and donor
2. Solid-phase assay to detect and define anti-HLA abs present in recipient serum
3. Perform CDC, flow, and virtual XMs

Crossmatch Test Interpretation

Crossmatch Interpretation (Nephrology 2011;16:125)	
(+) CDC T-cell XM (+) CDC B-cell XM	DSA to HLA class I, +/– class II High risk of AMR and is a contraindication to transplant, unless DSA can be reduced with desensitization protocols
(–) CDC T-cell XM (+) CDC B-cell XM	DSA to HLA class II OR low level class I DSA OR non-HLA Abs High risk of AMR and is a contraindication to transplant, unless DSA can be reduced with desensitization protocols
(+) CDC T-cell XM (–) CDC B-cell XM	Possible false (+); test should be repeated
(+) flow XM	Poses an intermediate risk of AMR→ may benefit from pre-txp desensitization and require ↑ post-txp immunosuppression and/or monitoring (AJT 2004;4:1033)
(+) DSA by solid-phase assay (–) flow and CDC XM	↑ Risk of AMR and graft failure compared with negative DSA (JASN 2012;23:2061)

Crossmatch Pitfalls and Limitations
- False-positive flow XMs may be caused by nonspecific Ig binding to Fc receptors on donor lymphocytes. Rituximab therapy in recipients may also cause false-positive flow XM.
- Antigens such as MHC class I-related chain A (MICA) and angiotensin II type I receptor (AT1R) have been implicated in graft failure but are not routinely detected by traditional XM platforms

POST-TRANSPLANT IMMUNE MONITORING

- Presence of DSA, whether formed prior to or after txp, is a/w inferior graft outcomes.
- De novo DSA formation (after transplant) occurs in 13–30% of previously nonsensitized pts.
- De novo DSA formation associated with late acute AMR, chronic AMR, transplant glomerulopathy, and ↓ graft survival (AJT 2012;12:1157; CJASN 2018;13:182)
- Risk factors for de novo DSA: high HLA mismatches (especially DQ), inadequate immunosuppression, and graft inflammation of any cause (CJASN 2018;13:182)
- Post-transplant DSA monitoring (using solid phase assays such as Luminex®), with protocol biopsies for high immunologic risk patients, is recommended to guide immunotherapy and permit early intervention (Transplantation 2013;95:19)

Post-transplant DSA Monitoring	
High-risk: pts with preexisting DSA	Months 1, 3, 6, 12, annually thereafter Protocol biopsies are recommended in the first yr to screen for subclinical AMR.
Low-risk: nonsensitized, 1st txp	At least once 3–12 mo post-txp, and/or whenever a significant change in maintenance immunosuppression is considered, suspected nonadherence, graft dysfunction, or before transfer of care to another transplant center

KIDNEY ALLOCATION

- Deceased donor transplantation provides a significant survival advantage over dialysis
- There are large regional variations in the median time to transplantation
- While pre-emptive listing prior to starting dialysis is preferred given outcomes for pre-emptive transplantation, only a minority of patients are pre-emptively waitlisted
- Discards are higher on the weekend even after adjusting for organ quality (*KI* 2016;90:157)
- Inappropriate unilateral kidney discards is common (*CJASN* 2018;13:118)

Kidney Allocation System (KAS) (*Transplant Rev* 2017;31:61)

- The new KAS was implemented to improve organ utilization, reduce racial disparities in waitlisting, introduce longevity matching and prioritization for the most sensitized patients
- Allocation time starts from start of dialysis or when added to the waitlist, whichever is earlier. Can be pre-emptively listed if the measured or calculated **GFR or CrCl ≤20**
- Kidney Donor Risk Index (KDRI): estimate of the relative risk of post-transplant graft failure Variables: age, height, weight, ethnicity/race, HTN, DM, cause of death, Cr, HCV, donation after circulatory death (DCD)
- **Kidney Donor Profile Index** (KDPI): simple mapping of the KDRI to a cumulative % scale using all kidneys procured for txp in the preceding calendar year in the US eg, KDPI 85% has higher graft failure risk than 85% of all donated kidney
- **Estimated Post-Transplant Survival** (EPTS) score: assigned to all waitlisted patients Variables: age, dialysis vintage, DM, number of all previous transplant 0–100%; lower scores a/w longer survival; pts w/ ≤20% are prioritized to KDPI <20%
- Calculated panel reactive antibody (CPRA) score: the percentage of antibodies in the recipient serum to the donor pool. This is monitored on a monthly basis.

New Kidney Allocation System (KAS)	
Sequence (KDPI)	**Priorities and Comments**
A (0 ~ ≤20%)	CPRA ≥98; 0-ABDRmm (EPTS ≤20%); prior living donor; local pediatrics; local EPTS ≤20%; all 0-ABDRmm (EPTS >20%); all local; regional pediatrics; regional EPTS ≤20%; all regional; national pediatrics; national EPTS ≤20%; all national
B (>20 ~≤35%)	CPRA ≥98; 0-ABDRmm; prior living donor; local pediatrics; local adults; regional pediatrics; regional adults; national pediatrics; national adults
C (>35% ~≤85%)	CPRA ≥98; 0-ABDRmm; prior living donor; local; regional; national
D (>85%)	CPRA ≥98; 0-ABDRmm; local + regional; national Only w/ signed informed consent

Priorities within sequences:
- Higher CPRA given priority w/ geographic prioritization (1st DSA, 2nd region, 3rd national)
- 0-ABDRmm: zero antigen mismatch
Pediatric recipients are prioritized for kidneys with KDPI <35% (Share 35 policy)

- Sensitizing events: blood transfusions, pregnancies, prior transplant

Allocation Points for Adult Transplantation Candidate	
Characteristics	**Points Given**
Allocation time	1/d
Prior living donor	4
Sensitization (CPRA, %)	0.08 (≥20,<30), 0.21 (≥30,<40),…,17.30 (≥97,<98), 24.40 (≥98,<99), 50.09 (≥99,<100), 202.1 (100%)
Single HLA–DR mismatch	1
Zero HLA–DR mismatch	2

- Priority was also established for blood group B candidates to accept blood group A2

Outcomes of KAS

- KAS has resulted in a significant decrease in racial disparities in access to transplantation
- ↑ shipping times d/t more national sharing for high KDPI kidneys → ↑ cold ischemia time, DGF
- Despite prioritization, candidates with CPRA ≥98% continue to have long wait list times
- The discard rate continues to rise and is approximately 20% post KAS

Reference
https://optn.transplant.hrsa.gov/learn/professional-education/kidney-allocation-system/
  ✓ Policy 8: allocation of Kidneys and Frequently asked questions

ALLOGRAFT DYSFUNCTION

Definition and Background

- After excluding volume depletion: >25% rise in serum Cr and/or new proteinuria >1 g
- Cr >1.5, or ΔCr between 6 mo → 1 yr a/w graft failure regardless of cause (KJ 2002;62:311)
- Improvement w/ empiric reduction in CNI is insufficient (unless extremely elevated) since many patients have more than 1 diagnosis (ie, AMR + CNI toxicity)
- Most surgical complications (ie, subcapsular hematomas, lymphoceles) are only seen early and can usually be detected on U/S

Causes and Workup

Differential Diagnosis of Allograft Dysfunction	
Time After txp	**Possible Causes**
0–3 mo	**Parenchymal:** ATN, acute cellular rejection (ACR), antibody-mediated rejection (AMR), drug-induced TMA, AIN, CNI toxicity, pyelonephritis, Recurrent FSGS, subcapsular hematoma **Urologic:** bladder outlet obstruction (BPH, blood clot), ureteral (ischemic stricture, blocked stent, blood clot, extrinsic compression from lymphocele), urine leak **Vascular:** transplant renal artery stenosis (TRAS), anastomotic edema, technical, fibrous contraction, vascular compression from lymphocele, pseudo-TRAS, iliac vascular disease, venous stenosis
3–12 mo	**Parenchymal:** ACR, AMR, BK virus nephropathy, recurrent glomerular disease, CNI toxicity (acute or chronic), TMA, pyelonephritis, viral interstitial nephritis, AIN **Urologic:** ureteral strictures (ischemic or BK viruria related), kidney stones (frequently asymptomatic) **Vascular:** TRAS or pseudo-TRAS
>12 mo	**Parenchymal:** chronic AMR, mixed ACR/AMR, recurrent glomerular disease, chronic CNI toxicity, BK virus nephropathy Dominant role of noncompliance (AJT 2012;12:388)

Workup

- CBC, BMP, LFTs, IS levels, BKV DNA PCR, LDH, haptoglobin, donor-specific antibody (DSA) via Luminex® or Flow crossmatch, urine protein/creatinine, U/A with urine culture, and appropriate serologies if original disease was GN
- Renal transplant U/S with dopplers of renal artery and vein
- Renal bx: usually required unless U/S diagnostic; LM, IF +C4d staining (marker of C' activation in AMR), EM helpful for recurrent disease and some cases of AMR

Treatment and Prognosis

- Depends in underlying cause of dysfunction (covered individually in these pages), reversibility, and degree of interstitial fibrosis
- Each 0.5 change in Cr a/w a 2.5 fold ↑ RR of graft failure (KJ 2002;62:311)
- Later changes in Cr (>1 yr out) are less likely to be reversible than earlier changes since degree of fibrosis tends to be worse and the causes of dysfunction may be less likely to respond to treatment

DELAYED GRAFT FUNCTION (DGF)

Definition

- DGF: need for dialysis within 7 d of transplantation for any reason
- Slow graft function: dysfunction that does not require dialysis. Has inconsistent definition in studies ↓ 25% in serum Cr between POD 1 and 2 or serum Cr >3 on d 5. Similar mechanism to DGF but less severe.
- Primary nonfunction: dialysis never stopped or eGFR <20 at 3 mo

Background

- 20–25% of deceased donor recipients
- 5–6% of live donor recipients. Associated with ~25% graft failure at 1 yr, usually related to severe event, ie, allograft thrombosis
- Associated with 40% increase in relative risk of allograft failure, increased rejection risk and 6 fold increase in risk of Chronic Allograft Nephropathy (AJT 2011;11:2279)

Pathogenesis and Risk Factors

- Donor factors: pre-existing ATN—prehospital down time, hypotension/hypovolemia a/w brain death, donor DIC, ↑ terminal Cr, DCD, age
- Ex vivo factors: prolonged cold ischemia time (CIT), perfusate solution choice, pump versus off pump transport (particularly if CIT >24 hr or DCD donor) (Br J Surg 2013;100:991)
- Recipient factors: age, DM, obesity, ↑ PRA, African American, males (AJT 2010;10:298)
- Pre-existing donor quality with ischemia reperfusion injury related to redox species, followed by abnormal local C' regulation, release of DAMPs → activation of innate immunity → cellular infiltrates, tubular degeneration with apoptosis/necrosis

Clinical Manifestations

- Oliguria–anuria, persistent elevation in Cr, fluid overload
- ↑ K: from ↓ K excretion, absorbing blood in surgical bed, tissue destruction

Workup

- Daily CBC, LFTs, BMP, and IS levels
- Renal U/S q3–4 d initially; as UOP increases during recovery occasionally unmasks ureteral or bladder outlet obstruction, evaluate renal arterial velocities for stenosis
- Renal biopsy after 7–10 d (earlier in patients with DSA) for rejection, TMA due to IS, early recurrence of FSGS

Treatment

- Induction with thymoglobulin versus no induction or basiliximab may reduce risk slightly but allows for delayed introduction of CNI (JASN 2009;20:1385)
- Delayed administration of CNI has no impact on DGF rate, but may shorten duration of HD dependence (Transplantation 2009;88:1101)
- For persistent DGF, reasonable to attempt conversion to belatacept, avoid conversion to rapamycin/mTOR inhibitor; prolongs recovery (Transplantation 2003;14:1037)
- Preoperative dialysis ineffective at preventing DGF (Transplantation 2009;88:1377)

Prognosis

- ↑ Graft failure 2.5 fold in standard donors (AJT 2006;6:1153)
- ↑ Both ACR and AMR, persists beyond duration of ATN, likely due to both allograft factors and expansion of alloimmune response during what was initially non-specific innate immune activation (KI 2015;84:851)

RECURRENT GLOMERULAR DISEASE

Background

- Nearly all glomerular diseases can recur in the allograft. For most, the rate of recurrence and allograft failure from recurrence is lower than allograft causes from other causes (ie, rejection, drug toxicity) (NEJM 2002;347:103)
- Impact of GN recurrence increases over time: 1–3% of biopsies in the first 6 mo but 16% of all biopsies beyond first yr (AJT 2012;12:388)
- Risk factors for recurrence: younger recipient age, DDRTx, steroid-free regimen (predominantly for IgA), more HLA mismatches reduces recurrence risk (KI 2017;92:461)

Recurrent Glomerular Disease After Transplantation (NDT 2014;29:15; KI 2017;92:461)		
GN Type	Clinical Recurrence	Graft Failure 5–10 yr After Recurrence
IgAN	10–15% (>50% histologically)	10–40%
MN	5–30%	5–40%
FSGS	20–40%	20–40%
MPGN type 1	20–50%	30–70%
C3GN/DDD	>80%	30–70%
Lupus	5–30%	<10%
ANCA	20%	7%
Anti-GBM	Extremely rare	Unknown

IgA Nephropathy (IgAN)

- Histologic recurrence is more common than clinical disease and early graft failure is rare. However, recurrence leads to worse outcomes beyond 10–15 yr
- Earlier age of onset and crescent are a/w recurrence *(Am J Nephrol 2017;45:99)*
- Steroid withdrawal a/w an ↑ rate of recurrent disease in several studies. In US-UNOS data, maintenance steroid use a/w ↓ risk of allograft loss due to recurrent IgAN (RR 0.66) but no difference in overall patient or graft survival *(Transpl Int 2018;31:175)*
- Thymoglobulin induction a/w ↓ recurrence in single center studies *(Transplantation 2008;85:1505)*

Membranous Nephropathy (MN)

- Presence of anti-PLA2R Ab in serum pretransplant increases risk of recurrence 3–4 fold, with 73% recurrence if positive, 33% if negative serologies *(Transplantation 2016;100:2710)*
- In those with recurrence, adding rituximab (with continued maintenance immunosuppression) resulted in complete or partial remission in 75% *(AJT 2009;9:2800)*

Focal Segmental Glomerulosclerosis (FSGS)

- Risk factors for recurrence: younger age, rapid time to progression to ESRD, white race > non-white race, and prior recurrence in allograft >80% chance if first allograft failed from recurrent disease *(NDT 2010;25:25)*
- Recurrent cases suspected to be related to soluble factor. ~2/3 will have partial or complete response to plasmapheresis and plasmapheresis use associated with better long-term outcomes *(J Transplant 2015;2015:639628)*
- Prophylactic PLEX or RTX did not reduce recurrence *(Transplantation 2018;102:e115)*
- ApoL1 risk variants recipient do NOT predispose to recurrent disease, but deceased donor carriers of risk alleles associated with increased risk of graft failure *(AJT 2012;12:1924)*
- De novo FSGS after transplantation: a/w viral infections (CMV, Parvovirus B19, HIV), ischemia (ie, transplant renal artery stenosis), and CNI toxicity

Complement-Mediated (Atypical) Hemolytic Uremic Syndrome (aHUS)

- Unlike diarrhea-HUS, aHUS associated with genetic abnormalities in alternate complement cascade has a high recurrence and graft failure rate, depending on mutation. Eculizumab prophylaxis may prevent recurrences in some cases *(AJT 2010;10:1517)*

Recurrence and Graft Failure Rate of aHUS *(AJT 2010;10:1517)*				
Mutation	CFH	C3	CFI	MCP
Recurrent disease	76%	57%	92%	20%
Graft failure	86%	80%	85%	17%

DE NOVO THROMBOTIC MICROANGIOPATHY

Background

- De novo TMA in patients whose original kidney disease was not related to TMA
- 0.8–3% of KTR, most commonly in the 1st several mo after transplant *(AJKD 2003;42:1058)*
- Approximately 30% have renal limited disease which has a better prognosis but can only be diagnosed by renal biopsy *(AJKD 2003;41:471)*

Pathogenesis

- Similar to native disease though etiology of injury different; endothelial injury and swelling with detachment from basement membrane leads to localized thrombosis, hemolysis, and platelet consumption. Progresses to mucoid edema and onion skin appearance of vessel walls. With time, glomeruli develop thickened endothelium, mesangial interposition, and double contours (nonimmunologic MPGN changes).
- Calcineurin inhibitors (Cyclosporine > Tacrolimus) contribute to endothelial injury. mTOR inhibitor use associated with TMA as well but less frequently
- Sirolimus have been rarely a/w TMA, particularly in combination with cyclosporine
- AMR, ischemia-reperfusion injury, DCD also risk factors *(AJT 2010;10:1517)*
- Infection: work as triggers; CMV, Parvo B19, HCV, in addition to the diarrheal associated HUS forms more common in native renal TMA *(Curr Opin Organ Transplant 2014;19:283)*

Clinical Manifestations

- Systemic form: renal dysfunction, thrombocytopenia, anemia, low haptoglobin, elevated LDH, fevers, hypertension
- Renal limited form: renal dysfunction, hypertension, elevation in resistive index on U/S, no-minimal evidence of hemolysis on blood tests

Workup

- Anti-HLA ab screen, crossmatch with donor, anti-cardiolipin ab, lupus anticoagulant, ADAMTS13 level, CMV PCR, Parvo B19 PCR

- Renal biopsy is diagnostic. Presence of C4d staining in peritubular capillaries strongly suggests AMR, presence of tubular vacuolization or arteriolar hyalinosis in nonaffected vessels suggestive of CNI-mediated injury

Treatment
- CNI-mediated TMA: controversial. Cessation of CNI adequate in most cases but places patient at risk for rejection. PLEX has been used while excluding other causes. Switching CNI to an mTOR inhibitor has been reported. Careful monitoring for renal toxicity is recommended. Belatacept has been used as a replacement for CNI (AJT 2009;9:424)
- AMR related: treat underlying rejection with steroids, PLEX, +/– rituximab, proteasome inhibitor. Some refractory cases have responded to eculizumab (NEJM 2009;360:542)

Prognosis
- Renal limited has better prognosis than systemic TMA (0% vs 38% graft failure)
- From 1990s, de novo TMA has 50% graft failure rate at 3 yr (AJKD 2003;42:1058), though the advent of belatacept has increased therapeutic options
- In contrast, recurrent TMA has graft survival rate of only 20% at 1 yr

---

SURGICAL AND UROLOGIC COMPLICATION

Background
- ~6% of renal transplants, most occur within first 6 mo after surgery
- Ureteral stents reduce incidence of urine leaks and obstruction but may increase cost of transplant and require cystoscopy for removal 3–6 wk post-transplant

Urinoma/Urine Leaks: 1–3% of Transplants
- Pathogenesis: most common site of leak is ureter–bladder anastomosis, though leaks from mid-ureter and renal pelvis also seen
- Renal failure accompanied by enlarging fluid collection (usually adjacent to allograft and bladder), chemical peritonitis and ileus are frequent, occasionally leakage from wound. May only manifest as delayed graft function or immediately after ureteral stent removal
- Diagnosis: (1) sample fluid collection for electrolytes and creatinine. If urine leak, then creatinine and K^+ will be higher than serum. (2) nuclear medicine renal scan can also be diagnostic in cases where fluid inaccessible
- Treatment: the majority of urinary leaks require surgical correction. Distal leaks with minimal extravasation and clinical stability may respond to Foley insertion for 5–7 d.

Lymphocele: 1–16% of Transplants
- Pathogenesis: inadequate ligation of lymph vessels near iliac vessels or hilum → lymph collection accumulates between the transplanted kidney and bladder
- Small lymphoceles are frequent but usually asymptomatic. Larger collections present few wk to mo after transplantation. A bulge near the surgical wound sometimes with extravasation of lymph and edema of lower limb ipsilateral to the graft may be seen. Rarely, compressive symptoms such as urinary urgency or hydronephrosis and allograft dysfunction may occur
- Diagnosis: renal ultrasound showing the collection with associated compressive effects. Fluid sampling to rule out urinoma (serum creatinine/potassium are similar to serum).
- Tx: expectant treatment for small lymphoceles. Drainage or laparoscopic/open surgery ("marsupialization") for larger and recurrent collections.

Ureteral Stricture: 3–6% of Transplants
- Pathogenesis: usually ischemia due to inadequate distal blood flow in ureter, though fibrosis from local BK virus replication and rejection is also suggested (AJT 2006;6:352)
- Risk factors: donor age, DGF, abnormal vasculature
- Renal insufficiency with hydronephrosis on U/S despite decompressed bladder
- Diagnosis: renal U/S or CT urogram usually suffice. If the diagnosis is uncertain, and antegrade pyelogram needs to be performed
- Tx: decompress collecting system with nephrostomy to reverse AKI and perform pyelogram. Stent placement can temporize, dilatation with stents or balloons frequently ineffective; success 28–80%. Most need surgical reimplantation (Clin Transplant 2015;29:26)

Allograft Pyelonephritis: 10–15% of Transplants in First Year
- Pathogenesis: reflux from surgical bladder anastomosis. RF: Female sex, diabetes, UTIs prior to transplant, immunosuppression, ureteral stent
- AKI, fever, pain over allograft, frequently h/o UTI symptoms preceding allograft pain. Occasionally asymptomatic, found on biopsy done for graft dysfunction
- Diagnosis: usually made clinically, confirmed with urine culture, blood cultures frequently positive as well. CT A/P can suggest diagnosis but not specific as perinephric stranding is common after all renal transplant surgeries.

- Tx: broad spectrum IV Abx pending sensitivities, continued treatment for 2–3 wk. Patients with 2 episodes in 6 mo or 3 episodes in 1 yr should be investigated further by urology. Many benefit from suppressive antibacterials, such as methenamine 1 g BID plus vitamin C
- Prognosis: single episode of pyelonephritis does not impact long-term allograft function (Transp Infect Dis 2016;18:647). Pyelonephritis may predispose to subsequent rejection and recurrent episodes can lead to allograft failure.

Asymptomatic Bacteriuria: 35–40% of Transplants
- UTIs and episodes of pyelonephritis frequently preceded by periods of asymptomatic bacteriuria but most do not progress to symptomatic disease
- Randomized trial of treating asymptomatic bacteriuria NOT associated with reduction in UTIs, hospitalizations, or pyelonephritis (AJT 2016;16:2943)

TRANSPLANT RENAL ARTERY STENOSIS

Background
- Different etiologies than native RAS and more likely to respond to treatment with improvement in renal function and BP control
- Incidence: 2% in US transplant population by 3 yr (reported range 1–20%) with risk factors: donor age, recipient age, h/o DM, ischemic heart disease (Am J Nephrol 2009;30:459)
- Pseudo-TRAS: similar presentation to TRAS but location of vascular obstruction in vasculature proximal to anastomosis; common iliac or early external iliac artery

Etiology by Location of Stenosis (AJT 2014;14:133)		
RAS Type	Location of stenosis	Mechanism
A	Anastomosis	Surgical error—sewn too tightly, fibrous contraction
B	Bend/kink in artery at any point	Malpositioning of kidney leads to a kink (like a bent straw) causing reduction in blood flow, may be missed if only do fluoroscopy in one orientation
P	Post-Anastomosis	Atherosclerotic disease, compression from fluid collection, twist in artery related to orientation during sewing, weak association with rejection
Pseudo-TRAS	Proximal to arterial anastomosis	Iliac artery atherosclerotic disease, clamp injury

Pathogenesis
- Goldblatt 1 Kidney: 1 clip model of hypertension
- Reduction in lumen size by >50% (usually >70%) WITH a mean arterial pressure gradient >10 mmHg across lesion. Renal hypoperfusion → ↓ GFR and sodium retention/volume expansion → HTN. Renin, angiotensin, aldosterone levels usually in normal range

Clinical Manifestations
- Graft dysfunction out of proportion to biopsy findings; delayed graft function
- Hypertension requiring multiple drugs to control; Edema w/o proteinuria/hypoalbuminemia
- Audible bruit over allograft (low sensitivity and specificity)

Workup
- Renal U/S with Doppler: operator dependent, sensitivity/specificity ~85% Anastomosis >200 cm/s, acceleration time >0.1 s, iliac to renal artery gradient >1.8
- Nuclear medicine: sensitivity/specificity ~70–80%
  - Separation in rate of appearance of tracer in allograft vs artery (Hilson Index)
- CTA and MRA: sensitivity/specificity ~95% but require contrast
- Angiography: gold standard

Treatment
- Angioplasty alone—patency rate 30–69% at 10 yr (J Vasc Surg 2013;57:1621)
- Angioplasty with stent—patency rate >80%, DES = BMS
- Vascular reconstruction—best treatment if within first 1–2 wk of operation when stent placement could rupture anastomosis and cannot wait. Late attempts at surgical correction associated with graft loss

Prognosis
- Untreated TRAS associated with high rates of graft failure (AJT 2014;14:133)
- Creatinine decreased 2.9-> 1.6 when angioplasty done for graft dysfunction
- Angioplasty for HTN without graft dysfunction and/or fluid retention unlikely to lead to clinical improvement (ie, if no graft dysfunction, it is unlikely that stenosis is physiologic) (J Vasc Surg 2013;57:1621)

ACUTE CELLULAR REJECTION (ACR)

- As immunosuppression has intensified, cellular rejection rates have been decreasing for past 30 yr; now consistently below 15% for living donor recipients *(AJT 2004;4:378)*
- Early detection and treatment are crucial, as complete reversal of rejection can improve prognosis to level of nonrejectors

Pathogenesis

- Migration of passenger dendritic cells (or native immune cells having processed alloantigens) migrate to 2° lymphoid organs, stimulating immune cells via direct- (or indirect-) allorecognition. Many become circulating effector T cells that infiltrate the allograft → interstitial inflammation/tubulitis/rejection *(NEJM 2010;363:1451)*
- Innate immunity respond to tissue "damage associated molecular patterns (DAMPs)" including redox species, nucleic acids, extracellular matrix components among others leading to macrophage and dendritic cell activation as well as upregulation of adhesion molecules → attraction of adaptive immune cells and milieu for cell activation rather than anergy *(AJT 2016;16:3338)*

Biopsy-Based Definition

- Recommended adequacy: 2 separate cores (~90% concordance among samples), ≥10 glomeruli, and ≥2 arteries
- Minimal adequacy: 7–9 glomeruli and 1 artery

Acute T-cell Mediated Rejection *(Banff Criteria AJT 2018;18:293)*	
Grade	Histologic Criteria
Borderline	Foci of tubulitis (t>0) + minor interstitial inflammation (i0–1), or moderate–severe interstitial inflammation (i2–3) + mild tubulitis (t1)
IA	Interstitial inflammation involving >25% of nonscarred cortex (≥i2) + moderate tubulitis (t2)
IB	Interstitial inflammation involving >25% of nonscarred cortex (≥i2) + severe tubulitis (t3)
IIA	Mild to moderate intimal arteritis (v1) ± any i/t
IIB	Severe intimal arteritis (v2) ± any i/t
III	Transmural arteritis and/or fibrinoid necrosis (v3) ± any i/t

Additional Notes

- Gene expression profiles suggest that not all borderline inflammation is alloimmune in nature *(Nat Rev Nephrol 2016;12:534)*
- Arteritis lesions may also be related to antibody-mediated rejection

Treatment

- Borderline: it is not clear that all patients need to be treated, though most centers will treat borderline rejection associated with allograft dysfunction using methylprednisolone 500 mg IV × 3, followed by corticosteroid taper
- IA: methylprednisolone 500 mg IV × 3, 250 mg IV × 1, then oral CS taper
- IB: center dependent—many use Thymoglobulin at 10.5 mg/kg total dose in addition to CS. However, in select patients, IV corticosteroids as above may be adequate depending on comorbidities and infectious risk.
- IIA/IIB: thymoglobulin 10.5 mg/kg in divided doses with IV CS
- III: thymoglobulin 10.5 mg/kg in divided doses with IV CS

Prophylaxis

- Mucosal candidiasis: nystatin SS TID–QID, clotrimazole troches 10 mg TID (N.B. drug interaction with calcineurin inhibitors) for 1–3 mo
- Pneumocystis: trimethoprim–sulfamethoxazole 1 SS QD or 1 DS TIW for 1–3 mo, or dapsone 100 mg QD for 1–3 mo or atovaquone 1,500 mg QD for 1–3 mo
- CMV: valganciclovir adjusted for renal function for 1–3 mo in intermediate and high-risk

Prognosis

- Severity: direct correlation between the severity of rejection and long term graft survival at 8 yr (control = 97.6%, borderline = 93.3%, IA/B = 79.6%, IIA/B + III = 73.6%) *(Transplantation 2014;97:1146)*
- Reversibility: if creatinine returns to baseline after treatment, long-term outcomes equal those without rejection (though more severe rejections less likely to reach baseline) *(Transplantation 1997;63:1739)*
- Time: late rejections have a worse prognosis than early rejections. Usually have more advanced fibrosis and less likely to be reversible *(Transplantation 2014;97:1146)*
- Repeat rejection is common, particularly when associated with noncompliance

ANTIBODY-MEDIATED REJECTION (AMR)

- Early AMR (<3 mo): 10% of for cause biopsies done in the first 6 wk after surgery, almost always in sensitized patients. If donor specific ab (DSA) at time of transplant, risk is 20–40% depending on strength. If no h/o sensitizing events, risk is <5% (AJT 2012;12:388)
- Late AMR (>3 mo): usually from *de novo* DSA formation, frequently presents as chronic active AMR (CAAMR) with slowly progressive rise in creatinine, and progressive proteinuria from transplant glomerulopathy/glomerulitis. CAAMR make up majority of renal biopsy results beyond first yr after transplant.

Pathogenesis

- Circulating antibodies bind to target on endothelial cells. The most frequent targets of antibodies are HLA molecules (MHC classes I and II), though anti-angiotensin receptors, anti-MICA Ab, endothelial Ab, and others have been described (Nat Rev Nephrol 2016;12:484). Antibody then cause injury through changing intracellular signaling, local activation of complement, and attraction of inflammatory cells.
- Endothelial injury can be sufficient to lead to local thrombus generation (TMA) though chronic activation leading to increase matrix deposition and multilayering of peritubular capillaries is more common
- Concomitant cellular rejection is common (30–40%); a/w rapid ↓ renal function

Definition

- Recommended adequacy: 2 separate cores of tissue, ≥10 glomeruli, and ≥2 arteries
- Minimal adequacy: 7–9 glomeruli and 1 artery

Antibody-Mediated Rejection: all 3 criteria must be met for diagnosis
(Banff Criteria AJT 2018;18:293)

Active Antibody-Mediated Rejection

1. Histologic evidence of acute tissue injury (≥1)
   - Microvascular inflammation: glomerulitis (g>0) and/or peritubular capillaritis (ptc>0)
   - Arteritis (v>0)
   - Acute thrombotic microangiopathy without other apparent cause
   - Acute tubular injury without other apparent cause
2. Evidence of antibody interaction with endothelium (≥1)
   - Linear C4d staining in peritubular capillaries (C4d≥2 by IF, C4d≥0 by IHC)
   - At least moderate microvascular inflammation (g + ptc ≥2; g must be ≥1 if TCMR)
3. Serologic evidence of donor-specific antibodies

Chronic Antibody-Mediated Rejection

1. Histologic evidence of chronic tissue injury (≥1)
   - Transplant glomerulopathy (cg>0)
   - Severe peritubular capillary BM multilayering (EM)
   - Arterial intimal fibrosis w/o other apparent cause
2. Evidence of antibody interaction with endothelium (≥1)
   - Linear C4d staining in peritubular capillaries (C4d≥2 by IF, C4d≥0 by IHC)
   - At least moderate microvascular inflammation (g + ptc ≥2; g must be ≥1 if TCMR)
3. Serologic evidence of donor-specific antibodies

Clinical Manifestations

- Active AMR: rapid decline in kidney function (or lack of recovery from DGF) with fluid retention and ↓ UOP, occasionally a/w thrombocytopenia/anemia and features of TMA
- Chronic AMR: slow progressive decline in kidney function associated with proteinuria

Measuring DSA

- **Complement-Dependent Cytotoxicity Crossmatch (CDC-XM):** recipient sera + donor lymphocytes + complement + anti-human IgG Ab. Technician uses a vital dye to determine if cell death has occurred. With +CDC-XM, >90% risk of hyperacute rejection and precludes transplantation
- **Flow Crossmatch (FXM):** recipient sera + donor lymphocytes, run through a flow cytometer with fluorescent marker antibodies against human IgG, T cells (usually anti-CD3), and B cells (usually anti-CD19) to assess presence–absence of binding as well as cell type. Strength of antibody can be assessed by dilution or expressed at "mean channel shift"—a measure of brightness compared to background. +FXM at time of transplant predicts a higher risk of AMR (20–50%) and ACR (20–50%) as well as higher risk of graft failure at 5 yr (AJT 2014;14:1573)

- Limitation: does not tell target specificity (which HLA antigen is target) and many false positives. Requires donor cells which may not be available during post-transplant phase, particularly if deceased donor
- Bead-based Multiplex (eg, **Luminex® Assay**): recipient sera + polystyrene beads coated with HLA peptides, place in flow cytometer with fluorescent anti-IgG antibodies. Read out is expressed as mean fluorescence intensity—"MFI" that is semiquantitative assessment of Ab concentration. Allows identification of Ab but may detect levels that are not clinically significant. Modification of assay to include complement C1q binding or generation of C4d may lead to better discrimination of high risk Ab *(NEJM 2013;369:1215)*

Treatment
- Reverse inflammation: high-dose intravenous corticosteroids +/– Thymoglobulin
- Antibody reduction strategies:
  - Plasmapheresis daily or every other day is effective, many centers replace with IVIg after treatments to prevent hypogammaglobulinemia. Duration is determined by level of antibody assessed from FXM or Luminex® testing
  - High-dose IVIg (2 g/kg in divided doses) has been used with some success
  - Rituximab: anti-CD20 Ab to depletes B-cells in hopes of reducing DSA—randomized trial showed no difference in graft survival at 1 yr compared to control but did low DSA *(Transplantation 2016;100:391)*
  - Proteasome inhibition (bortezomib × 2 cycles of 4 doses) was no different from placebo in a European trial *(JASN 2018;29:591)*
- Limit complement-mediated injury:
  - Terminal complement blockade with Eculizumab prevents membrane attack complex formation. Many case reports suggest utility for treating refractory AMR, and reduced AMR rates when given prophylactically to high-risk patients but 1 yr outcomes show significant chronic Ab-mediated injury *(AJT 2011;11:2405)*
  - C1 esterase inhibition has also been successful *(AJT 2016;16:1596)*
- Anticytokine therapy: tocilizumab blocks IL-6, a key component in maturation of T-, B-, and plasma-cells, all of which are involved in progression of AMR. Use in transplant patients has led to increased transplantation rates in sensitized waitlisted patients as well as patients with AMR post-transplant *(AJT 2017;17:2381)*

Prognosis
- Overall: 1-yr graft survival: 80–96%, 5-yr graft survival: 65–75%
- C1q binding: anti-HLA Ab that bind to C1q (thus activating complement locally) are associated with a worse 5-yr graft survival: 54% vs 93% *(NEJM 2013;369:1215)*
- Time to rejection: early AMR (<3 mo) has a better prognosis than late AMR (>3 mo), 4-yr graft survival of 75% vs 40% *(Transplantation 2013;96:79)*
- Proteinuria, transplant glomerulopathy, and presence of interstitial inflammation/concomitant cellular rejection have all been associated with more rapid disease progression *(Transplant Immunology 2014;31:140)*

INFECTION AFTER KT

Background
- Infectious complications occur in >2/3 of patients in the 1st yr with UTIs and viral infections are the most common causes
- Infections are the 2nd leading cause of death in KTR (USRDS Annual Report 2010)
- Risk factors for infection after transplant: donor exposures, prior and recent recipient exposures, prior and current immunosuppression (IS) regimens, recent treatment for rejection (AJT 2017;17:856)

Timeline of Common Infections After Kidney Transplantation (KT)		
<1 mo	1–12 mo	>12 mo
Wound infection, UTI, Dialysis-access infection, C. difficile colits	BK polyoma virus	Community-acquired pneumonia
Multidrug-resistant organisms: MRSA, VRE, ESBL	Herpes viruses: CMV, EBV, HSV, VZV	UTI
Donor-derived infections (uncommon)	PJP	Fungal infections
	Cryptococcus	Late reactivation of herpes viruses

DONOR-DERIVED INFECTIONS
- Unexpected transmission of infections from donor is rare, and may be a/w significant morbidity and mortality. May occur with living or deceased donors (AJT 2013;13 Suppl 4:22)
- Kidneys from deceased donors with premorbid bacteremia can be used for transplantation with minimal risk for disease transmission if prophylactic antibiotics are used. Kidneys from bacteremic donors have an increased risk of DGF but similar patient and graft survival (Transplantation 1999;68:1107; Clin Transplant 2016;30:415)
- Kidneys from donors w/ bacterial meningitis may be used (AJT 2011;11:1123)
- Rabies, parasites, lymphomas, and leukemias (via lymphotropic viruses) when donors w/ encephalitis w/o a proven cause were accepted as organ donors

Possible Transmission from Donors
- *Strongyloides stercoralis* from donors who lived in endemic areas (ie, Central and South America). Serologic screening of donors at-risk and prophylaxis with ivermectin in recipients when donors test (+) can prevent transmission (AJT 2015;15:1369)
- *Trypanosoma cruzi* from donors who lived in endemic areas (ie, Central and South America). In donors who test (+), regular testing of recipient by PCR, hemoculture, and serology can identify disease transmission early (reported in 13%), and prompt treatment with benznidazole can ↓ morbidity a/w Chagas disease (AJT 2013;13:2418)

CYTOMEGALOVIRUS (CMV) INFECTION
- Risk of CMV disease is related to donor/recipient serologic match:
  - High-risk: D+/R–, intermediate risk: D+/R+, and D–/R+, low-risk: D–/R–
- A/w ↑ acute/chronic rejection, graft failure, EBV-associated PTLD, other opportunistic infections (Transplantation 2013;96:333)

Clinical Manifestations
- **CMV syndrome:** fevers, malaise, weight loss, diarrhea, arthralgias, leukopenia, thrombocytopenia, transaminitis
- **Tissue-invasive disease:** GI (m/c tissue-invasive disease in KTR; colitis > gastritis; CMV viral load may be negative; if clinical suspicion is high, need biopsy with staining for CMV), pneumonitis, nephritis, hepatitis, retinitis (Clin Infect Dis 2008;46:840)

Prophylaxis
- Valganciclovir (900 mg QD, adjusted for CrCl) significantly reduces risk of CMV post-transplant. Also a/w ↓ in other viral (HSV, VZV) and bacterial infections
- Duration: minimum 6 mo if high-risk; 3 mo if intermediate risk, consider 3 mo if low-risk (Transplantation 2013;96:333)
- Longer duration (200 d vs 100 d) a/w ↓ CMV infection in high-risk (AJT 2010;10:1228)
- Risk of infection after stopping prophylaxis, esp in 1st 3 mo and high risk; ✓ CMV titer

Treatment

- PO valganciclovir (900 mg BID, adjusted for CrCl) and IV ganciclovir (5 mg/kg q12, adjusted for CrCl) equivalent; consider IV if tissue-invasive disease or significant GI symptoms. Treat until viral load undetectable × 2 wk, then start secondary prophylaxis. Consider dose-reduction of antimetabolite during/after treatment of CMV *(AJT 2007;7:2106)*

Resistant CMV Infection *(Transplantation 2011;92:217; Clin Infect Dis 2017;65:57)*

- Occurs in 1–2% of kidney transplant recipients
- Risk factors for resistant CMV include D+/R−, longer duration of antiviral exposure
- Treatment: cidofovir and foscarnet; mortality rate up to 11% in resistant CMV

VARICELLA ZOSTER VIRUS (VZV) INFECTION *(AJT 2009;9:S108)*

- Disseminated infection: vesicles and crusts not limited to a dermatome; 2/3 had visceral involvement; mortality (a/w AZA and visceral involvement) 17% *(Transplant Proc 2012;44:2814)*
- Visceral involvement: DIC, hepatitis, pneumonitis, pancreatitis, meningoencephalitis, vasculopathy; may develop w/o skin lesion *(NDT 2011;26:365)*
- Antivirals for CMV prophylaxis reduce risk of VZV reactivation
- Tx: acyclovir IV if disseminated, visceral or facial involvement; valacyclovir PO if limited to single dermatome; Consider decreasing or holding antimetabolite until all lesions healed

---

EPSTEIN–BARR VIRUS (EBV) INFECTION

- EBV mismatched (D+/R−) recipients have higher risk of EBV viremia, up to 67% in 1st yr. It may be asymptomatic, may be a/w mononucleosis-like symptoms, or may progress to PTLD. Late persistent EBV viremia may be a/w ↑ risk of solid cancers *(AJT 2013;13:656; Transplantation 2017;10:1473)*
- Risk of PTLD 24× higher in EBV-seronegative recipients *(Clin Infect Dis 1995;20:1346)*
- Monitoring in EBV D+/R−: ✓ viral replication at least monthly for 3–6 mo, then every 3 mo until the end of the 1st yr. Resume after acute rejection tx *(KDIGO AJT 2009;9 suppl3:S1)*
- EBV D+/R− recipients with increasing EBV viral load should have immunosuppression reduced, which is a/w ↓ risk of developing PTLD *(AJT 2013;13 suppl3:41)*
- Use of rituximab in EBV D+/R− recipients with asymptomatic increasing EBV viral load may reduce risk of developing PTLD *(AJT 2011;11:1058)*
- Antiviral prophylaxis for CMV does not reduce the risk of developing PTLD *(AJT 2017;17:770)*

BK POLYOMAVIRUS INFECTION

- Ubiquitous polyomavirus; establishes latency in GU tract and can reactivate in setting of IS
- BK viruria occurs in ~30%, BK viremia in 15–20%, and BK nephropathy in 1–10%. BK viruria can cause hemorrhagic cystitis (more common after HSCT) or irritative voiding symptoms. Only sign of BK viremia/nephropathy typically ↑ creatinine *(NEJM 2002;347:488; Transplantation 2013;95:949; BMT 2008;41:363)*
- Viral replication in urine and blood is most common in 1st yr post-transplant
- Risk factors: ↑ IS (most important), ↑ age, male gender, diabetes, Caucasian, ureteral stent, donor/recipient serologic mismatch
- BK nephropathy is an early complication that adversely affects allograft survival *(KI 2006;69:655; NEJM 2002;347:488)*
- Kidney Bx: intranuclear viral inclusions, interstitial infiltrates, and lymphocytic tubulitis (may be difficult to distinguish from acute rejection); immune staining +SV40. ↑ Severity of BK nephropathy by Banff criteria a/w worse graft survival *(JASN 2018;29:680)*
- Screening for BK viremia, with ↓ in IS if persistent viremia, can ↓ risk of nephropathy. Screening: minimum q3mo in 1st 2 yr, then annually through 5th yr. Screening should be resumed after treatment for rejection *(AJT 2013;13 suppl4:179)*
- Despite ↓ in IS if viremic, development of BK viremia a/w ↑ risk of allograft failure *(Transplantation 2013;15:949)*
- Tx: first-line treatment is ↓ in IS. Typically, ↓ /eliminate antimetabolite, then ↓ CNI trough if viremia persists. Other therapies include switch from tacrolimus to cyclosporine, switch from CNI to mTORi, switch MMF to leflunomide, add cidofovir *(AJT 2013;13 suppl4:179; CJASN 2014;9:583; AJT 2015;15:1014)*

HEPATITIS C INFECTION VIRUS (HCV)

- Hepatitis C infected patients who remains on dialysis are at higher risk of death than those who receive a kidney transplant (Transplantation 2013;95:943)
- Anti-HCV antibody positive KTR have lower allograft survival rates and ↑ risk of death compared to anti-HCV antibody negative recipients (AJT 2005;5:1452)

Management of HCV (+) KTR: Liver Biopsy and Portal Pressure Help Guide	
No significant fibrosis (stage 0–2), no live donor	DDRT w/ HCV+ or HCV–, then DAA post-transplant
No significant fibrosis, has live donor	DAA then transplant with HCV– kidney
Significant fibrosis (stage 3–4), portal HTN	SLK. Not a candidate for KT alone.
Significant fibrosis, no portal HTN	DAA and KT w/ HCV– kidney vs SLK (JASN 2016;27:2238)
	In patients w/ compensated HCV cirrhosis and hepatoportal venous gradient <10 mmHg, KT alone may be performed with similar patient and graft survival c/w HCV+ recipients w/o cirrhosis (Transplantation 2012;15:250)

- Historically, the use of interferon-based regimen to treat hepatitis C in KT patients was a/w increased risk of acute humoral rejection and should be avoided (AJT 2003;3:74)
- Post-transplant treatment with DAA for 12 or 24 wk achieves sustained virologic response at 12 wk in most HCV+ KTR and is well tolerated, with an acceptable safety profile (Ann IM 2017;166:109)
- Transplantation of kidneys from HCV-positive deceased donors into HCV-negative recipients, followed by the use of DAA, has been performed as a way to address the organ shortage. Short-term results show 100% sustained virologic response with excellent allograft function (NEJM 2017;376:2394; Ann IM 2018;168:533)

HIV INFECTION

- In selected HIV+ pts w/ ESRD (CD4 >200/mL^3, viral load undetectable on stable antiretroviral regimen), pt and graft survival are high at 3-yr (88% and 74%), although slightly lower than among all US recipients. HIV infection remained well controlled and there were few HIV-associated complications (NEJM 2010;363:2004). The slightly lower survival in HIV+ recipients may be due to HCV co-infection, as HIV+ and HCV– recipients have similar patient and allograft survival compared with HIV– recipients (KI 2015;88:341)
- Protease inhibitors: interaction with Tac and CsA, and dose and frequency of antirejection medications may need to be reduced. ↑ allograft loss, especially during the 1st yr post-transplant, and are a/w ↑ death. A nonprotease-inhibitor-based ART regimen is preferred in potential KTR if feasible (AJT 2017;17:3114)
- KT from HIV-positive deceased donors may be an acceptable treatment option for HIV-infected patients, with patient survival of 84% at 1 yr, 84% at 3 yr, and 74% at 5 yr, and allograft survival of 93%, 84%, and 84% (NEJM 2015;37:613)

PNEUMOCYSTIS JIROVECII PNEUMONIA (PJP)

- Can occur anytime post transplantation, though it is rare in patients who remain on PJP prophylaxis. Low eGFR and lymphopenia are risk factors (Am J Infect Control 2016;44:425).
- PJP transmission post-transplant can be nosocomial. Standardized prophylaxis protocol and airborne droplet precautions on transplant units and clinics may help decrease nosocomial transmission (KI 2013;84:240)
- Unexplained PTH-independent hypercalcemia in a renal transplant patient who presents with subacute respiratory complaints should raise concern for PJP (KI 2015;88:1207)

FUNGAL INFECTIONS

- Invasive fungal infections: occur in ~1.3% of KTR in the 1st yr post-transplant. Invasive candidiasis and aspergillosis are the most frequent cause (Clin Infect Dis 2010;50:1101)
- Candiduria in KTR is a/w reduced patient survival rate. However, treatment of asymptomatic candiduria does not appear to improve outcomes (Clin Infect Dis 2005;40:1413)

URINARY TRACT INFECTION (UTI)

- m/c infectious complication, all UTIs in transplant recipients are complicated UTIs
- Risk factors: female, ↑ age, ESRD due to reflux, DDRT, ↑ immunosuppression
- For patients with allograft pyelonephritis, fevers/allograft tenderness may persist for several days despite appropriate antibiotic choice
- Recurrent UTIs defined as >3 in 12 mo or >2 in 6 mo, can occur in up to 32% of patients. Recurrent UTIs typically treated with longer course of antibiotics and require evaluation for structural/functional abnormalities (AJT 2015;15:1021)
- High prevalence of ESBL organisms, especially if recurrent (Transpl Infect Dis 2012;14:595)
- No RCTs to guide duration of therapy: 7–10 d for first UTI (longer if ureteral stent in place), 14–21 d for allograft pyelonephritis or UTI with bacteremia
- Asymptomatic bacteriuria develops in ~50% of transplant recipients (KI 2010;87:774)
- Treatment does not ↓ rate of UTI, nor improve renal function (AJT 2016;16:2943)

INFECTIOUS DIARRHEA

- Diarrhea is a frequent post-transplant. Two m/c etiologies are medications (mycophenolate > tacrolimus) and infections. Evaluate for infection before ↓ mycophenolate dose as ↓ mycophenolate dose → ↑ risk of rejection/graft failure (Transplantation 2006;82:102)
- Common causes of infectious diarrhea: viral (CMV, EBV, adenovirus, Norovirus), bacterial (C. difficile), parasitic. Infectious etiology identified up to 70% of cases with molecular testing (Transplantation 2014;98:806)
- C. difficile: 3.5–16% of hospitalized KTRs, 8–33% will have at least 1 relapse. Initial Rx 10–14 d; if on Abx for co-infection with other organism, continue for 1 wk after other antibiotic stopped. Consider longer duration with relapses/vanco taper. Consider prophylaxis if h/o C. diff and requiring new course of antibiotics (Transplantation 2014;98:806)
- Norovirus: 17–26% of severe diarrhea, may have significant weight loss. Main treatment if transient ↓ in IS. Nitazoxanide may be effective in some cases. If viral shedding and symptoms persist, mycophenolate may need to be d/ced (Transplantation 2014;98:806)

METABOLIC COMPLICATION AFTER KT

NEW-ONSET DIABETES AFTER TRANSPLANT (NODAT)

Epidemiology and Clinical Implication
- 20–30% in the 1st yr after kidney transplantation (KT); Risk attributable to KT alone is highest in the 1st 6 mo after txp
- ↓ Patient and long-term allograft survival, ↑ risk of major CV events, infection, and sepsis

Diagnosis and Post-Transplant Screening
- Symptoms of diabetes plus random plasma glucose ≥200
- Fasting glucose ≥126 ×2, weekly × 4, at 3 mo, then annually post-txp
- A1c ≥6.5% (test only valid after 3 mo post-txp; A1c cannot be used in conditions that change RBC turnover); ✓ at 3 mo, q3mo for 1st yr, and at least annually thereafter

Risk Factors and Pathogenesis
- Traditional: age >40, BMI ≥30, AA, Latino, FHx of DM, personal hx gestational DM, IGT
- Transplant-specific: infection (CMV, HCV), postop hyperglycemia (fasting glucose >200), ↓ Mg, deceased donor, increased HLA-mismatch, PCKD, immunosuppressive agents

Immunosuppressive Drugs and Risk of NODAT		
	NODAT Risk	**Mechanism**
Corticosteroids	↑↑	Reduce peripheral insulin sensitivity
CNIs	Tac ↑↑ CsA ↑	Direct toxicity to pancreatic β-cells
Sirolimus	↑	Reduce peripheral insulin sensitivity

Treatment
- Lifestyle modification: first-line therapy
- 2nd-gen sulfonylureas, repaglinide, and DPP-4 inhibitors have proven efficacy in KTRs
- SGLT-2 inhibitor: appears safe and ↓ A1c and weight (Diabetes Care 2019;42:1067)
- Metformin: limited data; appears to be safe in stable KTRs with eGFR >45
- Insulin as needed to attain A1c <7%
- Prednisolone reduction to 5 mg/d a/w improved glycemia (NDT 2001;16:829)
- Mixed data re: benefit of complete/early steroid withdrawal on risk of NODAT
- Belatacept-based regimens a/w a lower incidence of NODAT (Transplantation 2011;91:976)

LIPID ABNORMALITIES AFTER KT

Background and Effect of Immunosuppressive Drugs
- High prevalence: total chol >240 (60%), LDL >130 (60%), TG >200 (35%) (NDT 2006;21:iii3)
- CV disease is the leading cause of death with a functioning graft in KTRs
- Corticosteroids ↑, Cyclosporine ↑, Tacrolimus ↔, Sirolimus (predominantly TG) ↑↑↑

Treatment
- Statins ↓ MACE by 21% and cardiac death or nonfatal MI by 29% (ALERT AJT 2005;5:2929)
- Statins for all adult KTR. If <30 w/o DM, CVD, individualized decision (KDIGO Lipid 2013)
- CsA (but not tacrolimus) inhibits hepatic metabolism of statins, raising levels
- Goal is to attain a target statin dose rather than a specific LDL value (see table)
- Ezetimibe is probably effective in statin-intolerant KTRs, but data is limited
- Avoid fibrates: ↑ adverse events, a/w graft dysfunction (AJKD 2004;44:543)

Starting and Target Doses of Statins in KTR (KDIGO Lipid 2013)		
	Starting Dose (and Target Dose if pt Taking Cyclosporine)	**Target Dose if No Cyclosporine**
Fluvastatin	40 mg	80 mg
Atorvastatin	10 mg	20 mg
Rosuvastatin	5 mg	10 mg
Pravastatin	20 mg	40 mg
Simvastatin*	20 mg	40 mg

*2011 FDA: concomitant use of CsA and simvastatin is contraindicated; however, if statin cannot be changed d/t cost and patient is stable, may monitor CPK and LFTs q6–12mo

CKD-MBD ABNORMALITIES AFTER KT

Pathophysiology
- Regression of structural changes in the parathyroid gland (hyperplasia, adenoma) can take mo to yr; resolution of uremia improves end-organ resistance to PTH
- Persistently ↑ PTH + PTH responsiveness/healthy allograft → ↓ P, ↑ Ca: similar to 1° hyperparathyroidism (HPT)
- ↑ FGF-23 levels in the early post-txp period also promotes phosphaturia
- CS: ↓ bone formation of osteoblasts, ↑ bone resorption of osteoclasts, ↑ RANKL

Epidemiology and Clinical Implication
- Persistent HPT is common after KT: >80% of patients have PTH > 65 and >40% have PTH >130 at 1 yr post-txp, despite good renal function (Transplantation 2016;100:184)
- High pretransplant PTH level is a/w graft failure (Transplantation 2006;82:362)
- ↓ PO₄: 40–90% of pts during the first 3 mo, gradually improves thereafter (NDT 2004;19:1281)
- ↑ PO₄: A/w txp failure and mortality (AJKD 2017;70:377)
- ↑ Ca: approx 1/3 of patients during 1st yr, usually within the 1st 3 mo
- ↓ 25-OH vit D is a/w interstitial fibrosis progression and low graft function (JASN 2013;24:831)
- Post-txp CKD-MBD abnormalities are a/w ↑ fracture, allograft dysfunction/loss, progression of vascular calcification, and mortality

Monitoring
- ✓ Ca, Phos w/ routine labs; ✓ PTH, 25-vit D q3mo for 1st yr, then q6–12 mo thereafter (more frequently if abnormalities or if receiving vitamin D/calcimimetic therapies)

Treatment
- Consider parathyroidectomy before txp if iPTH ≥800 despite adequate medical therapy
- Avoid PO₄ supplementation unless severe (<1.0, or symptomatic <1.5), as it may ↑ PTH
- ↑ PTH w/o ↑ Ca: replete 25-OH vit D to >20 (KI 2009;75:646)
  - If PTH remains elevated, treat with activated vit D
- ↑ PTH w/ ↑ Ca:
  - Cinacalcet: may ↓ tac level (NDT 2008;23:1048)
  - Parathyroidectomy: superior Ca and PTH reduction to cinacalcet (JASN 2016;27:2487)

HYPERTENSION AFTER KT

Background
- >90% of CNI-treated transplant recipients have HTN (<5% normotensive w/o medications)
- Risk factors: male, recipient age, donor age, DM, obesity, presence of native kidneys, delayed graft function, previous acute rejection, CNIs and steroids, CKD in transplant
- Complications: increased risk of CVD, graft failure, and death
- Risk of graft loss ↑ by ~15% with each 10 ↑ in SBP at 1 yr post-Tx (JAMA 2000;283:633)
- Lowering SBP to ≤140 by 3 yr is a/w significantly improved 10-yr graft survival (RR 0.79) and ↓ risk of CV death (RR 0.73) (AJT 2005;5:2725)

Pathogenesis
- Immediate post-Tx period: volume overload, graft dysfunction, ischemia, CNI toxicity
- CNIs (CsA > Tac) → activate SNS, upregulate endothelin, inhibit NO oxide → systemic and renal (afferent arteriolar) vasoconstriction; ↑ NCC activity (Nat Med 2011;17:1304)
- Glucocorticoids (ie, prednisone >10 mg/d): sodium and water retention due to partial activation of mineralocorticoid receptors
- Activation of the RAS in the native kidneys and/or a failing allograft

Evaluation
- ✓ graft dysfunction, CNI toxicity, recurrence of primary disease, post-bx AVF

Transplant Renal Artery Stenosis (TRAS): Important to Identify
- Presentation: worsening or refractory HTN and/or unexplained graft dysfunction, HF, flash pulmonary edema
- Risk factors: operative trauma, atherosclerosis of transplant renal artery or iliac artery, CMV infection, delayed graft function
- Diagnosis: PRA may be relatively low due to volume expansion and high PRA is non-specific; Doppler U/S has 87–94% sensitivity and 86–100% specificity; spiral CT; MRA; arteriography (risk of AKI due to contrast or thromboembolism)
- Treatment: conservative therapy w/ ACEi; PTA +/− stenting (can restore perfusion in 70–90% but may recur in up to 10%); surgery if PTA unsuccessful or stenosis inaccessible to PTA (successful in 63–92% but recurrence rate up to 12% and high risk of complications, should be reserved for refractory HTN) (JASN 2004;15:134)

Treatment
- Target BP is based on presence of proteinuria and additional comorbidities (DM, CVD, HF)

Guidelines for Target BP

Guideline	Recommendation
KDOQI	<130/80; if proteinuria, ↓ goal may be appropriate (AJKD 2004;43:S1)
KDIGO	≤130/≤80, irrespective of the level of urine albumin (KI 2013;83:377)
EBPG	<130/85 w/o proteinuria, <125/75 w/ proteinuria (NDT 2002;17:25)

- Choice of drug class should be based on time after Txp, use of CNIs, presence/absence of persistent albuminuria, and comorbidities

Drug Treatment

DHP CCBs (amlodipine, nifedipine)	May ameliorate vasoconstriction induced by CNIs CCB a/w ↓ graft loss (RR 0.75) and ↑ GFR (mean Δ 4.45) c/w placebo/no Rx (Transplantation 2009;88:7) Nifedipine ↑ GFR at 1 and 2 yr c/w lisinopril (Transplantation 2001;72:1787)
Non-DHP CCBs (diltiazem, verapamil)	Potent inhibitors of CYP3A4, cause ↑ plasma levels of Tac, CsA, and sirolimus; effect occurs in 48–72 hr; close monitoring of CNI or mTOR inhibitor levels is required
ACEi, ARBs	Cause Δs in GFR which may interfere with dx of acute rejection (esp. in first 6 mo post-Tx); can exacerbate hyperkalemia (RR 3.76 for incidence of hyperkalemia w/ ACEi c/w CCB), esp. in Pts on CNIs; can exacerbate anemia (Transplantation 2009;88:7) Losartan can lower plasma uric acid levels in Pts with gout Despite beneficial effects on proteinuria and HTN, no long-term benefit on graft, patient survival has been shown in RCTs Wait 3–6 mo post-Tx before starting ACEi or ARB, if indicated

MALIGNANCY AFTER KT

Background
- Overall cancer risk rate is elevated in solid organ transplant (SOT) patients
- Standardized incidence Ratio (SIR) c/t general population is 2.1 (JAMA 2011;306:1891)

SIR of Malignancies in Transplant Recipients (JAMA 2011;306:1891)			
Infection Related		**Noninfection Related**	
Kaposi sarcoma	61.46	Nonmelanoma skin	13.85
Liver	11.56	Kidney	4.65
Vulva	7.6	Thyroid	2.95
Non-Hodgkin lymphoma	7.54	Melanoma	2.38
Anus	5.84	Lung	1.97
Hodgkin lymphoma	5.84	Urinary bladder	1.52
Penis	4.13	Pancreas	1.46
Oropharynx including tonsil	2.01	Colorectum	1.24
Stomach	1.67	Prostate	0.92
Cervix	1.03	Breast	0.85

- Cancer (20%) is 2nd leading cause of death after CVD (24%) (JAMA Oncol 2016;2:463)
- Cancers may occur de novo (eg, NMSC and Kaposi sarcoma), donor-related (eg, RCC, melanoma, or choriocarcinoma), and recurrent cancers
- Impaired immune surveillance is thought to be the major underlying pathogenesis coupled with higher rates of oncoviral infections

Risk Factors and Pathogenesis
- Smoking History: cancer-related death ↑ 1.4× if quit before txp, ↑ 2.6× if continued smoking (Transplantation 2016;100:227)
- History of prior cancer
- Kidney and thyroid cancers a/w kidney allograft failure (JASN 2016;27:1495)

General Screening and Prevention Strategies
- Smoking cessation
- Updating pretransplant recipient malignancy screening
- Screening post-transplant for skin, breast, colorectal, cervical cancer per USPSTF
- EBV IgG seronegative recipients of seropositive organ should have protocol EBV PCR monitoring throughout first year and beyond

General Treatment
- ↓ IS; Chemotherapy; Radiation; Removal of affected organ as indicated
- Pembrolizumab (anti-PD-1 Ab) caused cell-mediated rejection (NEJM 2016;374:896); CTLA-4 inhibitor, ipilimumab, did not (J Clin Oncol 2014;32:e69)

NONMELANOMA SKIN CANCERS (NMSC)

Background
- Basal cell carcinoma (BCC) and squamous cell carcinoma (SCC) are the most common malignancies in solid organ transplant recipients (Dermatol Surg 2012;38:1622–1630)
- Although mortality risk is low, it has the highest incremental risk of death compared to general population (×29.8) (JAMA Oncol 2016;2:463)

Risk Factors
- Cumulative ultraviolet radiation exposure. Age at txp (>50 yr 3× ↑ risk). Duration of txp.
- Immunosuppression: type (AZA has 1.5× risk of SCC) and Dose: high accumulated dose of AZA, CNI, and steroids ↑ risk of SCC 4.6× (Am J Clin Dermatol April 2018)
- Type of organ transplanted: higher risk of NMSC if utilize more intense immunosuppression such as combined heart and kidney transplant compared to kidney alone
- History of previous NMSC increases risk for subsequent NMSC

Screening and Prevention
- Self-exam AND Health care provider skin exam annually (KDIGO Transplantation 2009)
- Sun protection education (Use of high-SPF sunscreen decreases SCC, BCC)
- Sirolimus ↓ 56% risk NMSC vs CNI (BMJ 2014;349:g6679). But a/w higher mortality (CJASN 2016;11:1845)

- In aggressive SCC, reduction of immunosuppression
- Consider change to MMF from AZA, or mTOR inhibitor from CNI, systemic retinoids
  (Am J Clin Dermatol April 2018)

POST-TRANSPLANT LYMPHOPROLIFERATIVE DISORDER (PTLD)

Background
- Incidence 1% at 10 yr post-transplant, with majority (>80%) occurring in first yr post-transplant *(Pediatr Nephrol 2014;29(9):1517)*
- Cumulative incidence over 5 yr is 1–3% in kidney transplants
- The majority are EBV-driven; up to 30% are EBV negative

Risk Factors
- IS after SOT is a/w marked ↑ risk of malignancy *(JAMA 2006;296:2823)*
- Negative EBV serostatus of the recipient at the time of kidney transplant
- Prior malignancy
- Time Post-Transplant, EBV naïve occur early, whereas EBV IgG seropositive recipients develop ~10 yr post-transplant *(Transplantation 2013;5:470)*

Clinical Presentation
- Nonspecific constitutional symptoms; B symptoms (fever, weight loss, night sweat)
- Lymphadenopathy and organ dysfunction: extranodal masses (>1/2), CNS disease (20–25%), infiltrative lesions of the allograft (20–25%)
- ↓ Hb, Plt, WBC, ↑ LDH, Ca, uric acid, monoclonal protein in urine or serum
- Allograft dysfunction: hydronephrosis, renal vessel stenosis, graft infiltration

Prevention
- No role of antiviral prophylaxis *(AJT 2017;17:770)*

Workup and Management of EBV Reactivation *(AJT 2013;13:41)*
- Initial reactivation with elevated EBV PCR over 2 wk
  Reduce immunosuppression, monitor EBV PCR once weekly until negative
- In the following settings of EBV viremia, r/o PTLD via CT imaging or PET scan, and pursue excisional biopsy when appropriate:
  Persistent EBV viremia, or high asymptomatic EBV viremia w/wo ↓ IS
  Any EBV viremia with associated symptoms

Treatment *(BJH 2010;149:693; National Comprehensive Cancer Network Guidelines)*
- Goals: eradication of PTLD and preservation of graft function
- Tumor histologic staging with WHO criteria
- EBV status of tumor established (EBV+ tumor may respond best to reduction of IS, EBV-negative lymphomas unlikely to respond)
- Reduction of IS (where alternative organ supports possible, eg, dialysis)
- Immunotherapy with CD20 monoclonal antibody rituximab (Effective in CD20+ PTLD)
- Chemotherapy:
  Anthracycline-based: CHOP (cyclophosphamide, doxorubicin, vincristine, prednisone)
  - Care must be taken in patients with impaired cardiac function
  Platinum drugs are nephrotoxic and even in normal renal function, care should be taken
  Fludarabine is renally excreted, monitor renal function
- Radiotherapy
- Surgical management
- CNS Involvement: radiation therapy, surgical removal, and methotrexate (if renal function preserved)

Prognosis *(J Clin Oncol 2013;10:1302)*
- Patients with PTLD had 5-yr survival rate of 53%, 10-yr survival rate of 45%
- Multivariable analyses revealed that age >55 yr, serum creatinine >1.5 mg/dL, ↑ LDH, disseminated lymphoma, brain localization, invasion of serous membranes, monomorphic PTLD, and T-cell PTLD were independent prognostic indicators of poor survival

CKD after Nonrenal Solid Organ Transplantation (NRSOT)

- CKD is a known complication post NRSOT
- CKD prevalence reported at 5 yr after transplantation was 21.3% for intestine recipients, 18.1% for liver recipients, 15.8% for lung recipients, 10.9% for heart recipients, and 6.9% for heart-lung recipients
- ESRD occurred at a rate of 1–1.5%/yr among NRSOT recipients (NEJM 2003;349:931)

Risk Factors for CKD Post NRSOT (NEJM 2003;349:931; JASN 2007;18:3031; Transplant Rev 2015;29:175)	
Pretransplant factors	Older age, ♀, pre-existing CKD, DM, HTN, HCV
Peritransplant factors	Renal hypoperfusion: LV dysfunction, hepatorenal syndrome
	Perioperative AKI: hypotension, hypovolemia, iodine contrast, nephrotoxic medications, atheroembolic disease
Post-transplant factors	Calcineurin inhibitor toxicity
	Acute: vasoconstriction of afferent arterioles;
	Chronic: interstitial fibrosis, nodular arteriolar hyalinosis, glomerulosclerosis, thrombotic microangiopathy
	Nephrotoxic antibiotics, ongoing transplant organ dysfunction, BK nephropathy (rare)

Treatment

- NRSOT recipients with eGFR <30, proteinuria >500 mg/d or rapidly declining GFR should be referred for renal evaluation. Management of complications of CKD (eg, anemia, metabolic acidosis, bone and mineral disease) should follow guidelines for nontransplant pts (J Heart Lung Transplant 2010;29:914; Liver Transpl 2013;19:3).
- BP targets and management should follow those for the general population. CCBs are most commonly used, but ACEI/ARB should be used if proteinuria and may be preferred in DM. In patients on mTORi, ARB may be preferred to ACEI due to lower risk of angioedema (J Heart Lung Transplant 2010;29:914; Liver Transpl 2013;19:3; CJASN 2010;5:703).

Conversion from CNI to mTORi

- a/w ↑ GFR. However, conversion to mTORi also a/w ↑ acute rejection in liver transplant and high discontinuation rate due to side effects.
- mTORi conversion associated with improved GFR in heart and lung transplant recipients. mTORi may slow progression of cardiac allograft vasculopathy (Transplantation 2016;100:621; 2016;100:2558)
- Patients with preexisting proteinuria or CKD may have worsening renal function after conversion to an mTORi (BMC Gastroenterol 2017;17:58; J Heart Lung Transplant 2009;28:564)

Dialysis after NRSOT

- HD is the most common RRT modality in NRSOT patients who develop ESRD
- PD has been used in heart and lung transplant recipients, who might be very sensitive to volume changes and fluid shifts associated with hemodialysis
- In thoracic transplant recipients showed higher rate of hospitalization with HD vs PD (231.4 vs 72.7/100 patient yr), higher rate of dialysis-related infections with PD (0.36 vs 0.08/patient yr), and no difference in mortality (Perit Dial Int 2015;35:98)

Kidney Transplantation (KT) after NRSOT

- Early referral for KT evaluation is essential given high mortality rate while on dialysis
- KT is a/w small ↑ mortality peritransplant in NRSOT. However, the mortality rate is ↓ significantly after 141 d and remains sustained for 5 yr postrenal transplant (NEJM 2003;349:931)
- 5-yr overall graft survival for KT in heart or lung recipients is lower than with primary KT. However, death-censored graft survival is comparable and KT ↓ risk of death compared with dialysis by 43% in heart and 54% in lung recipients. Liver transplant recipients with ESRD have a 44–60% reduction in mortality compared with remaining on dialysis (AJT 2009;9:578; Liver Transpl 2013;19:3)

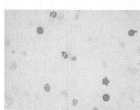

Dysmorphic RBCs. RBCs of different size, shape, hemoglobin content, with fragmentation and budding. Seen in glomerular bleeding. Hansel stain.

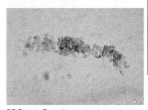

RBC cast. Typically seen in glomerulo-nephritis or vasculitis.

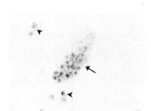

WBC cast (KI 2008;73:980). Frequently seen in interstitial nephritis, presence of eosino-phils suggests allergic origin. May also be seen in glomerulonephritis. Hansel stain.

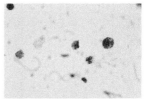

Renal epithelial cell in AKI. Multiple vac-uolated renal epithelial cells in foscarnet nephrotoxicity (ATN). Hansel stain.

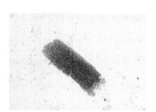

Muddy brown granular cast (AJKD 2005;46:820). Muddy brown cast typically seen in ATN.

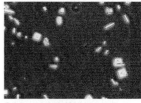

Calcium oxalate (CaOx) crystals. Multiple envelope-shaped (CaOx dihydrate) and needle-shaped (CaOx monohydrate) crystals seen in Ethylene Glycol poisoning.

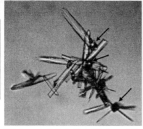

Calcium phosphate (brushite) crystals *(Int J Surg 2016;36:624)*. Asymmetrical rod-shape aggregate of calcium phosphate (brushite) crystals intermingled with calcium oxalate dihydrate crystals (*arrows*), seen in hypercalciuria and hyperoxaluria.

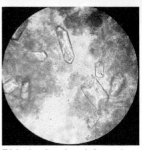

Triple phosphate (struvite) crystals *(KI 2015;88:205)*. Coffin-lid shaped Triple (ammonium-magnesium) phosphate crystals (struvite) seen in infected alkaline urine with urease-producing bacteria.

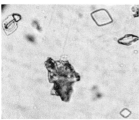

Urate crystals *(KI 2012;81:1281)*. Rosettes and rhomboid-shaped crystals of uric acid in pink urine after recurrent seizure; after propofol anesthesia. Also seen in heat stress–related Mesoamerican nephropathy.

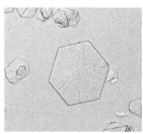

Cystine crystals *(Semin Nephrol 2008;28:99)*. Hexagonal crystals seen in stone former with cystinuria.

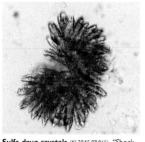

Sulfa drug crystals *(KI 2015;87:865)*. "Shock of wheat" appearance of Sulfamethoxazole crystals seen in acute kidney injury following high dose Sulfamethoxazole–Trimethoprim therapy.

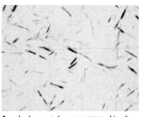

Acyclovir crystals *(KI 2011;79:574)*. Needle-shaped acyclovir crystals seen in acute valacyclovir overdose with AKI.

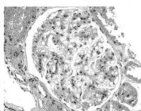

Mesangial proliferative GN, H&E

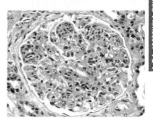

Endocapillary proliferative GN, H&E

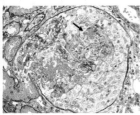

Crescentic GN with fibrinoid necrosis (*arrow*), JMS

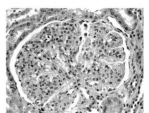

MPGN, H&E

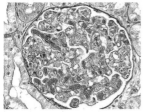

Immune thrombi in cryoglobulinemic GN, PAS

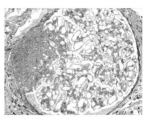

FSGS, NOS type, PAS

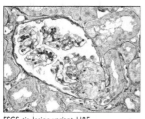

FSGS, tip lesion variant, H&E

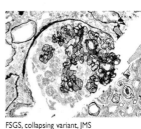

FSGS, collapsing variant, JMS

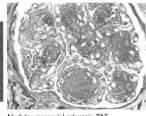

Nodular mesangial sclerosis, PAS

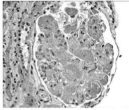

Acute thrombotic microangiopathy in glomerulus, H&E

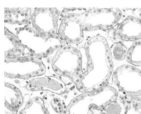

Acute tubular necrosis, PAS

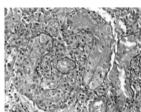

Acute interstitial nephritis, PAS

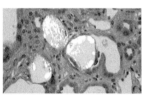

Strongly birefringent calcium oxalate crystals, H&E, polarized light

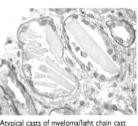

Atypical casts of myeloma/light chain cast nephropathy, PAS

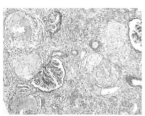

Granulomatous interstitial nephritis, PAS

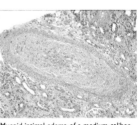

Mucoid intimal edema of a medium-caliber artery; scleroderma renal crisis H&E

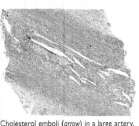

Cholesterol emboli (*arrow*) in a large artery, H&E

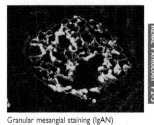

Granular mesangial staining (IgAN)

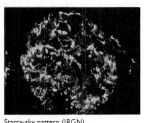

Granular mesangial and GCW (subendothelial) staining (MPGN)

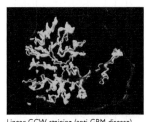

Granular GCW (subepithelial) staining (MN)

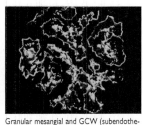

Starry-sky pattern (IRGN)

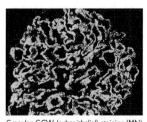

Linear GCW staining (anti-GBM disease)

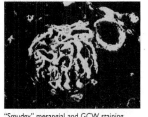

"Smudgy" mesangial and GCW staining (amyloidosis)

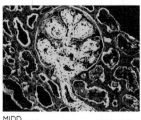

MIDD

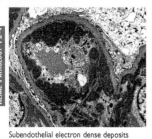

Subendothelial electron dense deposits

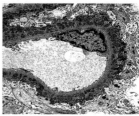

Subepithelial electron dense deposits

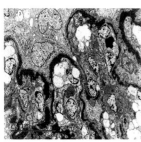

Dense deposition disease

Amyloid fibrils (8–10 nm)

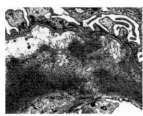

Fibrillary deposits (16–20 nm)

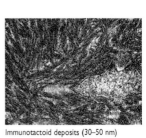

Immunotactoid deposits (30–50 nm)

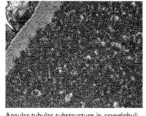

Annular-tubular substructure in cryoglobuli-nemic GN

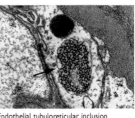

Endothelial tubuloreticular inclusion

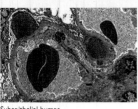

Subepithelial humps

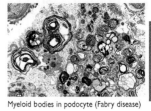

Myeloid bodies in podocyte (Fabry disease)

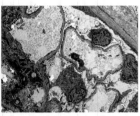

Diffuse podocyte foot process effacement
(MCD)

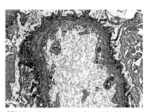

GBM lamellation in Hereditary Nephritis
("basket weaving")

Units Used and Omitted in This Book (Blood and Urine if not Specified)	
CrCl, eCrCl	mL/min
GFR, eGFR	mL/min/1.73 m^2
Na, K, Cl, CO$_2$, HCO$_3^-$ (serum, plasma, and urine)	mmol/L
BUN, Cr, Ca, PO$_4$, Mg, uric acid, glucose, cholesterol, triglycerides; urine protein, urine albumin	mg/dL
Hemoglobin, serum protein, serum albumin	g/dL
Iron, TIBC	µg/dL
Ferritin, 25-OH vit D, cyclosporine (CsA) and tacrolimus (Tac) level	µg/L = ng/mL
PTH	pg/mL
Osmolality, osmolal gap	mOsm/kg
SBP, DBP, MAP, CVP, PCWP	mmHg

Unit Conversion

Unit Conversion: × Factor Below				
Substance (MW)	Conventional Unit	SI Unit	Conventional to SI	SI to Conventional
BUN (14 × 2 = 28)	mg/dL	mmol/L	0.357	2.8
Urea (60)*	mg/dL	mmol/L	0.167	6
Creatinine (113)	mg/dL	µmol/L	88.4	0.0113
Calcium (40)	mg/dL	mmol/L	0.25	4
Phosphorous (31)	mg/dL	mmol/L	0.3229	3.1
Magnesium (24.3)	mg/dL	mmol/L	0.41	2.43
Glucose (180)	mg/dL	mmol/L	0.055	18
Uric acid (168)	mg/dL	µmol/L	59.485	0.0168
PTH	pg/mL	pmol/L	0.106	9.4
Total cholesterol	mg/dL	mmol/L	0.026	38.67
25-OH vit D	ng/mL	nmol/L	2.496	0.4
1,25-(OH)$_2$ vit D	pg/mL	pmol/L	2.6	0.38
UPCR	g/g cr	mg/mmol	113.6	0.0088
UACR	g/g cr	mg/mmol	113.6	0.0088

*Urea 1 mmol/L = BUN 1 mmol/L; BUN 1 mg/dL = Urea 2.14 mg/dL

Sodium Chloride 58.44 g/mol: Na$^+$ 22.99 g/mol + Cl$^-$ 35.45 g/mol
NaCl 3% = 30 g/L = 513 mEq/L; 3% 100 mL = 3 g = 51.3 mEq Na + 51.3 mEq Cl
NaCl 2% = 20 g/L = 342 mEq/L; 2% 100 mL = 2 g = 34.2 mEq Na + 34.2 mEq Cl
NaCl 5.1 g = 87 mEq (2 g) Na + 87 mEq (3.1 g) Cl
NaCl 5.8 g (1 teaspoon) = 100 mEq (2.3 g) Na + 100 mEq (3.5 g) Cl
NaCl 1 g = 17.1 mEq (393 mg) Na + 17.1 mEq (606 mg) Cl

Sodium Bicarbonate 84.01 g/mol: Na$^+$ 22.99 g/mol + HCO$_3^-$ 61.02 g/mol
NaHCO$_3$ 8.4% = 84 mg/mL = 1 mEq/mL: 23 mg Na + 61 mg HCO$_3$ per mL
  50 mL = 50 mEq Na + 50 mEq HCO$_3$: almost same Na contents with 3% 100 mL
NaHCO$_3$ 650 mg = 7.7 mEq Na + 7.7 mEq HCO$_3$
NaHCO$_3$ 4.8 g (1 teaspoon) = 57 mEq (1.3 g) Na + 57 mEq (3.5 g) HCO$_3$

Potassium Chloride 74.55 g/mol: K 39.10 g/mol + Cl$^-$ 35.45 g/mol
KCl 1 g = 13.6 mEq (530 mg) K + 13.6 mEq (470 mg) Cl

Protein Size

Protein Size (kDa)			
Albumin	68	β2 microglobulin	11.8
Myoglobin	17.8	Cystatin C	13.3
Hemoglobin	68.8	κ light chain	22.5
IgG	150	λ light chain	45

ABBREVIATIONS

1°	primary
2°	secondary
βB	beta-blocker
ΔMS	change in mental status
11βOHSD2	11beta-hydroxysteroid dehydrogenase type 2
18F-FDG	fludeoxyglucose F 18
6-MP	6-mercaptopurine
a/w	associated with
AA	amino acid
AAMI	Association for the Advancement of Medical Instrumentation
Ab	antibody
ABG	arterial blood gas
ABMR	antibody-mediated rejection
abnl	abnormal
ABPM	ambulatory blood pressure monitoring
abx	antibiotics
ACCP	American College of Chest Physicians
ACE	angiotensin converting enzyme
ACEi	angiotensin converting enzyme inhibitor
ACL	anticardiolipin antibody
ACR	acute cellular rejection
ACS	acute coronary syndrome
ACTH	adrenocorticotrophic hormone
AD	autosomal dominant
ADAMTS13	a disintegrin and metalloproteinase with a thrombospondin type 1 motif, member 13
ADH	antidiuretic hormone
ADTKD	autosomal dominant tubulointerstitial kidney disease
AFB	acid-fast bacilli
Afib	atrial fibrillation
AG	anion gap
Ag	antigen
AGMA	anion gap metabolic acidosis
aHUS	atypical hemolytic uremic syndrome
AIDS	acquired immunodeficiency syndrome
AIHA	autoimmune hemolytic anemia
AII	angiotensin II
AIN	acute interstitial nephritis
AJT	American Journal of Transplantation
AKI	acute kidney injury
AKI-D	dialysis requiring acute kidney injury
alb	albumin
aldo	aldosterone
ALI	acute lung injury

Allo-HSCT	allogenic hematopoietic stem cell transplantation
ALT	alanine aminotransferase
AME	apparent mineralocorticoid excess
AML	acute myelogenous leukemia
AMR	antibody mediated rejection
ANA	antinuclear antibody
ANCA	antineutrophilic cytoplasmic antibody
Ann IM	Annals of Internal Medicine
APC	antigen-presenting cell
APD	automated peritoneal dialysis
APLA	antiphospholipid antibody
APOL1	apolipoprotein L1
APS	antiphospholipid syndrome
AR	autosomal recessive
ARB	angiotensin receptor blocker
ARDS	acute respiratory distress syndrome
ARNi	angiotensin Receptor Neprilysin Inhibitor
ARV	antiretroviral
ASA	aspirin
ASCVD	atherosclerotic cardiovascular disease
AST	aspartate aminotransferase
asx	asymptomatic
ATI	acute tubular injury
ATN	acute tubular necrosis
Auto-HSCT	autologous hematopoietic stem cell transplantation
AV	arteriovenous, aortic valve
AVB	atrioventricular block
AVF	arteriovenous fistula
AVG	arteriovenous graft
AVM	arteriovenous malformation
AZA	azathioprine
Aφ	alkaline phosphatase
b/c	because
BCx	blood culture
BJP	Bence Jones protein
BK	maxi-K channel
BKV	BK virus
BM	bone marrow
BMD	bone mineral density
BMI	body mass index
BMP	basic metabolic panel
BNP	B-type natriuretic peptide
BP	blood pressure
BPH	benign prostatic hypertrophy
BT	bleeding time
BUN	blood urea nitrogen

bx	biopsy	CO	carbon monoxide/cardiac output
c/t	compared to		
c/w	compared with/consistent with	COPD	chronic obstructive pulmonary disease
C′	complement	COX	cyclo-oxygenase
C3G	C3 glomerulopathy	CPPD	calcium pyrophosphate crystal deposition
C3GN	C3 glomerulonephritis		
CA	carbonic anhydrase	CPRA	calculated panel reactive antibody
CABG	coronary artery bypass grafting		
		CR	complete remission, complete response
CAD	coronary artery disease		
CAI	carbonic anhydrase inhibitor	Cr	creatinine
		CrCl	creatinine clearance
CAKUT	congenital anomalies of the kidney and urinary tract	CRP	C-reactive protein
		CRRT	continuous renal replacement therapy
CaOx	calcium oxalate		
CaP	calcium phosphate	CRT	cardiac resynchronization therapy
CAPD	continuous ambulatory peritoneal dialysis		
		CS	corticosteroids
CaSR	calcium-sensing receptor	CsA	cyclosporine A
CBC	complete blood count	C-section	cesarean section
CCB	calcium channel blocker	CSF	cerebrospinal fluid
CCD	cortical collecting duct	CT	computed tomogram
CD	collecting duct	CTA	computed tomography angiogram
CDC	complement-dependent cytotoxicity		
		CTD	connective tissue disease
CDI	central diabetes insipidus	CTLA-4	cytotoxic T-lymphocyte associated antigen-4
ceph.	Cephalosporin		
CF	cystic fibrosis	CV	cardiovascular
CFB	complement factor B	CVA	cerebrovascular accident
CFH	complement factor H	CVD	cardiovascular disease
CFTR	cystic fibrosis transmembrane conductance regulator	CVP	central venous pressure
		CVS	cardiovascular system
		CVVH	continuous veno-venous hemofiltration
CFU	colony forming units		
CH50	total complement activity	CVVHD	continuous veno-venous hemodialysis
		CVVHDF	continuous veno-venous hemodiafiltration
CHF	congestive heart failure		
CHO	carbohydrate	cx	culture
CI	cardiac index	CXR	chest radiograph
CIAKI	contrast-induced AKI	CyBorD	cyclophosphamide, bortezomib, dexamethasone
CIN	contrast induced nephropathy		
		CYC	cyclophosphamide
CIT	cold ischemia time	CYP	Cytochromes P450
CK	creatine kinase	cys	cystatin C
CKD	chronic kidney disease	d	day
CKD 5D	dialysis-dependent chronic kidney disease	d/c	discontinue, discontinuation
		d/t	due to
CKD ND	non-dialysis dependent chronic kidney disease	DA	dopamine
		DAA	direct-acting antiviral
CKD T	non-dialysis dependent chronic kidney disease with a kidney transplant	DAH	diffuse alveolar hemorrhage
		DAMPs	damage-associated molecular patterns
CKD-EPI	Chronic Kidney Disease-Epidemiology Collaboration		
		DBP	diastolic blood pressure
CLL	chronic lymphocytic leukemia	DCD	donation after circulatory death
		dcSSc	diffuse cutaneous systemic sclerosis
CML	chronic myelogenous leukemia		
		DCT	distal convoluted tubule
CMP	cardiomyopathy	DDAVP	1-desamino-8-D-arginine vasopressin
CMS	Centers for Medicare & Medicaid Services		
		DDD	dense deposition disease
CMV	cytomegalovirus	DDKT	deceased donor kidney transplantation
CNI	calcineurin inhibitors		
CNT	connecting tubule		

Ddx	differential diagnosis	**EIA**	enzyme-linked immunoassay
def	deficiency		
DES	drug-eluting stent	**ELISA**	enzyme-linked immunosorbent assay
dFLC	difference between the involved and uninvolved light chain	**EM**	electron microscopy
		ENaC	epithelial sodium channel
		EP	electrophysiology
DGF	delayed graft function	**Epo**	erythropoietin
DHP	dihydropyridine	**EPS**	encapsulating peritoneal sclerosis
dHUS	diarrhea associated hemolytic uremic syndrome		
		EPTS	Estimated Posttransplant Survival
DI	diabetes insipidus	**ERBP**	European Renal Best Practice
DIC	disseminated intravascular coagulation		
		ESA	erythropoiesis stimulating agent
DKA	diabetic ketoacidosis		
DLCO	diffusion capacity of the lung	**ESR**	erythrocyte sedimentation rate
DM	diabetes mellitus	**ESRD**	end-stage renal disease
DMARD	disease-modifying anti-rheumatic drug	**ESRD-HD**	hemodialysis dependent end-stage renal disease
DN	diabetic nephropathy		
DOAC	direct oral anticoagulant	**ET-1**	endothelin-1
DOE	dyspnea on exertion	**EtOH**	alcohol
DPGN	diffuse proliferative glomerulonephritis	**EU**	endotoxin units
		EULAR	the European League Against Rheumatism
DRESS	drug reaction with eosinophilia & systemic symptoms		
		f/u	follow-up
		FDA	U.S. Food and Drug Administration
DRI	direct renin inhibitor		
dRTA	distal renal tubular acidosis	**FFP**	fresh frozen plasma
		FGF-23	fibroblast growth factor 23
ds	disease		
DSA	donor specific antibody	**FGN**	fibrillary glomerulone-phritis
DVT	deep vein thrombosis		
DW	dry weight	**FHx**	family history
dx	diagnosis	**FLC**	free light chain
DXA	dual energy x-ray absorptiometry	**FMD**	fibromuscular dysplasia
		FMF	familial Mediterranean fever
e/o	evidence of		
EAV	effective arterial volume	**FQ**	fluoroquinolone
EBPG	European Best Practice Guidelines	**FRAX**	fracture risk assessment tool
		FRC	functional residual capacity
EBV	Epstein-Barr virus		
ECF	extracellular fluid	**FSG**	fasting serum glucose
ECG	electrocardiogram	**FSGS**	focal segmental glomeru-losclerosis
ECMO	extracorporeal mem-brane oxygenation		
		FTT	failure to thrive
EDD	electron dense deposit	**G6PD**	glc-6-phosphate dehy-drogenase
EDTA	ethylenediaminetet-raacetic acid		
		GBM	glomerular basement membrane
EDW	estimated dry weight		
EF	ejection fraction	**GCA**	giant cell arteritis
EGD	esophagogastroduode-noscopy	**G-CSF**	granulocyte colony stimulating factor
EGFR	epidermal growth factor receptor	**GCW**	glomerular capillary wall
		GERD	gastroesophageal reflux disease
eGFR	estimated glomerular filtration rate		
		GFR	glomerular filtration rate
eGFRcreat-cys	estimated glomerular filtration rate using creatinine and cystatin C	**GGT**	γ-glutamyl transpeptidase
		GI	gastrointestinal
		GIB	gastrointestinal bleed
		glc	glucose
eGFRcys	estimated glomerular filtration rate using cystatin C	**glom**	glomeruli
		GLP-1	glucagon-like-peptide-1
		GMCSF	granulocyte-macrophage colony-stimulating factor
EGPA	eosinophilic granuloma-tosis with polyangiitis		

GN	glomerulonephritis	**I&D**	incision & drainage
GNR	gram-negative rods	**IABP**	intra-aortic balloon pump
GnRH	gonadotropin-releasing hormone	**IBD**	inflammatory bowel disease
GOF	gain of function	**IBW**	ideal body weight
GP	glomerulopathy	**ICa**	ionized calcium
GPA	granulomatosis with polyangiitis	**ICD**	implantable cardiac defibrillator
GPC	gram-positive cocci	**ICP**	intracranial pressure
GRA	glucocorticoid-remediable aldosteronism	**ICU**	intensive care unit
		IDA	iron deficiency anemia
GS	global sclerosis	**IDWG**	interdialytic weight gain
GU	genitourinary	**IE**	infective endocarditis
GVHD	graft-versus-host disease	**IF**	Immunofluorescence
h	hour	**IF/TA**	interstitial fibrosis and tubular atrophy
HA	headache		
hapto	haptoglobin	**IFN**	interferon
H&E	hematoxylin & eosin stain	**Ig**	Immunoglobulin
		IgAN	Immunoglobulin A nephropathy
H&P	history and physical examination	**IgAV**	Immunoglobulin A vasculitis
h/o	history of	**IGF-1**	Insulin-like growth factor 1
H2RA	H2-receptor antagonist		
Hb	hemoglobin	**IgG4-RD**	Immunoglobulin G4-related disease
HBcAb	hepatitis B virus core antibody	**IGRA**	interferon-γ release assay
HBeAg	hepatitis B virus envelope antigen	**IGT**	impaired glucose tolerance
		iHD	intermittent hemodialysis
HBsAb	hepatitis B virus surface antibody	**IIFT**	indirect immunofluorescence testing
HBsAg	hepatitis B virus surface antigen	**IKMG**	the International Kidney and Monoclonal Gammopathy Research Group
HBV	hepatitis B virus		
HC	Heavy chain		
HCC	hepatocellular carcinoma		
HCDD	heavy chain deposition disease	**IL2RA**	interleukin-2 receptor antagonist
hCG	human chorionic gonadotropin	**ILD**	interstitial lung disease
		IMCD	inner medullary collecting duct
HCQ	hydroxychloroquine		
Hct	hematocrit	**IMI**	inferior myocardial infarction
HCV	hepatitis C virus		
HD	hemodialysis	**IN**	intranasal
HDL	high-density lipoprotein	**ING**	idiopathic nodular glomerulosclerosis
HELLP	hemolysis, abnl LFTs, low plts		
		INH	isoniazid
HF	heart failure, hemofiltration	**INR**	international normalized ratio
HHS	hyperosmolar hyperglycemic state	**IP**	intraperitoneal
		IRGN	infection-related glomerulonephritis
HIF	hypoxia induced factor		
HIT	heparin-induced thrombocytopenia	**IS**	immunosuppression
		ISPD	International Society for Peritoneal Dialysis
HLH	hemophagocytic lymphohistiocytosis		
		ITGN	immunotactoid glomerulonephritis
HoTN	hypotension		
hpf	high power field	**ITP**	idiopathic thrombocytopenic purpura
HPT	hyperparathyroidism		
HR	heart rate	**IUGR**	intrauterine growth restriction
HSCT	hematopoietic stem cell transplantation		
		IV	intravenous
HSP	Henoch–Schönlein purpura	**IVC**	inferior vena cava
		IVDU	intravenous drug use(r)
HSV	herpes simplex virus	**IVF**	intravenous fluids
HTN	hypertension	**IVIg**	intravenous immunoglobulin
HUS	hemolytic uremic syndrome		
hx	history		

ABBREVIATIONS: 13-5

NAGMA	non-anion gap metabolic acidosis	**PCOS**	polycystic ovary syndrome
NaPi	sodium phosphate cotransporter	**PCP**	*Pneumocystis jiroveci* pneumonia
NASH	non-alcoholic steatohepatitis	**PCR**	protein catabolic rate, polymerase chain reaction
NCC	sodium chloride cotransporter	**PCSK9-I**	proprotein convertase subtilisin/kexin type 9 inhibitor
NCX	sodium calcium exchanger	**PCT**	proximal convoluted tubule
NDI	nephrogenic diabetes insipidus	**PCV13**	13-valent pneumococcal conjugate vaccine
NFAT	nuclear factor of activated T cells	**PCWP**	pulmonary capillary wedge pressure
NGT	nasogastric tube	**PD**	peritoneal dialysis
NHANES	the National Health and Nutrition Examination Survey	**PE**	pulmonary embolism
		PET	positron emission tomography
NHE	sodium hydrogen exchange	**PEx**	physical examination
NHL	non-Hodgkin lymphoma	**PFO**	patent foramen ovale
NKCC	sodium potassium chloride cotransporter	**PFT**	pulmonary function test
nl	normal	**PG**	prostaglandin
NMSC	non-melanoma skin cancer	**PGNMID**	proliferative glomerulonephritis with monoclonal immunoglobulin G deposits
NNRTI	non-nucleoside reverse transcriptase inhibitor		
NODAT	new-onset diabetes after transplant	**PHPT**	primary hyperparathyroidism
NPO	nothing by mouth	**PHS**	Public Health Service
Npt	NaPi cotransporters	**PI**	protease inhibitor
NPV	negative predictive value	**PICC**	peripherally inserted central catheter
NR	no response		
NRSOT	non-renal solid organ transplantation	**PiT**	inorganic phosphate transporter
NRTI	nucleoside/nucleotide reverse transcriptase inhibitor	**PJP**	*Pneumocystis jiroveci* pneumonia
		PKD	polycystic kidney disease
NS	normal saline; nephrotic syndrome	**PLEX**	plasma exchange
		plt	platelet
NSAID	nonsteroidal anti-inflammatory drug	**PMHx**	past medical history
NSF	nephrogenic systemic fibrosis	**PML**	progressive multifocal leukoencephalopathy
NYHA	New York Heart Association	**PMN**	polymorphonuclear leukocyte
OAT	organic anion transporter	**PNA**	pneumonia
OCT	organic cation transporter	**PND**	paroxysmal nocturnal dyspnea
OG	osmolal gap	**PNH**	paroxysmal nocturnal hemoglobinuria
OPTN	Organ Procurement and Transplantation Network	**PNS**	peripheral nervous system
OSA	obstructive sleep apnea	**PO**	oral intake, by mouth
OTC	over-the-counter	**POD**	postoperative day
p/w	present(s) with	**PPD**	purified protein derivative
PA	primary aldosteronism		
PAC	plasma aldosterone concentration	**PPI**	proton pump inhibitor
PAD	peripheral artery disease	**PPSV23**	23-valent pneumococcal polysaccharide vaccine
PAH	pulmonary arterial hypertension	**PPV**	positive predictive value
PAN	polyarteritis nodosa	**Ppx**	prophylaxis
PAS	periodic acid–Schiff stain	**PR**	partial remission, partial response
PASP	PA systolic pressure		
PCI	percutaneous coronary intervention	**PRA**	plasma renin activity, panel reactive antibody
PCN	penicillin		

PRBCs	packed red blood cells	**RZV**	recombinant zoster vaccine
PRES	posterior reversible encephalopathy syndrome	**s/e**	side effect
		s/p	status post
pRTA	proximal renal tubular acidosis	**s/s**	symptoms and signs
		SAH	subarachnoid hemorrhage
PSGN	post streptococcal glomerulonephritis	**SBP**	spontaneous bacterial peritonitis/systolic blood pressure
pt	patient		
PT	proximal tubule, prothrombin time	**SC**	subcutaneous
		SCC	squamous cell carcinoma
PTA	percutaneous transluminal angioplasty	**SCD**	sickle cell disease/sudden cardiac death
PTH	parathyroid hormone	**SCLC**	small cell lung cancer
PTH-rP	parathyroid hormone-related protein	**SCT**	stem cell transplantation
		Se	sensitivity
PTLD	posttransplant lymphoproliferative disease	**sFLC**	serum free light chain
		SGLT	sodium glucose cotransporter
PTT	partial thromboplastin time		
		SIADH	syndrome of inappropriate ADH
PVR	pulmonary vascular resistance		
		SIEP	serum immunoelectrophoresis
q	every		
qac	before every meal	**SIFE**	serum immunofixation electrophoresis
qd	daily		
qhs	every bedtime	**SIR**	standardized incidence ratio
qod	every other day		
QoL	quality of life	**SJS**	Stevens-Johnson syndrome
r/i	rule in		
r/o	rule out	**SLE**	systemic lupus erythematosus
RA	rheumatoid arthritis, right atrium		
		SLED	slow low efficiency dialysis
RAAS	renin–angiotensin–aldosterone system		
		SLK	simultaneous liver kidney transplantation
RAASi	renin–angiotensin–aldosterone system inhibition		
		SMA	superior mesenteric artery
RANKL	receptor activator of nuclear factor kappa-β ligand		
		sMAC	soluble membrane attack complex
		SMM	smoldering multiple myeloma
RAS	renal artery stenosis		
RBC	red blood cell	**SMX**	sulfamethoxazole
RBF	renal blood flow	**SNGFR**	single nephron glomerular filtration rate
RCT	randomized controlled trial		
		SNRI	serotonin-norepinephrine reuptake inhibitors
RF	rheumatoid factor, risk factor		
		SNS	sympathetic nervous system
RI	resistive index, renal insufficiency		
		SOS	sinusoidal obstruction syndrome
ROMK	renal outer medullary potassium channel		
		Sp	specificity
ROS	reactive oxygen species, review of systems	**SPEP**	serum protein electrophoresis
		SRC	scleroderma renal crisis
RP	retroperitoneal	**SS**	supersaturation
RPGN	rapidly progressive glomerulonephritis	**SS**	Sjögren syndrome
		SSc	systemic sclerosis
RR	relative risk, respiratory rate	**SSRI**	selective serotonin reuptake inhibitor
RRF	residual renal function		
RRT	renal replacement therapy	**SVC**	superior vena cava
		SvO$_2$	mixed venous oxygen saturation
RT	radiation therapy		
RTA	renal tubular acidosis	**SVT**	supraventricular tachycardia
RTE	renal tubular epithelial		
RTX	rituximab	**sx**	symptom(s), symptomatic
RVT	renal vein thrombosis		
Rx	therapy	**synd**	syndrome
RYGB	Roux-en-Y gastric bypass	**T1DM**	type 1 diabetes mellitus

T2DM	type 2 diabetes mellitus	**UCl**	urine chloride
Tac	Tacrolimus	**UCx**	urine culture
TAL	Thick ascending limb of the loop of Henle	**UF**	ultrafiltration
TB	tuberculosis	**UFH**	unfractionated heparin
TBM	tubular basement membrane	**UGIB**	upper gastrointestinal bleed
TBMN	thin basement membrane nephropathy	**UIFE**	urine immunofixation electrophoresis
TCA	tricyclic antidepressant	**UK**	urine potassium
TCC	transitional cell carcinoma	**ULN**	upper limit of normal
Tdap	tetanus, diphtheria, pertussis	**UNa**	urine sodium
TEE	transesophageal echo	**UNOS**	United Network for Organ Sharing
temp	temperature	**UOP**	urine output
TG	triglycerides	**UPCR**	urine protein to creatinine ratio
TGF	tubuloglomerular feedback	**UPEP**	urine protein electrophoresis
TIA	transient ischemic attack	**Uprot**	urine protein
TIBC	total iron binding capacity	**URI**	upper respiratory tract infxn
TIN	tubulointerstitial nephritis	**USPSTF**	U.S. Preventive Services Task Force
TINU	tubulointerstitial nephritis and uveitis	**USRDS**	United States Renal Data System
TIW	three times a week	**UTI**	urinary tract infection
TKV	total kidney volume	**UTO**	urinary tract obstruction
TLS	tumor lysis syndrome	**VBG**	venous blood gas
TMA	thrombotic microangiopathy	**Vd**	volume of distribution
TMP	trimethoprim	**VDRL**	venereal disease research laboratory (test for syphilis)
TNF	tumor necrosis factor		
TP	total protein		
TPN	total parenteral nutrition	**VEGF**	vascular endothelial growth factor
TRALI	transfusion-related acute lung injury	**VF**	ventricular fibrillation
TRAS	transplant renal artery stenosis	**VHL**	Von Hippel–Lindau
		vit	vitamin
TRI	tubuloreticular inclusion	**VKA**	vitamin K antagonist
TRP	transient receptor potential	**VOD**	veno-occlusive disease
		VT	ventricular tachycardia
Tsat	transferrin saturation	**VTE**	venous thromboembolus
TSH	thyroid stimulating hormone	**VUR**	vesicoureteral reflux
		vWF	von Willebrand factor
TTE	transthoracic echo	**VZV**	varicella zoster virus
TTKG	transtubular potassium gradient	**w/**	with
		w/o	without
TTP	thrombotic thrombocytopenic purpura	**w/u**	workup
		WBC	white blood cell (count)
TURP	transurethral resection of the prostate	**WHO**	World Health Organization
Tx	treatment	**wk**	week
txp	transplantation	**WM**	Waldenström macroglobulinemia
TZD	thiazolidinediones		
U/A	urinalysis	**WRF**	worsening renal function
U/S	ultrasound	**WRT**	water restriction test
UA	uric acid		
UACR	urine albumin to creatinine ratio	**wt**	weight
		XL	X-linked
UAG	urine anion gap	**XO**	xanthine oxidase
Ualb	urine albumin	**XOI**	xanthine oxidase inhibitor
UAPR	urine albumin to protein ratio		
		y	year
UC	ulcerative colitis	**y/o**	year old
UCa	urine calcium	**ZVL**	zoster vaccine live

Note: Page numbers followed by f and t denote figure and table respectively.